Helliwell.

PROGNOSIS IN THE RHEUMATIC DISEASES

PROGNOSIS IN THE RHEUMATIC DISEASES

Edited by
Nicholas Bellamy,
MD, MSc, FRCP(Glas), FRCP(Edin), FRCP(C), FACP
*Associate Professor of Medicine, Epidemiology and Biostatistics,
University of Western Ontario, London, Ontario, Canada;
Director, Division of Rheumatology, Victoria Hospital,
London, Ontario, Canada*

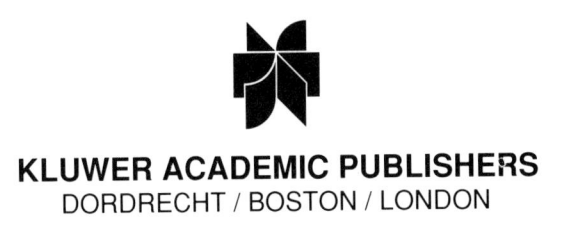

KLUWER ACADEMIC PUBLISHERS
DORDRECHT / BOSTON / LONDON

Distributors

for the United States and Canada: Kluwer Academic Publishers, PO Box 358, Accord Station, Hingham, MA 02018-0358, USA
for all other countries: Kluwer Academic Publishers Group, Distribution Center, PO Box 322, 3300 AH Dordrecht, The Netherlands

British Library Cataloguing in Publication Data

Prognosis in the rheumatic diseases.
 1. Man. Rheumatic diseases
 I. Bellamy, Nicholas 1950–
 616.723

 ISBN 0-7923-8958-1

Library of Congress Cataloging in Publication Data

Prognosis in the rheumatic diseases/edited by Nicholas Bellamy.
   p. cm.
  Includes bibliographical references and index.
  ISBN 0-7923-8958-1 (casebound)
  1. Rheumatism—Prognosis. 2. Arthritis—Prognosis. I. Bellamy, Nicholas, 1950–
   [DNLM: 1. Prognosis. 2. Rheumatic Diseases. WE 544 P964]
RC927.P685 1991
616.7'23—dc20
DNLM/DLC
for Library of Congress   90-15602
                                                                      CIP

Copyright

© 1991 by Kluwer Academic Publishers

All rights reserved. No part of this publication may be reproduced, stored in a retrieval system, or transmitted in any form or by any means, electronic, mechanical, photocopying, recording or otherwise, without prior permission from the publishers, Kluwer Academic Publishers BV, PO Box 17, 3300 AA Dordrecht, The Netherlands.

Published in the United Kingdom by Kluwer Academic Publishers, PO Box 55, Lancaster, UK

Kluwer Academic Publishers BV incorporates the publishing programmes of D. Reidel, Martinus Nijhoff, Dr W. Junk and MTP Press.

Printed in Great Britain by Butler and Tanner, Ltd., Frome and London.

Contents

	List of Contributors	vii
	Foreword J. L. Decker	xi
	Preface N. Bellamy	xiii
1	Introduction J. F. Fries and N. Bellamy	1
2	Osteoarthritis K. D. Brandt and D. Flusser	11
3	Rheumatoid arthritis F. Wolfe	37
4	Juvenile arthritis B. M. Ansell	83
5	Crystal-associated arthropathies B. T. Emmerson	97
6	Ankylosing spondylitis P. S. Helliwell and V. Wright	133
7	Psoriatic arthritis D. D. Gladman	153
8	Reiter's syndrome W. F. Kean and D. W. MacPherson	167
9	Systemic lupus erythematosus R. Roubenoff and M. C. Hochberg	193

CONTENTS

10	Systemic sclerosis (scleroderma) V. D. Steen and T. A. Medsger	213
11	Polymyositis-dermatomyositis C. V. Oddis and T. A. Medsger	233
12	Vasculitis F. J. Barbado, J. J. Vasquez, M. Khamashta and G. R. V. Hughes	251
13	Polymyalgia rheumatica and giant cell arteritis L. A. Healey	269
14	Arthritis in pregnancy N. Bellamy, R. R. Grigor and R. P. Naden	279
15	Fibromyalgia F. Wolfe	321
16	Low back pain I. K. Y. Tsang	333
17	Prediction of the clinical efficacy of and intolerance to antirheumatic drug therapy P. M. Brooks and W. W. Buchanan	347
18	Prediction of organ system toxicity with anti-rheumatic drug therapy W. W. Buchanan and P. M. Brooks	403
19	New concepts in prognosis of rheumatic diseases for the 1990s T. Pincus	451
	Index	

List of Contributors

BARBARA M. ANSELL, CBE, MD, FRCS, FRCP

Consultant Paediatric Rheumatologist, Previously Head of Division of Rheumatology, Clinical Research Centre, Northwick Park Hospital, Harrow, Middlesex, UK

Juvenile Arthritis

FRANCISCO J. BARBADO, MD

Assistant Professor of Medicine, Universidad Autonoma de Madrid; Consultant Physician, Department of Internal Medicine, Hospital 'La Paz', Madrid, Spain

Vasculitis

NICHOLAS BELLAMY, MD, MSc, FRCP(Glas), FRCP(Edin), FRCP(C), FACP

Associate Professor of Medicine, Epidemiology and Biostatistics, University of Western Ontario, London; Associate Professor of Clinical Epidemiology and Biostatistics, McMaster University, Hamilton; Director, Division of Rheumatology, Victoria Hospital, London, Canada

Preface
Introduction
Arthritis in Pregnancy

KENNETH D. BRANDT, MD

Professor of Medicine and Head, Rheumatology Division, Indiana University School of Medicine; Director, Indiana University Multipurpose Arthritis Center and Director, Indiana University Specialized Center of Research in Osteoarthritis, Indianapolis, Indiana, USA

Osteoarthritis

PETER M. BROOKS, MB, BS, MD, FRACP, FACRM

Florance and Cope Professor of Rheumatology, University of Sydney and Head, Department of Rheumatology, Royal North Shore Hospital, Sydney, Australia

Prediction of the Clinical Efficacy of and Intolerance to Antirheumatic Drug Therapy
Prediction to Organ System Toxicity with Antirheumatic Drug Therapy

LIST OF CONTRIBUTORS

W. WATSON BUCHANAN, MD, FRCP(Glas, Edin, and C), FACP

Professor of Medicine, McMaster Faculty of Health Sciences, 1200 Main Street West, Hamilton, Ontario, Canada, L8N 3Z5

Prediction of Organ System Toxicity with Antirheumatic Drug Therapy
Prediction of the Clinical Efficacy of and Intolerance to Antirheumatic Drug Therapy

BRYAN T. EMMERSON, MD, PhD

Professor of Medicine and Head of the Department of Medicine, University of Queensland; Princess Alexandra Hospital, Brisbane, Queensland, Australia 4102

Crystal-associated Arthropathies

DANIEL FLUSSER, MD

Rheumatology Fellow, Indiana School of Medicine, Indianapolis, Indiana, USA

Osteoarthritis

JAMES F. FRIES, MD

Associate Professor of Medicine, Stanford University School of Medicine, Stanford, California, USA

Introduction

DAFNA D. GLADMAN, MD

Associate Professor of Medicine, University of Toronto, Rheumatic Disease Unit, Wellesley Hospital, Toronto, Ontario, Canada

Psoriatic Arthritis

ROBERT R. GRIGOR, MB, FRACP

Chairman, Department of Rheumatology, Auckland Hospital; Clinical Lecturer, School of Medicine, University of Auckland, Auckland, New Zealand

Arthritis in Pregnancy

LOUIS A. HEALEY, MD

Clinical Professor of Medicine, University of Washington School of Medicine; Head, Section of Immunology and Rheumatic Disease, Virginia Mason Clinic, Seattle, Washington, USA

Polymyalgia Rheumatica and Giant Cell Arteritis

PHILIP HELLIWELL, MA, DM, MRCP

Senior Registrar in Rheumatology, Leeds General Infirmary and Royal Bath Hospital, Harrogate, UK

Ankylosing Spondylitis

MARC C. HOCHBERG, MD, MPH

Associate Professor of Medicine, Welch Center for Prevention, Epidemiology and Clinical Research, The Johns Hopkins University School of Medicine; Joint Appointment in Epidemiology, The Johns Hopkins University School of Hygiene and Public Health, Baltimore, MD, USA

Systemic Lupus Erythematosus

LIST OF CONTRIBUTORS

GRAHAM R. V. HUGHES, MD, FRCP

Head, Lupus Research Unit, The Rayne Institute; Consultant Rheumatologist, St Thomas' Hospital, London, UK

Vasculitis

WALTER F. KEAN, MD(Glas), FRCP(C), FACP

Associate Clinical Professor of Medicine and Associate Department of Chemistry, McMaster University, Hamilton, Ontario, Canada

Reiter's Syndrome

MUNTHER A. KHAMASHTA, MD

Deputy Director, Lupus Research Unit, The Rayne Institute; Honorary Consultant Physician, St Thomas' Hospital, London UK

Vasculitis

DOUGLAS W. MACPHERSON MD, MSc(CTM), FRCP(C)

Assistant Clinical Professor of Medicine and Medical Microbiology, McMaster University, Hamilton, Ontario, Canada

Reiter's Syndrome

THOMAS A. MEDSGER, Jr., MD

Professor of Medicine and Chief, Division of Rheumatology and Clinical Immunology, University of Pittsburgh School of Medicine, Pittsburgh, PA, USA

Systemic Sclerosis (Scleroderma)
Polymyositis-dermatomyositis

RAYMOND P. NADEN, MD, ChB, FRACP

Senior Lecturer, Department of Medicine and Obstetrics, School of Medicine, University of Auckland; Physician, National Womens Hospital, Auckland, New Zealand

Arthritis in Pregnancy

CHESTER V. ODDIS, MD

Assistant Professor of Medicine, Division of Rheumatology and Clinical Immunology, University of Pittsburgh School of Medicine, and Associate Chief of Staff for Education, Oakland Veterans Administration Medical Centre, Pittsburgh, PA, USA

Polymyositis-dermatomyositis

THEODORE PINCUS, MD

Professor of Medicine and Microbiology, Division of Rheumatology and Immunology, Department of Medicine, Vanderbilt University School of Medicine, Nashville, TN, USA

New Concepts in Prognosis of Rheumatic Diseases for the 1990s

LIST OF CONTRIBUTORS

RONENN ROUBENOFF, MD, MPH

Postdoctoral Fellow, USDA Human Nutrition Research Center on Aging, Tufts University, Boston, MA; Former Postdoctoral Fellow in Clinical Epidemiology and Medicine (Rheumatology), The Johns Hopkins University School of Medicine, Baltimore, MD, USA

Systemic Lupus Erythematosus

VIRGINIA D. STEEN, MD

Associate Professor of Medicine, Division of Rheumatology and Clinical Immunology, University of Pittsburgh School of Medicine, Pittsburgh, PA, USA

Systemic Sclerosis (Scleroderma)

IAN K. Y. TSANG, MB, FRCPC

Associate Dean, Clinical Associate Professor of Medicine, Faculty of Medicine, University of British Columbia; Head, Division of Rheumatology, University Hospital, Shaughnessy Site, Vancouver, British Columbia, Canada

Low Back Pain

JUAN J. VÁZQUEZ, MD

Professor of Medicine, Universidad Autonoma de Madrid; Head, Department of Internal Medicine, Hospital 'La Paz', Madrid, Spain

Vasculitis

FREDERICK WOLFE, MD

Clinical Professor of Medicine, University of Kansas School of Medicine – Wichita, and Director, Arthritis, Center, Wichita, Kansas, USA

Rheumatoid Arthritis
Fibromyalgia

VERNA WRIGHT, MD, FRCP

Professor of Rheumatology, University of Leeds, Leeds, UK

Ankylosing Spondylitis

Foreword

Seer, forecaster, prophet, geomancer, or tout — all predict future events as physicians must. The medical activity is *prognosis* from the Greek *pro* (forward) and *gnosis* (special knowledge), thus foreknowledge, and the practitioner is the *prognosticator*, a sobriquet which falls unhappily upon the ear. Like it or not, there is nothing more critical in the management of chronic rheumatic conditions than a reasonably clear picture of what time and disease will bring. The knowledge is so much a part of ordinary medical thinking that we rarely grace it with the label prognosis. But, like so much of "ordinary medical thinking" (an oxymoron, perhaps), quantitative data are very thin and the chestnuts of personal observation and authority figure assertion loom large. Unlike several books I have seen or written, this one on prognosis needs no justification.

The entirety of a person's life contributes to and confounds what the future holds. The ingredients include education level, income, support structures such as family, housing, occupation, availability of medical services, diagnosis, treatment, rate of disease progression, age, gender, race, marital status, and others too numerous to mention or too arcane to be recognized. One would think the task of estimating prognosis impossible. And yet there is light on the horizon – we do know a few things such as the effect of high rheumatoid factor titers on the prognosis of RA or the likely outcome of certain kidney lesions in SLE. There are really two elements of the act of prognosticating: early and late, predictors and outcome. These, systematically studied and leashed with an appreciation of the difficulties of probability, should bring us much closer to divining the future of any given patient.

First, outcome, something that follows as a result or consequence. One should not think of outcome as a splendid day at the end of something; the situation today *is* the outcome of yesterday and yesteryear. The measurements you perform and the facts that you record at any patient visit are an outcome and are likely to be in the same descriptive terminology you will use 10 and 20 years hence. It has been shown that big league joint involvement in RA is a predictor of big league joint involvement in the future. Here the predictor and the outcome are identical, emphasizing the fact that the observations of any one day may be either.

The words *big league* also illustrate the degree to which we lack quantitative measures of status. When it comes to numbers of joints inflamed, the sedimentation rate, and the grip strength we are in good shape but, let's face it, those measures are fit for circumstances very much shorter than 10, 15, or 20 years of disease. Of merit in testing NSAIDs or for thinking of the next month's treatment, they are only a part, and a small part at that, of wellness measured 10 years later, for example. The conviction that rheumatologists have a contribution to make must be buttressed by improvement in outcomes assessable in the longer frame.

So much for outcome, what about predictors? Assuming that a predictor is recorded on any given day, it is to be measured precisely as if it were an outcome. Admittedly one can do a better job of predicting, given assessments of the rate of progression over 6 months or so. But each visit has its own predictors. And, of course, some predictors, such as schooling or family support, are not likely to be changing very fast. The critical issue is, "What are we to measure in quantitative fashion today which might be meaningful if repeated 10 years hence?" The answer must come from ascertaining the patient's relationship to life, a tall order but one which is being surmounted by the use of self-administered questionnaires such as HAQ and AIMS, themselves based upon earlier efforts to define good health or wellness. A big advantage of these carefully constructed and validated scales is that the patient can prepare them in brief order without assistance. Given the record-keeping potential of personal computers, you can rapidly collect a vast amount of data allowing quantitative statements about patients and comparing them to normative data or to the patients of your colleagues.

Admittedly these methods, as with any method, will need more research, studies by the way which are unglamorous and slow in the doing. It can be carried on in the offices of individual practitioners, most effectively in circumstances of continuing care given over many years. Insofar as a journey of a thousand miles must begin with a single step, the installation of one of these questionnaire methods in your office now has much to recommend it.

If you don't believe me, read this book. Even if you do, it would be well to read this book.

John L. Decker, M.D.
National Institutes of Health
Bethesda, MD,
USA
June 1990

Preface

Patients with rheumatic disease frequently request information regarding their future health status and the probability of a beneficial or adverse response to antirheumatic drug therapy. Health policy planners, senior hospital administrators, insurance adjudicators and members of the legal profession involved in litigation medicine also require some knowledge of the prognosis of the rheumatic diseases in making judgments regarding certain individuals or groups of patients. While thoroughly discussing the etiology, pathogenesis, pathology, clinical, serologic and radiographic features and management of the rheumatic diseases, most standard texts give a superficial treatment to the area of prognosis. Although prognostication is highly individualized and has dynamic qualities which vary over time, there have been a large number of prognosis studies conducted in different musculoskeletal conditions. However, this information is scattered over many different journals and has been published over several years. Furthermore the relevant material is difficult to locate and has not been adequately appraised to date. In order to bring these diverse sources of important information together, we have invited the international collaboration of physicians experienced in the assessment and management of patients with musculoskeletal disease. Their critical, but constructive, reviews have created a very informative text which will be of interest to clinicians managing patients with musculoskeletal disease, as well as to agencies, and individuals who have a professional responsibility for dealing with the consequences of this group of disorders.

Nicholas Bellamy
London, July 1990

1
Introduction

J. F. FRIES and N. BELLAMY

This book is about prognosis in the rheumatic diseases. By establishing what is currently known about the long-term outcomes of rheumatologic conditions and what is not, we hope that this volume will assist in the development of improved management plans and in the development of a long-range view of treatment. In addition, the high levels of chronic morbidity underscore the necessity for musculoskeletal disease to be emphasized in undergraduate and postgraduate medical education, and in the planning of health care services. In spite of its key importance to patients, clinicians, hospital administrators, insurance agencies, central government, and the legal profession[1], prognosis has been relatively neglected even in major textbooks of medicine and rheumatology[2,3]. Possibly this is due to the complexity of prognosticating and the dynamic nature of disease, which may modify the original prognosis over time. Alternatively it may be because the term "prognosis" lacks adequate definition. It is not always clear what one does when one "gives a prognosis."

A prognosis is in fact a prediction. It is a prediction of an expected future clinical outcome based on some selected current information. Like all predictions, it is inherently probabilistic and inherently uncertain. Prognosis takes place not only in the clinical dynamic of a patient's disease but also in the face of changing therapy and possibly in the face of a changing natural history. Despite these problems, the ability to estimate prognosis is essential to rational clinical decision-making. A rational clinical decision can be made by estimating the outcomes that would occur under two or more alternative types of management, and then selecting the alternative that is most likely to lead to the best patient outcome. If outcomes for different alternatives cannot be estimated accurately or are not forecast optimally, then the clinical decision is likely to be incorrect or even inappropriate. This issue is equally relevant to several commonly recurring decisions: (1) which treatment program to recommend to a patient; (2) what advice to give a patient, employer, or insurer regarding a patient's future employability; (3) how to organize and if necessary rationalize health care delivery to optimize the cost-effectiveness with which health care funds are expended; and (4) whether a patient's current clinical status is due entirely to a pre-existing musculoskeletal condition, or is partly or entirely due to an intercurrent traumatic event (e.g., MVA). Error in any of these four areas has far-reaching consequences, particularly for the patient, but also for relatives; employers and other employees; insurers, politicians, and other health planners; third parties involved in litigation; and society at large.

In general the literature that pertains to musculoskeletal prognosis is diverse and widely scattered in subspeciality journals or contained with in a handful of structured databases. Before commenting on these sources of information it is appropriate to consider the nature of the prognosis, i.e. what are the characteristics of "a prognosis."

1. While overall prognosis for a group of patients with, say, rheumatoid arthritis is interesting and important in many ways, it is not directly relevant to the clinical situation. The clinical decision has to be based on *individual* prognostic factors. In essence, therefore, prognosis is primarily for an individual. There is mild disease and there is severe; there is early disease and late disease; disease happens in young and old; in men and women; and in different racial groups. Certain constellations of symptoms and outcomes cluster together. The presence of some findings nearly excludes certain future events, and may nearly ensure others. On the other hand, prognosis cannot be individualized to the level of the anecdote. We need experience with certain numbers of patients in order to be confident that particular outcomes are likely to follow. Thus, prognostic predictions require stratification by different variables, such as those above, and use of any other characteristics that might serve to define a patient as a member of a reasonably small and relatively homogeneous subgroup.

2. To be useful, prognosis must be *quantified* as much as possible. "Good prognosis" or a "poor prognosis" are terms with very limited clinical value. Thus, data from large patient populations stored in computer data banks or from relevant studies in the literature are needed to develop numerical estimates. Life table statistics are often particularly appropriate to this task and have been employed by some but not all investigators.

3. Prognosis for a chronic illness must include estimation of *distant* event probabilities as well as proximate. Short-term (weeks or months) or even intermediate-term (1–5 years) predictions are not entirely sufficient. With rheumatic diseases, or for that matter any chronic diseases, emphasis upon short-term outcomes can be misleading and often is ultimately detrimental to care. A typical course of rheumatoid arthritis, diagrammed in Figure 1, serves as an example. The patient with rheumatoid arthritis has an average 21-year disease course[4]. Death occurs typically some 4–12 years

INTRODUCTION

prematurely; disability increases slowly through the course, with the most rapid rises in the early years; discomfort fluctuates throughout the period of disease; iatrogenic effects from medicine or surgery occur sporadically; and massive economic impact is felt, with costs generally increasing over the course of the illness. The therapeutic goal, to improve outcome, consists of reducing the stippled areas in Figure 1, being interested at once in the area under the curve and at the final point at the end of illness[5]. Presentation of prognosis in terms of "disability-years" or lifetime medical cost is also appropriate.

4. Prognosis must proceed from a *specific point* in the course, represented by the parameters of the individual patient. For describing the "natural" history of a disease, an "inception cohort" of individuals followed from the onset of symptoms is appropriate. In the clinical setting, however, it is more usual for prognostic questions to arise later in the disease course; indeed, the need for prognostic estimates occurs with every clinical decision throughout the course of illness. For these questions the past is past, and it is the future from that point that must be predicted. Thus, the patient who originally has seronegative nonerosive rheumatoid arthritis may in a matter of months have seropositive nodular erosive disease. It is the need to deal with such dynamic changes that makes prognostication difficult but not impossible.

5. Prognosis must encompass *all* meaningful outcomes. With the rheumatic diseases in particular, one cannot focus solely on mortality rates. Indeed, many of the conditions discussed in this book have negligible effects upon mortality. Nor is it ethically or practically possible to derive a single number to represent prognosis. To do so would require setting a cost equal to a year of life, a year of life equal to a degree of disability, a degree of disability equal to an amount of pain, and so forth. In prediction of rheumatic disease outcomes there are frequently conflicts between outcomes in different dimensions and erroneous decisions may be made if all dimensions are not considered. For example, a drug might reduce disability but carry a certain risk of death. A strong analgesic might be quite successful at reducing pain but might impede function.

In this volume we define "outcome" as consisting of five dimensions: Death, Disability, Discomfort, Iatrogenic Effects, and Economic Impact (Figure 1). We have attempted to define these dimensions so that they are mutually exclusive yet collectively exhaustive. Thus, discomfort includes concepts such as depression or patient dissatisfaction as well as physical pain or fatigue, iatrogenic effects can be "medical" or "surgical," and economic impacts "direct" or "indirect."

In the following chapters, authors have taken these considerations into account in their discussions. They have discussed the differing

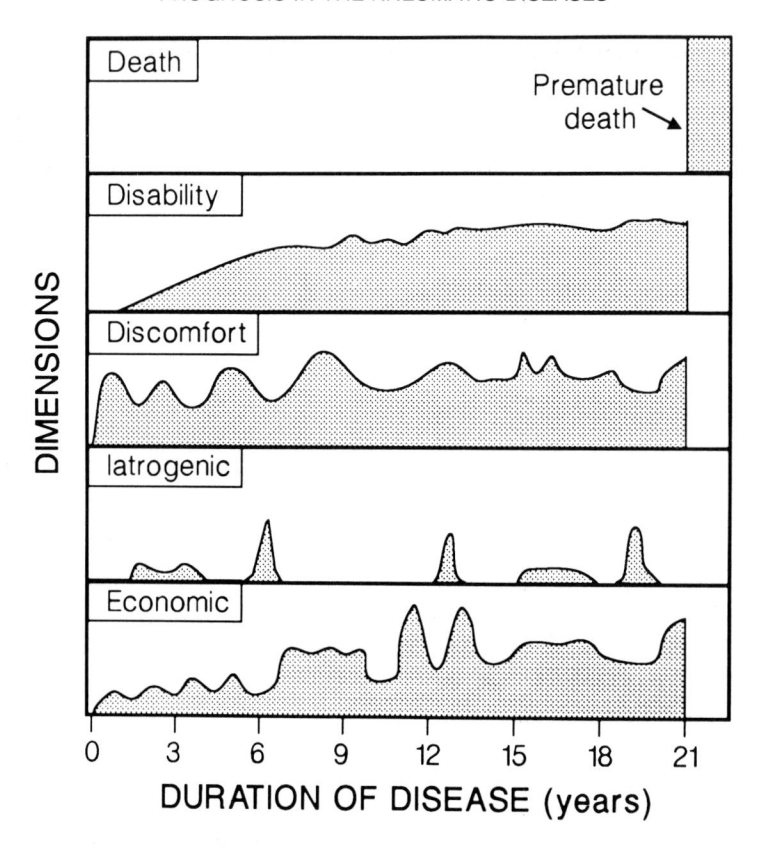

Figure 1 Prototype individual patient outcome

predictions among different clinical subgroups, quantified information whenever possible, considered long-term and cumulative outcomes, and discussed separately, where applicable, death, disability, discomfort, iatrogenic effects, and economic impact. They have attempted to identify areas of present ignorance as well as the weaknesses and strengths of currently available data. Their estimates and interpretations are based on an in-depth knowledge of the literature as well as personal experience, and in some cases direct or indirect access to established databases that are currently being used to track large numbers of patients with musculoskeletal disease. In assessing prognosis studies many authors have employed criteria based on those formalized by clinical epidemiologists for critically appraising the literature[6].

Assessment of clinical outcomes

The primary task of medicine is to make people better. Unfortunately, this straightforward directive contains hidden pitfalls, some discussed

INTRODUCTION

above. We must know what "better" is, and we must be able to tell when we have achieved it. With short-term illness such as appendicitis or pneumococcal pneumonia, the answers are almost self-evident. But with the rise of chronic diseases as the dominant health threat in developed nations, the answers have become far more complex. Based on social science research techniques we and others have been able to develop instruments that reflect patient preferences: to be alive, to have full function, to be free of symptoms, to be free of side-effects, and to remain solvent[7]. It has been possible to develop instruments that obtain direct quantitative assessments in patient-oriented terms, such as disability, rather than in doctor-oriented terms, such as reduction of sedimentation rate[8].

There has been gradual acceptance of a framework within which these assessments can be made. This framework, elaborated above and demonstrated in Figure 1, encompasses five disease dimensions (mortality, and four measures of morbidity-disability, discomfort, iatrogenic adverse reactions, and economic impact)[9]. Defining the medical task as that of improving long-term cumulative health outcomes implies a new emphasis in our investigative approaches, medical literature, and education processes. Changes are needed, conceptually and practically. Implicit in such change is a decision, not only what to measure, but also how to measure it. We have previously reviewed the principal practical alternatives[9] but four conceptual issues in outcome assessment deserve reiteration.

1. An important first step has been to shift the focus from measures of "process" to measures of "outcome." "Process" measures include such variables as sedimentation rate, latex titer, or level of antibody to DNA. Process measures have no intrinsic value to the patient; they are of clinical value only to the extent that they serve as accurate surrogates for "outcome" measurements. Thus, if the sedimentation rate accurately quantitated "fatigue," and "fatigue" is part of patient discomfort, and patient discomfort is an outcome, then the sedimentation rate would have value as a surrogate outcome measurement, conveniently ascertained. However, since these traditional tests are only loosely correlated with ultimate outcome, they are extremely limited in value and clinically represent false endpoints.

2. An important second step has been to rethink our use of the terms "hard data" and "soft data." "Hard data" have generally been thought to be those obtained from a laboratory test, such as hemoglobin values. Hard data are easily quantitated, continuous on a long scale, relatively reproducible, and reassuringly numeric. Because variables such as "hemoglobin" have these attributes, we have come to believe that so do all numbers that emerge from the laboratory such as serum complement, sedimentation rates, or levels of antibody to DNA. We have tended to use the word "hard" for data that are essentially "process" variables as discussed above.

More properly, we should have reserved use of the term "hard" to represent data with good measurement characteristics of reliability and validity. A dilemma for the clinician in this old formulation was that the variables that were "hard" were largely irrelevant to patient status, while those that were clearly relevant (e.g., quality of life measures) were considered "soft." Fortunately, in the new science of clinical metrology, the distinction between "hard" and "soft" data is itself a "soft" one. The carefully developed new measures of patient outcome, such as the Health Assessment Questionnaire (HAQ)[5,7,10] or the Arthritis Impact Measurement Scales (AIMS)[8] provide data that have far more robust measurement characteristics than many laboratory data[11,12].

Had we applied tests of measurement characteristics to laboratory values, such as erythrocyte sedimentation rates, we would have become disillusioned with these measures somewhat earlier. Essentially, no relevant published data are available for sedimentation rates with split samples sent to separate laboratories or for repeat measurements in the same individual on successive days. It has seldom been asked whether the sedimentation rate is an important endpoint (face validity) or whether it correlates well with measures that are important (convergent construct validity). When tests such as level of antibody to DNA or serum complement have been subjected to such examination, their measurement characteristics have been found wanting[11]. Large laboratory errors, 20% or more, are frequently encountered[11]. In contrast, test–retest correlations of the new disability scales, for example, may be as high as 0.98[13-16]. We believe that the role of patient-relevant measures in outcome assessment is increasingly recognized. Indeed, a recent survey in Canada of international clinical trial experts revealed the five most valued endpoints for rheumatoid arthritis were global assessment by the physician, joint count, self-report of pain, self-report of morning stiffness, and grip strength in that order[17]. None of these is a "hard" measure in the traditional sense. A second meeting in England called for the HAQ to be one of the measures to be used in serial annual assessments in RA[18].

Thus, the terms "hard" and "soft" must now be used to refer to the actual measurement characteristics of a variable rather than to the point of origin of the data. On many of the central characteristics that define "hard" data (precision, quantitability, reproducibility, interobserver variability, face validity, convergent validity, responsiveness), many laboratory test results currently used in evaluating an arthritis patient are far inferior to the questionnaire outcome assessment instruments. It is timely to adopt the general use of high-performance patient-relevant measures in the future assessment of all musculoskeletal patients.

3. Long-term observations (over 5 years) are clearly needed for evaluation of long-term diseases. Health status at any one time

INTRODUCTION

represents a combination of present disease activity and accumulated past damage. Obviously, an optimal therapy must be one that minimizes the impact of the disease over time, neither disregarding the early symptoms nor neglecting the long-term complications. A clinician managing a patient with rheumatoid arthritis is frequently aided by a long-term flow sheet that displays sedimentation rate, grip strength, hemoglobin, latex fixation titer, and other values over time. From the discussion above, it is clear that the physician will be even better served by flow sheets that include assessment of outcome status at intervals, perhaps every 6 months, suitable for evaluation of intermediate-term (1-5 years) and long-term (over 5 years) outcomes. If we wish to reduce the cumulative impact of disease, then we must be able to define and measure cumulative impact. Chart forms meeting these specifications have been developed by the American Rheumatism Association Medical Information System (ARAMIS) and are available from ARAMIS offices at 701 Welch Road, Suite 3301, Palo Alto, CA 94304.

4. A final basic consideration refers to the disturbingly multivariate world of chronic illness. Nonbiologic inputs clearly affect outcome. Yet, our medical system teaches biologic mechanisms almost exclusively. In the rheumatic diseases, patient motivation and compliance, educational level, socioeconomic status, availability of community resources, payment mechanisms, public and patient education, family support, level of depression, and other factors may be more important determinants of disability than the biologic activity of the disease or the effect of medication. These multiple influences on patient outcome require a broader model of health. The traditional univariate experiment that has formed the basis of biologic science and its clinical analog, the randomized controlled clinical trial, are of only limited use in approaching problems of this complexity. Such experiments necessarily study single factors in isolation. In comparison, multivariate problems involving multiple "risk factors" and many interactions are not susceptible to reductionist forms of analysis. The newer broader concept of patient outcome, however, requires that clinical knowledge be developed within this more complex framework.

The current state of the art

There are relatively few prospective large-volume structured databases of musculoskeletal patients. The American Rheumatism Association Medical Information System (ARAMIS) was first developed in 1975 as part of a concerted effort to structure the accumulation of high-quality data on a variety of musculoskeletal disorders, facilitate the determination of long-term outcome, and identify factors of prognostic importance. The Stanford Arthritis Center Health Assessment Questionnaire (HAQ) is a standard part of ARAMIS Outcome Assessment Protocols and has been modified for use in the United States Health and Nutrition Survey (NHANES-I Follow-up, NHANES-II, and NHANES-III). The HAQ was 7 years in development and testing and the resulting questionnaire has been administered in more than one hundred settings, with computer-stored data available in over 100 000 administrations on 20 000 patients. During that time[5,7,10,12-17,19-22] similar values have been observed in rheumatoid arthritis populations as diverse as Stanford, Phoenix, Witchita, and Saskatoon[13]. It appears that the mean disability values and rate of increase in disability in RA patients differ from OA patients (mean disability value RA=1.2, OA=0.4, rate of increase in disability <50% compared with RA) as measured by the HAQ instrument. The ability of this and a few other instruments to measure change in terms such as increase in disability per year of disease (RA=0.08 units)[5], is an obvious advantage in attempts to quantitate prognosis and predict the future outcome of patients belonging, at a specified point in time, to a particular subgroup of diseased individuals. Recent progress is further underscored by the fact that the HAQ disability index can predict 4-year outcomes more accurately than can measures of morning stiffness, number of involved joints, sedimentation rate, and latex fixation titer[13,20]. In addition, this instrument can be used to quantify the economic consequences of disease. For example, the medical costs for those in the fourth quartile of disability are more than 9 times those in the first quartile[21]. Such information is critical for rational decision making. This is not to say that other conventional measures of joint tenderness, upper or lower limb performance, dolorimeter scores, or joint circumference are irrelevant, but to emphasize the point that the patients' level of discomfort and disability, their mortality rates, the treatment-related side-effects they experience, and the economic consequences of their disease represent the true impact of disease on the individual and his or her society.

Although the preceding paragraphs are focused on overall outcome another component of prognostication is the identification of the clinical, serologic, radiographic, or other variables that predict the outcome of interest. Such predictor variables are diverse and may include some of the following: age, gender, extent or severity of articular disease, presence or absence of major organ involvement, normality or abnormality of specific serologic tests (e.g., RF, anti-Ro), and the presence or absence of radiographic signs of bone damage (e.g., erosion). In addition, the severity of disease as measured by a health status instrument at one point in time may be predictive of the patient's future health status. Of course, as new therapeutic modalities appear, the prognosis may either improve as a result of enhanced therapeutic benefit or worsen as a result of previously unexpected drug toxicity or surgical misadventure. Finally, it should be acknowledged that the opportunity of a new rheumatoid arthritis patient achieving a favorable long-term outcome is at least in part dependent on the diligent skill of the attending health professionals. That is to say, the outcomes published in the literature often represent the effects of exemplary patient care. It follows, therefore, that the education of undergraduates and the continued education of postgraduate health care providers as well as the further enlightenment of patients is critical to achieving the best prognosis possible.

The development of outcome assessment and prognostication is in an exciting stage. The new concepts challenge traditional views about the role of medical care, the importance of strictly biologic inputs and the role of the patient in deciding what should or should not be done. There is a tremendous opportunity to further the science of prognosis by utilizing structured protocols and flow sheets to track patients over time. Health outcome measurements are an essential part of such flow sheets and may well prove to be the most important part of such serial observations.

The existence of a combination of large epidemiologic databases, scientifically rigorous randomized controlled trials, case control studies, and precedent-setting case reports provide vitally important sources of information. It is hoped that the remaining chapters of this book have brought together much of the relevant information and placed it in a context whereby the reader can usefully apply the information in clinical decision making, and will in addition stimulate clinical investigators to supplement current sources and fill in the remaining deficiencies in our knowledge.

References

1. Fries, J. F. and Ehrlich, G. E. (eds.) (1985). *Prognosis: Contemporary Outcomes of Disease.* (Menlo Park, Calif.: Addison-Wesley)
2. Kelley, W. N. *et al.* (1989). *Textbook of Rheumatology*, 3rd edn. (Philadelphia: W. B. Saunders)
3. Wyngarten, J. B. and Smith, L. B. (eds.) (1988). *Cecil Textbook of Medicine.* (Philadelphia: W. B. Saunders)
4. Mitchell, D. M., Spitz, P. W., Young, D. Y., Bloch, D. A., McShane, D. J. and Fries, J. F. (1986). Survival, prognosis, and causes of death in rheumatoid arthritis. *Arthritis Rheum.*, **29**, 706–714
5. Fries, J. F. (1983). The assessment of disability. From first to future principles. *Br. J. Rheumatol.* **22**(suppl.), 48–48
6. Tugwell, P. (1981). How to read clinical journals; 3. To learn the course and progress of disease. *Can. Med. Assoc. J.*, **124**, 869–872
7. Fries, J. F., Spitz, P., Kraines, R. G. and Holman, H. R. (1980). Measurement of patient outcome in arthritis. *Arthritis Rheum.*, **23**, 137–145
8. Meenan, R. F., Gertman, P. M. and Mason, J. H. (1980). Measuring health status in arthritis: The arthritis impact measurement scales. *Arthritis Rheum.*, **23**, 146–152
9. Bellamy, N. and Buchanan, W. W. (1988). Clinical evaluation in rheumatic diseases. In: McCarty, D. (ed.) *Arthritis and Allied Conditions*, 11th edn. pp. 158–186. (Philadelphia: Lea and Febiger)
10. Fries, J. F. (1983). Toward an understanding of patient outcome measurement. *Arthritis Rheum.*, **26**, 697–704
11. Feigenbaum, P. A., Medsger, Jr, T. A., Kraines, R. G. and Fries, J. F. (1982). The variability of immunologic laboratory tests. *J. Rheumatol.*, **9**, 408–414

12. Fries, J. F., Spitz, P. W. and Young, D. Y. (1982). The dimensions of health outcomes: The health assessment questionnaire, disability and pain scales. *J. Rheumatol.*, **29**(6), 789-793
13. Mitchell, D. M., Spitz, P. W., Young, D. Y., Bloch, D. A., McShane, D. J. and Fries, J. F. (1986). Survival, prognosis, and causes of death in rheumatoid arthritis. *Arthritis Rheum.*, **29**(6), 706-714
14. Kirwan, J. R. and Reeback, J. S. (1986). Stanford Health Assessment Questionnaire modified to assess disability in British patients with rheumatoid arthritis. *Br. J. Rheumatol.*, **25**, 206-209
15. Pincus, T., Summey, J. A., Soraci, S. A. *et al.* (1983). Assessment of patient satisfaction in activities of daily living using a modified Stanford Health Assessment Questionnaire. *Arthritis Rheum.*, **26**, 1346-1353
16. Sullivan, F. F., Eagers, R. C., Lynch, K. and Barber, J. H. (1987). Assessment of disability caused by rheumatic diseases in general practice. *Ann. Rheum. Dis.*, **46**, 598-600
17. Bombardier, C., Tugwell, P., Sinclair, A., Dok, C., Anderson, G. and Buchanan, W. W. (1982). Preference for endpoint measures in clinical trials: results of structured workshops. *J. Rheumatol.*, **9**, 798-801
18. Symmons, D. P. M. and Dawes, P. T. (1988). Summary and consensus view. *Br. J. Rheumatol.*, **27**(suppl. I), 76-77
19. Peck, J. R., Ward, J. R., Smith, T. W. *et al.* (1987). Convergent/discriminant validity of the HAQ disability index in rheumatoid arthritis using a multitrait-multimethod matrix. *Arthritis Rheum.*, **30**, S193 (abstract)
20. Wolfe, F., Kleinheksel, S. M., Cathey, M. A., Hawley, D. J., Spitz, P. W. and Fries, J. F. (1988). The clinical value of the Stanford Health Assessment Questionnaire Functional Disability Index in patients with rheumatoid arthritis. *J. Rheumatol.*, **15**, 1480-1488
21. Nevitt, M. C., Yelin, E. H., Henke, C. J. *et al.* (1986). Risk factors for hospitalization and surgery in patients with rheumatoid arthritis: Implications for capitated medical payment. *Ann. Intern. Med.*, **105**, 421-428
22. Bombardier, C., Ware, J., Russell, I. J. *et al.* (1986). Auranofin therapy and quality of life in patients with arthritis, results of a multicenter trial. *Am. J. Med.*, **81**, 565-578

2
Osteoarthritis

K. D. BRANDT and D. FLUSSER

THE MAGNITUDE OF THE PROBLEM

It is difficult to give an accurate figure for the prevalence of osteoarthritis (OA). While the radiograph may be the "gold standard" for the diagnosis of OA, it is not practical to obtain radiographs of all the joints in a large, representative sample. Hence, prevalence figures based on radiographic changes must be limited to specific joints. Depending on whether mild changes are included, or only more severe changes, the prevalence rate will vary.

While prevalence for specific joints may be determined radiographically, estimates of *overall* prevalence must be based on clinical information. However, many people who have no symptoms have radiographic evidence of OA.

Based upon the National Health and Nutrition Examination Survey I (NHANES-I), considering the medical history, radiographs, and physical examination, 12% of the US population between the ages of 25 and 74 years (nearly 16 million people) have OA[1]. Based on radiographic changes alone, regardless of symptoms, if all degrees of severity of OA are included, for adults aged 25-74 the overall prevalence estimates are approximately 32% for the hands, 22% for the feet, 4% for the knees, and 1% for the hips (considering males only, since hip radiographs were not obtained in women less than 50 years of age). If only people with moderate/severe OA are considered, the corresponding estimates are about 8% for the hands (10.3 million people), 2% for the feet (3 million people), 1% for the knees (117 000 people) and 0.5% for the hips (males only, 29 000). By the age of 75 years almost all people have radiographic evidence of OA in their hands and about 50% in their feet. At younger ages, males have radiographic evidence of OA more frequently than females. In older age groups, females show OA changes more often than males, and their changes are more severe.

When symptomatic OA is considered, the highest prevalence rates for OA with pain are found in the hands: 2.4% of males and 3.8% of females had pain of some severity associated with radiographic changes of OA[1]. Obviously, many people with radiological evidence of OA do not have pain, especially in the hands and feet. In contrast, in the NHANES-I survey 10-30% of people with knee OA, and 21-39% of those with hip OA, were currently receiving treatment for their joint complaints[2]. In another study, 21% of patients with OA reported difficulty in the performance of daily activities[3].

Socioeconomic impact of OA

Analysis of the direct and indirect costs incurred by ambulatory patients with rheumatoid arthritis and with OA, in terms of 1979 dollars, showed that patients spent an average of $147 for arthritis medications, aids and devices, and $207 for outpatient visits. In addition to these direct dollar costs, they averaged nearly 7 days of restricted activity per month. Among working patients, 2.5 work days per month were lost because of arthritis, and 30% reported that they were unemployed or retired because of poor health. Notably, costs were similar whether the patient had rheumatoid arthritis or OA, except for outpatient charges, which were much higher for those with rheumatoid arthritis[4].

Kramer et al.[5] found that people with OA utilized outpatient physician services approximately 3.5 times in 1 year; this was half the rate for patients with rheumatoid arthritis.

In people aged less than 65 who were considered to have OA, earnings losses and work disability were almost as great as in those considered to have rheumatoid arthritis[6]. Approximately 67% of men and 36% of women with presumed OA, and 56% of men and 31% of women with symmetric polyarthritis (presumably rheumatoid arthritis) were working. In contrast, for people without arthritis, employment rates were 90% for men and 62% for women. The rate of work disability in people presumed to have OA involving only one knee or one hip was about the same as that for people with symmetric polyarthritis involving two knees or two hips. Earnings of women and men with presumed OA were only 30% and 63%, respectively, of those for people with no arthritis. Less than one-third of the earnings losses in the OA group were explained by the presence of arthritis, however, since higher age, lower education level, and comorbidity had significant effects on earning power in this group.

OA has an impact on how patients spend their time and on their level of activity over time. Patients with OA experienced more losses in the performance of household chores, shopping, and errands than controls who were matched for age, sex, and community of residence[7]. In addition, the OA patients slept longer and spent more time shopping and in personal care, although they were similar to controls with respect to the amount of time spent dressing and taking medicines.

PROBLEMS IN DETERMINING THE PROGNOSIS OF OA

Data concerning the natural history of OA and its progression are remarkably scanty. The general impression is that, at least once symptoms appear, OA is inexorably progressive. However, for any individual patient, whether the disorder will progress, at what rate, or, indeed, whether it will improve, are all very difficult to predict. This difficulty can be attributed to several factors:

First, no satisfactory definition of OA exists. There is general agreement that the main pathologic characteristics include breakdown of articular cartilage, proliferation of bone and cartilage at the joint margins, and remodeling of subchondral bone. However, at a recent international workshop on OA, at which the clinical, pathologic, histologic, biomechanical, and biochemical features of OA were consolidated into a comprehensive definition, the participants agreed unanimously that the definition was inadequate[8].

Second, the radiographic interpretation of OA presents problems. While all would agree that osteophytes are a radiographic hallmark of OA, the presence of osteophytes *alone* — in the absence of joint space narrowing, geodes, or subchondral sclerosis — may reflect aging, rather than OA[9,10]. If this is not recognized, OA will be overdiagnosed radiographically.

Third, the prognosis varies with the site of involvement. Clinical studies have often lumped together patients with OA at various sites. Clearly, this is not valid; the outlook for interphalangeal joint OA is very different from that for knee or hip OA.

Fourth, most of our information concerning the prognosis of OA is based only on radiographs. Longitudinal studies examining the effects of OA at various sites on symptoms and function, as well as on radiographic changes, are badly needed. Risk factors for progression of OA, and for pain and disability, need to be much better defined.

Finally, what do we mean by prognosis? Are we speaking about prognosis with respect to progression of pathology? Or pain? Mobility? Disability?

No standard method exists for evaluating patients with OA clinically. Current methods of clinical assessment show a high degree of variability. To address this issue Bellamy and Buchanan[11] have recently developed a multidimensional outcome measure for use in patients with hip and knee OA that probes the severity of discomfort and disability and defines the clinical importance of component items.

Pain and function. Pain in OA may be due to several causes (e.g., synovial inflammation, stretching of nerve endings in the periosteum at the site of bony spurs, microfracture of subchondral bone, medullary hypertension, capsular distension, muscle spasm)[12]. However, the discrepancy between pain severity and severity of pathologic changes is often striking; one patient with radiographic evidence of advanced OA may have no complaints. Another, with only mild changes, may complain of severe discomfort. Why? What factors determine whether a patient with OA has joint pain?

Periarticular muscle weakness may be one of the determinants of pain in OA. While rheumatologists and orthopedic surgeons commonly recommend isometric exercises to strengthen the quadriceps femoris muscle in patients with knee OA, the benefits of such an exercise program have received very little study. However, a controlled investigation of patients with knee OA found that joint pain was significantly reduced by such exercises[13]. Exercises produced subjective and objective improvement also in patients with OA of the hip, but outpatient hydrotherapy produced no additional benefit over that achieved by the exercise regimen alone[14]. Whether muscle weakness is a risk factor for pain or disability in patients who have pathologic changes of OA but no symptoms remains to be determined. If so, muscle strengthening might play a preventative, as well as a therapeutic, role.

Psychologic factors (e.g., feeling in low spirits) were found to be associated with knee pain in white women with OA[15]. In another study, anxiety was associated with total amount of pain while depression was associated with pain severity in OA[16].

When factors predisposing to knee pain in 55-year-old people in Sweden were analyzed, it was found that 10% of the population had knee pain. Only 1% (all males) had radiographic signs of knee OA, however. Women with knee pain more often had varus knees, while men with knee pain tended to be heavier than those without pain. Those with pain had been less successful in a childhood intelligence test, had had a shorter period of education, were less satisfied with their current working conditions, had jobs with heavier physical demands, and had a lower average income than subjects without knee pain. When interactions between these measured variables were eliminated, two variables — body weight and job satisfaction — remained independent in men. In women, none of the variables was independent[17].

In another study, disability support status predicted functional impairment in patients with OA with chronic knee pain. Those receiving disability payments were much more functionally limited than those not receiving such financial support[18]. Obese patients showed a higher level of pain behaviors, e.g., guarded movements, than nonobese patients and were more impaired with respect to mobility and physical activity.

Disability. What are the risk factors for disability in OA? In an analysis of NHANES-I data, in which musculoskeletal impairments (not specifically OA) were considered in comparison with those who were not disabled, those who were disabled with musculoskeletal symptoms tended to be older, nonwhite, of lower education and income, and either widowed, separated, or divorced. Disability was increased in those who attributed their symptoms to an accident or injury and those who had musculoskeletal symptoms in multiple sites[19].

The association of disability with separated/divorced marital status may be related to the lack of social support. In a randomized control trial involving chiefly black female patients of lower socioeconomic class attending a general medicine clinic, provision of health information on a regular basis resulted in improved physical health, decreased pain, and enhanced functional status[20]. Indeed, an interaction as simple as a telephone interview appeared to provide OA patients with sufficient social support to improve their functional status[21]. In similar patients with OA, hassles (minor stressors) were better predictors of health status than major life-change events and correlated strongly with functional status[22].

It is worth noting that the critical determination for institutionalization in the elderly is lack of social support, not functional impairment[23]. Furthermore, intensification of rehabilitation services for homebound elderly patients with musculoskeletal disability did not significantly improve functional scores, frequency of institutionalization, or quality of life, even though a majority of patient goals were met[24].

Who is the better judge of health status — patient or doctor? When functional status was measured in a group of elderly people with arthritis, scores for dependence, difficulty, and pain correlated with the patients' report of their joint condition and ability to cope with the arthritis, but not with the opinion of the patients' medical staff concerning the status of the joint or the patients' ability to deal with their arthritis[25].

Other data suggest that OA may not contribute significantly to the objective decline in function in the aged but that the patient's awareness of the presence of OA might contribute to a *perception* of disability[26]. Thus, when hand function was measured objectively in subjects over 60 years of age, results were related to age, coordination, and hand strength, but not to the extent or severity of OA. However, subjective hand disability, measured with the Stanford Health Assessment Questionnaire, correlated with radiographic evidence of OA, joint tenderness, and hand strength.

Mortality in OA. In a large cohort of patients with OA in Boston, mortality was 11% greater than that occurring from all causes in the general population[27]. In particular, deaths from respiratory and gastrointestinal causes were increased. Similarly, in the NHANES-I follow-up survey, excess mortality and decreased survival were noted for women with knee OA[28]. It may be speculated that the higher than normal mortality from gastrointestinal causes was related to side-effects of treatment with NSAIDs. Indeed, an association between knee OA and peptic ulcer disease has been demonstrated[29]. After adjustment for severity of radiographic changes, subjects with knee pain had a twofold greater risk of ulcer disease than those without knee pain. In contrast, the risk of ulcer disease was no greater in people with asymptomatic knee OA than in those with normal radiographs and no knee pain. The association between treatment with NSAIDs and ulcer disease is well recognized.[30,31]

The increased mortality of OA may relate not only to iatrogenic factors but to comorbid conditions. In population samples in Great Britain and Jamaica, generalized OA was more common in older males with a high diastolic blood pressure than in those with low blood pressure[32]. Knee OA in women also was associated with hypertension.

HOW PROGRESSIVE IS OA?

While the common view of both lay people and physicians is that OA is inevitably progressive, clinical observations and basic research suggest that this is overly pessimistic. The widespread belief that nothing can be done to arrest its progress can be attributed to the fact that, until recently, loss of articular cartilage — the hallmark of OA — was thought to be due principally to *nonbiologic* "wear-and-tear" and/or aging. It is difficult, without surgical intervention, to halt wear-and-tear and impossible to halt aging. Given that view, how can progression of OA not be inevitable?

It is highly significant — and a basis for optimism — that our concept of the pathogenesis of OA today focuses as much on the *biology* of articular cartilage as it does upon mechanical factors. Although cartilage breakdown may be driven by mechanical factors, metabolic alterations — including a striking biosynthetic ("repair") response as well as heightened matrix catabolism — are readily discernible in OA cartilage. This suggests that pharmacologic agents might be devised to modify the course of OA. Even in the absence of such therapy, however, progressive joint degeneration in OA is not inevitable.

Evidence for reversibility of OA. In OA of the hip, spontaneous recovery of the joint space has been documented radiographically[33-37]. In these cases the joint usually undergoes resurfacing with fibrocartilage. Perry concluded that the presence of substantial osteophytes favored spontaneous recovery of the joint space and reduction in joint pain, whereas the presence of only small osteophytes, or absence of osteophytes, was associated with radiographic and clinical deterioration[33].

Spontaneous recovery of radiographic joint space in OA joints other than the hip appears to be much less common. However, in the knee, osteotomy, in addition to relieving pain, can arrest cartilage degeneration and lead to cartilage healing if the contact area is increased and/or stresses are lowered[37]. Fibrocartilaginous repair may restore the joint space[38-40] and lead to disappearance of subchondral bony sclerosis[38,41,42] and geodes[26,39,43]. Healing occurs via metaplasia of extrinsic cells, derived principally from the subchondral bone.

Insight into the ability of the chondrocyte to limit the progression of cartilage breakdown in OA is provided by recent experiments in dogs subjected to transection of the anterior cruciate ligament (ACL). In this model, metabolic, biochemical, biomechanical and morphologic changes occur in articular cartilage of the unstable knee that mimic those of human OA; however, in contrast to the findings in humans with advanced OA, full-thickness loss of articular cartilage is rare.

A recent study of this model showed that a progressive *increase* occurs in the amount of articular cartilage in the unstable knee after ACL transection[44]. The total amount of proteoglycan (PG) and, commonly, the PG concentration of the OA cartilage were increased, and the rate of PG synthesis was commonly elevated, in comparison with that in cartilage from the contralateral knee. Thus, knee instability did not lead to loss of articular cartilage but to an active synthetic response by the chondrocyte, resulting in hypertrophic cartilage repair.[44].

Although the lack of progression of cartilage breakdown in this model had been noted previously, it had been attributed to buttressing of the unstable knee by large osteophytes and capsular fibrosis[45]. However, radiographs nearly 4 years after ACL transection show only minimal limitation of flexion and extension of the OA knee[46] and forces generated by the OA limb, measured by a force plate, were no smaller at that time than only 6 months after ACL transection (O'Connor, B. and Brandt, K., unpublished). Furthermore, when joint loading was reduced by application of an orthopedic cast to the unstable knee of dogs subjected to ACL transection, cartilage atrophy — with a *decrease* in PG synthesis — ensued, not OA[47].

The significance of the above observations lies in the fact that they demonstrate that preservation of articular cartilage in the OA knee in this model is not due principally to mechanical factors, but to an increased rate of PG synthesis that can maintain — or even lead to an increase in — the amount of cartilage in the joint. Recent magnetic resonance imaging studies have shown that the cartilage in the unstable canine joint remains thicker than normal nearly 4 years after ACL transection[46]. How much longer the increase in PG synthesis in the OA cartilage will support good joint function remains to be seen.

In humans with OA, cartilage PG synthesis also is elevated, at least until the late stages of the disease[48]. In man, however, depletion of matrix PGs and loss of cartilage are hallmarks of OA. The accelerated breakdown of cartilage in OA has been attributed to mechanical factors and/or enzymatic degradation[49,50]. However, consistent with our observations in dogs, Thompson *et al.* noted that the PG concentration in relatively unaffected areas of cartilage from femoral heads of patients with advanced OA also was increased[51]. Similarly, in knees of Rhesus monkeys with early spontaneous OA, the hexosamine content of the cartilage was elevated[52].

RISK FACTORS FOR CLINICAL PROGRESSION OF OA

Crystals of calcium pyrophosphate dihydrate (CPPD) and calcium hydroxyapatite (HA). The occurrence of crystals of CPPD or HA in synovial fluid from OA hips and knees has been associated with rapid progression (i.e., > 50% narrowing of the joint space within 1 year). In a study in which patients with severe joint space narrowing were excluded (since the subchondral bone would have been a confounding source of apatite), 8 of 10 fluids from patients with rapidly progressive OA, but only 19 of

84 fluids from patients with "ordinary" OA contained such crystals[53]. In the subset with rapidly progressive disease, CPPD was present in 6 cases, HA in 1, and both types of crystal in 1. Several other recent reports have also drawn an association between crystal deposition and rapidly progressive OA[54,55]. The prognostic value of synovial fluid crystals and their pathogenetic significance in rapidly progressive OA, however, remain to be determined.

Primary OA. Underlying primary OA appears to affect the prognosis for secondary OA, as shown by a study of hands and knees of patients who had undergone unilateral meniscectomy a mean of nearly 25 years earlier[56]. Clinical and radiographic features of OA were more frequent and more severe in operated than in unoperated knees. Patients who had had radiographic changes of primary generalized OA showed more frequent and more severe knee OA, judged clinically and radiographically, in both the operated and unoperated knees than patients without hand OA. The increased frequency of OA in the operated knees remained significant even after exclusion of the patients with OA in the unoperated knee.

Synovial inflammation. It has been considered that synovitis, in addition to being a source of joint pain, may drive the progression of articular cartilage breakdown in OA. In a canine model of OA[57], cytokines (e.g., interleukin-1, tumor necrosis factor) that may mediate chondrocytic chondrolysis have been shown to be produced by inflamed synovium. Neutral proteases capable of causing tissue damage also may be produced by the OA synovium[58]. The clinical significance of these matrix-degrading enzymes and cytokines in OA, however, remains to be demonstrated. Indeed, when synovial inflammation was virtually eliminated in a canine model of OA, changes in articular cartilage biochemistry and PG metabolism were no different from those seen in the presence of marked synovial inflammation, suggesting that these cartilage changes are due chiefly to mechanical factors, rather than to synovitis (Myers, S., O'Connor, B., and Brandt, K., unpublished observations).

Adrenal glucocorticoids. Moskowitz et al.[59] demonstrated nuclear degeneration and cyst formation in articular cartilage following injection of triamcinolone acetonide into the knees of normal rabbits. In the only published investigation in nonhuman primates[60], one knee of macaca irus monkeys was injected with 20 mg of methylprednisolone once, twice, or six times over a 12-week period, while the opposite knee was injected with the drug vehicle. At the close of the study, examination of cartilage from both knees showed cartilage clefts, cloning of chondrocytes, and hypocellularity, but changes in the joints injected with steroids were not significantly different from those in the control joints.

In man, intra-articular steroids are widely used for symptomatic relief in patients with osteoarthritis, although limited control studies show that they produce only short-term relief or are of no benefit[61]. In addition, concern exists that repeated intra-articular injections of steroid may accelerate joint breakdown and lead to Charcot-like arthropathy.

What is the basis for this concern? In 1958, Chandler and Wright[62] described 18 patients with rheumatoid arthritis, each of whom was treated with repeated injections of intra-articular hydrocortisone over a 48-week period. Radiographic deterioration of the injected joints was observed that the authors attributed to sustained relief of pain, with consequent overuse of the damaged joint. In 1959, the same group reported a 66-year-old woman whose osteoarthritic hip was injected with 50 mg of hydrocortisone acetate monthly for 18 months[63]. The patient experienced symptomatic relief of pain for 3 weeks after each injection. However, radiographs showed progressive destruction of the hip that the authors attributed to the treatment with hydrocortisone.

Although other studies have failed to show development of progressive joint breakdown after multiple steroid injections[64,65], the early reports by Chandler[62,63], even though they represent only uncontrolled observations, have left lingering concerns about the potential adverse effects of intra-articular steroid injections on the course of osteoarthritis.

More recently, however, with the growing understanding that articular cartilage breakdown in osteoarthritis is mediated by collagenase and metalloproteinases that degrade matrix proteoglycans[66,67], that these enzymes are produced and secreted by chondrocytes; that stimulation of the chondrocyte to produce and release these matrix-degrading enzymes may be mediated by cytokines derived from the inflamed synovium, e.g., interleukin-1 and tumor necrosis factor[68], and that production of these cytokines is exquisitely sensitive to inhibition by very low concentrations of glucocorticoids[69], interest has arisen in the possibility that steroids might have a *favorable* effect on the progression of cartilage breakdown in osteoarthritis.

Williams and Brandt[70] showed that a single intra-articular injection of triamcinolone hexacetonide protected against iodoacetate-induced cartilage breakdown in guinea pigs and markedly reduced osteophyte formation in this model. Similarly, in a rabbit model of osteoarthritis, oral and intra-articular steroid therapy both ameliorated the severity of osteoarthritis[71,71].

Following anterior cruciate ligament transection, Pelletier and Martel-Pelletier[73] treated six dogs with oral prednisone, 0.25 mg kg^{-1} d^{-1} until the animals were sacrificed 8 weeks later. At the time of sacrifice, cartilage erosions were found in only 8% of the steroid-treated animals, but in 25% of dogs that underwent cruciate ligament transection but did not receive steroids. Furthermore, knee cartilage from the dogs given prednisone showed less severe histologic changes of osteoarthritis than the controls.

Although the authors considered the prednisone regimen they employed (0.25 mg kg^{-1}d^{-1}) to be "a low dose," it is equivalent to 17 mg/d of prednisone in a 70-kg human – so high as to be prohibitive for treatment of osteoarthritis in man because of the side-effects it would produce. Notably, in an essentially identical study, a lower dose of prednisone, 0.1 mg kg^{-1} d^{-1} (i.e., the equivalent of only 7 mg/d in a 70-kg human), did not reduce the severity of osteoarthritis in dogs (Myers, S. and Brandt, K., unpublished observations).

Obesity. In cross-sectional studies an association between obesity and knee OA has long been recognized[74-77]. These analyses, however, provided no insight into which was cause and which was effect. In a recent analysis of data from the Framingham study, Felson et al.[78] found that the presence of obesity in subjects in 1948-1952 (when they were, on average, 37 years old) increased the risk that they would have radiographic and symptomatic evidence of OA during a follow-up evaluation in 1983-1985 (when the subjects were, on average, 73 years old). In NHANES-I, obesity was a stronger predictor of bilateral knee OA than was prior knee injury, which was a much stronger predictor of unilateral knee OA[79]. Whether, once symptoms of OA appear, weight reduction will decrease pain, improve mobility or retard the progression of joint breakdown, is unknown.

Muscle contraction. Although periarticular muscle weakness may be a risk factor for pain in established OA (see above), based upon pathoanatomic studies showing predominant sites of wear in human femoral heads, Barrie has suggested that increased muscle tone (spasm), by increasing the loading of OA articular cartilage, could be a risk factor for disease progression (the clenched hip).[80]

Stiffness of subchondral bones. It has been suggested that stiffening of subchondral bone (manifest as subchondral sclerosis on the radiographs) contributes to the progression of OA[81]. Stiffening of subchondral bone *in vivo* results in breakdown of overlying articular cartilage[82]. Subchondral bone has been shown to be stiffer than normal.[83]

Age. While age is probably the most powerful risk factor for OA, there are no data to indicate that, once OA is present, age affects prognosis (except, perhaps, in the distal interphangeal joints, see below). Indeed, in a cross-sectional study in Sweden, radiographic and clinical evidence of knee OA was less prevalent with advancing age.[84]

FACTORS SHOWN EXPERIMENTALLY TO ACCELERATE JOINT DESTRUCTION IN OA

Given that cartilage loss is the result of an imbalance between catabolic and anabolic activities of the chondrocyte and that a marked capacity for synthesis of matrix ("repair") exists in OA cartilage that may prevent, or retard the progression of, cartilage breakdown, it is reasonable to ask whether factors might exist that could "tip the scales" and accelerate cartilage loss in OA. Recent experimental work provides insight into two such factors: (i) certain antirheumatic drugs and (ii) impairment of sensory nerve input from the limb containing the OA joint.

OSTEOARTHRITIS

Nonsteroidal anti-inflammatory drugs. A substantial body of evidence from this laboratory and others indicates that some, but not all, nonsteroidal anti-inflammatory drugs (NSAIDs) suppress PG biosynthesis in normal articular cartilage *in vitro*. The effect has been shown to occur with salicylates, fenoprofen, tolmetin sodium, and ibuprofen[85,86]. In contrast, indomethacin, sulindac sulfide, diclofenac sodium, piroxicam, tiaprofenic acid[87], and naproxen sodium (Brandt, K., unpublished observations) had no significant effects on net PG synthesis; benoxaprofen significantly increased the rate of synthesis over control levels[88]. Suppression of PG metabolism was noted with concentrations of NSAID in the culture medium that approximated those in serum and/or synovial fluid of patients treated with anti-inflammatory doses of the drug.

The suppressive effects on PG synthesis were concentration-dependent, reversible, and independent of changes in prostaglandin biosynthesis[85,86,89]. The rate of PG catabolism in both normal and OA knee cartilage was unaffected by the above NSAIDs, except for fenoprofen, which minimally retarded the rate of PG breakdown[86].

Notably, the inhibitory effect on PG synthesis of salicylate and most other NSAIDs was much more marked in OA cartilage than in normal cartilage[90]. However, neither piroxicam nor diclofenac were found to affect PG synthesis in OA cartilage.

Consistent with its *in vitro* inhibition of PG biosynthesis, aspirin has been shown to exacerbate cartilage degeneration also *in vivo*; other NSAIDs have not yet been similarly tested. *In vivo* studies with aspirin were carried out in a canine model of OA induced by unilateral ACL transection. Articular cartilage from the unstable knee a few months later exhibited fibrillation, PG depletion and an increased rate of PG synthesis. In contrast, cartilage from the contralateral knee was grossly, histologically, histochemically, and biochemically normal[91].

When aspirin was administered orally in daily doses sufficient to maintain a serum salicylate concentration of 20–25 mg/dl the PG concentration in cartilage from the experimental knee fell significantly below that seen in degenerating cartilage of animals treated similarly but not given aspirin. No augmentation of PG synthesis was seen in the OA cartilage of dogs that had received aspirin, indicating that aspirin feeding had abrogated repair activity of the chondrocyte. Notably, no *in vivo* effect of salicylate on PG biosynthesis or on the PG content of normal cartilage was seen[91].

The effects of aspirin and other NSAIDs on articular cartilage *in vivo* may be related to the concentration of drug present in the synovial fluid bathing the cartilage. In clinical situations, this concentration is related to the amount of drug administered, which, in turn, is determined by the relative antirheumatic "potency" of the NSAID and its toxicity. Extrapolation of the *in vitro* data would suggest that, to the extent that the effective antirheumatic dose of an NSAID is lower than that of salicylate, it may have less marked effects than salicylate on degenerating cartilage[92]. If the effects of salicylate and other NSAIDs on articular cartilage in man are similar to those seen in animal models of OA, these compounds, while they may produce symptomatic relief, could accelerate the progression of OA.

On the other hand, despite a lack of clinical evidence, it has been suggested that NSAIDs may be "chondroprotective[93]." Such claims are based largely on *in vitro* evidence that they may modify PG or collagen metabolism, cytokine-mediated matrix degeneration, release or activity of neutral proteases, and/or actions of toxic oxygen metabolites[93-103]. No clinical evidence exists to support the contention that NSAIDs favorably influence the progression of joint degeneration in man.

Prediction of the *in vivo* effects of an NSAID based on its *in vitro* effects on cartilage is naive. Synovial inflammation itself may alter the integrity of articular cartilage in the OA joint. The relative importance of the effect of the NSAID on synovitis, of its direct effect on chondrocyte metabolism, and of its analgesic action — perhaps permitting overloading of an already damaged joint — cannot be predicted from *in vitro* studies. Indeed, several clinical studies have implicated NSAIDs in the acceleration of joint destruction in man. In 1977, "indomethacin hips" were described[104]. Aspirin too, has been considered to aggravate joint damage in OA and, more recently, a variety of NSAIDs were considered to have contributed to destruction of acetabular bone in a small number of patients with OA of the hip[105].

In a randomized, but not blinded, prospective clinical trial, azapropazone, a weak prostaglandin-synthetase inhibitor with no effects on PG synthesis, was compared with indomethacin, a potent prostaglandin synthetase inhibitor, in 105 patients with hip OA who were awaiting arthroplasty[106]. Patients in the indomethacin group took 50% less time to reach arthroplasty and showed more rapid radiologic deterioration than those receiving azapropazone. Notably, compared to azapropazone, indomethacin enhanced the rate of cartilage loss in both the OA hip and the contralateral hip.

A number of factors other than effects on PG or prostaglandin synthesis could have accounted for the apparently enhanced rate of destruction of the OA joints in patients taking indomethacin. Overuse was not considered likely, however, since the doses of azapropazone and indomethacin that were employed provided comparable pain relief.

A double-blind control comparison of naproxen sodium versus acetaminophen is currently in progress to examine the influence of the NSAID on the natural history of knee OA (Ward, J., personal communication). Unfortunately, the dropout rate has been so high that it will be difficult to generalize the results.

Neurogenic acceleration of OA. A number of years ago experiments were initiated in this unit to define the role of peripheral sensory innervation in development of OA. Unilateral hind limb deafferentation, achieved by L4-S1 ganglionectomy, produced no abnormalities in the ipsilateral knees of dogs maintained for up to 64 weeks after the neurosurgical procedure. However, when destabilization of the knee — achieved by ACL transection — was superimposed upon the deafferentation procedure, osteophytes, cartilage ulceration and osteochondral fracture developed within 3 weeks(!) and the articular cartilage showed extensive fibrillation, chondrocyte cloning, and acellularity.

In contrast, in neurologically intact dogs no morphologic abnormalities were seen this soon after ACL transection. Thus, ipsilateral deafferentation converted the essentially "nonprogressive" OA in this animal model (see above) into severe joint breakdown that progressed with galloping speed[107].

Of clinical relevance, we have recently described patients with long-standing insulin-dependent diabetes mellitus in whom neuropathic arthropathy developed within weeks after an episode of minor trauma to the foot or ankle. In these individuals, diabetic neuropathy served as the functional equivalent of dorsal root ganglionectomy in the canine model, and the minor trauma as the equivalent of ACL transection. The data suggest that a neurosensory deficit may adversely affect the prognosis of OA[108].

THE PROGNOSIS OF OA IN SOME SPECIFIC JOINTS

Knee. In 1977, Hernborg and Nilsson[109] published results of a prospective study of 71 Swedish patients who were selected on the basis of evidence of knee OA on a previous radiograph and on whom clinical data and repeat knee radiographs were obtained 10–18 years (mean = 13 years) after the initial radiograph. The course tended to be progressive and unfavorable. Fifty-six percent reported that their symptoms had worsened. Some had developed knee pain even at rest. In most cases, radiographic progression of OA was seen. In 25% of cases that initially showed only medial compartment disease, the second radiograph showed involvement also of the lateral compartment, but in most knees the changes remained confined to the compartment initially affected. Varus deformity and joint instability were significantly associated with worsening. For most patients, walking distance had become limited to less than 400 meters because of knee pain. Seventeen percent of patients, however, reported that their symptoms had *improved*.

Only one other longitudinal prospective study of knee OA exists. In 1989, Massardo et al.[110] described 31 patients with knee OA who underwent clinical and radiographic evaluation on two occasions, at an 8-year interval. Twenty patients (65%) had worsened. Many had incurred severe disability. In contrast to the findings of Hernborg and Nilsson[109], radiographic progression of OA changes was not apparent in the United Kingdom study[110] and four patients (17%) *improved* during the period of observation — similar to the proportion showing improvement in the Scandinavian series[109]. It was suggested that improvement was associated with the presence of chondrocalcinosis, with a hypertrophic bone response, and with continued physical activity. Thus, improvement in pain did not appear to be due to the fact that the patient bore less load on the OA knee. However, three of the four patients who improved symptomatically lost knee motion and developed more severe radiographic changes. A good outcome in hip OA also has been correlated with a hypertrophic bone reaction[111].

In most patients, additional joints, particularly in the hand, gradually became involved by OA during the 8-year period of observation ("monoarthritis multiplex"), so that by the end of the study all patients had oligoarticular disease[110]. A striking relationship was noted between hand OA and knee OA, suggesting a limited form of generalized OA.

Hip. Symptomatic OA of the hip is commonly bilateral. In 35 of 51 patients who underwent bilateral total hip arthroplasty, symptoms began simultaneously in both hips; in 13 the second hip became symptomatic within 4 years of the first[112].

Some cases of hip OA, however, may show spontaneous symptomatic and radiographic improvement[33-35,113]. In a series of 91 unoperated hips followed for 10 years by Danielsson[35], more than 60% reported a decrease in pain; some became painless. In 7%, a decrease in the severity of the radiographic changes was seen.

Seifert et al.[34] found no deterioration in 33% of 44 unoperated cases that were followed for 5 years. The absence of bony cystic change in the initial radiograph appeared to indicate a favorable prognosis. In view of the fact that obesity appears to be a risk factor for OA of the knee, but not necessarily for OA of the hip[114], it is interesting that no correlation was observed between excess weight and deterioration of established hip OA[33]. The number of obese patients in the series was small, however. In 14 of 31 unoperated cases (45%), Perry[33] reported recovery of the joint space on radiographs taken, on average, 10 years after the onset of symptoms.

In contrast to Seifert's observations that cystic change was an unfavorable prognostic sign[34], all 14 hips that underwent spontaneous improvement in Perry's series[33] had (pseudo)cystic degeneration and joint space recovery was related to development of osteophytes, which caused restriction in joint motion, with a decrease in pain and reduction in intake of analgesic drugs.

Interphalangeal joints. In contrast to the rate of progression observed in many patients with hip or knee OA, in a study limited to assessment of hand radiographs the rate of change in severity of OA of distal and proximal interphalangeal (DIP, PIP, respectively) joints was typically slow[115]. The maximum rate of degeneration was seen in DIP joints, where the average increase within an individual was 1.25 grades within 12-16 years. The rate of deterioration in DIPs was enhanced with increasing age. OA of PIP joints deteriorated less rapidly, and less predictably, than OA in DIP joints, and did not appear to be age-related.

Since the radiographic grading scale used in the above study[116] gives considerable weight to the presence of osteophytes, which may be a manifestation of aging, rather than of OA, it is unclear to what extent the observed "worsening" represents true disease progression, with loss of cartilage, development of subchondral cysts and bony sclerosis.

Furthermore, the relation of radiographic progression to symptoms and function was not considered.

However, when hand function was assessed by a standardized test of activities of daily living, only minor global impairment was seen among OA patients, although significant differences were noted between controls and patients[117]. Patients with erosive OA had poorer hand function than those with nodal generalized OA. Differences between controls and patients were most obvious in younger subjects; in the elderly, hand function in the two groups was essentially the same. In controls, increasing age was directly related to the time required to complete tasks and inversely related to power grip. In patients, correlations were similar but less marked. Thus, for patients with nodal generalized OA, functional outcome is good. OA appears to have little effect on hand function in the aged. These results are consistent with the data reported by Baron *et al.*, who also found that OA does not contribute to the objective decline in hand function in the elderly[26].

Elbow. OA of the elbow is uncommon and usually secondary to major occupational factors or major trauma. Thus, it is seen in pneumatic drill operators, grinders, and baseball pitchers. Occasionally, elbow OA occurs unrelated to trauma in patients with generalized nodal OA or pyrophosphate arthropathy[118]. Doherty and Preston[119] recently reported 16 patients with elbow OA (26 elbows) unrelated to nodal OA, crystal deposition, or trauma. Mean duration of symptoms at entry into the study was 7 years. Most had OA also at other sites and in 10 patients, OA was prevalent in the 2nd/3rd metacarpophalangeal joints. The 16 patients, 14 of whom were male, represented 7% of all patients referred to a rheumatology clinic over a 3-year period with nonnodal, large joint OA and no evidence of calcium crystal deposition disease.

The predominant symptom (100%) was pain on use, although morning and inactivity stiffness also were common. Elbow flexion was restricted in every case. Treatment included analgesics and NSAIDs and occasional intra-articular steroid injections. The duration of follow-up ranged from 1 to 4 years.

The clinical outcome for the affected elbows was favorable. In most cases, symptoms improved or disappeared completely; in only one case did they worsen. All patients continued to work and had only minor, usually episodic difficulties with daily activities. Notably, good symptomatic and functional outcome was seen also for the associated metacarpophalangeal joint disease.

EFFECTS OF JOINT REPLACEMENT SURGERY ON PROGNOSIS

Where medical management is inadequate for control of pain, or limitation of mobility interferes with quality of life, joint replacement surgery is being performed with increasing frequency. In 1982, approximately 150 000 total hip and knee arthroplasties were performed in the United States (mostly for OA). In 1985, the number had doubled![120]

Measurements of health status in patients after total hip or knee replacement showed highly significant gains in global health and function, compared with the preoperative assessment[121]. The costs of the surgery in monetary terms are high, however, and among working-age persons only about 30% of those who were totally work-disabled prior to total hip arthroplasty had returned to work 1 or 4 years after surgery. Clearly, work capacity is determined by a variety of factors. Neither elimination of pain nor restoration of function in a major joint predicts subsequent return to work by patients with OA[122].

ARTHROSCOPIC PROCEDURES: JOINT DEBRIDEMENT, CARTILAGE SHAVING, ABRASION ARTHROPLASTY

Arthroscopic debridement of the joint, with removal of loose bodies and degenerated tissue fragments, is employed in some patients with severe OA of the knee. Controlled studies showing that it has favorable effect on pain and function in patients with OA are largely lacking, however.

Prior to the advent of arthroscopy, it was noted that removal of loose bodies, torn menisci, and articular cartilage flaps could relieve the joint pain of patients with knee OA — sometimes for years[123-125]. Indeed, in cases of only moderately severe OA, not only was symptomatic relief achieved, but progression of OA was said to be favorably influenced. However, the procedure required arthrotomy with lengthy rehabilitation, significant postoperative pain, and the risk of other postsurgical complications, and was not widely employed.

It is, therefore, a major advance that arthroscopic techniques now permit debridement of OA joints without the morbidity of an arthrotomy. In uncontrolled studies, OA patients with symptoms related to internal derangements seem to benefit most from the procedure while those with moderate OA without internal derangement benefit less frequently[126]. Those with significant joint instability without an internal derangement seem to benefit least.

The shaving of fibrillated articular cartilage, leaving a smoother surface, is also advocated as a means of achieving symptomatic relief in patients with knee OA. No long-term clinical studies have been reported that support the efficacy of this procedure, however. In fact, in humans, shaving of damaged knee articular cartilage was considered possibly to have caused increased fibrillation and cell necrosis in cartilage adjacent to the original defect[127]. In rabbits, shaving of normal patellar cartilage did not lead to progressive deterioration; neither, however, did it stimulate cartilage repair[128].

Abrasion of exposed subchondral bone to cause bleeding, with formation of a fibrin clot and subsequent articular cartilage repair, is also used in treatment of knee OA. No randomized controlled trial of arthroscopic abrasion arthroplasty has been reported. Uncontrolled studies[129-131] indicate that it decreased symptoms of OA in 60–83% of patients, with only 6–15% showing worsening at follow-up. Furthermore, in many patients with radiographic evidence of severe joint space loss the joint space increased after abrasion arthroplasty[131]. However, none of the patients became asymptomatic after treatment and the procedure was considered to be palliative.

In the few published studies of the effects of abrasion arthroplasty in OA, follow-up periods have been brief, making it difficult to determine whether it alters progression of OA. In general, neither outcome measures nor patient selection criteria or evaluation are well described, and results are usually reported by the surgeon who performed the procedure.

TIDAL IRRIGATION OF THE JOINT

At least part of the improvement that may occur following arthroscopy may be due to removal of debris from the joint space by the saline lavage employed during the procedure[132,133]. Joint irrigation alone, similar to that performed at the time of abrasion arthroplasty, has been reported to improve the pain of patients with OA who have been refractory to other medical measures[134,135] although, as with arthroscopy, the placebo effect of joint irrigation may be considerable, and randomized, controlled double-blinded studies of this procedure have not been performed.

POTENTIAL PREDICTIVE TESTS FOR PROGNOSIS OF OA

Scintigraphy. Hutton et al.[136], in a study of 29 women with OA of the hand, showed poor correlation between radiographic changes of OA and scintigraphic abnormalities after intravenous injection of ^{99m}Tc-labeled methylene diphosphate. In a number of cases, scans were abnormal when the radiograph showed no abnormality in the "hot" joint. When approximately half of the original population was followed for 2–5 years, in several instances scan positivity preceded radiographic evidence of OA by months or years[137]. The number of patients studied is yet too small to provide assurance that an abnormal scintigram will predict subsequent development of OA and, if so, whether the findings can be generalized to other joints.

Immunologic tests. Enzymes, such as stromelysin, that cleave the core protein of PGs, function in the turnover of cartilage matrix. After enzymatic cleavage of the PG, degradation products are rapidly lost from the cartilage matrix and may be recovered from the synovial fluid. From the joint space they gain access to the circulation via the synovial lymphatics and are removed from the plasma by the liver and kidney.

The concentration of keratan sulfate in blood may be measured by immunoassay and has been reported to be higher in patients with OA than in controls[138], although the extent or severity of cartilage degeneration in the controls was not ascertained. Since the acute degradation of cartilage induced by injection of papain into an intervertebral disc[139] or into a diarthrodial joint[140] was followed by a marked increase in the serum keratan sulfate concentration, and activities of matrix-degrading enzymes are known to be increased in OA cartilage, it was presumed that the elevated serum levels in some patients with OA reflected increased catabolism of cartilage in the involved joint(s). Alternatively, the increase in serum keratan sulfate concentration may reflect escape of newly synthesized PG molecules from OA cartilage, due to a relative insufficiency of hyaluronate to aggregate all the PGs that are synthesized (Poole, A. R., personal communication).

More recent studies have shown that, in contrast to its utility in detecting massive cartilage breakdown in acute animal experiments, determination of the serum keratan sulfate concentration is *not* useful for monitoring the more gradual progression of cartilage damage in OA, or the response to therapeutic intervention[141,142].

However, while the serum concentration of keratan sulfate (or of other putative markers of articular cartilage metabolism) may not be useful for following progress of OA in a given joint, if the blood level reflects the rate of cartilage catabolism *throughout the body*[141] measurement of the serum concentration could serve to identify people at risk for the development of OA or those with preclinical or subclinical OA. If that is the case, an elevated serum keratan sulfate value could represent a risk factor for OA, just as hypercholesterolemia is a risk factor for coronary artery disease[142]. Prospective serial evaluations of subjects with high and low serum keratan sulfate concentrations will resolve this issue for that potential marker.

To ascertain whether the release of matrix macromolecules from cartilage of a joint that has suffered damage to a meniscus or crucite ligament will predict development of posttraumatic OA, samples of synovial fluid have been assayed for their content of PGs (or immunoreactive fragments thereof)[143]. Average levels in synovial fluid of such patients were high and similar to those in joint fluid from patients with pyrophosphate arthroplasty or reactive arthritis[144]. The values were nearly 4 times higher than those for age-matched controls with knee pain who did not have evidence of joint pathology. Notably, in cross-sectional studies, elevated synovial fluid levels of PG fragments were noted more than 4 years after the knee injury — perhaps because of increased release of PGs from cartilage as a result of persistent synovitis or mechanical instability. Unfortunately, the patients in the above study were not followed longitudinally and were not randomly selected from a group of patients incurring knee trauma of a specific type or severity. Controlled longitudinal studies will provide insight into whether immunoassay of synovial fluid for cartilage matrix molecules will predict development of OA after joint injury.

CAN THE PROGNOSIS OF OA BE FAVORABLY INFLUENCED PHARMACOLOGICALLY?

Recently, compounds that are not NSAIDs or analgesics have been shown to stimulate chrondrocyte metabolism and/or inhibit matrix-degrading enzymes. These have received attention as potential "disease-modifying" therapy in OA. In a rabbit model of surgically-induced OA, Arteparon®, (glycosaminoglycan polysulfuric acid ester) reduced the severity of morphologic changes even when treatment was initiated after the onset of OA[145]. Similar results were noted in a canine model of OA[146].

In a long-term study that did not include a placebo control, a large group of OA patients in Czechoslovakia were treated with Arteparon® or Rumalon® (an extract of calf bone marrow that has been characterized as a sulfated glycosaminoglycan-peptide complex), in addition to NSAIDs. These patients showed less progression of OA, required surgery less often, and had fewer symptoms than those treated only with NSAIDs[147]. Much more data from well-controlled studies in humans are required.

References

1. Lawrence, R. C., Hochberg, M. C., Kelsey, J. L., McDuffie, F. G., Medsger, T. A. Jr., Felts, W. R. and Shulman, L. E. (1989). Estimates of the prevalence of selected arthritis and musculoskeletal diseases in the United States. *J. Rheumatol.*, **16**, 427–440
2. Maurer, K. (1979). Basic data on arthritis of knee, hip, and sacroiliac joints in adults ages 25–74 years: United States, 1971–1975. *Vital and Health Statistics*, Series II, No. 213, DHEW Publication No. (PHS) 79-1661. (Hyattsville, MD: National Center for Health Statistics)
3. Fries, J. F., Spitz, P. W. and Young, D. W. (1982). The dimensions of health outcomes: The Health Assessment Questionnaire, disability and pain scales. *J. Rheumatol.*, **9**, 789–793
4. Liang, M. H., Larson, M., Thompson, M., Eaton, H., McNamara, E., Katz, R. and Taylor, J. (1984). Costs and outcomes in rheumatoid arthritis and osteoarthritis. *Arthritis Rheum.*, **27**, 522–529
5. Kramer, J. S., Yelin, E. H. and Epstein, W. V. (1983). Social and economic impacts of four musculoskeletal conditions. A study using national community-based data. *Arthritis Rheum.*, **26**, 901–907
6. Pincus, T., Mitchell, J. M. and Burkhauser, R. V. (1989). Substantial work disability and earnings losses in individuals less than age 65 with OA: Comparisons with rheumatoid arthritis. *J. Clin. Epidemiol.*, **42**, 449–457
7. Yelin, E., Lubeck, D., Holman, H. and Epstein, W. (1987). The impact of rheumatoid arthritis and osteoarthritis: the activities of patients with rheumatoid arthritis and osteoarthritis compared to controls. *J. Rheumatol.*, **14**, 710–717
8. Mankin, H. J., Brandt, K. and Shulman, L. E. (1986). Workshop on etiopathogenesis of osteoarthritis. *J. Rheumatol.*, **13**, 1130–1160
9. Danielsson, L. G. (1964). Incidence and prognosis of coxarthrosis. *Acta Orthop. Scand.*, **66**(suppl.), 9–114
10. Hernborg, J. and Nilsson, B. E. (1973). The relationship between osteophytes in the knee joint, osteoarthritis and aging. *Acta Orthop. Scand.*, **44**, 69–74
11. Bellamy, N. and Buchanan, W. W. (1986). A preliminary evaluation of the dimensionality and clinical importance of pain and disability in osteoarthritis of the hip and knee. *Clin. Rheumatol.*, **5**, 231–241
12. Brandt, K. D. (1989). Management of osteoarthritis. In Kelley, W. N., Harris, E. D. Jr, Ruddy, S. and Sledge, C. B. (eds.). *Textbook of Rheumatology*, 3rd edn., Chapter 32, pp. 1501–1512. (Philadelphia: W. B. Saunders)
13. Chamberlain, M. A., Care, G. and Harfield, B. (1982). Physiotherapy in osteoarthritis of the knee: A controlled trial of hospital versus home exercises. *Int. Rehabil. Med.*, **4**, 191–206

14. McKenna, F., Green, J., Redfern, E. J. and Chamberlain, M. A. (1988). The value of outpatient hydrotherapy for osteoarthritis of the hip. *Br. J. Rheumatol.*, **27**(suppl. 2), 18
15. Hochberg, M. C., Lawrence, R. C., Everett, D. F. and Coroni-Huntley, J. (1989). Epidemiologic association of pain in osteoarthritis of the knee: data from the National Health and Nutrition Examination Survey and the National Health and Nutrition Examination — I. Epidemiologic Follow-up Survey. *Semin. Arthritis Rheum.*, **18**, 4-9
16. Summers, M. N., Haley, W. E., Reveille, J. D. and Alarcon, G. S. (1988). Radiographic assessment and psychologic variables as predictors of pain and functional impairment in osteoarthritis of the knee or hip. *Arthritis Rheum.*, **31**, 204-209
17. Bergenudd, H., Nilsson, B. and Lindgarde, F. (1989). Knee pain in middle age and its relationship to occupational work load and psychosocial factors. *Clin. Orthop.*, **245**, 210-215
18. Keefe, F. J., Caldwell, D. S., Queen, K., Gil, K. M., Martinez, S., Crisson, J. E., Ogden, W. and Nunley, J. (1987). Osteoarthritis knee pain: a behavioral analysis. *Pain*, **28**, 309-321
19. Cunningham, L. S. and Kelsey, J. L. (1984). Epidemiology of musculoskeletal impairments and associated disability. *A.J.P.H.*, **74**, 574-579
20. Weinberger, M., Hiner, S. L. and Tierney, Wm M. (1986). Improving functional status in arthritis: The effect of social support. *Soc. Sci. Med.*, **23**, 899-904
21. Weinberger, M., Tierney, W. M., Booher, P. and Katz, B. P. (1989). Can the provision of information to patients with osteoarthritis improve functional status? *Arthritis Rheum.*, **32**, 1577-1583
22. Weinberger, M., Hiner, S. L. and Tierney, W. M. (1987). In support of hassles as a measure of stress in predicting health outcomes. *J. Behav. Med.*, **10**, 19-31
23. Bloom, M., Buchon, E., Frires, G., Hanson, H., Hurd, G. and South, V. (1971). Interviewing the ill aged. *Gerontologist*, **11**, 292-299
24. Liang, M. H., Partridge, A. J., Gall, V. and Taylor, J. (1986). Evaluation of a rehabilitation component of home care for homebound elderly. *Am. J. Prev. Med.*, **2**, 30-33
25. Deniston, D. L. and Jette, A. (1980). A functional status assessment instrument: Validation in an elderly population. *Health Serv. Res.*, **15**, 21-34
26. Baron, M., Dutil, E., Berkson, L., Lander, P. and Becker, R. (1987). Hand function in the elderly. Relation to osteoarthritis. *J. Rheumatol.*, **14**, 815-819
27. Monson, R. R. and Hall, A. P. (1976). Mortality among arthritics. *J. Chronic Dis.*, **29**, 459-467
28. Lawrence, R. C., Everett, D. F., Coroni-Huntley, J. and Hochberg, M. C. (1987). Excess mortality and decreased survival in females with osteoarthritis. *Arthritis Rheum.*, **30**(suppl.), S130
29. Hochberg, M. C., Lawrence, R. C., Everett, D. F. and Coroni-Huntley, J. (1988). Association of gastroduodenal ulcers with knee pain in persons with osteoarthritis of the knee. *Am. J. Epidemiol.*, **128**, 937-938
30. Carson, J. L., Strom, B. L., Soper, K. A., West, S. L. and Morse, M. L. (1987). The association of nonsteroidal anti-inflammatory drugs with upper gastrointestinal tract bleeding. *Arch. Intern. Med.*, **147**, 85-88
31. Griffin, M. R., Ray, W. A. and Schaffner, W. (1988). Nonsteroidal anti-inflammatory drug use and death from peptic ulcer in elderly persons. *Ann. Intern. Med.*, **109**, 359-363
32. Lawrence, J. S. (1975). Hypertension in relation to musculoskeletal disorders. *Ann. Rheum. Dis.*, **1**, 451-456
33. Perry, G. H., Smith, M. J. G. and Whiteside, C. G. (1972). Spontaneous recovery of the joint space in degenerative hip disease. *Ann. Rheum. Dis.*, **31**, 440-448
34. Seifert, M., Whiteside, C. G. and Savage, O. (1969). A 5-year follow-up of fifty cases of idiopathic osteoarthritis of the hip. *Ann. Rheum. Dis.*, **28**, 325
35. Danielsson, L. G. (1964). Incidence and prognosis of coxarthrosis. *Acta Orthop. Scand.*, **66**(suppl.), 1-114
36. Storey, G. O. and Landells, J. W. (1971). Restoration of the femoral heads after

collapse in osteoarthritis. *Ann. Rheum. Dis.*, **30**, 406-412
37. Radin, E. L. and Burr, D. B. (1984). Hypothesis: joints can heal. *Semin. Arthritis Rheum.*, **13**, 293-302
38. Radin, E. L., Maquet, P. and Parker, H. (1985). Rationale and indications for the "hanging hip" procedure. A clinical and experimental study. *Clin. Orthop.*, **30**, 112-221
39. Ferguson, A. B. (1977). The pathology of degenerative arthritis of the hip and the use of osteotomy in its treatment. *Clin. Orthop.*, **71**, 84-97
40. Weisl, H. (1980). Intertrochanteric osteotomy for osteoarthritis. A long-term follow-up. *J. Bone Joint Surg.*, **62B**, 37-42
41. Ferguson, A. B. (1964). High intertrochanteric osteotomy for osteoarthritis of the hip. A procedure to streamline the defective joint. *J. Bone Joint Surg.*, **46A**, 1159-1175
42. Koshino, T. (1982). The treatment of spontaneous osteonecrosis of the knee by high tibial osteotomy with and without bone-grafting or drilling of the lesion. *J. Bone Joint Surg.*, **64A**, 47-58
43. Harris, N. H. and Kirwan, E. (1964). The results of osteotomy for early primary osteoarthritis of the hip. *J. Bone Joint Surg.*, **46B**, 477-487
44. Brandt, K. D. and Adams, M. E. (1989). Exuberant repair of articular cartilage damage. Effect of anterior cruciate ligament transection in the dog. *Trans. Orthop. Res. Soc.*, **14**, 584
45. Marshall, J. L. and Olsson, S. E. (1971). Instability of the knee, a long term experimental study. *J. Bone Joint Surg.*, **53A**, 1561-1750
46. Braunstein, E. M., Albrecht, M. and Brandt, K. D. (1989). MR imaging of canine osteoarthritis shows sustained hypertrophic repair of articular cartilage. *Radiology*, **173(P)**, 171
47. Palmoski, J. J. and Brandt, K. D. (1982). Immobilization of the knee prevents osteoarthritis after anterior cruciate ligament transection. *Arthritis Rheum.*, **25**, 1201-1208
48. Mankin, H. J., Dorfman, H., Lipiello, L. and Zarins, A. (1971). Biochemical and metabolic abnormalities in articular cartilage from osteoarthritic human hips. *J. Bone Joint Surg.*, **52A**, 523-537
49. Radin, E. L. (1981). Mechanical factors in the etiology of osteoarthrosis. In J. G. Peyron (ed.) *Epidemiology of Osteoarthritis*, pp. 136-139. (Rueil-Malmaison: Ciba-Geigy)
50. Martel-Pelletier, J., Pelletier, J. P. and Malemud, C. J. (1988). Activation of neutral metalloprotease in human osteoarthritic knee cartilage: evidence for degradation in the core protein of sulphated proteoglycan. *Ann. Rheum. Dis.*, **47**, 801-808
51. Thompson, R. C. and Oegema, T. R. (1979). Metabolic activity of articular cartilage in osteoarthritis. *J. Bone Joint Surg.*, **61A**, 407-416
52. Chateauvert, J., Pritzker, K. P. H., Kessler, M. J. and Grimpas, M. D. (1989). Spontaneous arthritis in Rhesus macaques. I. Chemical and biochemical studies. *J. Rheumatol.*, **16**, 1098-1104
53. Bardin, T., Bucki, B., Lequesne, M., Kuntz, D. and Dryll, A. (1988). Crystals in the synovial fluid of osteoarthritic joints are associated with rapid disease progression. *Br. J. Rheumatol.*, **27**(suppl. 2), 94
54. Menkes, C. J., Decraemere, W., Postel, M. and Forest, M. (1985). Chondrocalcinosis and rapid destruction of the hip. *J. Rheumatol.*, **12**, 130-133
55. Pattrick, M. and Doherty, J. (1987). Rapidly destructive hip disease following ipsilateral hemiparesis: Report of two cases. *Ann. Rheum. Dis.*, **46**, 477-481
56. Doherty, M., Watt, I. and Dieppe, P. (1983). Influence of primary generalized osteoarthritis on development of secondary osteoarthritis. *Lancet*, **2**, 8-11
57. Pelletier, J. P., Martel-Pelletier, J., Ghandur-Mnaymnhe, L., Howell, S. and Woessner, J., Jr. (1985). The role of synovial membrane inflammation in cartilage matrix breakdown in the Pond-Nuki dog model of OA. *Arthritis Rheum.*, **28**, 554-561
58. Martel-Pelletier, J., Cloutier, J. M. and Pelletier, J. P. (1986). Neutral proteases in human OA synovium. *Arthritis Rheum.*, **29**, 1112-1121
59. Moskowitz, R. W., Davis, W., Sammarco, J., Mast, W. and Chase, S. W. (1970). Experimentally induced corticosteroid arthropathy. *Arthritis Rheum.*, **13**, 236-243

60. Gibson, T., Barry, H. C., Poswillo, P. and Glass, J. (1976). Effect of intra-articular corticosteroid injections on primate cartilage. *Ann. Rheum. Dis.*, **36**, 74–79
61. Gray, R. G. and Gottlieb, N. L. (1983). Intra-articular corticosteroids, an updated assessment. *Clin. Orthop.*, **177**, 235–263
62. Chandler, G. N. and Wright, V. (1958). Deleterious effects of intra-articular hydrocortisone. *Lancet*, **2**, 661–663
63. Chandler, G. N., Jones, D. T., Wright, V. and Hartfall, S. J. (1959). Charcot's arthropathy following intra-articular hydrocortisone. *Br. Med. J.*, **1**, 952–953
64. Balch, H. W., Gibson, J. M. C., El-Ghorbarey, A. F., Bain, L. S. and Lynch, M. A. (1977). Repeated corticosteroids injection into knee joints. *Rheumatol. Rehabil.*, **11**, 137–140
65. Keagy, R. D. and Kein, H. A. (1962). Intra-articular steroid therapy: repeated use in patients with chronic arthritis. *Am. J. Med. Sci.*, **253**, 75–81
66. Pelletier, J.-P., Martel-Pelletier, J., Howell, D. S., Ghandur-Mnaymneh, L., Enis, J. and Woessner, J. F., Jr. (1983). Collagenase and collagenolytic activity in human osteoarthritis cartilage. *Arthritis Rheum.*, **26**, 63–68
67. Ehrlich, M. G. (1985). Degradative enzyme systems in osteoarthritic cartilage. *J. Orthop. Res.*, **3**, 170–184
68. Saklatvala, J. and Sarsfield, S. J. (1988). How do interleukin-1 and tumour necrosis factor induce degradation of proteoglycan in cartilage? In Glauert, A. M. (ed.). *The Control of Tissue Damage*, pp. 97–106. (Amsterdam: Elsevier Science Publishers)
69. Steinberg, J. J. and Sledge, C. B. (1983). Synovial factors and chondrocyte-mediated breakdown of cartilage inhibition by hydrocortisone. *J. Orthop. Res.*, **1**, 13–21
70. Williams, J. and Brandt, K. (1985). Triamcinolone hexacetonide protects against fibrillation and osteophyte formation following chemically-induced articular cartilage damage. *Arthritis Rheum.*, **28**, 1267–1274
71. Colombo, C., Butler, M., Hickman, L., Selwyn, M., Chart, J. and Steinetz, B. (1983). A new model of osteoarthritis in rabbits. II. Evaluation of anti-osteoarthritic effects of selected antirheumatic drugs administered systemically. *Arthritis Rheum.*, **26**, 1132–1139
72. Butler, M., Colombo, C., Hickman, L., O'Byrne, E., Steele, R., Steinetz, B., Quintavalla, J. and Yokoyama, N. (1983). A new model of osteoarthritis in rabbits. III. Evaluation of anti-osteoarthritic effects of selected drugs administered intra-articularly. *Arthritis Rheum.*, **26**, 1380–1386
73. Pelletier, S. P. and Martel-Pelletier, J. (1989). Protective effect of corticosteroids on cartilage lesions and osteophyte formation in the Pond-Nuki dog model of osteo-arthritis. *Arthritis Rheum.*, **32**, 181–193
74. Acheson, R. and Collard, A. B. (1975). New Haven survey of joint diseases: XVII. Relationship between some systemic characteristics and osteoarthrosis in a general population. *Ann. Rheum. Dis.*, **34**, 379–387
75. Hartz, A. J., Fischer, M. E., Bril, G., Kelber, S., Rupley, D. Jr., Oken, B. and Rimm, A. A. (1986). The association of obesity with joint pain and osteoarthritis in the HANES data. *J. Chronic Dis.*, **39**, 311–319
76. Leach, R. E., Baumgard, S. and Broom, J. (1973). Obesity: its relationship to osteoarthritis of the knee. *Clin. Orthop.*, **93**, 271–273
77. Lawrence, J. S., Bremner, J. M. and Bier, F. (1966). Osteoarthrosis: prevalence in the population and relationship between symptoms and X-ray changes. *Ann. Rheum. Dis.*, **25**, 1–24
78. Felson, D. T., Anderson, J. J., Naimark, A., Walker, A. M. and Meenan, R. F. (1989). Obesity and knee osteoarthritis. The Framingham study. *Ann. Intern. Med.*, **109**, 18–24
79. Davis, M. A., Ettinger, W. H., Neuhaus, J. M., Cho, S. A. and Hauck, W. W. (1989). The association of knee injury and obesity with unilateral and bilateral osteoarthritis of the knee. *Am. J. Epidemiol.*, **130**, 278–288
80. Barrie, H. J. (1986). Unexpected sites of wear in the femoral head. *J. Rheum.*, **13**, 1099–1104
81. Radin, E. L. (1987). Osteoarthrosis. What is known about prevention. *Clin. Orthop.*, **222**, 60–65

82. Radin, E. L., Martin, R. B., Burr, D. B., Caterson, B., Boyd, R. D. and Goodwin, C. (1986). Mechanical factors influencing cartilage damage. In Peyron, J. G. (ed.) *Osteoarthrosis: Current Clinical and Fundamental Problems*, pp. 90-99. (Paris: Ciba-Geigy)
83. Radin, E. L. and Paul, I. L. (1971). Importance of bone in sparing articular cartilage from impact. *Clin. Orthop.*, **78**, 342-344
84. Bergström, G., Bjelle, A., Sundh, F. and Svanborg, A. (1986). Joint disorders at ages 70, 75 and 79 years — a cross-sectional comparison. *Br. J. Rheum.*, **25**, 333-341
85. Palmoski, M. J. and Brandt, K. D. (1979). Effect of salicylate on proteoglycan metabolism in normal canine articular cartilage *in vitro*. *Arthritis Rheum.*, **22**, 746-754
86. Palmoski, M. J. and Brandt, K. D. (1980). Effects of some nonsteroidal anti-inflammatory drugs on proteoglycan metabolism and organization canine articular cartilage. *Arthritis Rheum.*, **23**, 1010-1020
87. Muir, H., Carney, S. L. and Hall, L. G. (1988). Effects of tiaprofenic acid and other NSAIDs on proteoglycan metabolism in articular cartilage explants. *Drugs*, **35**(suppl. 1), 15-23
88. Palmoski, M. and Brandt, K. (1983). Benoxaprofen stimulates proteoglycan synthesis in normal canine knee cartilage *in vitro*. *Arthritis Rheum.*, **20**, 771-774
89. Palmoski, M. and Brandt, K. (1984). Effects of salicylate and indomethacin on glycosaminoglycan and prostaglandin E_2 synthesis in intact canine knee cartilage *ex vivo*. *Arthritis Rheum.*, **27**, 398-403
90. Palmoski, M. J., Colyer, R. A. and Brandt, K. D. (1980). Marked suppression by salicylate of the augmented proteoglycan synthesis (?matrix repair) in osteoarthritic cartilage. *Arthritis Rheum.*, **23**, 83-91
91. Palmoski, M. J. and Brandt, K. D. (1983). *In vivo* effects of aspirin on canine osteoarthritic cartilage. *Arthritis Rheum.*, **26**, 994-1001
92. Brandt, K. D. (1987). Effects of nonsteroidal antiinflammatory drugs on chondrocyte metabolism *in vivtro* and *in vivo*. *Am. J. Med.*, **83**(5A), 29-34
93. Doherty, M. (1989). 'Chondroprotection' by non-steroidal anti-inflammatory drugs. *Ann. Rheum. Dis.*, **48**, 619-621
94. Ghosh, P. (1988). Anti-rheumatic drugs and cartilage. *Clin. Rheumatol.*, **2**, 309-338
95. Herman, J. H., Appel, A. M. and Hess, E. V. (1987). Modulation of cartilage destruction by select nonsteroidal antiinflammatory drugs. In vitro effect on the synthesis and activity of catabolism-inducing cytokines produced by osteoarthritic and rheumatoid synovial fluid. *Arthritis Rheum.*, **30**, 257-265
96. McKenzie, L. S., Horsburgh, B. A., Ghosh, P. and Taylor, T. K. F. (1976). Effect of antiinflammatory drugs on sulphated glycosaminoglycan synthesis in aged human articular cartilage. *Ann. Rheum. Dis.*, **35**, 487-497
97. Kalbhen, D. A. (1984). Biochemically induced osteoarthritis in the chicken and rat. In Munthe, E. and Bjelle, A. (eds.) *Effects of Drugs on Osteoarthritis*, pp. 48-68. (Berne, Stuttgart: Huber)
98. Herman, J. H. and Hess, E. V. (1984). Nonsteroidal anti-inflammatory drugs and modulation of cartilaginous changes in osteoarthritis and rheumatoid arthritis: clinical implications. *Am. J. Med.* (suppl.), 16-25
99. Carlin, G., Djursärd, G. and Gerdin, B. (1985). Effect of anti-inflammatory drugs on xanthine oxidase and xanthine oxidase induced depolymerisation of hyaluronic acid. *Agents Actions*, **16**, 377-384
100. Lentini, A., Ternai, B. and Thosh, P. (1987). Inhibition of human leukoycte elastase and cathepsin G by non-steroidal antiinflammatory compounds. *Biochem. Int.*, **15**, 1069-1078
101. Burkhardt, D. and Ghosh, P. (1987). Laboratory evaluation of antiarthritic drugs as potential chondro-protective agents. *Semin. Arthritis Rheum.*, **17**(suppl. 1:3), 3-34
102. Shinmei, M., Kikuchi, T., Masuda, K. and Shimomura, Y. (1988). Effects of interleukin 1 and anti-inflammatory drugs on the degradation of human articular cartilage. *Drugs*, **35**(suppl. 1), 33-41
103. De Vries, B. J., Van Den Berg, W. B., Vittero, E. and Van de Putte, L. B. A. (1988). Effects of NSAIDs on the metabolism of sulphated glycosaminoglycans in healthy and post-arthritic articular cartilage. *Drugs*, **35**(suppl. 1), 24-32

104. Ronningen, H. and Langeland, N. (1977). Indomethacin hips. *Acta Orthop. Scand.*, **48**, 556
105. Newman, N. M. and Ling, R. S. M. (1985). Acetabular bone destruction related to non-steroidal anti-inflammatory drugs. *Lancet*, **2**, 11-14
106. Rashad, S., Revell, P., Hemingway, A., Low, F., Rainsford, K. and Walker, F. (1989). Effect of non-steroidal anti-inflammatory drugs on the course of osteoarthritis. *Lancet*, **2**, 519-522
107. O'Connor, B., Palmoski, M. and Brandt, K. (1985). Neurogenic acceleration of degenerative joint lesions. *J. Bone Joint Surg.*, **57-A**, 562-572
108. Slowman-Kovacs, S. and Brandt, K. D. (1990). Rapidly progressive Charcot arthropathy following minor joint trauma in patients with diabetic neuropathy. *Arthritis Rheum.*, **33**, 412-417
109. Hernborg, J. S. and Nilsson, B. E. (1977). The natural course of untreated osteoarthritis of the knee. *Clin. Orthop. Rel. Res.*, **123**, 130-137
110. Massardo, L., Watt, I., Cushnaghan, J. and Dieppe, P. (1989). Osteoarthritis of the knee joint: an eight year prospective study. *Ann. Rheum. Dis.*, **48**, 893-897
111. Solomon, L. (1985). Osteoarthritis and its variants. In Peyron, J. G. (ed.) *Osteoarthritis: Current Clinical and Fundamental Problems*, pp. 55-58. (Paris: Ciba-Geigy)
112. Macys, J. R., Bullough, P. G. and Wilson, P. D., Jr. (1980). Coxarthrosis: a study of the natural history based on a correlation of clinical, radiographic and pathologic findings. *Semin. Arthritis Rheum.*, **10**, 66-80
113. Pearson, J. R. and Riddell, D. M. (1962). Idiopathic osteoarthritis of the hip. *Ann. Rheum. Dis.*, **21**, 31-39
114. Felson, D. T. (1988). Epidemiology of hip and knee osteoarthritis. *Epidemiol. Rev.*, **10**, 1-28
115. Plato, C. C. and Norris, A. H. (1979). Osteoarthritis of the hand: longitudinal studies. *Am. J. Epidemiol.*, **110**, 740-746
116. Kellgren, J. H. (1963). *Atlas of Standard Radiographs of Arthritis*, Vol. II. *The Epidemiology of Chronic Rheumatism*. (Philadelphia: F. A. Davis Company)
117. Pattrick, M., Aldridge, S., Hamilton, E., Manhire, A. and Doherty, J. (1989). A controlled study of hand function in nodal and erosive osteoarthritis. *Ann. Rheum. Dis.*, **48**, 978-982
118. Dieppe, P. A., Alexander, G. J. M., Jones, H., Doherty, M., Scott, D. G. I., Manhire, A. and Watt, I. (1982). Pyrophosphate arthropathy: a clinical and radiological study of 105 cases. *Ann. Rheum. Dis.*, **41**, 371-376
119. Doherty, M. and Preston, B. (1989). Primary osteoarthritis of the elbow. *Ann. Rheum. Dis.*, **48**, 743-747
120. Felts, W. and Yelin, E. (1989). The economic impact of the rheumatic diseases in the United States. *J. Rheumatol.*, **16**, 867-874
121. Liang, M. H., Cullen, K. E., Larson, M. G., Thompson, M. S., Schwartz, J. A., Fossel, A. E., Roberts, W. N. and Sledge, C. B. (1986). Cost-effectiveness of total joint arthroplasty in osteoarthritis. *Arthritis Rheum.*, **29**, 937-943
122. Nevitt, M. C., Epstein, W. V., Masem, M. and Murray, W. R. (1984). Work disability before and after total hip arthroplasty. *Arthritis Rheum.*, **27**, 410-421
123. Magnuson, P. B. (1941). Joint debridement: Surgical treatment of degenerative arthritis. *Surg. Gynecol. Obstet.*, **73**, 1-9
124. Haggart, G. E. (1940). The surgical treatment of degenerative arthritis of the knee joint. *J. Bone Joint Surg.*, **22**, 717-729
125. Insall, J. (1974). The Pridie debridement operation of osteoarthritis of the knee. *Clin. Orthop.*, **101**, 61-67
126. Stulberg, S. D. and Keller, C. S. (1982). The principles and results of arthroscopic surgical treatment of osteoarthritis of the knee. *Arthritis Rheum.*, **25**(suppl.), S44
127. Schmid, A. and Schmid, F. (1987). Results after cartilage shaving studied by electron microscopy. *Am. J. Sports Med.*, **15**, 386-387
128. Coventry, M. B. (1973). Osteotomy about the knee for degenerative and rheumatoid arthritis: Indications, operative technique and results. *J. Bone Joint Surg.*, **55a**, 23-48
129. Friedman, M. J., Berasi, C. C., Fox, J. M., Del Pizzo, W., Snyder, S. J. and Ferkel,

R. D. (1984). Preliminary results with abrasion arthroplasty in the osteoarthritic knee. *Clin. Orthop.*, **182**, 200-205
130. Chandler, E. J. (1985). Abrasion arthroplasty of the knee. *Contemp. Orthop.*, **11**, 21-29
131. Johnson, L. L. (1986). Chondral condition. In *Arthroscopic Surgery, Principles and Practice*, 3rd edn., Chap. 9, pp. 669-787. (St. Louis, Mo; C. V. Mosby)
132. Burman, M. S., Finkelstein, F. H. and Mayer, L. (1934). Arthroscopy of the knee joint. *J. Bone Joint Surg.*, **16**, 255-268
133. Jackson, R. W., Silver, R. and Marans, H. (1986). Arthroscopic treatment of degenerative joint disease. *Arthroscopy: The Journal of Arthroscopic and Related Surgery*, **2**, 114
134. Arnold, W. J., Mather, S. E., Mostello, N. and Tongue, J. (1985). Tidal knee lavage in patients with chronic pain due to osteoarthritis of the knee. *Arthritis Rheum.*, **27** (suppl.), S66
135. Ike, R. W., Arnold, W. J., Simon, C. and Eisenberg, G. M. (1987). Tidal knee irrigation as an intervention for chronic pain due to osteoarthritis of the knee. *Arthritis Rheum.*, **30**, S17
136. Hutton, C. W., Higgs, E. R., Jackson, P. C., Watt, I. and Dieppe, P. A. (1986). ^{99M}Tc HMDP bone scanning in generalized osteoarthritis. I. Comparison of the standard radiograph and four hour bone scan image of the hand. *Ann. Rheum. Dis.*, **45**, 617-621
137. Hutton, C. W., Higgs, E. P., Jackson, P. C., Watt, I. and Dieppe, P. A. (1986). ^{99M}Tc HMDP bone scanning in generalized osteoarthritis. II. The four hour bone scan image predicts radiographic change. *Ann. Rheum. Dis.*, **45**, 622-626
138. Thonar, E. J.-M. A., Lenz, M., Klintworth, G. K., Caterson, B., Pachman, L. M., Guckman, P., Katz, R., Huff, Jr. and Kuettner, K. E. (1985). Quantification of keratan sulfate in blood as a marker of cartilage catabolism. *Arthritis Rheum.*, **28**, 1367-1376
139. Block, J. A., Schnitzer, T. J. and Andersson, G. B. J. (1987). Keratan sulfate release following chemonucleolysis. *Orthop. Trans.*, **12**, 304
140. Williams, J. M., Downey, C. and Thonar, E. J.-M. A. (1988). Increase in levels of serum keratan sulfate following cartilage proteoglycan degradation in the rabbit knee joint. *Arthritis Rheum.*, **31**, 557-560
141. Brandt, K. and Thonar, E. J.-M. A. (1989). Lack of association between serum keratan sulfate concentrations and cartilage changes of osteoarthritis after transection of the anterior cruciate ligament in the dog. *Arthritis Rheum.*, **32**, 647-651
142. Brandt, K. D. (1989). A pessimistic view of serologic "markers" for diagnosis and management of osteoarthritis. Biochemical, immunological and clinicopathological perspectives. *J. Rheumatol.*, **16**, 39-42
143. Lohmander, L. S., Dalhberg, L., Ryd, L. and Heinegard, D. (1989). Increased levels of proteoglycan fragments in joint fluid after knee injury. *Trans. Orthop. Res. Soc.*, **14**, 504
144. Saxne, T., Heinegard, D., Wollheim, F. A. and Petersson, H. (1985). Difference in cartilage proteoglycan level in synovial fluid in early rheumatoid arthritis and reactive arthritis. *Lancet*, **2**, 127-128
145. Howell, D. S., Carreno, M. R., Pelletier, J. P. and Muniz, O. (1986). Articular cartilage breakdown in a lapine model of osteoarthritis. *Clin. Orthop.*, **213**, 69-76
146. Altman, R. D., Dean, D. D., Muniz, O. E. and Howell, D. S. (1989). Therapeutic treatment of canine osteoarthritis in glycosaminoglycan polysulfuric acid ester. *Arthritis Rheum.*, **32**, 1300-1307
147. Rejholec, V. (1987). Long-term studies of antiosteoarthritic drugs: an assessment. *Semin. Arthritis Rheum.*, **17**(suppl. 1), 35-53

3
Rheumatoid arthritis

F. WOLFE

Interest in the course and prognosis of rheumatoid arthritis (RA) has seen several peaks and troughs over the course of this century. Successive waves of interest followed the identification of RA as a separate disease, the invention of major therapies, development of useful laboratory tests, the development of diagnostic criteria, the development of controlled clinical trials, the emergence of clinical epidemiology and statistics, the development of methods for functional assessment, and the development of computer databanks. It is hard to pick the most important of these factors, but it appears fair to say that it is clinical epidemiology and statistics through its emphasis on proper technique and inference that has become the backbone of our interest and knowledge of the course and prognosis of RA.

PROBLEMS IN CLASSIFICATION AND SELECTION

A major impediment to the understanding of RA lies in case definition. The early investigators of the syndrome were sometimes unaware of differences between RA (both seronegative and seropositive) and juvenile arthritis (JRA), the spondyloarthropathies, systemic lupus erythematosus, and similar disorders; or when they were aware of apparent differences, had no useful methods for differential classification. Indeed, it was not until 1956 that diagnostic criteria for RA were available that separated RA from other inflammatory conditions[1]. Revised in 1958 (Table 1)[2], these "ARA" criteria remained in effect for 30 years until they were suspended by current classification criteria (Table 2) promulgated by the ARA (now renamed the American College of Rheumatology)[3]. In spite of other proposed criteria, such as the "New York"[4] (Table 3), and the "Rome" criteria[5], the 1958 criteria were the major force in the definition and diagnosis of RA through the 1980s.

In essence the 1958 criteria conceived of "definite rheumatoid arthritis" as a (symmetrical) inflammatory polyarthritis of at least 6

Table 1 Rheumatoid arthritis diagnostic criteria (ARA 1958 Revision)

1. Morning stiffness.
2. Pain on motion or tenderness in at least one joint.
3. Swelling (soft-tissue thickening or fluid, not bony overgrowth alone) in at least one joint.
4. Swelling of at least one other joint.
5. Symmetrical joint swelling with simultaneous involvement of the same joint on both sides of the body. Terminal phalangeal joint involvement does not satisfy the criterion.
6. Subcutaneous nodules over bony prominences, on extensor surfaces or in juxta-articular regions.
7. Roentgenographic changes typical of rheumatoid arthritis (which must include at least bony decalcification localized to or greatest around the involved joints and not just degenerative changes).
8. Positive agglutination (antigammaglobulin) test.
9. Poor mucin precipitate from synovial fluid (with shreds and cloudy solution).
10. Characteristic histologic changes in synovial membrane.
11. Characteristic histologic changes in nodules.

A. Classic rheumatoid arthritis

This diagnosis requires seven of the following criteria. In criteria 1 through 5 the joint signs or symptoms must be continuous for at least 6 weeks. Any one of the features listed under Exclusions will exclude a patient from this and all other categories.

1. Morning stiffness.
2. Pain on motion or tenderness in at least one joint (observed by a physician).
3. Swelling (soft-tissue thickening or fluid, not bony overgrowth alone) in at least one joint (observed by a physician).
4. Swelling (observed by a physician) of at least one other joint (any interval free of joint symptoms between the two point involvements may not be more than 3 months).
5. Symmetric joint swelling (observed by a physician) with simultaneous involvement of the same joint on both sides of the body (bilateral involvement of proximal interphalangeal, metacarpophalangeal, or metatarsophalangeal joints is acceptable without absolute symmetry). Terminal phalangeal joint involvement will not satisfy this criterion.
6. Subcutaneous nodules (observed by a physician) over bony prominences, on extensor surfaces, or in juxta-articular regions.
7. Roentgenographic changes typical of rheumatoid arthritis (which must include at least bony decalcification localized to or most marked adjacent to the involved joints and not just degenerative changes). Degenerative changes do not exclude patients from any group classified as having rheumatoid arthritis.
8. Positive agglutination test — demonstration of the "rheumatoid factor" by any method that, in two laboratories, has been positive in not over 5% of normal controls, or positive streptococcal agglutination test.
9. Poor mucin precipitate from synovial fluid (with shreds and cloudy solution).
10. Characteristic histologic changes in synovium with three or more of the following: marked villous hypertrophy; proliferation of superficial synovial cells often with palisading; marked infiltration of chronic inflammatory cells (lymphocytes or plasma cells predominating) with tendency to form "lymphoid nodules"; deposition of compact fibrin either on surface or interstitially; foci of necrosis.
11. Characteristic histologic changes in nodules showing granulomatous foci with central zones of cell necrosis, surrounded by a palisade of proliferated mononuclear and peripheral fibrosis and chronic inflammatory cell infiltration.

RHEUMATOID ARTHRITIS

B. Definite rheumatoid arthritis

This diagnosis requires five of the above criteria. In criteria 1 through 5 the joint signs or symptoms must be continuous for at least 6 weeks.

C. Probable rheumatoid arthritis

This diagnosis requires three of the above criteria. In at least one of criteria 1 through 5 the joint signs or symptoms must be continuous for at least 6 weeks.

D. Possible rheumatoid arthritis

This diagnosis requires two of the following criteria and total duration of joint symptoms must be at least 3 months.

1. Morning stiffness.
2. Tenderness or pain on motion (observed by a physician) with history of recurrence or persistence for 3 weeks.
3. History or observation of joint swelling.
4. Subcutaneous nodules (observed by a physician).
5. Elevated sedimentation rate or C-reactive protein.
6. Iritis (of dubious value as a criterion except in juvenile arthritis).

E. Exclusions.
20 conditions that excluded a diagnosis of rheumatoid arthritis were listed. See reference 2.

---

weeks duration, and of "probable rheumatoid arthritis" as a slightly less certain, but similar disorder (Table 1). Substantial problems in our understanding of RA emanated from the case definitions inherent in these criteria. The criteria separated RA into four groups based on the number of criteria met. Two criteria constituted "possible RA," an entity that was largely ignored; 3-4 criteria constituted "probable RA"; 5 were "definite RA"; and 7 or more were "classical RA." In a series of important studies, Cathcart and O'Sullivan used these criteria to estimate the prevalence of RA in a sample of 4552 of 5976 eligible residents of Sudbury, Massachusetts in 1964[6,7]. In their reports they defined RA as being present when subjects met criteria for *either* "probable or definite" RA. A total of 3.8% of women and 1.3% of men satisfied the "probable or definite" definition used by these researchers. The authors also applied the more restrictive "New York criteria" to their population survey[4] (Table 3). By these criteria 0.55% of women and 0.14% of men had RA. The authors indicated that the "truer prevalence" of RA is better approximated by the New York criteria. They suggested further that, based on other studies[8], RA "may be a relatively benign disorder that is only occasionally disabling." In a follow-up study of the same cohort 3-5 years later, published in the *Annals of Internal Medicine*, they noted that only 36% of those meeting "definite" criteria and 9% of those meeting "probable" criteria had clinical evidence of disease. In all, "72 percent failed to meet either

Table 2 The 1987 revised criteria for the classification of rheumatoid arthritis

Criterion	Definition
1. Morning stiffness	Morning stiffness in and around the joints, lasting at least 1 hour before maximal improvement.
2. Arthritis of three or more joint areas	At least three joint areas simultaneously have had soft-tissue swelling or fluid (not bony overgrowth alone) observed by a physician. The 14 possible areas are right or left PIP, MCP, wrist, elbow, knee, ankle and MTP joints.
3. Arthritis of hand joints	At least one area swollen (as defined above) in a wrist, MCP, or PIP joint.
4. Symmetric arthritis	Simultaneous involvement of the same joint areas (as defined in 2) on both sides of the body (bilateral involvement of PIPs, MCPs, or MTPs is acceptable without absolute symmetry).
5. Rheumatoid nodules	Subcutaneous nodules, over bony prominences, or extensor surfaces, or in juxta-articular regions, observed by a physician.
6. Serum rheumatoid factor	Demonstration of abnormal amounts of serum rheumatoid factor by any method for which the result has been positive in <5% of normal control subjects.
7. Radiographic changes	Radiographic changes typical of rheumatoid arthritis on posteroanterior hand and wrist radiographs, which must include erosions or unequivocal bony decalcification localized in or most marked adjacent to the involved joints (osteoarthritis changes alone do not qualify).

*For classification purposes, a patient shall be said to have rheumatoid arthritis if he/she has satisfied at least 4 of these 7 criteria. Criteria 1 through 4 must have been present for at least 6 weeks. Patients with 2 clinical diagnoses are not excluded Designation as classic, definite, or probable rheumatoid arthritis is not to be made.

Table 3 Rheumatoid arthritis population survey criteria (New York, 1966)

1. History, past or present, of any episode of joint pain involving three or more limb joints without stipulation as to duration. The joints on either side shall count separately, but joints that occur in groups (e.g., the PIP or MCP joints) on one side shall count only as a single joint.
2. Swelling, limitation, subluxation, or ankylosis of at least three limb joints, including one hand, wrist, or foot with symmetry of at least one joint pair. (Joints excluded from criteria are the DIP, the fifth PIP, the first carpometacarpal (CMC) joints, the hips, and the first MTP. Subluxation of the lateral MTP must be irreducible.)
3. X-ray features of grade 2 or more erosive arthritis in the hands, wrists, or feet.
4. Positive serologic reaction for rheumatoid (antigammaglobulin) factor.

diagnosis at follow-up,"[7] but "only one third of those diagnosed by the New York clinical criteria" were normal on follow-up. The authors stressed "the benign nature of early rheumatoid arthritis," and concluded that "rheumatoid arthritis exists more frequently as a benign nondeforming condition."

The Cathcart and O'Sullivan studies[6,7], conceiving of RA as *either* probable *or* definite RA, suggested the benign and self-limiting nature of the illness. These reports had a profound influence on rheumatology. They were cited in major textbooks for two decades[9,10], and influenced a generation of clinicians and the construct of RA[11]. Even though most subsequent investigations (such as those relating to treatment or etiology) would require patients to have "definite" RA, "probable RA" could be regarded as an earlier and nonprogressive form of the illness. Rheumatoid arthritis, then, could be, and often was, considered to be a benign disorder, with frequent remissions in its early course, and one in which only a minority of patients progressed to disability.

But the case definition of "probable rheumatoid arthritis" as RA has not been sustained. When incident cases of inflammatory arthritis were evaluated between 1 week and 6 months of disease, 107 patients with "definite" RA and 161 with "probable" (i.e., nonspecific) RA were identified[12]. Three years later 6.5% of "definite" RA patients were symptom-free as were 59% of "probable" RA patients, suggesting that most "probable" cases do not progress to "definite RA," and that "definite" RA and probable RA are different conditions. From these data Isomäki estimated that the specificity of "probable" RA was 31%[13]. Thus, there appears to be a second interpretation to the Cathcart and O'Sullivan data: that ARA "probable" RA rather than identifying early or limited RA usually identifies self-limited forms of arthritis that are not rheumatoid arthritis.

Although "classical" RA was found to be a highly specific classification (specificity = 99%[13]), the category of "definite" RA when applied to early cases was not nearly so specific[7,13]. The 1958 criteria made no provision for transient polyarthritis of greater than 3 months duration, for what later would be recognized as reactive arthropathies (including some Reiter's syndrome *forme frustes*)[14], for limited joint (oligoarticular) arthritis[15], or for polymyalgia rheumatica[10]. These obvious problems with the ARA criteria resulted in many patients being classified by the clinician as having "atypical RA (actually not RA)" while still meeting the 1958 criteria for the disorder. In many studies, rheumatoid factor negative RA has been associated with an increased prevalence of HLA-B27[13] and in some (about half) a decreased prevalence of HLA-DR4[16], suggesting heterogeneity within the construct of seronegative RA and suggesting further that in many instances what is diagnosed as seronegative RA is actually a disorder different from seropositive disease[16,17] (Figure 1). Thus, the 30 years since the ARA criteria were made have witnessed a change in the construct of RA to exclude the mono- and oligoarthropathies, the spondyloarthropathies, and questioning of the appropriateness of seronegative RA in many instances[17,18].

An important consequence of the limitations of the 1958 diagnostic criteria in the decade of the 1980s is that RA has often appeared to be a relatively benign disorder with a more favorable mortality rate and a better overall prognosis than is actually the case[19,20]. A second con-

PROGNOSIS IN THE RHEUMATIC DISEASES

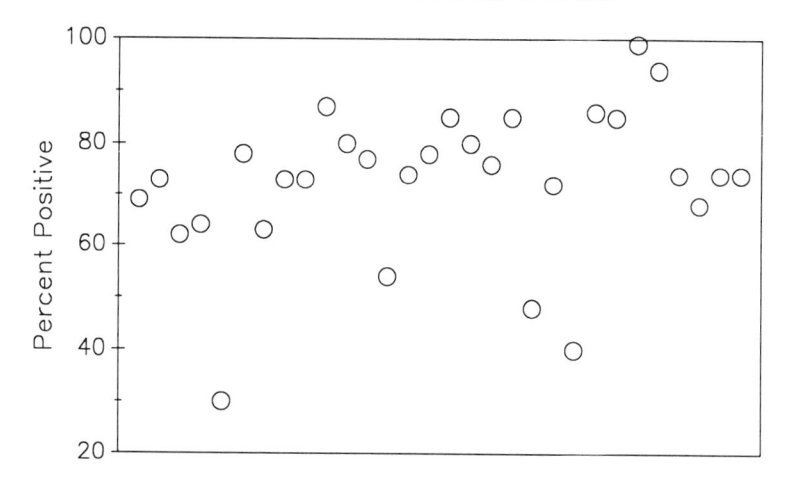

Figure 1 Percent of patients designated as rheumatoid factor positive by various methodologies in 30 studies of rheumatoid arthritis

sequence is that patients who did not have what we would recognize today as RA were entered into clinical trials of "disease modifying antirheumatic drugs" (DMARDs), with contamination of the trials. Such patients might have a better or worse outcome than those who would meet the 1987 criteria definition.

The 1987 American College of Rheumatology (ACR) criteria for the classification of RA (Table 2)[3] eliminated the probable, definite, and classical categories, but may not have entirely solved the misclassification problem since it is still possible that patients with three joints involved, provided two of those joints are wrists, can be classified as RA. It would be expected, however, that the misclassification rate will be much smaller.

An unappreciated problem of the 1958 and 1987 criteria at the clinical as opposed to the epidemiological level is that the criteria are exclusionary, being invoked by the investigator *after* the clinical diagnosis of RA has been made. For example, an investigator may identify a (seronegative) patient who meets 1987 criteria but who the investigator thinks has a "different" disorder and hence does not classify as having rheumatoid arthritis. It is difficult to know the consequences when criteria are used in this manner, but the varying percentages of rheumatoid factor positivity in reported series of RA patients (Figure 1) suggests that investigators have somewhat different conceptions of RA (and their different patients have different outcomes), criteria notwithstanding. No studies have been performed regarding this point, but it is likely that RA factor positive polyarthritis is almost always classified as RA, while the diagnosis has not been made as often or as soon when the RA factor is absent. A case has been made against seronegative RA[16,21] and a committee of the ACR has suggested that RA be subclassified as either seropositive or seronegative[22]. These suggestions have not been

Table 4 Factors important to patient outcome not usually reported in studies of rheumatoid arthritis

1. Education	7. Marital status
2. Ethnic origin	8. Living arrangements
3. Employment status	9. Comorbidity
4. Occupation	10. Medical insurance
5. Family income	11. Access to medical care
6. Social support	12. Pension status

acted upon generally for a number of reasons that include the facts that RA factor may be hidden[23,24], not IgM[25,26], and that it has not yet been shown that seronegative RA is not the same disorder as seropositive RA[3].

Socioeconomic factors

Recent efforts by Pincus and coworkers have stressed the importance of socioeconomic factors in the outcome of RA[27-29]. The designation and effect of these factors (Table 4) have been virtually ignored in most observational and intervention studies of RA in spite of the fact that they have been shown to influence outcome in most other acute and chronic medical disorders[30-35], and are of particular importance in chronic disease[36-42]. The socioeconomic status of patients, as determined by formal education level, occupation, pension status, and income, are rarely described in studies of RA and its outcome. These factors are likely to be very important[39,43-54], and may explain the differences in outcome noted in a number of observational studies[30,51,55].

Spectrum bias

Patients enrolled in clinical trials may not be representative of the spectrum of RA. Clinical trials often require exclusion of patients with mild disease as well as end-stage disease, the elderly, those with comorbidities, those of child-bearing potential, those with previous duodenal or gastric ulcers. For this review we analyzed the most recent visit of 1285 patients with RA seen in our clinic to see how many would be potentially eligible for pharmacologic studies. Using conservative criteria similar to those used in such studies, we defined activity as the presence of more than three of the following criteria: ESR > 28, presence of joint swelling, presence of fatigue, morning stiffness > 30 minutes, and number of tender joints > 4 (MCP, PIP, and MTP joints were each scored as a group). These criteria were satisfied by 48.6% of patients. But when we excluded patients because of ongoing therapy with second-line drugs or prednisone at doses greater than 10 mg only 36% qualified. Similarly, exclusion for age requirement (exclusion of patients over age 70) left 35.6%. When both age and concurrent therapy were considered, 25.5% remained. It is likely that if patients with other exclusions such as comorbidity, child-bearing potential, and previous GI disease were considered the percentage still eligible would fall below 20%. Pincus has reported that in two studies performed in his clinic 5% and less than 0.5% respectively met entry criteria[20].

Spectrum bias may also affect observational studies if patients do not return to clinic, are lost to follow-up, are noncompliant, have entered nursing homes, are too ill to participate, or lack sufficient education to complete assessments. In longitudinal studies of RA, patients with such characteristics have worse RA and have worse outcomes[56,57].

In general, then, and depending on the clinic and study, the effects of the biases noted above are to underestimate the severity of RA, to overemphasize the benefit of treatment, and to bias estimates of outcome toward the less severe.

The natural history of rheumatoid arthritis

There are few reliable data regarding untreated RA or RA that has been treated only with simple medications (e.g., salicylates) and nonpharmacologic therapies. As indicated above, earlier studies probably included patients (such as those with spondyloarthropathies) who would not be diagnosed as having RA today. Early studies also tended not to define RA precisely[58-60] or used imprecise outcome measures (e.g., "improved") or relatively insensitive measures (e.g., remission)[61,62]. None of these studies tracked a cohort of early RA patients. In 1962, Ragan and Farrington reported on 500 adult RA patients followed in an arthritis clinic of a metropolitan hospital in New York City for up to 16 years[63]. Approximately 50% of patients were employed during the observation period. Sixty percent were in ARA radiographic stage 3 or 4 (Table 5)[64] after 10 years. Only 45% of these patients were rheumatoid factor positive at the first visit, loss to follow-up continued throughout the study, and the number employed did not indicate the percentage of patients who had been working prior to disease onset, factors that limit the generalizability of the data. Steinbrocker, reviewing early data relating to employability, pointed out that "In 10% of individuals with RA, the disease early becomes disabling. From clinical observation it has been determined that another 10% develop cumulative and final disability at some time in the patient's life. The prognosis for employability appears to be good in 50–80% of RA patients according to the socioeconomic status and medical care, even with advancing rheumatoid involvement."[65]

Disability and function measurements in rheumatoid arthritis

The Steinbrocker classification (ARA Functional Class) (Table 6)[64], which has been the most widely used measure of functional capacity, is a physician assessment of the patient's functional capacity that takes

RHEUMATOID ARTHRITIS

Table 5 Classification of progression of rheumatoid arthritis

Stage I, Early
*1. No destructive changes on roentgenographic examination.
*2. Roentgenologic evidence of osteoporosis may be present.

Stage II, Moderate
*1. Roentgenologic evidence of osteoporosis, with or without slight subchondral bone destruction; slight cartilage destruction may be present.
*2. No joint deformities, although limitation of joint mobility may be present.
3. Adjacent muscle atrophy.
4. Extra-articular soft tissue lesions, such as nodules and tenosynovitis, may be present.

Stage III, Severe
*1. Roentgenologic evidence of cartilage and bone destruction, in addition to osteoporosis.
*2. Joint deformity, such as subluxation, ulnar deviation, or hyperextension, without fibrous or bony ankylosis.
3. Extensive muscle atrophy.
4. Extra-articular soft-tissue lesions, such as nodules and tenosynovitis, may be present.

Stage IV, Terminal
*1. Fibrous or bony ankylosis.
2. Criteria of stage III.

*Criteria prefaced by an asterisk are those that must be present to permit classification of a patient in any particular stage or grade.

Table 6 Classification of functional capacity in rheumatoid arthritis

Class I:	Complete functional capacity with ability to carry on all usual duties without handicaps.
Class II:	Functional capacity adequate to conduct normal activities despite handicap of discomfort or limited mobility of one or more joints.
Class III:	Functional capacity adequate to perform only few or none of the duties of the usual occupation or of self-care.
Class IV:	Largely or wholly incapacitated with patient bedridden or confined to wheelchair, permitting little or no self-care.

into account the ability to perform the patients' "usual occupation." The assessment bridges "functional capacity" and work disability. In the text below we will try to keep separate data that refer specifically to work disability from those that *estimate* such disability. Even so there will be an overlap.

Table 7 Work disability in rheumatoid arthritis

Able to work at:	5 years	10 years	15 years
Makisara & Makisara (1982) N=405			
All types of work	60	50	33
Light work	94	100	88
Moderately heavy work	60	44	28
Heavy work	31	21	18
Compulsory education only	56	46	29
More than compulsory education	89	92	64
No vocational training	51	38	23
Vocational training	72	72	48
Yelin, Henke, and Epstein (1987) N=306			
Able to work	68	50	40

Work disability (Table 7)

Makisara and Makisara[66] analyzed data from a cohort of 405 RA patients first seen at the Rheumatism Foundation Hospital between 1963 and 1968 and followed prospectively. Patients receiving pension from the Finnish National Pensions Act were considered unable to work. As noted in Table 7 an increasing proportion of patients became unable to work with longer duration of RA. At 10 years 50% could not work. The disability to work was related to the type of work patients performed. Patients doing light work were generally able to work (88-100% employed) regardless of the duration of disease. For those doing moderately heavy work 60% were able to work at 5 years duration, 44% at 10 years, and only 28% at 15 years duration. By contrast, of those doing heavy work 31%, 21%, and 18% were working at 5, 10, and 15 years after disease onset, respectively. Education played an important role in maintaining the ability to work. At 5, 10, and 15 years after onset of RA. 1.6, 2, and 2.2 times more patients who been educated beyond the compulsory minimum were still employed. Similar data were obtained regarding the effect of vocational training. Age at disease onset was also related to discontinuance of work. At the 5-, 10-, and 15-year follow-ups progressively fewer patients were still working in the age at onset groups of 16-30, 31-45, and 46-60, respectively.

Very similar results were obtained by Yelin and coworkers, who followed 822 patients recruited from a random sample of one-half of the board-eligible rheumatologists in northern California[67]. Of this sample, 353 patients (72% women) with a work history were assessed. As noted in Table 7, 50% of patients were work-disabled after 10 years of rheumatoid arthritis. The authors assessed the explanatory value of certain physical and laboratory variables measured over a 4-year period on the probability of work loss. Elevated ESR, RF positivity, and the count of erosions did not predict who would stop working after diagnosis. But the number of painful joints had a relative risk of 1.8, the

Stanford Health Assessment Questionnaire functional disability index (HAQ)[68] a 3.3 risk, and age a 1.7 relative risk on the probability of work loss. The type of work performed, however, had a profound effect on employment. Altering the characteristics of the workplace to make it more conducive to continuing employment increased by almost 100% the likelihood of continuing work. Service workers had more than twice the risk of stopping work as those in other employment capacities. Finally, as in the Makisara and Makisara study cited above[66], increasing the physical demands of the job adversely influenced employment.

It is much more difficult to obtain data regarding the effect of RA on the ability of homemakers to perform their usual work duties since the dichotomous work variable (working versus not working) is not as useful. Reisine et al. recruited 142 women with definite or classical RA from a university hospital clinic and five rheumatology practices to study the effect of RA on homemakers[60]. Patients all lived with their husbands, children, or both. The duration of disease was not stated. At the study onset their HAQ score was 0.6 (mild dysfunction). At least half the participants reported limitations in their usual role activities. Full-time homemakers as opposed to those employed out of the home were more impaired than those employed and had higher HAQ scores (0.7 vs. 0.4).

Functional capacity

Unlike work disability data, which tabulate fact (working or not), functional capacity data measure physician's and other health workers' opinions as to the capacity of the patients to perform various functional tasks including employment tasks. There are wide variations in the reported functional capacity of patients among the different reporting centers that may be related to non-disease-related factors. The ARA Functional Classification[64] is imprecise and subject to differing interpretation. Some observers will place patients who have pain but no or little functional limitation in Class I while others will place them in Class II. Similarly, the difference between Class II and III relies mostly on whether a patient can do more than "little or none of the duties of the usual occupation." Both "usual occupation" and "little or none" are subject to varying interpretations. Not only is the language imprecise, but placing the patient in the category calls for interpretations on the part of observers for which they may lack accurate data. A final problem with the ARA classification is that a patient may change jobs or retire because of RA and therefore improve his functional classification.

At a disease duration of about 10 years most studies indicate that 35–40% or more of patients are in Functional Class III or IV. These data, however, underestimate functional loss since by 10 and 20 years after disease onset many patients have died, usually those with higher functional class[70-72]. Data from Scott et al.[71] that place more than 75% of patients in Functional Class III or above when first seen (approximately 4.5 years after disease onset) and data from Sherrer et al.[72] at the opposite extreme (< 12% of patients in Class III or IV) are discrepant, and may reflect differing interpretations of Functional Class. In general, the ARA classification tends to score dysfunction in the homemaker who is not employed out of the home as being less severe. It seems likely that the objective "work disability" data[66,67] better describe work capacity than estimates of Functional Class.

Self-assessment health status measures and functional instruments

The crude nature of the Functional Class assessment, together with its insensitivity to change and biased assessment in part played a role in the development of a series of questionnaire instruments (Tables 8–10). In contradistinction to ARA Functional Class, which used a physician's assessment of functional ability, these instruments use the patients' assessment. As such they are more sensitive to the nuances of patient function; and they are sensitive enough to be used effectively in clinical trials[73,74].

The instruments that have been used most frequently in RA assessment are the HAQ (Stanford Health Assessment Functional Disability Index) (Table 8)[57,58], its modification the MHAQ (Modified Health Assessment Questionnaire) (Table 9)[75,76], and the AIMS (Arthritis Impact Measurement Scales) (Table 10)[77,78]. The HAQ instruments are scaled similarly to the Functional Class such that on the average 1 indicates some impairment in every area of daily function, 2 indicates more severe impairment or requiring assistance in all the areas, and 3 indicates being unable to perform these activities in spite of assistance. The HAQ scaling is from 0 to 3, and the MHAQ from 1 to 4. Since these instruments are derived from eight areas of function they are scored by totaling the eight individual domains and dividing by 8, yielding a continuous scale that can be expressed to two decimal places.

Pincus et al. used the MHAQ in 259 RA patients whose disease duration was 12.4 years. Fifty-eight percent of patients scored between 1 and 2; 33% between 2 and 3; and only 9% between 3 and 4[76]. MHAQ scores should be reduced by one unit to make them comparable with HAQ scores. In general, though, MHAQ scores are slightly lower than HAQ scores because of the shortened MHAQ scale. Wolfe et al.[57] reported HAQ scores on 400 patients with RA (mean disease duration 9.5 years). Forty-three percent scored between 0 and 1; 43% between 1 and 2; and 14% between 2 and 3. Only 7.8% had no functional disability (HAQ score = 0). Patients with scores of approximately 0.5, 1.5, and 2.5 had disease durations of 7.5, 9.8, and 14.2 years, respectively. Wolfe et al. in a second study[79] evaluated 1274 patients with RA. They used life-table methodology to estimate the probability of reaching HAQ scores of 1 ("moderate disability") for 800 patients, 2 ("severe disability") for 1141, and 2.5 for 1227 patients. The median

RHEUMATOID ARTHRITIS

Table 8 The Stanford Health Assessment Questionnaire

OVER THE PAST WEEK, were you able to:	With NO Difficulty	With SOME Difficulty	With MUCH Difficulty	UNABLE To Do
DRESSING & GROOMING				
Dress yourself, including tying shoelaces and doing buttons?	_____	_____	_____	_____
Shampoo your hair?	_____	_____	_____	_____
ARISING				
Stand up from an armless straight chair?	_____	_____	_____	_____
Get in and out of bed?	_____	_____	_____	_____
EATING				
Cut your meat?	_____	_____	_____	_____
Lift a full cup or glass to your mouth?	_____	_____	_____	_____
Open a new milk carton?	_____	_____	_____	_____
WALKING				
Walk outdoors on flat ground?	_____	_____	_____	_____
Climb up five steps?	_____	_____	_____	_____

PLEASE CHECK AIDS OR DEVICES THAT YOU USUALLY USE FOR ANY OF THESE ACTIVITIES

—Cane
—Walker
—Crutches
—Wheelchair

—Devices used for dressing (button hook, zipper pull, long-handled shoe horn, etc.)
—Built-up or special utensils
—Special or built-up chair
—Other (specify: _____)

PLEASE CHECK CATEGORIES FOR WHICH YOU USUALLY NEED HELP FROM ANOTHER PERSON:

—Dressing and Grooming   —Eating   —Arising   —Walking

OVER THE PAST WEEK, were you able to:	With NO Difficulty	With SOME Difficulty	With MUCH Difficulty	UNABLE To Do
HYGIENE				
Wash and dry your entire body?	_____	_____	_____	_____
Take a tub bath?	_____	_____	_____	_____
Get on and off the toilet?	_____	_____	_____	_____

OVER THE PAST WEEK, were you able to:

	With **NO** Difficulty	With **SOME** Difficulty	With **MUCH** Difficulty	**UNABLE** To Do
REACH				
Reach and get down a 5-pound object (such as a bag of sugar) from just above your head?	_____	_____	_____	_____
Bend down to pick up clothing from the floor?	_____	_____	_____	_____
GRIP				
Open car doors?	_____	_____	_____	_____
Open jars which have been previously opened?	_____	_____	_____	_____
Turn faucets on and off?	_____	_____	_____	_____
ACTIVITIES				
Run errands and shop?	_____	_____	_____	_____
Get in and out of a car?	_____	_____	_____	_____
Do chores such as vacuuming or yardwork?	_____	_____	_____	_____

PLEASE CHECK AIDS OR DEVICES THAT YOU USUALLY USE FOR ANY OF THESE ACTIVITIES

—Raised toilet seat
—Bathtub seat
—Jar opener (for jars previously opened)
—Long-handled appliances in bathroom)

—Bathtub bar
—Long-handled appliances for reach
Other (specify   )

PLEASE CHECK CATEGORIES FOR WHICH YOU USUALLY NEED HELP FROM ANOTHER PERSON:

—Gripping & opening things   —Hygiene

—Errands and chores   —Reach

---

time to reach a HAQ of 1 was 7.58 years (95% confidence limit 6.8–9.1); time to reach a score of 2 was 20.2 years (95% CL 18.8–21.9); but the risk of severe disability (HAQ = 2) was 25% at 9.6 years. Very few patients escaped dysfunction. At 17 years after the onset of RA, risk data indicated that 80% of patients would have HAQ scores of 1 or greater; and at 17 years 25% of patients would have scores of 2.5 or greater ("essential incapacity"). One-third of the patients who were examined for the risk of obtaining an HAQ score of 1 had already met

RHEUMATOID ARTHRITIS

Table 9 Activities and lifestyles index (First section is MHAQ)

The questions below concern your daily activities. The few minutes you spend answering these questions can provide a more complete picture of how a medical condition may affect your life, adding to information from standard medical tests such as blood tests and X-rays. Please try to answer each question, even if you do not think it is related to you or any condition you may have. Please answer exactly as you think or feel, as there are no right and wrong answers.

Please check the ONE best answer for your abilities.

At THIS MOMENT: are you able to:	Without ANY difficulty	With SOME difficulty	With MUCH difficulty	UNABLE to do
a. Dress yourself, including tying shoelaces and doing buttons?				
b. Get in and out of bed?				
c. Life a full cup or glass to your mouth?				
d. Walk outdoors on flat ground?				
e. Wash and dry your entire body?				
f. Bend down to pick up clothing from the floor?				
g. Turn regular faucets on and off?				
h. Get in and out of a car?				

How SATISFIED are you with your ability to:	VERY satisfied	SOME- WHAT satisfied	SOME- WHAT dissatisfied	VERY dissatisfied
a. Dress yourself, including tying shoelaces and doing buttons?				
b. Get in and out of bed?				
c. Lift a full cup or glass to your mouth?				
d. Walk outdoors on flat ground?				
e. Wash and dry your entire body?				
f. Bend down to pick up clothing from the floor?				
g. Turn regular faucets on and off?				
h. Get in and out of a car?				

How do you feel TODAY compared to most days during the past week?

Please check only **one**
—Much better today than most days
—Better today than most days
—The same today as most days
—Worse today than most days
—Much worse today than most days

Which of the following best describes you TODAY?

Please check only **one**
—I can do everything I want to do.
—I can do most of the things I want to do but have some limitations.
—I can do some, but not all, of the things I want to do, and I have many limitations.
I can do hardly any of the things I want to do.

How often is it PAINFUL for you to:	Never	Sometimes	Most of the time	Always
a. Dress yourself, including tying shoelaces and doing buttons?				
b. Get in and out of bed?				
c. Lift a full cup or glass to your mouth?				
d. Walk outdoors on flat ground?				
e. Wash and dry your entire body?				
f. Bend down to pick up clothing from the floor?				
g. Turn regular faucets on and off?				
h. Get in and out of a car?				

How much pain have you had because of your condition IN THE PAST WEEK?

NO PAIN _____ PAIN AS BAD AS IT COULD BE

that end-point at the study onset (left censoring) so it is likely that actual functional disability was underestimated in this analysis.

A cross-sectional study using the last available HAQ score was reported by Sherrer et al.[72] using data from the Saskatoon databank of ARAMIS[80]. They also showed an increase in HAQ scores over time in this separate study population. An HAQ score of approximately 1 was noted after 7.5 years of RA. At 17 years the mean HAQ score was approximately 1.75. In this study of 681 patients, data from an

RHEUMATOID ARTHRITIS

Table 10 The Arthritis Impact Measurement Scale (AIMS) questionnaire

Mobility

4	Are you in bed or chair for most or all of the day because of your health?
3	Are you able to use public transportation?
2	When you travel around your community, does someone have to assist you because of your health?
1	Do you have to stay indoors most or all of the day because of your health?

Physical activity

5	Are you unable to walk unless you are assisted by another person or by a cane, crutches, artificial limbs, or braces?
4	Do you have any trouble either walking one block or climbing one flight of stairs because of your health?
3	Do you have any trouble either walking several blocks or climbing a few flights of stairs because of your health?
2	Do you have trouble bending, lifting, or stooping because of your health?
1	Does your health limit the kind of vigorous activities you can do such as running, lifting heavy objects, or participating in strenuous sports?

Dexterity

5	Can you easily write with a pen or pencil?
4	Can you easily turn a key in a lock?
3	Can you easily button articles of clothing?
2	Can you easily tie a pair of shoes?
1	Can you easily open a jar of food?

Social role

7	If you had to take medicine, could you take all your own medicine?
6	If you had a telephone, would you be able to use it?
5	Do you handle your own money?
4	If you had a kitchen, could you prepare your own meals?
3	If you had laundry facilities (washer, dryer, etc.) could you do your own laundry?
2	If you had the necessary transportation, could you go shopping for groceries or clothes?
1	If you had household tools and appliances (vacuum, mops, etc.) could you do your own housework?

Social activity

5	About how often were you on the telephone with close friends or relatives during the past month?
4	Has there been a change in the frequency or quality of your sexual relationships during the past month?
3	During the past month, about how often have you had friends or relatives to your home?
2	During the past month, about how often did you get together socially with friends or relatives?
1	During the past month, how often have you visited with friends or relatives at their homes?

PROGNOSIS IN THE RHEUMATIC DISEASES

Activities of daily living

4	How much help do you need to use the toilet?
3	How well are you able to move around?
2	How much help do you need in getting dressed?
1	When you bathe, either a sponge bath, tub, or shower, how much help do you need?

Pain

4	During the past month, how often have you had severe pain from your arthritis?
3	During the past month, how would you describe the arthritis pain you usually have?
2	During the past month, how long has your morning stiffness usually lasted from the time you wake up?
1	During the past month, how often have you had pain in two or more joints at the same time?

Depression

6	During the past month, how often did you feel that others would be better off if you were dead?
5	How often during the past month have you felt so down in the dumps that nothing could cheer you up?
4	How much of the time during the past month have you felt downhearted and blue?
3	How often during the past month did you feel that nothing turned out for you the way you wanted it to?
2	During the past month, how much of the time have you been in low or very low spirits?
1	During the past month, how much of the time have you enjoyed the things you do?

Anxiety

6	During the past month, how much of the time have you felt tense or "high strung"?
5	How much have you been bothered by nervousness, or your "nerves" during the past month?
4	How often during the past month did you find yourself having difficulty trying to calm down?
3	How much of the time during the past month were you able to relax without difficulty?
2	How much of the time during the past month have you felt calm and peaceful?
1	How much of the time during the past month did you feel relaxed and free of tension?

Each group of items is listed in Guttman scale order with the scale level in the left column. Subjects failing an item also tend to fail all lower items in the group.

additional 281 patients were not used because they had died before HAQ administration was available. These patients had more severe RA and were in a higher ARA Functional Class, suggesting that the disability scores by virtue of the left censoring by death significantly underestimated functional disability. These workers also found a correlation of 0.65 between the HAQ scores and Functional Class. Using the MHAQ, Pincus reported a correlation of 0.60 with Functional Class in an assessment of 259 patients. Similarly HAQ scores were strongly associated with work disability and had large relative risks for future work disability (3.28[67] and 3.8[81]) in two studies.

Only limited longitudinal data are available for the AIMS instrument at this date. One study showed no worsening of arthritis impact over a 5-year period in patients who had been identified first as participants in a drug study[82]. A number of additional longitudinal studies are in progress.

Mortality

Most[83-94], but not all studies[95] have shown mortality to be increased in RA. Mitchell et al. found the median age of death in RA males and females to be 4 and 10 years earlier than in the general population, and an overall standardized mortality rate (SMR) of 151 (SMR = (observed deaths/expected deaths) × 100)[80]. The relative risk of mortality compared with controls was 2.73 for 57 men and 1.88 for 236 women with RA in Stockholm over an 11-year observation period[89]. Four hundred eighty-nine English RA patients were followed over an 11-year period with standardized mortality rates of 260 for men and 340 for women[91]. Relative risks of mortality were 2.6 for men and 3.4 for women in 489 RA patients first seen in hospital in Birmingham, UK[94]. One thousand RA patients and 1000 controls followed in Finland over a 10-year period demonstrated a relative risk of mortality of 1.4 for men and 2.0 for women[96]. These data indicate a substantial effect of RA on mortality.

A number of studies have investigated factors associated with mortality. In general, more severe arthritis as measured by factors such as functional disability, ARA diagnostic class, extra-articular disease, and side-effects of treatment, etc., have been found associated with increased deaths. After age, Mitchell et al.[80] found ARA Functional Class to be the most important predictor of mortality with a relative risk of 1.49. Similar associations with Functional Class were noted by Alleback et al.[89], Rasker and Cosh[84], and Pincus and coworkers[86]. Wolfe et al.[57] studied 400 patients every 6 months over 3 years with standard clinical and questionnaire assessments. Adjusting for the effect of other clinical and laboratory variables, after age and gender, only the HAQ functional disability index was predictive of mortality with a relative risk of 1.77 (95% CL 1.02-3.06).

Some studies have demonstrated the effect of other factors on mortality rates, including rheumatoid factor, ARA classical RA, joint count, and extra-articular manifestations of disease. Both Mitchell et al.[80] and Allebeck et al.[89] found associations between RA mortality and RF positivity. But such an association may reflect problems in case definition associated with the construct of seronegative arthritis, and the heterogeneity of patients carrying that diagnosis. Significant association between disease severity as defined by the number of extra-articular manifestations of RA has been found[97].

Although "rheumatoid arthritis" infrequently appears on the death certificate even among those clearly dying of RA[89], attempts have been made to identify excess mortality that can be directly related to the illness. "Attributable" deaths refer to those where RA was the cause of death, as in rheumatoid vasculitis and renal failure from amyloid. "Contributory" deaths are those where the RA or its treatment contributed to the death but was not the primary reason for death. Infection following surgery for RA is an example of this sort of death association. Accurate data about these categories may be difficult to obtain if autopsies are not obtained; for example, in cases when the cause of death is amyloid renal disease. Of 79 deaths considered "excess," 25% were directly attributable to rheumatoid disease, and 10% were "contributory" deaths related to side-effects of treatment in the Mitchell et al. series[80]. Rasker and Cosh found that "attributable" deaths reduced life expectancy by 15 years, "contributory" by 10, and "unrelated" by 5.

Pincus[83] has reviewed attributed causes of death of 2262 RA patients in 13 reported series and compared death rates with US data (Table 11). In this report the percent RA mortality was increased for infection (9.4 vs. 1), renal disease (7.8 vs. 1.1), respiratory disease (7.2 vs. 3.9), rheumatoid arthritis (5.3 vs. 0), and gastrointestinal disease (4.2 vs. 2.4); and decreased for cancer (14.1 vs. 20.4), CNS disease (4.2 vs. 9.6), accidents (1.0 vs. 5.4), and miscellaneous causes (6.4 vs. 15.2). Although cancer mortality was reduced in this compilation, data strongly indicate that hematologic and lymphoproliferative malignancies are increased in RA separately from increases that may be caused by the use of cytotoxic agents.[96,98].

Non-disease-related factors have been identified by Pincus, who found a strong association between formal education level and RA survival[27,29], thus extending the observations made in the nonrheumatologic literature as to the effect of social class, socioeconomic status, and education to rheumatoid arthritis.

In summary, mortality data indicate at least a two-fold increase in mortality among RA patients, with the most pronounced effect being observed in women. Life expectancy may be reduced by as much as 5 (men) to 15 years (women). The major increases in mortality come from infection, renal and respiratory causes. Rheumatoid arthritis is both directly and indirectly linked to mortality as an effect of the disease and of its treatment. Various markers of disease severity have been predictive of increased mortality, including extra-articular manifestations of disease, functional disability and rheumatoid factor status.

Table 11 Meta-analysis of causes of mortality in rheumatoid arthritis

Attributed cause of death	2262 RA deaths	1977 US population
Cardiovascular disease	42.1	41.0
Cancer	14.1	20.4
Infection	9.4	1.0
Renal disease	7.8	1.1
Respiratory disease	7.2	3.9
Rheumatoid arthritis	5.3	NL
Gastrointestinal disease	4.2	2.4
Central nervous system disease	4.2	9.6
Accidents	1.0	5.4
Miscellaneous	6.4	15.2
Unknown	0.6	NL

Adapted from Pincus, T.: Is mortality increased in rheumatoid arthritis? *The Journal of Musculoskeletal Medicine*, June 1988

Non-medical factors, particularly formal educational level, are associated with premature mortality. Even so, our knowledge of predictive markers of mortality remains crude. In a time-oriented, chronic disease, measures which are assessed over time such as prolonged dysfunction, pain, ESR, joint counts and similar clinical observations, radiographic changes, psychological and psychosocial status would be expected to have important effects on mortality. Current studies, however, have used cross-sectional data, often collected in the early stage of the illness, to predict outcome 20 years later. The use of chronic disease databanks with serial rather than cross-sectional observations can be expected to yield up additional information about mortality in RA.

The costs of rheumatoid arthritis

It has long been known that the societal costs of RA are high. Costs may be divided into direct medical costs and "indirect" costs that refer to lost wages and productivity. McDuffie[99] recently summarized annual RA costs using data from Kelsey. US indirect costs in 1983 for RA were $215 million and direct costs $777 million. Thus, the total RA cost approximated 1 billion US dollars. Several studies have been conducted that attempted to measure direct and indirect medical costs at the level of the patient rather than at the societal level. Lubeck et al. used the ARAMIS databank to assess these costs during 1981 in 940 patients with definite or classical RA[100]. Total costs, in 1981 dollars, were $2532 per patient. Of these costs, $1092 were outpatient costs, $913 inpatient costs, and $527 miscellaneous costs related to transportation, domestic assistance, etc. The largest single category of costs were for medications (16%), exceeding the costs for physician visits (8.1%). Wolfe et al. studied in detail hospitalizations in the same sample during 1981[56,101]. They noted that of nonsurgical hospitalizations, 46.6% were for diagnosis and treatment, 42.5% for treatment of adverse reactions to therapy, and 11% for complications of RA. During the study year 54.4% of hospitalizations were related to orthopedic surgery. Ninety-nine RA and 49 OA patients were studied by Liang and colleagues in 1984[102]. These workers combined costs of both diseases, but indicated that the outpatient costs for RA were much higher than for OA (exact figures not supplied). They estimated total yearly direct cost for the combined disorders of $683, of which $136 was said to be "out-of-pocket" costs. Total annual direct costs (RA and non-RA) to those receiving public assistance in California in 1981–1982 were estimated to be $2569 per year as opposed to those for non-RA patients receiving assistance of $782. (RA patients were older and a higher proportion were female. Data were not adjusted for these differences[103].) Two hundred ninety-three RA patients participating in a drug trial in 1982–1983 had annual costs of their RA determined before study participation[104]. Hospitalization costs were $1080 and total costs including nursing home care were $2374.

Indirect costs in stage 3[64] RA have been reported in several studies from the University of California at San Francisco[105,106]. Individuals with this condition lost 61% of their premorbid income, and families lost 37%. In 1976 dollars the mean income loss was $6830. Although these data apply to stage 3 RA, data from a larger sample of all RA patients (cited above) indicate that 50% of those employed at the onset of their illness will stop work because of RA within a decade of disease onset[67].

Stone used estimates of incidence of RA and published data relating to direct and indirect costs of the illness to estimate the lifetime direct and indirect costs of RA for disease with onset in 1977[107]. Lifetime direct costs were estimated at $4398 and indirect costs at $16 014. Although the direct costs appear high, they are substantially less than those that might be projected from the studies cited above[56,100-103].

Several studies have examined predictive factors associated with direct and indirect medical costs. The HAQ disability index was found to be an important predictor of direct[101,108,109] and indirect[67,81] medical costs in a number of studies. As noted above, the ability to maintain employment is related to workplace autonomy and physical demand of the job as well as to arthritis severity[67,81,105].

These data, then, stress the high direct medical costs and even higher indirect costs of RA. Both costs increase with increasing severity of disease, and direct medical costs increase with duration of disease since the major factor in hospitalization is the late need for joint replacement surgery. Employment is more likely to be maintained by those with workplace autonomy, better education, and less physically severe work.

Pain

It is likely that pain contributes more to the overall perceived severity of RA than any other feature of the illness. But unlike other measures of RA outcome (e.g., functional loss, work loss, and economic loss — outcomes that generally become progressively worse) it does not worsen with increasing duration of disease[110]. Indeed there is evidence that pain "levels" may decrease over time as patients learn to cope with this aspect of their illness. When patients with active RA have a remission of their arthritis (as defined by ACR criteria[111]) pain disappears entirely, even when RA has been present for many years. Pain is thus clearly a process measure, particularly if one looks at data in a cross-sectional way. Pain assumes the proper characteristics of an outcome measure when it is considered over time as, for example, an "area under the curve" measurement or as a "mean" measurement of a series of pain assessments over some period of time.

Although there is an extensive literature on pain assessment[112-125], most often pain is assessed in RA patients with a visual analog scale[122-125]. Surprisingly there are very few data that describe changes in pain scores *in the same patients* over periods in excess of a year. Wolfe et al.[110] however, studied RA pain in groups of patients seen for the first time at about 1, 5, 10, 15 and 20 years after the onset of RA. Pain decreased in the 1-year group over the next year, but did not change over more than 2 years follow-up in any of the subsequent time groups. In these assessments the authors tested whether the slopes of the pain scores in the individual observation periods were different from 0. Moreover, pain scores for the 5-20 year RA patients did not differ significantly. Meenan et al.[82] similarly found no change in pain scores in a 2-year follow-up of patients initially seen as part of a drug trial.

Mason et al. used the AIMS instrument[68] to assess RA and five nonrheumatic disorders[126]. As might be expected, pain scores (5.5 on 1-10 scale) were higher in RA patients than those with other chronic conditions. Wolfe used a (0-3) visual analog scale to measure pain in the following groups: rheumatoid arthritis (n=1285), low back pain (n=1068), osteoarthritis of the knee (n=744), fibromyalgia (n=572), and osteoarthritis of the hand (n=493)[127]. Mean plus SD pain scores for these respective groups were 1.7 (0.61), 1.9 (0.78), 1.8 (0.73), 1.8 (0.70), 1.6 (0.77).

The assessment of pain is a very sensitive process measure in short- and medium-term drug trials in RA, and it might be expected to be a sensitive outcome measure (it has a large potential effect size) when used to assess longitudinal trends in RA, including the long-term effects of remittive therapy. At present, pain as a longitudinal outcome measure has not been utilized significantly in RA research.

Psychological measurements

Although a count has not been done it would not be surprising if more has been written about the psychological aspects of RA than any other health status domain. Most of the early psychological studies were seriously flawed methodologically[128-130] and contributed little useful information about RA and psychological status. Recent trends in psychological studies of RA have included the use of disease markers of RA severity in multivariate analyses to assess the effect of RA on psychological status and, contrariwise, the effect of psychological status on RA outcome. Even so, most studies have examined the RA-psychological interaction cross-sectionally rather than longitudinally and thus measures such as "anxiety" and "depression" appear as process measures rather than outcome measures, a situation analogous to pain measurements noted above. Literally, millions of dollars have been spent trying to assess whether various measures of psychological health are impaired in RA and to what extent they are impaired compared with various control groups. The thrust of these studies has been to show that RA patients, like those with other chronic diseases, have some increase in depression and anxiety, with the degree of increase varying from center to center.

Several studies have examined psychological status longitudinally, however. Hawley and Wolfe[54] followed 400 patients with RA over a more than 3-year duration, assessing psychological status with the AIMS[77] anxiety and depression scales, the HAQ disability questionnaire, and standard clinical rheumatologic measurements. Twenty-five percent of the variance in initial psychological scores could be explained by pain, HAQ functional disability score, age, family income, and joint count. Over the follow-up period, worsening in depression scores was associated with socioeconomic but not clinical factors. Patients with high levels of anxiety and depression used more clinical services over the follow-up period, but did not have more severe disease. Changes in psychological scores showed weak correlations with clinical measure (HAQ, joint count, and grip strength). McFarlane and Brooks also studied RA over time, assessing psychological function and clinical activity in two assessments, 3 years apart[131]. They found few significant relationships between duration of illness, disease severity, and psychological measures. These studies suggest that severity of RA has a modest effect on psychological health, but that disease duration is generally unrelated to psychological status. Whether there are subgroups of RA patients on whom RA severity and duration has a profound effect has not yet been determined.

Adverse reactions

Adverse reactions to medical and surgical therapies range in severity from the trivial to those that are fatal. Although the risk of having an adverse reaction may be increased by various factors including, for example, age, concurrent medication, or comorbidity, one can assume that the risk of an adverse reaction at any one moment is relatively constant over the course of the illness, and that the cumulative risk is directly related to the duration of exposure. Since the average duration of RA is in excess of 20 years, almost all patients with this illness will experience at least one adverse reaction, and some will experience multiple reactions. The net impact to the RA patient, then, is dependent upon the number of adverse reactions and the severity of each, or the sum of the individual severities of the reactions.

In spite of the fact that adverse reactions are common, it is difficult to obtain useful data concerning such reactions. "Side-effects" are reported by patients at differing thresholds. Side-effect frequency elicited by observers differs according to whether the information is spontaneously elicited or deliberately requested. The offending drug is often administered with other drugs, making the determination of which drug is causing the effect difficult; the illness or other illnesses can be responsible for the apparent side-effect as well. In addition, it is difficult to accurately grade the "severity" of side-effects.

Some information about adverse reactions (ADRs) related to drug therapy can be gained by the cross-sectional tabulation of side-effects during placebo controlled trials. But from the point of view of outcome assessment the tabulation of these reactions yields little information about the impact of ADRs on the patients. *Such tabulations yield information about drugs, not patients.* Central mechanisms of obtaining adverse drug reaction information include direct reporting to regulatory authorities such as the US Food and Drug Administration (FDA) and the Committee on Safety of Medications in the United Kingdom. While useful for getting some estimates of serious ADRs, the FDA reporting system depends on the reporting interest of the physician who has to file the report. The actual numerator and denominator for the suspected ADRs are not known accurately, but it has been estimated that less than 10% of ADRs are reported[132]. In addition, data specifically relating to RA are not available.

The indirect mechanisms available by which the impact of ADRs on the RA patients can be estimated involve the assumption that certain side-effects by virtue of their prevalence, morbidity, cost, and potential associations with mortality, "impact" RA more than just trivially. The only ADR to satisfy these requirements is that of gastric and duodenal ulceration. The available epidemiologic reports, however, assess the effect of nonsteroidal anti-inflammatory drugs (NSAIDs) in general, rather than their specific effect in RA. It is then assumed that since RA patients are frequent users of such agents the data can be extrapolated to RA as well. NSAID use is generally associated with increased risks of bleeding, perforation, and death, with the relative risk of these events compared to controls being in the order of 2 to 4[132-138]. Even so, the actual risk of serious events (perforation, or GI bleeding, or death) is small when the data are examined cross-sectionally: approximately 1 per 10 000 person-months of NSAID treatment[132]. Such risk may not be small to the RA patient who receives daily NSAID therapy, and whose disease lasts, on the average, more than 20 years. Data from cross-sectional assessments cannot be applied simply to longitudinal outcomes of chronic diseases.

Data from Fries and associates[139] using the ARAMIS databank provide insight into the magnitude of GI hospitalization and the associated risk of NSAID therapy. In their longitudinal study (mean follow-up 3.5 years) the risk of upper GI hospitalization was 1 per 100 patient-years. The assessment included 6650 patient-years, approximately two-thirds of which occurred during NSAID therapy. The hazard ratio for use of NSAIDs on hospitalization was 6.45. Although number of hospitalizations related to perforation, bleeding, and death were not specified in this report, the 1 per 100 patient-years translates to 1 per 1200 patient-months, a figure that should be compared to the estimate of Langman for serious events, noted above[132].

In general the above data suggest that 1% of patients with RA will be hospitalized each year for reasons related to upper GI disease, and that from 1/2 to 5/6 (ARAMIS data) of those hospitalizations are related to NSAID therapy. In addition, as noted by Pincus in his meta-analysis of mortality, the overall mortality due to GI causes is increased by approximately 1.8% (4.2% rheumatoid arthritis vs 2.8% for controls)[83]. The above discussion suggests that a sizable proportion of that mortality can be expected to be attributable to NSAIDs.

Although the magnitude of the side-effects-related NSAID therapy is striking, it provides only a small insight into the cumulative impact of adverse reactions on persons with RA. The determination of this impact is no simple task, since comparing various adverse reactions must take into account multiple adverse reactions[140-142], including pain, psychological stress, cognitive problems[143], direct and indirect costs, worsening of RA, the production of new medical conditions, and the risk of death or comorbidity. Such outcomes are modified by the status of the patient, and the circumstances in which the reaction occurs. Recently, Fries and coworkers have described a side-effect index that accounts for many of the side-effect outcomes noted above and assigns "severity" ratings to each side-effect, thus allowing quantification of side-effect impact as well as investigations of the factors leading to side-effect severity. Such an index presages a more complete understanding of adverse reactions and their associated causes than has been available previously[144].

Radiographic outcome

Hand radiographs occupy a special place with the construct of outcome since they are unrelated, in the most direct sense, to what the patient experiences. Moreover, the results of the radiographic examination cannot be expressed in terms that relate to other patient outcomes, and a radiographic report has little meaning for an individual patient. Radiographs are generally modestly correlated with patient clinical status. Pincus et al. found the hand radiographic score to be inversely correlated with grip strength ($r=-0.51$), but less strongly related to the patients' self-report (Modified Health Assessment Questionnaire —

MHAQ) (r=0.28)[76]. However, Sharp noted a correlation coefficient of 0.51 between his radiographic scoring method and the HAQ functional disability index in cited but unpublished data[145]. Regan-Smith *et al.*, using the less sensitive Steinbrocker radiographic staging system[64] and the AIMS instrument[77], found no correlation between these assessment measures[146]. Regardless of the method of radiographic scoring, radiographic progression occurs inexorably over the course of RA[71, 147-150]. Sharp has suggested that radiographic progression is linear over the first 20 years of the illness, but later levels off[151]. However, unpublished observations from Sharp suggest that progression may be linear throughout the course of RA (personal communication). Radiographic abnormality is noted within the first 2 years of disease[150]. Hand radiographs are the most commonly applied assessment tool, but are less sensitive to change than radiographs of the feet[152-154].

The difficulty in linking patient outcome to radiographic outcome limits the usefulness of radiographs in assessing how the *patient* is doing. Radiographic abnormality is most closely linked to progressive inflammatory disease, correlating best with continuous disease activity[152]. But radiographic changes may progress in the face of quiescent disease as well[155-158]. Although radiographs represent a generally irreversible "outcome" of disease, the inability to represent them in human terms makes them most useful as a measure of clinical intervention in pharmocologic trials. As such they perform as an ongoing "process" measure.

ALTERATION OF PROGNOSIS

We have defined prognosis and outcome, as noted above, in terms of mortality, psychological ad functional disability, work disability, direct and indirect costs of illness, side-effects of treatment, and radiographs. The first five categories represent the 5 "Ds" (death, disability, dollar costs, discomfort, and drug side-effects) suggested by Fries[68,159]. These outcome categories, in addition, tend to require longitudinal observation for their best assessment. Most studies in RA have been cross-sectional or short-term rather than longitudinal, and many have used disease process measures, including radiographic changes, physical examination (e.g., articular index, grip strength, range of motion), symptom (e.g., morning stiffness), and laboratory (e.g., ESR) features as indicators of outcome.

Nonmedical factors

A number of nonmedical factors acting separately, but more usually in combination, exert influence on the prognosis of RA. These factors include education, social status, social support, income, race, access to medical care, medical insurance, gender, and employment.

Education. As noted above, it is likely that demographic and socioeconomic factors influence RA outcome. Pincus and coworkers have presented data from three sources, suggesting that education level influences outcome. In a national data set, rheumatoid arthritis (actually symmetrical polyarthritis) occurred more frequently in those with less education after controlling for confounding variables[51]. Disease severity markers and outcome markers such as ESR, joint counts, and radiographic changes, similarly, are worse in those less educated[27,51]. Finally, education was a strong predictor of mortality in 75 patients followed for 9 years[86]. The mechanism by which education level may exert this effect is uncertain. It is likely, however, that education may be a surrogate, measuring the combined effects of education, income, motivation, social class, lifestyle, compliance, etc.[27]. A number of other medical conditions are influenced by such factors, including cardiovascular disease and cancer[30-34]. The effects noted by Pincus were profound and possibly exceed the effect of treatment. Nevertheless they have not yet been examined in clinics outside of Tennessee. They require further confirmation.

Race and other socioeconomic factors. Race and socioeconomic status have not been studied as predictors of outcome in RA. We studied the age of death of *parents* of persons with RA[160]. We found that parents in a predominantly black, lower socioeconomic class area died 6 years earlier than parents in a middle-class, white, midwestern region. It is almost certain that similar effects on mortality will be noted on their children who have RA. The effect of race and socioeconomic status on mortality in general is well known (see socioeconomic section above), and whether these factors are entirely independent of RA or not is unknown.

It is likely that socioeconomic status may influence the results of therapeutic trials, but the socioeconomic status of patients in such trials is almost never described.

Income. Although it is known that income falls in families with RA, there are no data on the specific effects of income and its surrogates on RA prognosis. It seems likely, however, that income, independently, by virtue of providing entry to the medical system, and supporting the family economically, among other factors, may buffer and mitigate the effects of RA.

Access to care. Access to care is often tightly linked to other socioeconomic variables such as income and race[32,161]. Yelin has provided data that fee-for-service and Health Maintenance Organizations (HMO) provide equal levels of care[162], but investigations have not been performed among those without medical insurance or those with limited ability to pay. Anecdotally, we have noted a number of patients who declined medical treatments because of costs or did not have joint replacement surgery that would have profoundly improved functional status because of the economic effects on themselves and their families. Although it has been suggested recently that the economic status of the elderly has improved in comparison to younger persons[163], it is not uncommon to see elderly US rheumatoid arthritis patients spending almost all of their pension benefits on drugs for RA and other treatments. Liang[164] has shown that simple and often inexpensive changes made to the physical environment of elderly patients with arthritis can result in substantial improvement in living quality and arrangements. The major limitation to the accomplishment of such changes is the lack of a societal mechanism to implement the changes.

Social support. Few data are available that specifically detail the effect of social support on RA outcome. Short-term studies fail to show significant benefits from social support interventions[165], but it is possible that decreased utilization of services, reduced adverse reactions, better compliance, and reduced mortality might be effected by such interventions. Although this has not been studied longitudinally in RA, data from other chronic illnesses suggest that mortality is increased in those with decreased social contacts[41].

Employment. As noted above, a number of studies clearly demonstrate that the type of employment profoundly affects ability to work (and thus income) in persons with RA. Hard physical work and little workplace autonomy were factors associated with loss of employment and income[52,66,67,81,166]. Such data suggest that retraining or otherwise placing patients with RA into different types of employment will significantly improve the socioeconomic outcome of rheumatoid arthritis.

Genetic and disease severity factors. HLA-DR4, HLA-DR1, or both are found in 93% of RA patients[167]. While about half of the published studies have found HLA-DR4 inceased in seropositive RA compared with seronegative RA (or decreased in seronegative RA!)[16] most studies have failed to find important links between these HLA antigens and severity and outcome markers of RA such as radiographic erosions[152,168], and clinical and functional status[70,169-172]. HLA-Dw2 and B-27 predicted radiographic changes in the cervical spine in one report[168]; and certain studies have found worse outcomes in HLA-DR4 associated familial cases of RA[173,174]. We studied 985 RA patients for the presence of familial RA. No differences in the severity of familial and nonfamilial cases were found[175]; and the proportion of HLA-DR4 was similar in familial and nonfamilial RA[176]. Similar results were obtained by Sanders et al.[177]

HLA studies of RA appear to be confounded by the definition of RA (and the associated seronegativity/seropositivity) used within the reporting centers. The issue of the homogeneity of seronegative RA[16] and whether it usually represents "true rheumatoid arthritis" is critical to most prognostic indicators. The longer persons with seronegative RA have been followed the more often they are discovered to have other identifiable rheumatic disorders[13]. It would seem wiser to avoid diagnostic conundrums such as this by studying seropositive and seronegative RA separately.

One report has suggested that RA may be becoming milder, perhaps because of unknown environmental influences, based on the finding of decreased rheumatoid factor positivity and erosiveness in succeeding generations of RA patients[178]. The authors acknowledge potential biases that could have explained their results. One perplexing finding was that those patients diagnosed as having RA in their 1980 cohort were only 53.5% rheumatoid factor positive, a value much lower than is usually thought to be found in RA (75-85%). As with other prognostic variables, definition of RA may be critical.

Rheumatoid factor. Virtually all studies show a worse outcome for rheumatoid factor (RF) positive patients regardless of the outcome measure assessed[12,13,70,71,97,168,179-182]. These judgments may reflect problems within the construct of seronegative RA, as we have indicated above. The titer of RF factor, among those who are rheumatoid factor positive, might be expected to give a better estimation of the importance of this observation to the outcome of RA since it assesses a more homogeneous group. Higher titers of RF are found earlier and more frequently in those with extra-articular manifestations of RA[97]. Mitchell et al.[88] noted an association between the RF titer (a single measurement) and risk of mortality in their study of 805 patients, although the association was weak. High titers of RF $>$ 1 : 2560 (latex) are seen frequently (17-68%) in patients with rheumatoid vasculitis[183]. Westedt et al., in one of the few studies that evaluated RF longitudinally, noted strong correlations between the RF titer and the articular and joint swelling indices (r=0.43-0.65) using the latex test, but found RF not to be predictive of future "joint disease activity"[184]. Radiographic abnormalities were not correlated with RF in 201 patients studied by Kaye et al.[185], nor with rheumatoid positivity in other reports[158,186,187]. Reeback and Silman used the HAQ disability index and ROM at the wrist to assess outcome in 72 patients seen within 18 months of disease onset and followed for a subsequent 2 years[188]. Those with latex titers $>$ 1 : 40 had higher HAQ scores at follow-up, and there appeared to be a worsening trend of HAQ scores with higher titers of RF. RF subtypes, IgA, IgG, and IgM have been examined in a number of reports. In general, associations between various disease activity measures, including radiographic erosions, have been shown for IgG and IgA[25,189], but no longitudinal outcome data are available. In spite of these data, which identify higher titer RF in subsets of RA patients, the prognostic significance of RF titer (not RF positivity) remains uncertain. Positive RF titers change, are rarely assessed serially in research or clinical practice, and have not often been studied as a predictor of the outcomes of interest here. Overall, there are no convincing data that RF titers, as conventionally and clinically assessed and measured, contribute to functional or work disability, direct or indirect costs, pain, adverse reactions, or other outcome measures.

Gender. Although 65 to 75% of RA patients are women, rheumatoid vasculitis occurs about equally in both sexes[97,183]. Except for vasculitis, however, females are generally regarded as having a worse prognosis. Most studies, however, have considered outcome in terms of process measures or in terms of remittent vs. nonremittent disease, an issue that is confounded by the definition of RA. Feigenbaum et al.[181] noted that 5 years after the diagnosis of probable or definite RA of recent onset 100% of those with erosions and 91% of those with swelling were women, as opposed to 71% of those without swelling when assessed 5 years later. Using "clinical" and "laboratory" measures, Short and Bauer found that of 212 patients, 68.9% of women and 48.9% of men improved over a 12-year-plus period of follow-up[190]. Makisara and Makisara found no difference between the sexes in functional and work capacity in 405 RA patients, one-third of whom were seen 5, 10, and 15 years after disease onset[66]. Wolfe and Hawley studied remission in patients with definite or classical RA over 1131 patient-years[191]. Among those receiving second-line antirheumatic therapy, males constituted 35.7% achieving remission and 23.7% of those not achieving remission.

Clinical and laboratory measures of disease process. The effect of these measures has been assayed in three ways: in prognostic studies beginning in early RA, in prognostic studies beginning later in the course of RA, and in studies employing longitudinal data. The latter method is a recent development and is a powerful predictor of RA outcome for, as we will show, it is *sustained* disease activity that most affects RA prognosis. As noted in the discussions above, authors frequently describe other process measures as their *outcome*, adding confusion to an already difficult area.

Prognostic studies beginning in early rheumatoid arthritis

In two reports, Feigenbaum et al.[181] and Masi et al.[19] studied prognosis (5 years later) in 50 newly diagnosed probable and definite cases of RA. They categorized patients into three outcome classes based on no swelling, swelling, and radiographic erosions. Thus they were measuring the presence of ongoing disease activity, and the effect of disease activity as manifested by erosions. Among the data presented, the clinical measure of "2 or more swollen upper joints," grip strength in women, and the counts of tender and swollen joints separated the groups. ESR and hemoglobin were not significant in their analysis. It is difficult to interpret this study since it actually represents a "prognosis of early polyarthritis" rather than an RA prognosis study. In addition, a major implied endpoint is remission (no swelling), which was met by 36%, suggesting that the findings of the study related to the nature of the construct of RA more than to its outcome.

Rasker and Cosh reported a 20-year follow-up on 100 patients with definite or classical RA seen within the first year (average 4 months) of disease[70]. Initial functional status correlated with subsequent mortality, and with functional status when assessed at 11 or 15 years after disease onset. ESR was not a useful predictor of functional status.

Reeback and Silman's study of 72 RA patients seen within 18 months of disease onset utilized the Stanford HAQ[68] as one outcome measure at assessment 2 years later[188]. No association was found between initial values of ESR, CRP, morning stiffness, or physician or patient assessment of disease severity. Slight correlation was found with the articular index (r=0.35).

Prognostic studies beginning later in the course of rheumatoid arthritis

Scott and colleagues followed 112 patients with established RA (duration < 1.5 to > 10 years) for 20 years[71]. A sedimentation rate > 50 mm/h and Functional Class IV or V (British classification) were associated with worse outcome as assessed by functional classification and death, but the "predictive value of these laboratory measures was not strong." Other clinical and laboratory measures were not discussed in this report. In addition, the outcome measures were not adjusted for the effect of age or other covariates that might have been of influence.

Makisara and Makisara assessed 405 patients with definite or classical RA, measuring functional capacity with the Lee index[192] and assessing ability to work at various levels of physical stress[66]. ESR > 50 mm/h when first measured predicted functional outcome at 5 years but not 10 or 15 years. Radiographic erosions present at first examination predicted functional outcome at 10 and 15 years but not at 5 years. No other laboratory or clinical variables were reported, and no adjustments were made for differences in age and disease duration among patients at the first examination.

No association was found between first values of grip strength, joint count, radiographic erosions and ESR, and subsequent clinical remission for 458 patients with established RA (mean duration of 8 years) followed for 2.5 years, reported by Wolfe and Hawley[191].

Jacoby et al. reported no association between initial ESR and final functional status as measured by the ARA Functional Class for 100 patients followed over 11 years[186]. Functional assessment at 3 years was associated with functional outcome at 11 years (r=0.47).

Nevitt et al. followed 754 RA patients to assess factors related to hospitalization[108]. After adjusting for other variables, poor functional status as measured by the HAQ functional disability index was the most powerful predictor of surgical hospitalization during the follow-up year (odds ratio for 4th quartile HAQ score for any surgery = 6.3, and for total joint surgery = 13.0). For hospitalizations for medical reasons, the ESR odds ratio was 3.1, but the HAQ value did not contribute to the model for medical hospitalizations. Number of swollen or tender joints and other clinical and laboratory values were not significant in the model.

Yelin et al. studied factors relating to work disability in 270 patients with definite or classical rheumatoid arthritis[67]. No associations between erosions or ESR and work disability were noted, but symptoms of RA (number of painful joints) and HAQ functional score were associated with the risk of work loss. The relative risk for cross-sectional HAQ score was 3.28, and for predictive (change in HAQ score) HAQ score was 2.03. The relative risk for painful joints was 1.76.

Similar data were presented by Hansagi et al. who studied hospitalizations over a 13-year period for patients with RA[193]. The proportion of individuals with more than 300 days hospitalization was six times higher for those in ARA Functional Class 3 or 4 and three times higher for those reporting severe joint symptoms at the first assessment than for those not meeting the condition.

Functional impairment as measured by the HAQ disability index was shown to be associated with difficulty in the performance of homemaker tasks and roles for women with RA[69]. In another study from this group, Reisine et al. found confirmatory evidence in working women for the effect of functional loss on work disability[81].

Lubeck et al. determined annual costs and health service utilization for 940 RA patients[109]. HAQ functional disability and pain scores were predictive of these outcome measures over the 1-year follow-up. Clinical and laboratory measures were not studied.

Wolfe et al., studying the risk of hospitalization in a subset of the above group, found a HAQ disability to be strongly associated with hospital admission[101]. Wolfe et al. also studied prospectively 400 patients from their own center over a mean of 3.1 years[57]. ESR, pain, grip strength, and HAQ score predicted total medical cost over the study period. ESR explained 3% of the variance, pain 3.4%, grip strength 6.8%, and HAQ functional disability index 13%. Joint count and other clinical and laboratory values had no explanatory power. In a Cox regression analysis these authors studied the effect of demographic and clinical variables on mortality. Except for age and sex, only HAQ disability predicted mortality (relative risk 1.77).

Mitchell et al. examined the effect of multiple clinical variables on RA mortality for 805 patients followed for a mean of 12 years using the Cox proportional hazards model[88]. Clinical variables associated with mortality were Functional Class (relative risk (RR) 1.49), proteinuria (RR 1.35/⁺560 unit), and active joints (RR 0.12/joint).

Rasker and Cosh studied mortality in 100 RA patients over 18 years.[84] Functional Class at first assessment predicted mortality, but no association was found with Hb, ESR, joint score, or nodules.

Similarly Allenbeck et al. found Functional Class associated with mortality in their 11-year study of 293 RA patients[89]. Other clinical variables were not described.

Pincus et al. studied 75 patients with definite or classical RA over 9 years[85,86]. In Cox proportional hazards models, risk of mortality was associated with measures of functional capacity, but not with joint count, radiographs, grip strength, and morning stiffness.

Studies employing longitudinal data

Using data that represented mean values of four observations during a 1-year period in patients with early RA, Young et al. found that the clinical measures of grip strength, morning stiffness, functional grade, and joint score, and the laboratory measures, platelet count, hemoglobin, and ESR, predicted the development of erosions 3 years after the onset of disease[168]. The best single predictor among these measures was functional grade. In the 400-patient study of Wolfe et al. noted above, changes in the functional disability index score were not associated with increases in costs or utilization[57].

Mottonen studied 58 patients with early onset definite or classical RA every 6 months for 24 months to assess factors associated with radiographic abnormalities[152]. The *mean* values of most clinical and laboratory variables were associated with radiographic progress as measured by the Larsen index[194], and the increase in the number of new joints over the 2-year follow-up. The increase in new joints, for example, was correlated with the following variables: ESR, $r=0.413$; Hb, $r=0.361$; clinically active joints, $r=0.629$; morning stiffness, $r=0.428$; pain, $r=0.341$; grip strength, $r=0.400$. In addition, the more times a joint was noted to be swollen over the follow-up period the more likely it was to develop new erosions.

Treatment

The literature of clinical rheumatology is most devoted to treatment. Yet in spite of its importance and the length of its literature, the effects of treatment on the outcome of RA remain unclear. By the time RA has been present for more than a few years most patients have been treated with a multitude of drugs, and by the end of the disease course have received most first- and second-line therapies, physical and occupational therapies, and often surgical interventions. Such multiple therapies confound the understanding of therapeutic benefit. In addition, confounded or not, there are few studies of RA that extend beyond a year, and none that last 5 years or even begin to approximate the length of the illness. Long-term therapeutic outcome studies lack controls, are confounded by placebo effect, regression to the mean, disease severity, and treatment dropouts. While it is assumed that therapeutic intervention is beneficial, it is possible that this is not the case and that treatment may be harmful. Ineffective therapies are expensive to society and to individual patients at a time when they are ill-equipped to pay. In addition, patients may be physically harmed by both potentially effective and ineffective treatments.

Patient education and self-management programs increase knowledge regarding arthritis and its management, and variably reduce pain, psychological variables, and functional disability[195-198]. The effect is most obvious in pretest–posttest designs[197], and less often found in direct comparison with control patients[198]. Data are short-term. Effect on the long-term outcome of RA remains unknown, but some data from Lorig et al. suggest that benefit can be maintained[196].

There are no long-term data regarding the effect of physical therapy or occupational therapy programs. Short-term data indicate, as with education, variable benefit.

It is generally thought that therapy with nonsteroidal antiinflammatory drugs (NSAIDs) does not influence the course of RA. Yet there are no studies to show that this is the case. Salicylates have been available throughout this century, and few patients have dealt with their illness without them or without NSAIDs. All studies show such agents reduce pain, swelling, and tenderness, and it is quite possible that RA patients would be worse without them. Such drugs, however, may be responsible for considerable GI toxicity. As noted above, both hospitalization rates and mortality may be increased in RA patients because of adverse reactions to such agents.

The term "second-line therapy" has been given to drugs such as oral and injectable gold, penicillamine, hydroxychloroquine, sulfasalazine, methotrexate, azathioprine, and similar agents that are usually used after the "first-line" drugs (e.g., NSAIDs) have been started. Short-term trials have shown these agents to be superior to placebo, but questions about their long-term ability to alter the course of RA have been raised[199,200]. Several separate issues are of importance. First, can the agents retard the progression of RA for more than short periods of time (for example, for a year)? Second, can and will patients remain on the therapy? And third, will such therapy have long-term benefit? The second question is easiest to answer. Published data suggest that, regardless of the agent chosen, most patients discontinue a given second-line therapeutic agent less than 1.5 years after it is begun[201-203]. Data to answer the first question are limited by the generally short-term nature of clinical trials, and by the confounding effect of dropouts. Data concerning the third question are not directly available, but the outcome of the illness as detailed above suggests no reason to believe that therapy has been effective, and much reason to believe that it has failed to alter the course of RA[199,200].

It is almost certain that the most profound influence on RA prognosis has been total joint replacement surgery of the hip and knee. It is common to hear rheumatologists who have been in practice for 20 years state that they do not see as many "Class IV Stage 4" patients as they did previously; and it is likely that that observation derives from the effectiveness of total joint arthroplasty. Amor *et al.* compared patients with duration of disease of 10–15 years followed during two periods, 1966–1978, and 1948–1965[204]. They reported 16% in stage III and 4% in stage IV in the most recent period, half as many as were in those stages in the earlier period. The authors suggested that this reduction was the result of total joint arthroplasty. Synovectomy has not been found to alter RA outcome, and other common surgical interventions including upper extremity arthroplasties — arthroscopic surgery, for example — have not been studied in terms of the outcome considered here. Such studies are essential, both for total joint arthroplasty, and for the other surgical interventions.

The prognosis of rheumatoid arthritis

It is now clear that however the prognosis of rheumatoid arthritis is considered, it is bad. We have been held back in our unraveling of RA prognosis by including early polyarthritis (probable rheumatoid arthritis) in our calculations, and by mixing various seronegative and seropositive polyarthropathies into the RA brew together. In the end we have spent too much time measuring the effect of seropositivity on prognosis when, it seems likely, we have actually been comparing disparate disorders. Whether this is the case or not, much is to be gained by concentrating our attention on chronic polyarthritis. There is substantial evidence that RA that is present for 2 years is rarely remittent and is, indeed, the serious condition in which we are interested. Second, although the issue of whether seronegative and seropositive RA are often different disorders is not settled, we are likely to learn much more about both conditions if we consider them separately, and we will be in a much better position to compare studies from different centers with such a dichotomy.

The prognosis literature of RA has been hampered by the inaccurate use of language, including *prognosis, process, stage, outcome, status, disease activity, severity*, and *disease severity*. *Process measures* are those that reflect the inflammatory component of the arthritis, including ESR, Hb, platelet count, joint tenderness and swelling, morning stiffness, grip strength, pain and dysfunction. *Outcome measures* reflect the result of the ongoing arthritis activity, and include functional and work disability, economic consequence, pain, mortality, adverse reactions to therapy, and structural changes to joints (anatomically or radiographically), among others. Thus, the term "severity" or "severe RA" is confusing unless it is clear whether one is speaking about the "process" (the active disease) or the "outcome" (the result of the disease). Two items, functional disability and pain, fit into both categories. Pain, both physical pain and psychological distress, is essentially a process measure, but when it is assessed longitudinally it has aspects of a cumulative measure (an "area under the curve" measurement) that represents an outcome of the disease. Functional disability may be, likewise, an instantaneous process measure since it is responsive to pain and immediate flares of the disease. But, more importantly, it correlates with future functional measurements, and is almost always reflective of the outcome of the process of the illness. Both process and outcome measures are important in RA, but they represent different concepts.

The time over which the outcome is assessed is important. Studies of RA prognosis have come to conclusions about the outcome of RA on the basis of 3-year data and 20-year data, for example — time frames that do not allow for immediate comparison. We will increase our accuracy and our understanding if we qualify our outcomes with a time statement. Thus, the outcome of rheumatoid arthritis 1 or 2 years after the onset of a second-line drug is a useful construct, just as is the 10- and 20-year outcome.

Outcomes occur over time, and longitudinal studies are infinitely more powerful in their ability to describe outcome than cross-sectional investigations. The richness of the Scandinavian data and other longitudinal investigations cited above attests to this. Our ability to ascertain how much benefit accrues from second-line type therapy will only come with longitudinal, intermediate and long-term studies. Within such efforts, follow-up must be complete, and all patients must be accounted for.

Most prognostic studies followed patients from a starting point to a fixed endpoint or to death. But patients so followed were most often heterogeneous, with marked variation in age and duration of disease, such that reports of 10- or 20-year "outcome" were confounded by the deaths of older patients or the marked differences in severity at the first assessment. With increasing knowledge of these problems it now seems important to follow homogeneous groups, at least as to duration of disease.

Serial process measures are much more powerful predictors of outcome than are initial or random measurements. One of the reasons for our failure to identify "predictors" of RA outcome has been the reliance on a single "initial" measurement in early RA or a single measurement later in the course of the illness. Serial measures, means of a number of values over time, or slopes of values are likely to yield important information regarding RA prognosis.

In spite of the limitations noted above, the weight of evidence suggests that all aspects of rheumatoid arthritis outcome are driven most by sustained disease activity, and that improvement in the prognosis of RA will come when the inflammatory process is controlled. It is likely that such disease activity can be measured clinically by serial standard measurements of joint activity, ESR, etc. But by far the most powerful measure and predictor of future outcome is loss of function, as measured by the HAQ, the MHAQ, the AIMS, or similar instruments. We have suggested elsewhere that the power of functional measures as predictors results from the fact that they represent, at any given moment, the epitome of the various clinical and laboratory assessments and[57], in addition, reflect disability already present as an effect of the longitudinal aspects of the rheumatoid arthritis.

References

1. Ropes, M. W., Bennett, G. A., Cobb, S., Jacox, R. and Jessar, R. A. (1956). Proposed diagnostic criteria for rheumatoid arthritis. *Bull. Rheum. Dis.*, **7**, 121–124
2. Ropes, M. W., Bennett, G. A., Cobb, S., Jacox, R. and Jessar, R. A. (1959). 1958 Revision of diagnostic criteria for rheumatoid arthritis. *Arthritis Rheum.*, **2**, 16–20
3. Arnett, F. C., Edworthy, S. M., Bloch, D. A., McShane, D. J., Fries, J. F., Cooper, N. S., Healy, L. A., Caplan, S. R., Liang, M. H., Luthra, H. S., Medsger, T. A., Jr., Mitchell, D. M., Neustadt, D. H., Pinals, R. S., Schaller, J. G., Sharp, J. T., Wilder, R. L. and Hunder, G. G. (1988). The American Rheumatism Association 1987 revised criteria for the classification of rheumatoid arthritis. *Arthritis Rheum.*, **31**, 315–324
4. Bennett, P. H. and Burch, T. A. (1967). New York symposium on population studies in the rheumatic diseases: new diagnostic criteria. *Bull. Rheum. Dis.*, **17**, 453–458

5. Kellgren, J. H., Jeffrey, M. R. and Ball, J. (1963). Proposed diagnostic studies for use in population studies. In *The Epidemiology of Chronic Rheumatism*, p. 324. (Oxford: Blackwell Scientific Publications)
6. Cathcart, E. S. and O'Sullivan, J. B. (1976). Rheumatoid arthritis in a New England town: A prevalence study in Sudbury, Massachusetts. *N. Engl. J. Med.*, **282**, 421-424
7. O'Sullivan, J. B. and Cathcart, E. S. (1972). Follow-up evaluation of the effect of criteria on rates in Sudbury, Massachusetts. *Ann. Intern. Med.*, **76**, 573-577
8. Beall, G. and Cobb, S. (1961). The frequency distribution of episodes of rheumatoid arthritis as shown by periodic examination. *J. Chronic Dis.*, **14**, 291-310
9. Harris, E. D. Jr. (1985). Rheumatoid arthritis: The clinical syndrome. In Kelley, W. N., Harris, E. D. Jr., Ruddy, S. and Sledge, C. B. (eds.) *Textbook of Rheumatology*, 2nd edn., pp. 915-950. (Philadelphia: W. B. Saunders)
10. Medsger, T. A., Jr. and Masi, A. T. (1985). Epidemiology of the rheumatic diseases. In McCarty, D. J. (ed.) *Arthritis and Allied Conditions*, 10th edn, pp. 9-39. (Philadelphia: Lea & Febiger)
11. Healey, L. A. (1973). The prognosis in rheumatoid arthritis. *Med. Times*, **101**, 31-32
12. Nissila, M., Isomaki, H., Kaarela, K., Kiviniemi, P., Martio, J. and Sarna, S. (1983). Prognosis of inflammatory joint diseases. A three-year follow-up study. *Scand. J. Rheumatol.*, **12**, 33-38
13. Isomäki, H. (1987). An epidemiologically based follow-up study of recent arthritis. Incidence, outcome and classification. *Clin. Rheumatol.* **6**(suppl.), 53-59
14. Brewerton, D. A. and James, D. C. O. (1975). The histocompatibility antigen (HL-A 27) and disease. *Semin. Arthritis Rheum.*, **4**, 191-207
15. Schattenkirchner, M. and Kruger, K. (1987). Natural course and prognosis of HLA-B27-positive oligoarthritis. *Clin. Rheumatol.*, **6**, 83-86
16. Gran, J. T. and Husby, G. (1987). Seronegative rheumatoid arthritis and HLA-DR4: Proposal for criteria. *J. Rheumatol.*, **14**, 1079-1082
17. Calin, A. and Marks, S. H. (1981). The cases against seronegative rheumatoid arthritis. *Am. J. Med.*, **70**, 992-994
18. Husby, G. and Gran, J. J. (1988). What is seronegative rheumatoid arthritis? *Scand. J. Rheumatol.*, **17**(suppl. 75), 269-271
19. Masi, A. T., Maldonado-Cocco, J. A., Kaplan, S. B., Feigenbaum, S. L. and Chandler, R. W. (1976). Prospective study of the early course of rheumatoid arthritis in young adults: Comparison of patients with and without rheumatoid factor positivity at entry and identification of variables correlating with outcome. *Semin. Arthritis Rheum.*, **4**, 299-326
20. Pincus, T. (1988). Rheumatoid arthritis: disappointing long-term outcomes despite successful short-term clinical trials. *J. Clin. Epidemiol.*, **41**, 1037-1041
21. Wicks, I. P., Moore, J. and Fleming, A. (1988). Australian mortality statistics for rheumatoid arthritis 1950-81: analysis of death certificate data. *Ann. Rheum. Dis.*, **47**, 563-569
22. Decker, J. L. (1983). American rheumatism association nomenclature and classification of arthritis and rheumatism. *Arthritis Rheum.*, **26**, 1029-1032
23. Allen, J. C. and Kunkel, H. G. (1966). Hidden rheumatoid factors with specificity for native gamma globulin. *Arthritis Rheum.*, **9**, 758-768
24. Moore, T. L., Dorner, R. W., Osborn, T. G. and Zuckner, J. (1988). Hidden 19S IgM rheumatoid factors. *Semin. Arthritis Rheum.*, **18**, 72-75
25. Teitsson, I., Withrington, R. H., Seifert, M. H. and Valdimarsson, H. (1984). Prospective study of early rheumatoid arthritis. I. Prognostic value of IgA rheumatoid factor. *Ann. Rheum. Dis.*, **43**, 673-678
26. Tuomi, T., Aho, K., Palosuo, T., Kaarela, K., von Essen, R., Isomaki, H., Leirisalo Repo, M. and Sarna, S. (1988). Significance of rheumatoid factors in an eight-year longitudinal study on arthritis. *Rheumatol. Int.*, **8**, 21-26
27. Pincus, T. and Callahan, L. F. (1985). Formal education as a marker for increased mortality and morbidity in rheumatoid arthritis. *J. Chronic Dis.*, **38**, 973-984
28. Callahan, L. F. and Pincus, T. (1988). Formal education level as a significant marker of clinical status in rheumatoid arthritis. *Arthritis Rheum.*, **31**, 1346-1357
29. Pincus, T. (1988). Formal educational level — A marker for the importance of

behavioral variables in the pathogenesis, morbidity, and mortality of most diseases. *J. Rheumatol.*, **15**, 1457-1459
30. Syme, S. L. and Berkman, L. F. (1976). Social class, susceptibility and sickness. *J. Epidemiol.*, **104**, 1-8
31. Goodwin, J. S., Hunt, W. C., Key, C. R. and Samet, J. M. (1987). The effect of marital status on stage, treatment, and survival of cancer patients. *J. Am. Med. Assoc.*, **258**, 3125-3130
32. Woolhandler, S., Himmelstein, D. U., Silber, R., Bader, M., Hamly, M. and Jones, A. A. (1985). Medical care and mortality: racial differences in preventable deaths. *Int. J. Health Serv.*, **15**, 1-22
33. Rose, G. and Marmot, M. G. (1981). Social class and coronary heart disease. *Br. Heart J.*, **45**, 13-19
34. Maarmot, M. G., Shipley, M. J. and Rose, G. (1984). Inequalities in death-specific explanations of a general pattern? *Lancet*, **1**, 1003-1006
35. Kitagawa, E. and Hauser, P. (1973). *Differential Mortality in the U.S.* (Cambridge, Mass.: Harvard University Press)
36. Zambrana, R. E. (1987). A research agenda on issues affecting poor and minority women: a model for understanding their health needs. *Women Health*, **12**, 137-160
37. Cohen, S. and Wills, T. A. (1985). Stress, social support, and the buffering hypothesis. *Psychol. Bull.*, **98**, 310-357
38. Verbrugge, L. M. (1985). Gender and health: an update on hypotheses and evidence. *J. Health Soc. Behav.*, **26**, 156-182
39. Felton, B. J. and Revenson, T. A. (1984). Coping with chronic illness: a study of illness controllability and the influence of coping strategies on psychological adjustment. *J. Consult. Clin. Psychol.*, **52**, 343-353
40. Holmes, D., Teresi, J. and Holmes, M. (1983). Differences among black, Hispanic, and white people in knowledge about long-term care services. *Health Care Fin. Rev.*, **5**, 51
41. Orth-Gomér, K., Undén, A.-L. and Edwards, M.-E. (1988). Social isolation and mortality in ischemic heart disease. A 10-year follow-up study of 150 middle-aged men. *Acta Med. Scand.*, **224**, 205-215
42. Blaxter, M. (1987). Health and social class: evidence of inequality in health from national survey. *Lancet*, **2**, 30-33
43. Earle, J. R., Perricone, P. J., Maultsby, D. M., Perricone, N., Turner, R. A. and Davis, J. (1979). Psycho-social adjustment of rheumatoid arthritis patients from two alternative treatment settings. *J. Rheumatol.*, **6**, 80-70
44. Rogers, M. P., Liang, M. H. and Partridge, A. J. (1982). Psychological care of adults with rheumatoid arthritis. *Ann. Intern. Med.*, **96**, 344-348
45. Medsger, A. R. and Robinson, H. (1972). A comparative study of divorce in rheumatoid arthritis and other rheumatic diseases. *J. Chronic Dis.*, **25**, 269-275
46. Cornelissen, P. G., Rasker, J. J. and Valkenburg, H. A. (1988). The arthritis sufferer and the community: a comparison of arthritis sufferers in rural and urban areas. *Ann. Rheum. Dis.*, **47**, 150-156
47. Burchkardt, C. S. (1985). The impact of arthritis on quality of life. *Nurs. Res.*, **34**, 11-16
48. Lubeck, D. P. and Yelin, E. H. (1988). A question of value: measuring the impact of chronic disease. *Milbank Q.*, **66**, 444-464
49. Blalock, S. J., McEvoy de Vellis, B., de Vellis, R. F. and Van H. Sauter, S. (1988). Self-evaluation processes and adjustment to rheumatoid arthritis. *Arthritis Rheum.*, **31**, 1245-1251
50. Parker, J., McRae, C., Smarr, K., Beck, N., Frank, R., Anderson, S. and Walker, S. (1988). Coping strategies in rheumatoid arthritis. *J. Rheumatol.*, **15**, 1376-1383
51. Mitchell, J. M., Burkhauser, R. V. and Pincus, T. (1988). The importance of age, education, and comorbidity in the substantial earnings losses of individuals with symmetric polyarthritis. *Arthritis Rheum.*, **31**, 348-357
52. Meenan, R. F., Yelin, E. H., Nevitt, M. and Epstein, W. V. (1981). The impact of chronic disease: a sociomedical profile of rheumatoid arthritis. *Arthritis Rheum.*, **24**, 544-549

53. Nicassio, P. M., Wallston, K. A., Callahan, L. F., Herbert, M. and Pincus, T. (1985). The measurement of helplessness in rheumatoid arthritis. The development of the arthritis helplessness index. *J. Rheumatol.*, **12**, 462-467
54. Hawley, D. J. and Wolfe, F. (1988). Anxiety and depression in patients with RA: A prospective study of 400 patients. *J. Rheumatol.*, **15**, 932-941
55. Svensson, C. K. (1989). Representation of American blacks in clinical trials of new drugs. *J. Am. Med. Assoc.*, **261**, 263-265
56. Wolfe, F., Kleinheksel, S. M., Spitz, P. W., Lubeck, D. P., Fries, J. F., Young, D. Y., Mitchell, D. and Roth, S. (1986). A multicenter study of hospitalization in rheumatoid arthritis. *Arthritis Rheum.*, **29**, 614-619
57. Wolfe, F., Kleinheksel, S. M., Cathey, M. A., Hawley, D. J., Spitz, P. W. and Fries, J. F. (1988). The clinical value of the Stanford Health Assessment Questionnaire Functional Disability Index in patients with rheumatoid arthritis. *J. Rheumatol.*, **15**, 1480-1488
58. Thompson, H. E., Wyatt, B. L. and Hicks, R. A. (1938). Chronic atrophic arthritis. *Ann. Intern. Med.*, **11**, 1792-1805
59. Lewis-Fanning, E. and Fletcher, E. (1945). A statistical study of 1,000 cases of chronic rheumatism. Part III. *Postgrad. Med.*, **21**, 137-147
60. Fletcher, E. and Lewis-Fanning, E. (1945). Chronic rheumatic diseases. Part IV. A statistical study of 1,000 cases of chronic rheumatism. *Postgrad. Med.*, **21**, 176
61. Short, C. L., Bauer, W. and Reynolds, W. E. (1957). *Rheumatoid Arthritis*. (Cambridge, Mass.: Harvard University Press)
62. Short, C. L. (1968). Rheumatoid arthritis: types of course and prognosis. *Med. Clin. N. Am.*, **52**, 549-557
63. Ragan, C. and Farrington, E. (1962). The clinical features of rheumatoid arthritis: prognostic indices. *J. Am. Med. Assoc.*, **181**, 663-667
64. Steinbrocker, O., Traeger, C. H. and Batterman, R. C. (1949). Therapeutic criteria in rheumatoid arthritis. *J. Am. Med. Assoc.*, **140**, 659-662
65. Steinbrocker, O. (1969). Prognosis for employability in the major arthritides rheumatoid arthritis, osteoarthritis and gout. *Pa. Med.*, **72**, 82-85
66. Makisara, G. L. and Makisara, P. (1982). Prognosis of functional capacity and work capacity in rheumatoid arthritis. *Clin. Rheumatol.*, **1**, 117-125
67. Yelin, E., Henke, C. and Epstein, W. (1987). The work dynamics of the person with rheumatoid arthritis. *Arthritis Rheum.*, **30**, 507-512
68. Fries, J. F., Spitz, P. W. and Kraines, R. G. (1980). Measurement of patient outcome in arthritis. *Arthritis Rheum.*, **23**, 137-45
69. Reisine, S. T., Goodenow, C. and Grady, K. E. (1987). The impact of rheumatoid arthritis on the homemaker. *Soc. Sci. Med.*, **25**, 89-95
70. Rasker, J. J. and Cosh, J. A. (1987). The natural history of rheumatoid arthritis over 20 years. Clinical symptoms, radiological signs, treatment, mortality and prognostic significance of early features. *Clin. Rheumatol.*, **6**, 5-11
71. Scott, D. L., Symmons, D. P., Coulton, B. L. and Popert, A. J. (1987). Long-term outcome of treating rheumatoid arthritis: results after 20 years. *Lancet*, **1**, 1108-1111
72. Sherrer, Y. S., Bloch, D. A., Mitchell, D. M., Young, D. Y. and Fries, J. F. (1986). The development of disability in rheumatoid arthritis. *Arthritis Rheum.*, **29**, 494-500
73. Bombardier, C., Ware, J., Russell, I. J., Larson, M., Chalmers, A. and Read, J. L. (1986). Auranofin therapy and quality of life in patients with rheumatoid arthritis. Results of a multicenter trial. *Am. J. Med.*, **81**, 565-578
74. Meenan, R. F., Anderson, J. J., Kazis, L. E., Egger, M. J., Altz-Smith, M., Samuelson, C. O., Wilkens, R. F., Solsky, M. A., Hayes, S. P., Blocka, K. L., Weinstein, A., Guttadauria, M., Kaplan, S. B. and Klippel, J. (1984). Outcome assessment in clinical trials. *Arthritis Rheum.*, **27**, 1344-1352
75. Pincus, T., Summey, J. A., Soraci Jr., S. A., Wallston, K. A. and Hummon, N. P. (1983). Assessment of patient satisfaction in activities of daily living using a modified Stanford Health Assessment Questionnaire. *Arthritis Rheum.*, **26**, 1346-1353
76. Pincus, T., Callahan, L. F., Brooks, R. H., Fuchs, H. A., Olsen, N. J. and Kaye, J. J. (1989). Self-report questionnaire scores in rheumatoid arthritis compared with

traditional physical, radiographic, and laboratory measures. *Ann. Intern. Med.*, **110**, 259–266
77. Meenan, R. F., Gertman, P. M. and Mason, J. H. (1980). Measuring health status in arthritis: the arthritis impact measurement scales. *Arthritis Rheum.*, **23**, 146–152
78. Meenan, R. F., Gertman, P. M., Mason, J. H. and Dunaif, R. (1982). The arthritis impact measurement scales. *Arthritis Rheum.*, **25**, 1048–1053
79. Wolfe, F., Hawley, D. J. and Cathey, M. A. (1989). The risk of functional disability and the rate of its development in patients with rheumatoid arthritis. *Arthritis Rheum.*, **32**, S88 (Abstract)
80. Mitchell, D. M., Spitz, P. W., Young, D. Y., Block, D. A., McShane, D. J. and Fries, J. F. (1986). Survival, prognosis and causes of death in rheumatoid arthritis. *Arthritis Rheum.*, **29**, 706–714
81. Reisine, S. T., Grady, K. E., Goodenow, C. and Fifield, J. (1989). Work disability among women with rheumatoid arthritis: The relative importance of disease, social, work, and family factors. *Arthritis Rheum.*, **32**, 538–543
82. Meenan, R. F., Kazis, L. E. and Anderson, J. J. (1988). The stability of health status in rheumatoid arthritis: A five year study of patients with established disease. *AJPH*, **78**, 1484–1487
83. Pincus, T. (1988). Is mortality increased in rheumatoid arthritis? *J. Musculo. Med.*, **5**, 27–46
84. Rasker, J. J. and Cosh, J. A. (1981). Cause and age of death in a prospective study of 100 patients with rheumatoid arthritis. *Ann. Rheum. Dis.*, **40**, 115–120
85. Pincus, T., Callahan, L. F. and Vaughn, W., K. (1987). Questionnaire, walking time and button test measures of functional capacity as predictive markers for mortality in rheumatoid arthritis. *J. Rheumatol.*, **14**, 240–251
86. Pincus, T., Callahan, L. F., Sale, W. G., Brooks, A. L., Payne, L. E. and Vaughn, W. K. (1984). Severe functional declines, work disability, and increased mortality in seventy-five rheumatoid arthritis patients studied over nine years. *Arthritis Rheum.*, **27**, 864–872
87. Uddin, J., Kraus, A. S. and Kelly, H. G. (1970). Survivorship and death in rheumatoid arthritis. *Arthritis Rheum.*, **13**, 125–129
88. Mitchell, D. M., Spitz, P. W., Young, D. Y., Bloch, D. A., McShane, D. J. and Fries, J. F. (1986). Survival, prognosis, and causes of death in rheumatoid arthritis. *Arthritis Rheum.*, **29**, 706–714
89. Allebeck, P., Ahlbom, A. and Allander, E. (1981). Increased mortality among persons with rheumatoid arthritis, but where RA does not appear on death certificate: Eleven year follow-up of an epidemiological study. *Scand. J. Rheumatol.*, **10**, 301–306
90. Moesmann, G. (1969). Malignancy and mortality in subacute rheumatoid arthritis in old age. *Acta Rheum. Scand.*, **15**, 193–199
91. Prior, P., Symmons, D. P. M., Scott, D. L., Brown, R. and Hawkins, C. F. (1984). Cause of death in rheumatoid arthritis. *Br. J. Rheumatol.*, **23**, 92–99
92. Monson, R. R. and Hall, A. P. (1976). Mortality among arthritics. *J. Chronic Dis.*, **29**, 459–467
93. Koota, K., Isomaki, H. and Metru, O. (1977). Death rate and causes of death in RA patients during a period of five years. *Scand. J. Rheumatol.*, **6**, 241–244
94. Symmons, D. P. M., Prior, P., Scott, D. L., Brown, R. and Hawkins, C. F. (1986). Factors influencing mortality in rheumatoid arthritis. *J. Chronic Dis.*, **39**, 137–145
95. Linos, A., Worthington, J. W., O'Fallon, W. M. and Kurland, L. T. (1980). The epidemiology of rheumatoid arthritis in Rochester, Minnesota: A study of incidence, prevalence, and mortality. *Am. J. Epidemiol.*, **111**, 87–98
96. Larkku, L., Mutru, O., Isomaki, H. and Koota, K. (1986). Cancer mortality in patients with rheumatoid arthritis. *J. Rheumatol.*, **13**, 522–526
97. Gordan, D. A., Stein, J. L. and Broder, I. (1973). The extra-articular features of rheumatoid arthritis. A systematic analysis of 127 cases. *Am. J. Med.*, **54**, 445–452
98. Symmons, D. P. M. (1988). Neoplasia in rheumatoid arthritis. *J. Rheumatol.*, **15**, 1319–1321
99. McDuffie, F. C. (1985). Morbidity impact of rheumatoid arthritis on society. *Am. J. Med.*, **78**, 1–5

100. Lubeck, D. P., Spitz, P. W., Fries, J. F., Wolfe, F., Mitchell, D. M. and Roth, S. H. (1986). A multicenter study of annual health service utilization and costs in rheumatoid arthritis. *Arthritis Rheum.*, **29**, 488–493
101. Wolfe, F., Kleinheksel, S. M., Spitz, P. W., Lubeck, D. P., Fries, J. F., Young, D. Y., Mitchell, D. M. and Roth, S. H. (1986). A multicenter study of hospitalization in rheumatoid arthritis: effect of health care system, severity, and regional difference. *J. Rheumatol.*, **13**, 277–284
102. Liang, M. H., Larson, M., Thompson, M., Eaton, H., McNamara, E., Katz, R. and Taylor, J. (1984). Costs and outcomes in rheumatoid arthritis and osteoarthritis *Arthritis Rheum.*, **27**, 522–529
103. Jacobs, J., Keyserling, J. A., Britton, M., Morgan, G. J. Jr., Wilkenfeld, J. and Hutchings, H. C. (1988). The total cost of care and the use of pharmaceuticals in the management of rheumatoid arthritis: the Medi-Cal program. *J. Clin. Epidemiol.*, **41**, 215–223
104. Thompson, M. S., Read, J. L., Hutchings, H. C., Paterson, M. and Harris, E. D., Jr. (1988). The cost effectiveness of auranofin: results of a randomized clinical trial. *J. Rheumatol.*, **15**, 35–42
105. Meenan, R. F., Yelin, E. H., Henke, C. J., Curtis, D. L. and Epstein, W. V. (1978). The costs of rheumatoid arthritis. A patient-oriented study of chronic disease costs. *Arthritis Rheum.*, **21**, 827–833
106. Yelin, E. H., Feshbach, D. M., Meenan, R. F. and Epstein, W. V. (1979). Social problems, services and policy for persons with chronic disease: the case of rheumatoid arthritis. *Soc. Sci. Med. (Med. Econ.)*, **13**, 13–20
107. Stone, C. E. (1984). The lifetime economic costs of rheumatoid arthritis. *J. Rheumatol.*, **11**, 819–827
108. Nevitt, M. C., Yelin, E. H., Henke, C. J. and Epstein, W. V. (1986). Risk factors for hospitalization and surgery in patients with rheumatoid arthritis: implications for capitated medical payment. *Ann. Intern. Med.*, **105**, 421–428
109. Lubeck, D. P., Spitz, P. W., Fries, J. F., Wolfe, F., Mitchell, D. M. and Roth, S. H. (1986). A multicenter study of annual health service utilization and costs in rheumatoid arthritis. *Arthritis Rheum.*, **29**, 448–493
110. Wolfe, F., Hawley, D. J. and Cathey, M. A. (1989). Health status measures over time: serial assessments in 442 RA patients. *Arthritis Rheum.*, **82**, S64 (Abstract)
111. Pinals, R. S., Baum, J., Bland, J., Fosdick, W. M., Kaplan, S. B., Masi, A. T., Mitchell, D. M., Ropes, M. W., Short, C. L., Sigler, J. W. and Weinberger, J. J. (1981). Preliminary criteria for clinical remission in rheumatoid arthritis. *Arthritis Rheum.*, **24**, 1308–1315
112. Melzack, R. (1975). The McGill pain questionnaire. *Pain*, **1**, 277–299
113. Anderson, K. O., Bradley, L. A., McDaniel, L. K., Young, L. D., Turner, R. A., Agudelo, C. A., Gaby, N. S., Keefe, F. J., Pisko, E. J., Synder, R. M. *et al.* (1987). The assessment of pain in rheumatoid arthritis: disease differentiation and temporal stability of a behavioral observation method. *J. Rheumatol.*, **14**, 700–704
114. Badley, E. M. and Papageorgiou, A. C. (1989). Visual analogue scales as a measure of pain in arthritis: A study of overall pain and pain in individual joints at rest and on movement. *J. Rheumatol.*, **16**, 102–105
115. Kazis, L. E., Meenan, R. F. and Anderson, J. J. (1983). Pain in the rheumatic diseases: investigation of a key health status component. *Arthritis Rheum.*, **26**, 1017–1022
116. Burckhardt, C. S. (1984). The use of the McGill Pain Questionnaire in assessing arthritis pain. *Pain*, **19**, 305–314
117. Bushnell, W. J. (1986). The pain of rheumatoid arthritis. *Am. J. Med.*, **80**, 88–88
118. Callahan, L. F., Brooks, R. H., Summey, J. A. and Pincus, T. (1987). Quantitative pain assessment for routine care of rheumatoid arthritis patients, using a pain scale based on activities of daily living and a visual analog pain scale. *Arthritis Rheum.*, **30**, 630–636
119. Gracely, R. H., McGrath, P. and Dubner, R. (1978). Ratio scales of sensory and affective verbal pain descriptors. *Pain*, **5**, 5–18
120. Merskey, H. and International Association for the Study of Pain (1986). Classifica-

tion of chronic pain: Descriptions of chronic pain syndromes and definitions of pain terms. *Pain*, S1–S226
121. Parker, J., Frank, R., Beck, N., Finan, M., Walker, S., Hewett, J. E., Broster, C., Smarr, K., Smith, E. and Kay, D. (1988). Pain in rheumatoid arthritis: relationship to demographic, medical, and psychological factors. *J. Rheumatol.*, **15**, 433–437
122. Duncan, G. H., Bushnell, M. C. and Lavigne, G. J. (1989). Comparison of verbal and visual analogue scales for measuring the intensity and unpleasantness of experimental pain. *Pain*, **37**, 295–303
123. Huskisson, E. C., Jones, J. and Scott, P. J. (1976). Application of visual-analogue scales to the measurement of functional capacity. *Rheumatol. Rehabil.*, **15**, 185–187
124. Huskisson, E. C. (1974). Measurement of pain. *Lancet*, **2**, 1127–1131
125. Huskisson, E. C. (1975). Measurement of pain. *Lancet*, **2**, 1127–1131
126. Mason, J. H., Weener, J. L., Gertman, P. M. and Meenan, R. F. (1983). Health status in chronic disease: a comparative study of rheumatoid arthritis. *J. Rheumatol.*, **10**, 763–768
127. Wolfe, F. (1989). A brief health status instrument: CLINHAQ. *Arthritis Rheum.*, **32**, S99 (Abstract)
128. Baum, J. (1982). A review of the psychological aspects of rheumatic diseases. *Semin. Arthritis Rheum.*, **11**, 352–361
129. Anderson, K. O., Bradley, L. A., Young, L. D., McDaniel, L. K. and Wise, C. M. (1985). Rheumatoid arthritis: review of psychological factors related to etiology, effects, and treatment. *Psychol. Bull.*, **98**, 358–387
130. Bradley, L. A. (1985). Psychological aspects of arthritis. *Bull. Rheum. Dis.*, **35**, 1–12
131. McFarlane, A. C. and Brooks, P. M. (1988). An analysis of the relationship between psychological morbidity and disease activity in RA. *J. Rheumatol.*, **15**, 926–931
132. Langman, M. J. S. (1989). Epidemiologic evidence on the association between peptic ulceration and antiinflammatory drug use. *Gastroenterology*, **96**, 640–646
133. Bloom, B. S. (1989). Risk and cost of gastrointestinal side effects associated with nonsteroidal anti-inflammatory drugs. *Arch. Intern. Med.*, **149**, 1019–1022
134. Carson, J. L., Strom, B. L., Soper, K. A., West, S. L. and Morse, M. L. (1987). The association of nonsteroidal anti-inflammatory drugs with upper gastrointestinal tract bleeding. *Arch. Intern. Med.*, **147**, 85–88
135. Manniche, C., Malchow-Moller, A., Anderson, J. R., Pederrsen, C., Hansen, T. M., Jess, P., Helleberg, L., Rasmussen, S. N., Tage-Jensen, U. and Nielsen, S. E. (1987). Randomised study of the influence of non-steroidal anti-inflammatory drugs on the treatment of peptic ulcer in patients with rheumatic disease. *Gut*, **28**, 226–229
136. Bartle, W. R., Gupta, A. K. and Lazor, J. (1986). Nonsteroidal anti-inflammatory drugs and gastrointestinal bleeding. *Arch. Intern. Med.*, **146**, 2365–2367
137. Roth, S. H. (1986). Nonsteroidal anti-inflammatory drug gastropathy. We started it — Can we stop it? (editorial). *Arch. Intern. Med.*, **146**, 1075–1076
138. Skander, M. P. and Ryan, F. P. (1988). Non-steroidal anti-inflammatory drugs and pain free peptic ulceration in the elderly. *Br. Med. J.*, **297**, 833–834
139. Fries, J. F., Miller, S. R., Spitz, P. W., Williams, C. A., Hubert, H. B. and Bloch, D. A. (1989). Toward an epidemiology of gastropathy associated with nonsteroidal antiinflammatory drug use. *Gastroenterology*, **96**, 647–655
140. O'Brien, W. M. and Bagby, G. F. (1985). Rare adverse reactions to nonsteroidal antiinflammatory drugs. *J. Rheumatol.*, **12**, 13–20
141. O'Brien, W. M. and Bagby, G. F. (1985). Rare adverse reactions to nonsteroidal antiinflammatory drugs. *J. Rheumatol.*, **12**, 347–353
142. O'Brien, W. M. (1986). Adverse reactions to nonsteroidal anti-inflammatory drugs: diclofenac compared with other nonsteroidal anti-inflammatory drugs. *Am. J. Med.*, **80**(suppl. 46), 70–80
143. Goodwin, J. S. and Regan, M. (1982). Cognitive dysfunction associated with naproxen and ibuprofen in the elderly. *Arthritis Rheum.*, **25**, 1013–1015
144. Fries, J. F., Spitz, P. W., Bloch, D. A., Singh, G. and Hubert, H. B. (1990). A toxicity index for comparing side effects among different drugs. *Arthritis Rheum.*, **33**, 121–130
145. Sharp, J. T. (1989). Radiologic assessment as an outcome measure in rheumatoid arthritis. *Arthritis Rheum.*, **32**, 221–229

146. Regan-Smith, M. G., O'Connor, G. T., Kwoh, C. K., Brown, L. A., Olmstead, E. M. and Burnett, J. B. (1989). Lack of correlation between the Steinbrocker staging of hand radiographs and the functional health status of individuals with rheumatoid arthritis. *Arthritis Rheum.*, **32**, 128-133
147. Scott, D. L. and Bacon, P. A. (1985). Joint damage in rheumatoid arthritis: radiological assessments and the effects of anti-rheumatic drugs. *Rheumatol. Int.*, **5**, 193-199
148. Trentham, D. E. and Masi, A. T. (1976). Carpal:metacarpal ratio: A new quantitative measure of radiologic progression of wrist involvement in rheumatoid arthritis. *Arthritis Rheum.*, **19**, 939-944
149. Weisman, M. H. (1987). Use of radiographs to measure outcome in rheumatoid arthritis. *Am. J. Med.*, **83**, 96-100
150. Fuchs, H. A., Kaye, J. J., Callahan, L. F., Nance, E. P. and Pincus, T. (1989). Evidence of significant radiographic damage in rheumatoid arthritis within the first 2 years of disease. *J. Rheumatol.*, **16**, 585-591
151. Sharp, J. T. (1983). Radiographic evaluation of the course of articular disease. *Clin. Rheum. Dis.*, **9**, 541-557
152. Mottonen, T. T. (1988). Prediction of erosiveness and rate of development of new erosins in early rheumatoid arthritis. *Ann. Rheum. Dis.*, **47**, 648-653
153. Isomäki, H., Kaarela, K. and Martio, J. (1988). Are hand radiographs the most suitable for the diagnosis of rheumatoid arthritis. *Arthritis Rheum.*, **31**, 1452-1453
154. Brook, A. and Corbett, M. (1977). Radiographic changes in early rheumatoid disease. *Ann. Rheum. Dis.*, **36**, 71-73
155. Scott, D. L., Grindulis, K. A., Struthers, G. R., Coulton, B. L., Popert, A. G. and Bacon, P. A. (1984). Progression of radiographical changes in rheumatoid arthritis. *Ann. Rheum. Dis.*, **43**, 8-17
156. Scott, D. L., Coulton, B. L., Bacon, P. A. and Popert, A. J. (1958). Methods of X-ray assessment in rheumatoid arthritis: a re-evaluation. *Br. J. Rheumatol.*, **24**, 31-39
157. Scott, D. L., Coulton, B. L. and Popert, A. J. (1986). Long term progression of joint damage in rheumatoid arthritis. *Ann. Rheum. Dis.*, **45**, 373-378
158. Dawes, P. T., Fowler, P. D., Jackson, R., Collins, M., Shadforth, M. F., Stone, R. and Scott, D. L. (1986). Prediction of progressive joint damage in patients with rheumatoid arthritis receiving gold or D-penicillamine therapy. *Ann. Rheum. Dis.*, **45**, 945-949
159. Fries, J. F., Spitz, P. W. and Young, D. Y. (1982). The dimensions of health outcomes: the health assessment questionnaire, disability and pain scales. *J. Rheumatol.*, **9**, 789-793
160. Wolfe, F. (1989). Age of death of parents of patients with rheumatoid arthritis: data from a middle class sample. *J. Rheumatol.*, **16**, 735-739
161. Wenniker, M. B. and Epstein, A. M. (1989). Racial inequalities in the use of procedures for patients with ischemic heart disease in Massachusetts. *J. Am. Med. Assoc.*, **261**, 253-257
162. Yelin, E. H., Henke, C. J., Kramer, J. S., Nevitt, M. C., Shearn, M. and Epstein, W. V. (1985). A comparison of the treatment of rheumatoid arthritis in health maintenance organizations and fee-for-service practices. *N. Engl. J. Med.*, **312**, 962-967
163. Hurd, M. D. (1989). The economic status of the elderly. *Science*, **244**, 659-664
164. Liang, M. H., Partridge, A. J., Larson, M. G., Gall, V., Taylor, J., Berkman, C., Master, R. and Feltin, M. (1984). Evaluation of comprehensive rehabilitation services for elderly homebound patients with arthritis and orthopedic disability. *Arthritis Rheum.*, **27**, 258-266
165. Shearn, M. A. and Fireman, B. H. (1985). Stress management and mutual support groups in rheumatoid arthritis. *Am. J. Med.*, **78**, 771-775
166. Yelin, E., Meenan, R., Nevitt, M. and Epstein, W. (1980). Work disability in rheumatoid arthritis: effects of disease, social, and work factors. *Ann. Intern. Med.*, **93**, 551-556
167. McDermott, M. and McDevitt, H. O. (1988). The immunogenetics of rheumatic diseases. *Bull. Rheum. Dis.*, **38**, 1-10

168. Young, A., Corbett, M., Winfield, J., Jaqueremada, D., Williams, P., Papasavvas, G., Hay, F. and Roitt, I. (1988). A prognostic index for erosive changes in the hands, feet, and cervical spines in early rheumatoid arthritis. *Br. J. Rheumatol.*, **27**, 94-101
169. Silman, A. J., Reeback, J. and Jaraquemada, D. (1986). HLA-DR4 as a predictor of outcome three years after onset of rheumatoid arthritis. *Rheumatol. Int.*, **6**, 233-235
170. Gran. J. T., Husby, G. and Thorsby, E. (1983). The association between rheumatoid arthritis and the HLA antigen DR4. *Ann. Rheum. Dis.*, **42**, 292-296
171. (1986). HLA-DR antigens in rheumatoid arthritis. A Swiss collaborative study; final report. Swiss Federal Commission for the Rheumatic Diseases, Subcommission for Research. *Rheumatol. Int.*, **6**, 89-92
172. Quieros, M. V., Sanch, M. R. H. and Caetano, J. M. (1982). HLA Antigens and rheumatoid arthritis. *J. Rheumatol.*, **9**, 370-373
173. Walker, D. J., Griffeths, M., Dewer, P., Coates, E., Dick, W. C., Thompson, M. and Griffiths, I. D. (1985). Association of MHC antigens with susceptibility to and severity of rheumatoid arthritis in multicase families. *Ann. Rheum. Dis.*, **44**, 519-525
174. Brackertz, D. and Wernet, P. (1981). A hereditary basis for rheumatoid arthritis. HLA-D/DR-alloantigens and disease severity: Population and family studies. In Paulus, H. E., Erlich, G. E. and Linnenlaub, E. (eds.), *Controversies in the Clinical Evaluation of Analgesic-Antiinflammatory-Antirheumatic Drugs*, pp. 453-462. (Stuggart: Schatteur)
175. Wolfe, F., Kleinheksel, S. M. and Khan, M. A. (1988). Familial vs sporadic rheumatoid arthritis: a comparison of the demographic and clinical characteristics of 956 patients. *J. Rheumatol.*, **15**, 400-404
176. Khan, M. A., Wolfe, F., Kleinheksel, S. M. and Molta, C. (1987). HLA DR4 and B27 antigens in familial and sporadic rheumatoid arthritis. *Scand. J. Rheumatol.*, **16**, 433-436
177. Sanders, P. A., Grennan, D. M., Dyer, P. A., Thomson, W. and deLange, G. G. (1987). A comparison of clinical and immunogenetic features in familial and sporadic rheumatoid arthritis. *J. Rheumatol.*, **14**, 718-722
178. Silman, A., Davies, P., Currey, H. L. and Evans, S. J. (1983). Is rheumatoid arthritis becoming less severe? *J. Chronic Dis.*, **36**, 891-897
179. Isomaki, H., Martio, J., Sarna, S., Kiviniemi, P., Akimova, T., Ievleva, L., Mylov, N. and Trofimova, T. (1984). Predicting the outcome of rheumatoid arthritis. A Soviet-Finnish co-operative study. *Scand. J. Rheumatol.*, **13**, 33-38
180. Luukkainen, R., Kaarela, K., Isomaki, H., Martio, J., Kiviniemi, P., Rasanen, J. and Sarna, S. (1983). The prediction of radiological destruction during the early stage of rheumatoid arthritis. *Clin. Exp. Rheumatol.*, **1**, 295-298
181. Feigenbaum, S. L., Masi, A. T. and Kaplan, S. B. (1979). Prognosis in rheumatoid arthritis. A longitudinal study of newly diagnosed younger adult patients. *Am. J. Med.*, **66**, 377-384
182. Kaarela, K. (1985). Prognostic factors and diagnostic criteria in early rheumatoid arthritis. *Scand J. Rheumatol.*, **S57**(suppl.), 5-50
183. Schneider, H. A., Yonker, R. A., Katz, P., Longley, S. and Panush, R. S. (1985). Rheumatoid vasculitis: experience with 13 patients and review of the literature. *Semin. Arthritis Rheum.*, **14**, 280-286
184. Westedt, M. L., Daha, M. R., Baldwin, W. M., III, Stijnen, T. and Cats, A. (1986). Serum immune complexes containing IgA appear to predict erosive arthritis in a longitudinal study in rheumatoid arthritis. *Ann. Rheum. Dis.*, **45**, 809-815
185. Kaye, J. J., Callahan, L. F., Nance, E. P. Jr., Brooks, R. H. and Pincus, T. (1987). Rheumatoid arthritis: explanatory power of specific radiographic findings for patient clinical status. *Radiology*, **165**, 753-758
186. Jacoby, R. K., Jayson, M. I. and Cosh, J. A. (1973). Onset, early stages, and prognosis of rheumatoid arthritis: a clinical study of 100 patients with 11-year follow-up. *Br. Med. J.*, **2**, 96-100
187. Amos, R. S., Constable, T. J. and Crockson, R. A. (1977). Rheumatoid arthritis: relation of serum C-reactive protein and erythrocyte sedimentation rates to radiographic changes. *Br. Med. J.*, **1**, 195-197
188. Reeback, J. and Silman, A. (1984). Predictors of outcome at two years in patients

with rheumatoid arthritis. *J. R. Soc. Med.*, **77**, 1002–1005
189. Withrington, R. H., Teitsson, I. and Vladimarrison, H. (1984). Prospective study of early rheumatoid arthritis: association of rheumatoid factor isotypes with fluctuations in disease activity. *Ann. Rheum. Dis.*, **43**, 679–685
190. Short, C. L. and Bauer, W. (1948). The course of rheumatoid arthritis in patients receiving simple medical and orthopedic measures. *N. Engl. J. Med.*, **238**, 142–148
191. Wolfe, F. and Hawley, D. J. (1985). Remission in rheumatoid arthritis. *J. Rheumatol.*, **12**, 245–252
192. Lee, P. (1978). Measurement in rheumatoid arthritis. *Aust. NZ. J. Med.*, **8**, 114–115
193. Hansagi, H., Allebeck, P. and Allander, E. (1985). Utilization of hospital care among persons with rheumatoid arthritis compared with controls. *Scand. J. Rheumatol.*, **14**, 403–410
194. Larsen, A. (1973). Radiological grading of rheumatoid arthritis. *Scand. J. Rheumatol.*, **2**, 136–138
195. Mullen, P. D., Laville, E. A., Biddle, A. K. and Lorig, K. (1987). Efficacy of psychoeducational interventions on pain, depression, and disability in people with arthritis: a meta-analysis. *J. Rheumatol.*, **14**, 33–39
196. Lorig, K., Seleznick, M., Lubeck, D., Ung, E., Chastain, R. L. and Holman, H. R. (1989). The beneficial outcomes of the arthritis self-management course are not adequately explained by behavior change. *Arthritis Rheum.*, **32**, 91–95
197. Goeppinger, J., Arthur, M. W., Baglioni, A. J., Jr., Brunk, S. E. and Brunner, C. M. (1989). A reexamination of the effectiveness of self-care education for persons with arthritis. *Arthritis Rheum.*, **32**, 706–716
198. Cohen, J. L., Sauter, S. V., deVellis, R. F. and deVellis, B. M. (1986). Evaluation of arthritis self-management courses led by laypersons and by professionals. *Arthritis Rheum.*, **29**, 388–393
199. Gabriel, S. E. and Luthra, H. S. (1988). Rheumatoid arthritis: can the long-term outcome be altered? *Mayo Clin. Proc.*, **63**, 58–68
200. Iannuzzi, I., Dawson, N., Zein, N. and Kishner, I. (1983). Does drug therapy slow radiographic deterioration in rheumatoid arthritis? *N. Engl. J. Med.*, **309**, 1023–1028
201. Wolfe, F., Hawley, D. J. and Cathey, M. A. (1989). Length of time on slow acting anti-rheumatic drugs (SAARDs): evidence for methotrexate effectiveness. *Arthritis Rheum.*, **32**, S99(Abstract)
202. Sambrook, P. N., Browne, C. D., Champion, G. D., Day, R. O., Vallance, J. B. and Warwick, N. (1982). Terminations of treatment with gold sodium thiomalatae in rheumatoid arthritis. *J. Rheumatol.*, **9**, 932–934
203. Richter, J. A., Runge, L. A., Pinals, R. S. and Oates, R. P. (1980). Analysis of treatment termination with gold and antimalarial compounds in rheumatoid arthritis. *J. Rheumatol.*, **7**, 153–159
204. Amor, B., Herson, D., Cherot, A. and Delbarre, F. (1981). Polyarthrites rheumatoides evoluant depuis plus de 10 an (1966–1978). *Ann. Med. Interne (Paris)*, **132**, 168–173
205. Liang, M. H. and Cullen, K. E. (1984). Evaluation of outcomes in total joint arthroplasty for rheumatoid arthritis. *Clin. Orthop.*, **182**, 41–45

4
Juvenile arthritis

B. M. ANSELL

Early reviews of the prognosis of juvenile arthritis varied considerably in accuracy and precision of prediction, possibly owing to differences in the homogeneity of the patients studied. Thus, Barkin, reporting from an orthopedic hospital, suggested a very gloomy picture[1]. In contrast, Edstrom noted that three-fifths of his 161 patients observed over a 20-year period had recovered without defect, one-fifth had healed, and only one-fifth were crippled or dead[2]. Similar results came from Finland[3] and our early work at the Juvenile Rheumatism Unit, Taplow, England, agreed with these views[4,5]. It was noted that early referral and the pattern of disease were important in determining outcome. In our study 50% of those who had had systemic onset of the disease had recovered, but 29% ended up severely disabled; this is in contrast to the optimistic outcome suggested by Calabro and Marchesano in 1968[6].

There have been few population studies aimed at incidence[7]. Hospital-based studies on prognosis have often mixed early with late referrals, while nomenclature and classification have varied. The problem of classification of children with chronic arthritis, to say nothing of nomenclature, cannot be overemphasized[8]. Some years ago there was not even agreement about the age of onset: it varied from 12 to 16 years. Attempts have been made to try to standardize criteria, with suggested criteria for juvenile rheumatoid arthritis (JRA)[9,10], while in Europe a workshop also attempted this task[11]. There is now agreement about the age of onset, notably under 16 years, and the modes of onset, namely systemic, polyarticular with more than five joints, and pauci-articular with fewer than five joints, but the duration of illness varies from 6 weeks in the United States to 3 months in Europe. Current studies coordinated by A. M. Prieur for the pediatric group of the European League against Rheumatism considering the mode of onset in relation to course, suggest that 6 months is a better onset period. Subtyping is certainly important in determining course, but the three agreed designated groups remain heterogeneous so that course classification may well be desirable for basic studies. At a workshop on genetics during the International Rheumatology Congress in Sydney in

1985, it was suggested that a minimum of 2 years should elapse before inclusion of patients in such studies so as to allow time for their pattern of disease to declare itself.

One of our main prognosis studies was based on 243 children seen between 1947 and 1958 in whom management was conservative with (a) regular physiotherapy to maintain joint and muscle function, (b) preservation of optimum joint position by appropriate splints including the conservative correction of joint deformities as soon as possible after they had developed, and (c) drug therapy mainly with either codeine phosphate or aspirin[12]. By today's standards other drugs were minimal; thus, only 2% received an antimalarial and a further 2% gold; 36%, however, had received corticotrophin or cortisone at some time, the majority of such patients having had a systemic onset. As follow-up proceeded, it was possible to characterize syndrome profiles.

Systemic onset disease was most common under the age of 5 years, in which age group there was a similar sex incidence; over that age it was more frequent in girls. Intermittent fever is the hallmark of this subgroup, which takes on a characteristic swinging pattern and is usually associated with a maculopapular eruption seen at the height of the fever. Generalized lymphadenopathy occurred in half the children and hepatomegaly and splenomegaly were common, but clinical evidence of pericarditis was infrequent (about 10%) in this series.

Chronic iridocyclitis, recognized as being relatively frequent in chronic childhood arthritis, occurred in children, particularly girls, aged 1–5 years and was associated with a mono- or pauciarticular onset that tended to remain restricted, certainly for a few years. It was noted in a separate study that in such children the presence of antinuclear antibodies characterized the majority with chronic iridocyclitis[13].

A monoarticular onset was noted in approximately 18%. These were particularly young girls between the age of 1 and 5 years and at risk for iridocyclitis, as well as a small group of girls aged 7–11 years whose disease was restricted to the knee, and a few older boys who went on to juvenile spondylitis.

Juvenile spondylitis had a male predominance but an older age of onset and tended to present as a lower limb arthropathy that was usually pauciarticular; bouts of acute iridocyclitis had occurred in 26% by the 10-year follow-up. While sacroiliitis could be seen within 5 years of onset, back limitation was much later[14]. Subsequently a high incidence of HLA-B27 was demonstrated[15] and in more recent studies a family history of ankylosing spondylitis was not uncommon (25%).

Seropositive JRA had a female predominance affecting particularly girls aged 10 or more and with a tendency to erosive changes in hands and feet within a year of onset and followed by progressive joint destruction. The value of IgM rheumatoid factor as a marker for a variant had previously been recorded in a prospective study of 110 children, a disease onset between the age of 12 and 16 years accounting for almost 80% of those with positive tests for rheumatoid factor; seropositivity also correlated closely with the presence of nodules[16].

Similarly, a cross-sectional review of 110 patients commencing under 14 years of age noted a significant correlation between the serological reaction, age of onset, presence of nodules, and bone erosions[17].

Twenty-six percent did not fit into any specific subgroup, all had polyarthritis, but were probably not homogeneous.

The long-term outcome was closely associated with the pattern of disease present. Taking the group as a whole, 1 in 6 children was severely limited and likely to be a chronic attender at clinics, requiring support from social services and other agencies (Figure 1). This was most likely if there had been a systemic onset in early childhood. In general, the older the patient, with the exception of seropositive juvenile rheumatoid arthritis, the less disability was found at the 15-year follow-up. The most favorable prognosis was in those presenting as monoarticular disease[12].

A later follow-up study (median 10 years) of 33 patients with systemic onset[18] noted cardiac involvement, usually pericarditis, in 42% and, although myocarditis was rare, it was more serious and did account for one death. Amyloidosis was seen in 3 patients (9%). Severe growth retardation was seen in 39%. Clinical remission occurred in half, with an average of 5.9 years duration. Those patients who had an onset of disease over the age of 5 years and those who had little radiological change in the first 5 years of illness did best.

The cause of death in children with JRA who had been seen in recognized clinics in Europe, the United States, and the Pacific area showed that the European series had the highest incidence of deaths, possibly related to their longer follow-up[19]. Most of the children who had died had presented in the youngest age group, 51% being between 1 and 5 years. There was some increase in death rate with an onset from 6 to 10 years and then it gradually fell off. A significant proportion of those who died did so within 5 years of onset and the majority within 10 years of onset. The most common cause of death was renal failure, usually due to amyloidosis, and the next most frequent cause of death was infection. The children who died of infection tended to die early and it was usually seen in association with systemic disease, while those who died from amyloidosis died later, 10.8 years from onset of disease. The higher frequency of death in children with JRA in Europe is probably because of the higher frequency of amyloidosis. Rarer causes included heart disease, adrenal failure, blood dyscrasias, cerebral hemorrhage, and trauma.

In a 15-year follow-up study of 433 children from Garmisch Partenkirchen[20], mortality was 13.8% in the systemic group in contrast to 1% in the polyarthritic and 0% in the pauciarticular groups. Severe limitation occurred in 13.4% of the systemic and 11.4% of the nonsystemic, but 82.5% of those with pauciarticular onset had no or minimal limitation. Hepatic dysfunction was also noted to be a cause of death. It was considered that the liver of a child with systemic JCA appears to be particularly vulnerable. Thus, hepatic necrosis has been seen after infectious hepatitis[21]. Some of the deaths associated with

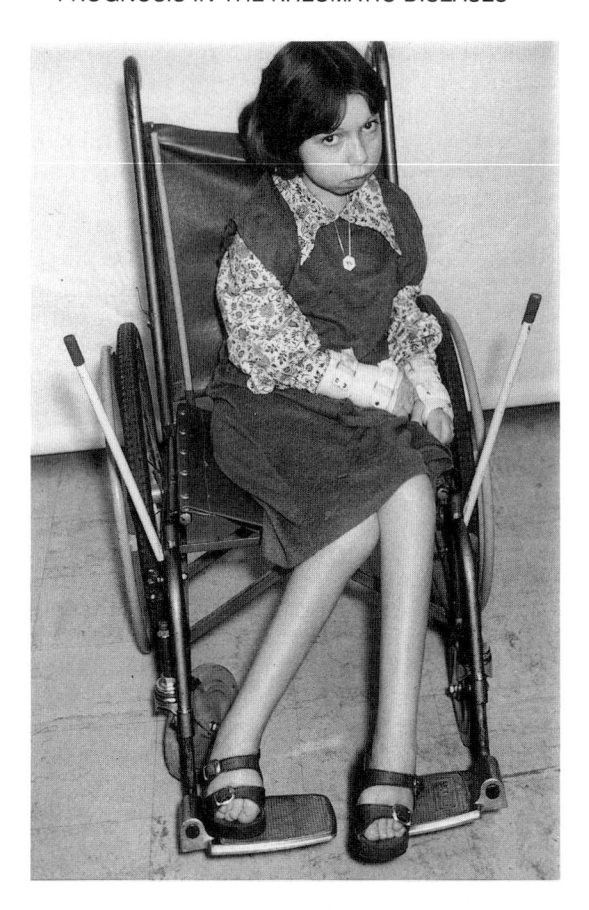

Figure 1. Reliance on a wheelchair early with little physiotherapy, and here at 10 years of disease, little activity but severe deformity with torticollis, flexed hips, valgus flexed R knee and foot deformity: most of these could be avoided by appropriate physical means.

liver failure resulted from drug therapy, and here aspirin and indomethacin are particular culprits. Our own studies also showed this excess mortality, particularly with early-onset disease, with amyloidosis and infection being the major causes[12].

Realizing that a child is susceptible to infection, one is more alert for its development and a reduction in death rate due to infection has certainly occurred. In our last follow-up, which was performed on early cases, there had been no deaths related to either the disease or infection over a 10-year period[22]. There had, however, been two severe hepatic incidents that had been managed better than in bygone years. A new complication appears to have been recognized: consumption coagulopathy, often in association with a second injection of gold, in the systemic group or intercurrent infection and requires intensive therapy[23,24]. Although amyloidosis was present in two patients in our study, their disease activity appeared to be controlled with cytotoxic therapy and progression was not evident at the 10-year follow-up. At this 10-year follow-up of 147 patients originally seen personally within 3 months of onset, of those with systemic disease, 50% were in remission at the 5-year follow-up (Figure 2), but by 10 years only a further 7% had remitted. Persistent systemic features together with an elevated IgA level and thrombocytosis after 1 year of disease was present in almost all who were still active at the 10-year follow-up. Such patients had tended to have recurrent exacerbations, often in association with intercurrent infections, without ever going into remission. They showed marked stunting of growth, presumably as a result of chronic active disease, with its associated poor nutritional status and also the effects of corticosteroids. Associated with this was abnormal development of joints, in particular the hips, with persistent anteversion of the femoral head and poor development of the acetabulum[25]. Those teenagers with seropositive disease tended to remain active despite slow-acting drugs such as gold and penicillamine and to have progressive joint damage so that nearly half of them had undergone a hip or knee replacement arthroplasty by the 10-year follow-up[22]. The patients who did best were children with early-onset pauciarticular disease that did not spread, 70% of whom were in remission at the 10-year follow-up. These constituted 46% of the whole group. Of those with older-onset pauciarticular disease, nearly half were inactive, but of the remainder a few had gone on to develop definitive ankylosing spondylitis with spinal involvement, although at this point the majority only had sacroiliitis. Criteria for remission have not been established: we used no joint activity, no drug therapy, and a normal ESR. However, the absence of disease activity does not necessarily mean normal function, and this was particularly noticeable in those who had had systemic disease when the Arthritis Impact Measurement Scale was used to assess outcome[26].

Pattern recognition has highlighted the complications likely to be encountered in any particular child. Amyloidosis is seen particularly in the systemic onset group and is now watched for carefully so that acute phase responses, e.g., C-reactive protein, can be reduced by appropriate medication[27]. Children with young-onset pauciarticular disease, and having a positive antinuclear antibody, should have very much better monitoring of the eye and therefore uveitis should be picked up early and treated accordingly, with hopefully less ultimate impairment of vision than the 33% on the blind register[28]. The realization that glaucoma has played a big role in the development of blindness has led to its earlier detection and better management.

Although eye involvement was first described in 1910[29], the exact incidence of iridocylitis has been difficult to determine, largely because of the special selection of referral cases. Thus, incidences as low as 2% and as high as 36% have been recorded[28]. The characteristic chronic

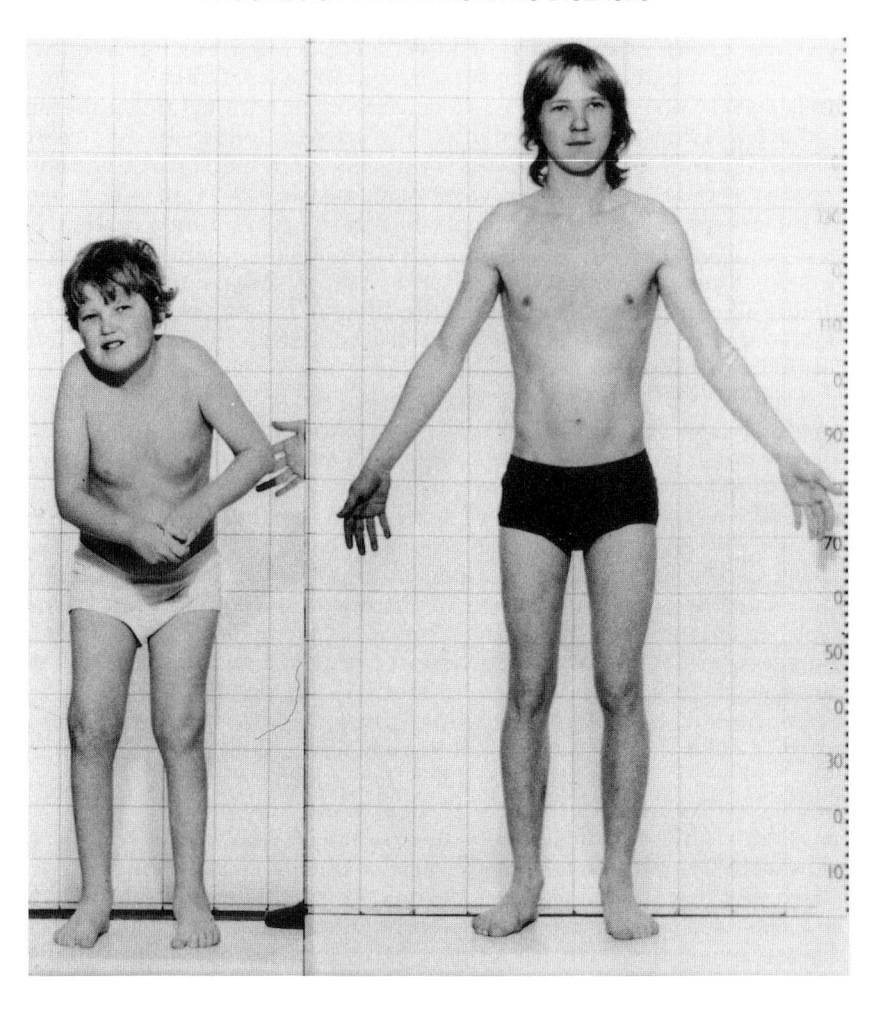

Figure 2. Systemic onset disease aged 5 years followed by severe arthritis. Treated by intensive physiotherapy, splinting, alternate-day steroid and naprosyn. Note recovery and good functional position over a 3-year period.

anterior uveitis tends to follow the arthritis, but can occasionally precede it and occurs particularly in young children, usually girls. The signs of eye involvement are inflammatory cells floating in the aqueous humor and adherent to the cornea and endothelium as keratic precipitates; these can only be detected by slit-lamp microscope examination. Complicated cataract developed in some 50% of Smiley's patients[28] and secondary glaucoma in 25% with 60% developing the corneal band opacity; this is not unique to juvenile chronic arthritis, but can occur in any chronic iridocyclitis. Fifty percent of all the eyes recorded by

Smiley[28] in his longitudinal study had less than 6/8 vision and, as already noted, 33% qualified for the blind register.

More recent studies suggest that the incidence of uveitis is about 20%; the mean age of onset was 6 years and it was usual to present before 8 years and affect girls in particular. It was bilateral in 71%[30].

From 103 patients seen early in the course and followed prospectively for some 14 years, 25% had a good visual prognosis and these divided into those with a very mild uveitis and those with one attack of severe uveitis lasting less than 4 months when treated energetically with local therapy. Another 50% had moderate to severe uveitis for more than 4 months and required, from time to time, intensive local therapy and 25% had severe prolonged uveitis that responded poorly to topical corticosteroids. It was among these that the complications of cataract (31% in the whole group) and secondary glaucoma (14% in the whole group) were seen[30].

Wolf *et al.*, reviewing 89 eyes with uveitis from 51 patients with a mean follow-up of 12.7 years, noted that 22% had severe visual loss, 46% had cataracts, 37% band keratopathy, and 27% glaucoma[31]. If posterior synechiae were present at the initial examination then the outlook was much worse. Those patients who presented with eye involvement had a particularly poor visual outcome, 67% being severely afflicted. Thus, uveitis remains a serious problem which requires early recognition and appropriate management.[32] Other ocular complications include keratoconjunctivitis sicca, which in Kanski's group was asymptomatic but not so in those previously described by Chylack *et al*[33]. Chorioretinal scars and severe unilateral corneal thinning may also occur.

Combined clinics where ophthalmologists and pediatric rheumatologists work in communicating rooms are a practical way of arriving at a complete assessment of the individual child, so that the management required can be discussed and appropriate general and local treatment needs agreed. It is essential to perform regular expert examination of all children with pauciarticular chronic arthritis at least every 2-3 months, particularly if ANA positive. Other children should also be assessed, but at less frequent intervals, probably 6 monthly for the polyarthritic and 12 monthly for the systemic. In view of the long-term management required and despite the dislocation this type of illness can bring to family life, complete cooperation of the parents is a prime necessity. Support for patient and parent will be required over a long period in an atmosphere of confidence born of knowledge and experience.

GROWTH RETARDATION

Prior to corticosteroid therapy, the duration of disease activity was an important factor in determining failure to grow in height[34]. Treatment with corticosteroids intensified this, even when disease activity was well controlled. A dosage as low as 5 mg/m^2 daily of prednisone over a 6-month period significantly reduced growth and this does not appear to have been overcome by the addition of human growth hormone[35]. One investigation suggested that even at presentation more children with juvenile arthritis were below the 3rd centile than normal and that growth retardation in the arthritic child was significantly greater in those with a systemic onset and who had been treated with corticosteroids. Indeed, corticosteroid therapy had had a more profound effect on growth and height in arthritic children than in those with systemic lupus erythematosus[36]. Efforts to alter corticosteroid regimes, aiming to reduce suppression of the hypothalamic pituitary adrenal axis, include giving a corticosteroid preparation every 48 hours. Certainly in patients who can tolerate this, growth does appear to proceed, albeit at a slower rate[37,38]. However, in some patients, usually those with systemic disease, this is not practical and daily therapy is required with all its attendant problems, including severe osteoporosis with collapse of vertebrae[39], which can occasionally cause compression of the spinal cord as well as further reduction in height.

LOCAL GROWTH DISCREPANCIES

Local lengthening of the metaphysis as well as overgrowth of the epiphysis occurs in children with monoarticular knee involvement, presumably due to increased vascularity resulting from the active arthritis, while wasting of the muscles causes the legs to be thin[40]. If inflammation in the knee can be controlled by means of local long-acting corticosteroid preparations (achievable in three-quarters) it appears that growth discrepancy does not progress[41]. Overgrowth of the tibial epiphysis is also seen in monoarticular ankle involvement, but this is much less common than in the knee. In children aged 8 years and over, premature fusion of epiphyses, particularly of the ulna styloid, metatarsophalanges, and metacarpophalanges, presumably as a result of local inflammation, causes growth anomalies in the form of short bones. In young children, periosteal reaction along the phalanges tends to consolidate with widening of the whole phalanx.

Growth disturbances of the hip are very frequent in children whose disease starts before the age of 8 years, and occurs even in the absence of hip involvement if normal walking patterns are not developed[25]. This leads to persistence of the infantile pattern of valgus of the femoral neck with a tendency towards overgrowth of the femoral head in the presence of inflammation and subsequent subluxation. Maldevelopment of the lower jaw causing micrognathia is seen in 14% of cases[33].

PSYCHOSOCIAL PROBLEMS

Although the need for family support is well recognized, the emotional and social problems of children and young people with arthritis have received less attention than the physical aspects. An early review of adolescents with severe residual deformities showed social isolation to be a real problem, with lack of opportunity for sexual contact[42]. The young people's anxieties centered on self-image (which was usually poor), failure of growth, and their dependence. These correlated particularly with an early age of onset, poor height attainment, and restricted mobility; broken families were an additional stress factor. Following a study comparing 43 children with severe and 52 with mild disease against 93 healthy children, Billings et al.[43] commented on the need to assess risk and resistance factors predictive of psychologic and social dysfunction. In general the severe group missed more time from school and participated in fewer social activities.

A research study aimed at identifying determinants of psychosocial adjustment in children and young adults in Australia noted that even at primary school some children tended to spend their leisure time alone[44]. The level of disability was associated with overall adjustment in this group. In a high-school group, the overall adjustment, indexed by the total self-concept score, was more obvious. Thus those with the lowest self-concept scores tended to spend their leisure time with the family and had a much smaller network of friends. In young adults, social functioning showed no relation to self-concept development. Sexual relationships were fewer than one would have expected and many young people had an arthritic friend as a close friend. The problem of family adjustment was also assessed, but the range was somewhat limited as these tended to be intact families. Nevertheless, problems reported by parents included financial concern and emotional strain as well as the time required for physical care. It was also noted that the impact of disease severity may not be seen clearly until the child enters adolescence.

MANAGEMENT

From the literature it is difficult to know what, if anything, has influenced the natural history of the disease[2] and there may be differences in manifestations in different parts of the world. Thus, in a follow-up study in Auckland of 78% of 55 children with a mean disease duration of 9.3 years, the outcome of those with a polyarticular course was poorer with respect to both ongoing disease activity and functional disability[45]. Only one case of mild uveitis was detected, i.e., a much lower incidence than is usually reported; a similar low incidence of iridocyclitis has also been recorded in Australia[46]. There is a remarkably low incidence of amyloidosis in Australia and the United States and juvenile spondylitis is rare in Japan. There is still a need for good basic epidemiologic studies worldwide.

Although there have been many drug studies, particularly involving the newer nonsteroidal anti-inflammatory drugs, there appears to be no one that is better than any other[47]. Dose has to be adjusted according to size and it is wise to continue for a minimum of 8–12 weeks, provided no side-effects occur, before saying the drug is ineffective[48]. The use of nonsteroidal anti-inflammatory drugs other than aspirin is increasing because of the risk of Reye's syndrome, particularly in young children. The failure of long-acting drugs in the group as a whole emphasizes the need for multicenter studies in the subgroups[49].

The major improvements have been in the development of children's arthritis programs, in association with special centers. Maintaining the position and function of joints by appropriate physiotherapy and splinting and the use of surgery is very important. Local steroid injections and soft-tissue release operations at hip and knee are playing an important part in the maintenance of function. Total joint replacement arthroplasty is important in maintaining function and nowadays, once the hip joint is completely destroyed, it is reasonable to suggest this, although usually a special small prosthesis may have to be prepared[50]. Other joints such as the knee may ultimately require replacement.

FUTURE PERSPECTIVE

Although clinical subsets have been described and HLA antigens support a genetic basis for the different subtypes[51], studies on better-defined larger groups are required. Thus, looking at seronegative polyarthritic onset, those patients commencing under age 5 had a high incidence of HLA-DRw8, suggesting that the genetic basis for susceptibility is similar to that of early onset pauciarticular disease[52].

Although the association of HLA-B27 with spondyloarthropathy in childhood is established[15], it is now being considered that this represents a symptom complex[53]. At times, other diseases such as ulcerative colitis and regional enteritis may be associated. It is suggested that this group accounts for 20% of children with arthritis and that the course of these children is extremely varied, some having just an episode of polyarthritis, others going on to sacroiliitis over a variable period of time[14,15] but only some ultimately developing spondylitis. Thus, of 36 children reviewed after a mean follow-up of 8.9 years, only 2 had developed definite ankylosing spondylitis[54]. The relationship of this group to the syndrome described by Rosenberg and Petty, frequently known as the "SEA" syndrome, is still uncertain[55]. The criteria for adult spondylitis are entirely unsatisfactory in children and criteria need to be established for the juvenile disease. These may well have to be in two parts: definite and probable. However, assessment in a number of centers is essential. The whole role of inflammation of the bowel, including that due to infection, is still uncertain and, while reactive arthritis is apparently relatively rare in children[56], its role needs further assessment. Similarly, juvenile psoriatic arthropathy, which is usually put into the spondyloarthropathy group, needs better criteria and reappraisal. Indeed, whether it should be a feature of the spondyloarthropathy group is even in question, since only a small proportion of such young patients carry HLA-B27 and develop sacroiliitis and even fewer spondylitis. The majority of such children start as pauciarticular and may even have the complication of iridocyclitis, but asymmetric polyarthritis eventually develops in a large proportion[57] so that course classification is necessary. The HLA profile of this subgroup also requires further reappraisal.

Meaningful basic studies require appropriate clinical data. There is a relative paucity of scientific data on the different forms of arthritis in childhood and this needs to be remedied. It would appear that corticosteroids will continue to play a major role in managing systemic JCA and a more minor role in other types. The use of intravenous methylprednisolone given at infrequent intervals, which allows maintenance of the hypothalamic pituitary adrenal axis as well as other immunologic parameters, needs further exploration. Similarly, the corticosteroid, deflazacort, which is currently under study, appears to be of benefit in reducing osteoporosis and when available may be the steroid of choice for these young people. The possible role of synthetic growth hormone in overcoming the growth failure associated with the disease and therapy needs careful appraisal.

Adult rheumatology does not provide a model for juvenile rheumatology as there are many differences between the clinical characteristics of the connective-tissue diseases in adults and children[58], and nowhere is this more obvious than in juvenile arthritis.

Children with rheumatic diseases face special problems of physical and psychological growth as well as sexual and social maturation. There is a lack of public awareness about arthritis in children and such children are not handled sympathetically. Personal and peer-group problems relating to self-image, social image, educational objectives, and maintenance of educational process are extremely important and require further assessment as well as sympathetic understanding. Physical modalities of treatment have been insufficiently tested to assess their value.

Introduction of patients into a good system of medical care is still inadequate in most countries. Any program must have the capability of comprehensive patient care and be closely related to clinical and basic research; it should also participate in the training of pediatric rheumatologists and allied health professionals at all levels. This should produce the personnel for research and patient care to upgrade what is currently available in both numbers and in quality. It is important that it relates effectively to community resources and it will need to provide a problem-based and solution-orientated continuum of care incorporating the views and skills of a multidisciplinary group. Physicians involved with such children should possess good collective expertise in pediatric and adolescent medicine, rheumatology, orthopedic surgery, and ophthalmology, and they should relate systematically to the patient and to each other. Attention must be given to the patients' physical, psychological, and social functioning with long-range planning from early in the course of management. Carefully evaluated activities of a daily living program need to be related to the home, school, or later work setting and corrective action coordinated within the community. The role of a nurse coordinator is an important one that could well be further expanded.

Future drug studies should take into account the pattern of disease present. Although a pilot study may be required to establish dosage and early side-effects, every effort should be made to have a comparative controlled study with adequate numbers. In order to get adequate numbers, these studies will need to be multicentered if the role of methotrexate, and intravenous gammaglobulin in systemic onset disease, is to be sorted out.

It is important to look at slow-acting drugs in polyarthritic onset groups by age of onset, while the possible role of methotrexate in extended young-onset pauciarticular disease patients who add on joints and become polyarthritic needs special attention. Similarly, the possible role of sulfasalazine in older onset pauciarticular disease (with particular reference to those with HLA-B27), requires further assessment. These are but a few examples. Surgical expertise needs concentrating in special centers as only some 10% of children will require this. Protocols should be prepared and carefully followed to assess the clinical results and cost-effectiveness of procedures undertaken. More studies are required with respect to psychosocial aspects, integration into society, and long-term prognosis as regards secondary joint degeneration and mortality.

References

1. Barkin, R. E. (1952). Clinical course of juvenile rheumatoid arthritis. *Bull. Rheum. Dis.*, **3**, 19–20
2. Edstrom, G. (1958). Rheumatoid arthritis and Still's disease in children — a survey of 161 cases. *Arthritis Rheum.*, **1**, 497–504
3. Laaksonen, A. L. (1966). A prognostic study of juvenile rheumatoid arthritis. *Acta Paediat. Scand.*, **166** (suppl.), 1–163
4. Ansell, B. M. and Bywaters, E. G. L. (1959). Prognosis in Still's disease. *Bull. Rheum. Dis.*, **9**, 189–192
5. Ansell, B. M. (1969). Still's disease followed into adult life. *Proc. R. Soc. Med.*, **62**, 912–913
6. Calabro, J. and Marchesano, J. M. (1968). The early natural history of juvenile rheumatoid arthritis. *Med. Clin. N. Am.*, **52**, 567–691
7. Kunnamo, I., Kallio, P. and Pelkonen, P. (1986). Incidence of arthritis in urban Finnish children. *Arthritis Rheum.*, **29**, 1232–1238
8. Holt, P. J. L. (1990). The classification of juvenile chronic arthritis. *Clin Exp. Rheumatol.*, **8**, 331–333
9. Brewer, E. J., Bass, J., Baum, J., Cassidy, J. T., Fink, C., Jacobs, J., Hanson, V., Levinson, J. E., Schaller, J. and Stillman, J. S. (1977). Current proposed revision of juvenile rheumatoid arthritis criteria. *Arthritis Rheum.*, **20**, 195–199
10. Cassidy, J. T., Levinson, J. E., Bass, J. C., Baum, J., Brewer, E. J., Fink, C. W., Hanson, V., Jacobs, J. C., Masi, A. T., Schaller, J. G., Fries, J. F., McShane, D. and Young, D. (1986). A study of classification criteria for a diagnosis of juvenile rheumatoid arthritis. *Arthritis Rheum.*, **29**, 274–281

11. Munthe, E. (1978). Special meeting on nomenclature and classification of arthritis in children. (Basle: EULAR Publication)
12. Ansell, B. M. and Wood, P. (1976). Prognosis in juvenile chronic arthritis. *Clin. Rheum. Dis.*, **2**, 397-412
13. Schaller, J. G., Johnson, G. D., Holborow, L. J., Ansell, B. M. and Smiley, W. K. (1974). The association of antinuclear antibodies with the chronic iridocyclitis of juvenile rheumatoid arthritis. *Arthritis Rheum.*, **17**, 409-416
14. Ansell, Barbara M. (1980). Juvenile spondylitis and related disorders. In Moll, J. M. H. (ed.) *Ankylosing Spondylitis*, pp. 120-136. (Edinburgh: Churchill Livingstone)
15. Edmonds, J., Morris, R. I. and Metzger, A. L. (1974). Follow-up study of juvenile chronic polyarthritis with particular reference to the histocompatibility antigen W2 in Still's disease. *Ann. Rheum. Dis.*, **33**, 289-292
16. Hanson, V., Drexler, E. and Kornreich, H. (1969). The relationship of rheumatoid factor to age of onset in juvenile rheumatoid arthritis. *Arthritis Rheum.*, **12**, 82-86
17. Cassidy, J. T. and Valkenburg, H. A. (1967). A five year prospective study of rheumatoid factor tests in juvenile rheumatoid arthritis. *Arthritis Rheum.*, **10**, 83-90
18. Svantesson, H., Akesson, A., Eberhardt, K. and Elborgh, R. (1983). Prognosis in juvenile rheumatoid arthritis with systemic onset — a follow-up study. *Scand. J. Rheumatol.*, **12**, 139-144
19. Baum, J. and Gutowska, G. (1976). Death in juvenile rheumatoid arthritis. *Arthritis Rheum.*, **20** (suppl.), 253-255
20. Stoeber, E. (1981). Prognosis in juvenile chronic arthritis. *Eur. J. Pediat.*, **135**, 225-228
21. Boone, J. E. (1976). Hepatic disease and mortality in juvenile rheumatoid arthritis. *Arthritis Rheum.*, **20** (suppl.), 257-258
22. Ansell, B. M. (1987). Juvenile chronic arthritis. *Scand. J. Rheumatol.*, **66** (suppl.), 47-50
23. De Vere Tyndall, A., Macauley, D. and Ansell, B. M. (1983). Disseminated intravascular coagulation complicating systemic juvenile chronic arthritis ("Still's disease"). *Clin. Rheumatol.*, **2**, 415-418
24. Silberman, E. D., Miller III, J. J., Bernstein, B. H. and Shalat, T. (1983). Consumption coagulopathy associated with systemic juvenile arthritis. *J. Pediat.*, **103**, 872-876
25. Gallino, L., Pountain, G., Mitchell, M. and Ansell, B. M. (1984). Developmental aspects of the hip in juvenile chronic arthritis. *Scand. J. Rheumatol.*, **13**, 310-318
26. Doherty, E., Rooney, M., Conroy, R. and Bresnihan, B. (1988). Health status of functionally independent young adults with chronic arthritis since childhood. *J. Orthop. Rheumatol.*, **1**, 51-58
27. Schnitzer, T. J. and Ansell, B. M. (1977). Amyloidosis in juvenile chronic polyarthritis. *Arthritis Rheum.*, **20**, 245-252
28. Smiley, W. K. (1976). The eye in juvenile chronic polyarthritis. *Clin. Rheum. Dis.*, **2**, 413-428
29. Ohm, J. (1910). Bandformige Hornhauttrubung bei einem neunjahrigen Madchen und ihre Behandlung mit subkonjunktivalen Jodkaliumeinspritzungen. *Klinische Monatsblatter fur Augenheilkund*, **48**, 243-246
30. Kanski, J. J. (1988). Uveitis in juvenile chronic arthritis: incidence, clinical features and prognosis. *Eye*, **2**, 641-645
31. Wolf, M. D., Lichter, P. R. and Ragsdale, C. G. (1987). Prognostic factor in the uveitis of juvenile rheumatoid arthritis. *Ophthalmology*, **94**, 142-148
32. Kanski, J. J., Shun-Shin, Adrien, G. (1984). Systemic uveitis syndromes in childhood: an analysis of 340 cases. *Ophthalmology*, **91**, 1247-1252
33. Chylack, L. T. Jr., Bienfore, D. C., Bellow, A. R. and Stillman, J. S. (1975). Ocular manifestations of juvenile rheumatoid arthritis. *Am. J. Ophthalmol.*, **79**, 1026-1033
34. Ansell, B. M. and Bywaters, E. G. L. (1956). Growth in Still's disease. *Ann. Rheum. Dis.*, **15**, 295
35. Ward, D. J., Hartog, M. and Ansell, B. M. (1966). Corticosteroid induced dwarfism in Still's disease are treated with human growth hormone. *Ann. Rheum. Dis.*, **25**, 416-421
36. Bernstein, B., Stobie, D., Singsen, H. H., Koster-King, K., Kornreich, H. K. and Hanson, V. (1977). Growth retardation in juvenile rheumatoid arthritis. *Arthritis Rheum.*, **20**(2), 212-226
37. Sturge, R. A., Beardwell, C., Hartog, M., Wright, D. and Ansell, B. M. (1970).

Cortisol and growth hormone secretion in relation to linear growth: patients with Still's disease on different therapeutic regimes. *Br. Med. J.*, **3**, 547-551
38. Byron, M. A., Jackson, J. and Ansell, B. M. (1983). Effect of different corticosteroid regimes in hypothalamic pituitary adrenal axis and growth in juvenile chronic arthritis. *J. R. Soc. Med.*, **76**, 452-457
39. Varonos, S., Ansell, B. M. and Reeve, J. (1987). Vertebral collapse in juvenile chronic arthritis — its relationship with glucocorticoid therapy. *Calcified Tissue Int.*, **41**, 75-78
40. Vostreys, Mary R. P. T. and Hollister, J. R. (1988). Muscle atrophy and leg length discrepancies in pauci-articular juvenile rheumatoid arthritis. *Am. J. Dis. Child.*, **142**, 343-345
41. Earley, A., Cuttica, G., McCullough, C. and Ansell, B. M. (1988). Triamcinolone into the knee joint in juvenile chronic arthritis. *Clin. Exp. Rheumatol.*, **6**, 153-155
42. Wilkinson, Vera, A. (1980). Juvenile chronic arthritis in adolescence: facing the reality. *Int. Rehabil. Med.*, **3**, 11-17
43. Billings, A. G., Moos, R. H., Miller, J. J. III and Gottlieb. (1987). Psycho-social adaptation in juvenile rheumatic disease — a controlled evaluation. *Health Psychol.*, **6**, 343-359
44. Ungerer, J. A., Chaitow, J. and Chammin, G. D. (1988). Psycho-social functioning in child and young adults with juvenile arthritis. *Pediatrics*, **81**, 195-202
45. McGill, N. W. and Gow, P. J. (1987). Juvenile rheumatoid arthritis in Auckland. A long term follow-up with particular reference to uveitis. *Aust. N.Z. J. Med.*, **17**, 305-308
46. McDougal, P. and Hill, D. J. (1981). Juvenile chronic arthritis. *Med. J. Aust.*, **2**, 89-92
47. Leak, A. M., Richter, M. R., Clemens, L. E., Hall, M. A. and Ansell, B. M. (1988). A crossover study of naproxen, diclofenac and tolmetin in seronegative juvenile chronic arthritis. *Clin. Exp. Rheumatol.*, **6**, 157-160
48. Lovell, D. J., Giannini, E. H. and Brewer, E. J. (1984). The course of response to non-steroidal anti-inflammatory drugs in JRA. *Arthritis Rheum.*, **27**, 1433-1437
49. Giannini, E. H., Brewer, E. J., Kuzmina, L. and Alekseev L. Shokh. (1988). Characteristics of responders and non-responders to slow acting anti-rheumatic drugs. *Arthritis Rheum.*, **31**, 15-20
50. Ansell, B. M. and Swann, M. (1983). The management of chronic arthritis of children. *J. Bone Joint Surg.*, **65-B**, 536-543
51. Forre, O., Doublong, J. H., Hoyeraal, H. M. and Thonsley, E. (1983). HLA antigens in juvenile arthritis: genetic basis for the different subtypes. *Arthritis Rheum.*, **26**, 35-38
52. Hall, P. J., Burman, S. J., Barash, J., Briggs, D. C. and Ansell, B. M. (1989). HLA and complement C4 antigens in polyarticular onset seronegative juvenile chronic arthritis: association of early onset with HLA-DRw8. *J. Rheumatol.*, **16**, 55-59
53. Jacobs, J. C., Berdon, W. E. and Johnston, A. D. (1982). HLA B27 associated spondyloarthropathy and enthesopathy in childhood clinical pathological and radio-logical observation in 58 patients. *J. Pediat.*, **100**, 521-528
54. Sheerin, K. A., Giannini, E. H., Brewer, E. J. and Barron, K. S. (1988). HLA B27 associated arthropathy in childhood — long term clinical and diagnostic outcome. *Arthritis Rheum.*, **31**, 1165-1170
55. Rosenberg, A. M. and Petty, R. E. (1982). A syndrome of seronegative enthesopathy and arthropathy in children. *Arthritis Rheum.*, **25**, 1041-1047
56. Singsen, B. H., Bernstein, B., Koster-King, K., Glovsky, M. M. and Hanson, V. (1977). Reiter's syndrome in childhood. *Arthritis Rheum.*, **20**, 402-407
57. Shore, A. and Ansell, B. M. (1982). Juvenile psoriatic arthritis: an analysis of 60 cases. *J. Pediat.*, **100**, 529-535
58. Leak, A. M. and Isenberg, D. (1989). Auto-immune rheumatic diseases in childhood — a comparison with adult onset disease. *Q. J. Med.*, **73**, 875-893

5
Crystal-associated arthropathies

B. T. EMMERSON

Three types of crystal are associated with joint inflammation — namely, monosodium urate monohydrate (MSUM or urate); calcium pyrophosphate dihydrate (CPPD or pyrophosphate); and basic calcium phosphate (BCP or apatite; a combination of carbonate-substituted hyroxyapatite, octacalcium phosphate and tricalcium phosphate). Two of these crystal types, MSUM and CPPD, will consistently induce an acute arthritis when injected into a joint. The role of basic calcium phosphate in joint disease is less clear and its etiologic role in joint inflammation less well defined. The associated clinical patterns of these crystal-associated arthropathies are more clearly defined, however, and in this chapter these conditions will be considered separately as urate crystal arthropathy or gout, as pyrophosphate-deposition disease, and as apatite-associated arthritis.

URATE CRYSTAL ARTHROPATHY

Problems in determining the prognosis of gout

Although the clinical pattern of an acute attack of gouty arthritis is reasonably characteristic and clinically homogeneous, the factors that contribute to the development of hyperuricemia and gout are almost as heterogeneous as the patients who suffer from this condition. This occurs because the development of the chief manifestation of gout, namely, acute gouty arthritis, depends upon the degree of elevation of the serum urate and upon the duration and extent of fluctuation of the hyperuricemia. It is now recognized that the serum urate concentration is subject to many influences, some of which are genetic in origin and others of which are modified by the environment and pattern of living. Moreover, the degree of hyperuricemia fluctuates in most patients and this will modify the prevalence of its complications. This means that the prognosis may be very variable in the individual. Accordingly, attempts will be made to analyze the various factors that modify the serum urate concentrations and that therefore determine the prognosis in each individual patient.

Gouty arthritis is also intimately associated with other conditions that in themselves can modify the prognosis for a particular patient. Thus, the manifestations of gout in a patient with preexisting renal disease may be quite different from those in a patient with normal renal function. Likewise, the presence of hypertension and/or vascular disease will have a profound effect upon the prognosis in a gouty patient, particularly insofar as mortality is concerned.

Gout secondary to proliferation of bone marrow elements is well known to cause excessive production of uric acid, which may ultimately lead to severe hyperuricemia and gout. A similar problem is seen during the chemotherapy of malignancy. Such types of gout of hemopoietic origin were commonly referred to as secondary gout[1]. However, as we have become able to identify increasing numbers of factors that result in hyperuricemia in patients with what was previously called "primary gout," the term "secondary gout" has lost its specific significance and is now best not used. In the case of gout due to excessive nuclear turnover in the bone marrow, the prognosis is determined more by the underlying disease causing the excessive production of uric acid than by the associated gout. Accordingly, this chapter will not deal further with the prognosis of gout due to neoplastic disease or proliferative change in the bone marrow.

Identification of factors contributing to hyperuricemia in primary gout

Urate is produced at a relatively constant rate in all individuals in a stable metabolic state, provided they are taking a diet essentially free of purines. The amount produced and excreted remains relatively constant for each individual and this is increased in proportion to the purine content of the diet[2]. However, a variety of situations can arise in which there is excessive degradation of adenine nucleotides and these can lead to the excessive production of purine bases, which are degraded to uric acid[3]. Factors that can cause this increased adenine nucleotide (AMP) degradation include the fructose content of the diet[4] and exercise[5]. Nonetheless, basal purine metabolism is relatively stable in the resting state and most increases and fluctuations are due to exogenous factors, some of the more important of which are listed here.

(1) *Diet*. Dietary nucleoprotein and other purines are ultimately degraded to cause an increase in the amount of uric acid produced. Thus, most purines consumed in the diet constitute a purine load that the body needs to eliminate either by the renal route (which accounts for approximately two-thirds) or by extra-renal excretion, usually into the small intestine by a process that is probably largely dependent upon the serum urate concentration. Any urate in the colon is completely degraded by bowel bacteria.

(2) *Alcohol consumption*. Alcohol contributes to elevation of the serum urate in several ways[6]. As already mentioned[7,8] it leads to degradation of adenine nucleotides to purine bases, which are degraded to uric acid. In addition, in its metabolism, there is an increase in lactate production and this acts at the renal tubule to reduce renal excretion of urate. Alcoholic beverages containing yeast, such as beer, may also contain considerable amounts of purines, often in the form of guanosine. Accordingly, the consumption of beer also functions as a purine load, the excretion of which is delayed by any associated lactic acidosis.

(3) *Obesity and hypertriglyceridemia*. While it was recognized over the centuries that many people with gout were obese, scientific support for an association between obesity and hyperuricemia has only recently been forthcoming[9,10]. However, as long ago as the nineteenth century cases were recorded in whom the tendency to gout remitted when the patient's obesity was corrected, often by the advent of hard times. In many Western societies, there is often now no lack of food and alcohol and such opulence of lifestyle often leads to obesity. Epidemiologic studies have confirmed a close correlation between body weight and the serum urate[11,12,13], although there is still some controversy concerning which measure of obesity correlates best with the serum urate concentration. Most studies support the use of the body mass index (weight/height^2).

Hypertriglyceridemia is also a very common association with gout. While in some patients this may be primary, in most cases the hypertriglyceridemia is intimately associated with both obesity and regular alcohol consumption. Other studies have suggested that the hypertriglyceridemia is independent of the patient's diet and body weight. Whatever the final mechanism of this association, which will be considered in more detail subsequently, hypertriglyceridemia is extremely common in Western-style societies in patients with gout.

(4) *Renal excretory capacity*. The normal renal clearance of urate is given as 8.7 ± 2.5 ml/min by Gutman and Yu[14]. This gives a range of urate clearance in 95% of the healthy population between approximately 3.7 and 13.7, which is an extremely wide clearance range ($>$ 3-fold). (In contrast, the clearance of creatinine in normal subjects ranges only about 10% to 15% on either side of the mean value.) Thus, a healthy normal subject with a urate clearance of 5 ml/min will have a much poorer renal excretory capacity for urate than one with a urate clearance of 15 ml/min. Factors that determine the level of the renal clearance of urate in normal subjects in a stable state are not well understood, but genetic factors are likely to be important in determining such a wide range of the normal clearance. Thus, persons with a low urate clearance may be considered as genetic underexcretors of urate. If such persons consume a low-purine diet, their renal excretory capacity for urate can cope with the urate load and maintain a normal serum urate concentration. However, once the environment provides a

significant purine load, the ability of the kidneys to eliminate this load is such that this can only be achieved at a higher serum rate concentration.

In addition to the intrinsic renal excretory capacity for urate, many drugs and metabolites can modify renal excretion of urate[6]. Plasma volume contraction from any cause promotes an increase in proximal tubular reabsorption of urate, as well as other ions, and several normal metabolites such as lactate and ketones and several hormones such as angiotensin and vasopressin are known to reduce renal excretion of urate. However, the most noted group of drugs that affect urate excretion and that are commonly used comprise the benzothiadiazine diuretic drugs, all of which result in hyperuricemia. The mechanism of the hyperuricemia is not precisely defined but is probably a combination of the volume contraction resulting from the diuretic together with some specific inhibition of urate excretory processes.

(5) *Renal disease*. The above consideration of renal excretory processes refers to a healthy kidney. However, most types of renal disease also result in a reduced capacity of the kidney to excrete urate as well as other nitrogenous products[15]. This results in a reduced total excretion of urate per 24 h[16] and there is some evidence that this is achieved in part by a reduction in urate production and in part by an increase in extrarenal elimination of urate. Tubulointerstitial varieties of renal disease often result in a greater increase in the serum urate concentration for any particular glomerular filtration rate than does primary glomerular disease. Chronic lead nephropathy is one variety of tubulointerstitial disease in which such excessive hyperuricemia is well documented[17]. However, there are many other varieties of chronic tubulointerstitial renal disease, such as analgesic nephropathy in which undue hyperuricemia seems likely. Hyperuricemia is also seen in reversible renal insufficiency.

(6) *Genetic urate overproduction*. Mutations in the enzymes hypoxathine-guanine phosphoribosyltransferase or of PRPP synthetase result in genetic overproduction of urate of considerable degree. Such overproduction of urate can be excreted by the kidney while it is healthy without the development of significant hyperuricemia. However, once there is any reduction in the ability of the kidney to handle this urate load, hyperuricemia results and there is the propensity for the development of renal disease caused by the deposition of crystals of either urate or of uric acid[16].

(7) *Hyperuricemia* is also a frequent finding in patients with myxedema or hyperparathyroidism, and is also found in patients with a chronic respiratory acidosis or in tissue damage such as occurs after myocardial infarction[6]. These are less commonly seen as primary factors causing hyperuricemia and gout but may contribute sufficiently to provoke this problem in patients in whom other contributory factors are operating.

The natural history of untreated gout

With several effective therapies available that can correct the hyperuricemia that is intrinsic to the development of gouty arthritis and its various complications, the natural history of untreated gout can now only be studied in subjects whose treatment has been neglected, either by themselves or by their physicians. It was as recently as 1955 that an article could be written which was titled "Gout — Now Amenable to Control"[18]. This was able to present some of the findings following treatment with probenecid, which was found to normalize the serum urate concentration and thereby prevent the development of acute gouty arthritis. It is, however, salutary to see another article in 1962[19] in which it is noted that "It is discouraging to report that a high percentage of patients fail to continue the now well-established long-term urate diuretic programme and therefore the challenge and therapy of gout today lies in the practical application of proven therapeutic measures." Despite this, the pattern of effective treatment is today sufficient for acute gouty arthritis to be no longer the foretaste of chronic gouty arthritis, which was so disabling prior to 1950. We must therefore principally seek evidence prior to the mid-1950s to determine the natural history of untreated gout.

The distinctive clinical pattern of attacks of gouty arthritis

That gout was able to be separated as a distinctive variety of arthritis by Hippocrates is well established[20]. This emphasizes the classical clinical pattern, namely an attack of acute monoarticular arthritis that remits completely and then recurs and then remits for progressively shorter periods. These acute attacks come on with considerable rapidity and severity and indeed it is informative to compare the Hippocratic description with the clinical criteria for the classification of the acute arthritis of primary gout as set out by the American Rheumatism Association[21]. This emphasizes that maximum inflammation develops within the first day, that relatively few joints are involved and that there is a special predilection for the first metatarsophalongeal joint to be affected.

Two aphorisms of Hippocrates are of particular relevance to the natural history, namely, (i) that an athlete could win a race in the Olympic Games in the interval between his acute attacks of gout, and (ii) that a woman does not develop gout until her menses be stopped. This is a clear forerunner of the current appreciation that the serum urate rises in the female after the menopause. Thus, the clinical pattern of acute gouty arthritis in the early stages has been very similar throughout the centuries. Acute attacks would recur unpredictably and would involve particularly the distal joints, especially of the lower limbs. They were regarded as occurring with increasing frequency until the patients passed into a stage of chronic gouty arthritis. Cartoons and caricatures of persons affected by gout have been recorded in "A Gallery of Gout" prepared by Rodnan[22] and these cover a selection of cartoons from the sixteenth century to the present day. Of the 32 figures included, all but three show a person with one or both feet swollen and elevated and too painful to walk on. Often they are pictured bound up and heavily padded to avoid even minor trauma. Patients so troubled are rarely seen today. It is notable also that most of the pictures in this gallery suggest a close association between chronic gouty arthritis and gluttony, obesity, and heavy alcohol consumption.

In 1941, Brochner-Mortensen[23] described the clinical features of 100 gouty patients. He was a particularly careful and reliable observer who had made a special study of gout and urate metabolism in Copenhagen prior to World War II. Of his 100 patients, 97 were males with an average age of 48 years and 71% of them were overweight. He reported moderate abuse of alcohol in 22% of patients and severe abuse in another 48%. This was mostly due to beer consumption. The gout affected the first metatarsophalangeal joint in 70% of patients and was polyarticular in 14%. Tophi were present in one-third and radiologic changes in one-half. Insofar as the kidneys were concerned, 21% demonstrated proteinuria and in 14% nephritis was detected that followed the development of acute gouty arthritis. He also reported five patients in whom chronic renal disease had preceded the gouty arthritis. Hypertension was found in 55% of his patients. These findings do not appear to be particularly different from those that could currently be seen today in patients with untreated gout.

Further observations were made on over 500 gouty patients from the San Francisco area of California in 1955[24]. In this group, there were three times as many males as females, whereas it is usually accepted there is a much greater male preponderance. The maximum incidence of gout was in the fifth decade in males and in the sixth decade in females. They also classified their patients into two categories, namely acute intermittent gout and chronic gout, the former being those with acute attacks and asymptomatic intervals, whereas the chronic gouty arthritis referred to those with constant musculoskeletal symptoms that required regular medication. The majority of their patients were classified as being chronic. Such chronic gout is now extremely rare. They found that only 10% of their patients demonstrated tophi, whereas 25% of the males and 36% of the females suffered from hypertension. Renal insufficiency was present in 5% of the males and 4% of the females and the chief cause of death was myocardial infarction. They commented that 50% of their patients were obese and noted a much higher incidence of hyperlipidemia in their gouty group. They found less alcoholism (6% of males and 3% of females) than is usually reported and less renal insufficiency. At that time, the authors were able to comment that effective treatment of acute gout included colchicine, ACTH, and phenylbutazone and that, in the management of hyperuricemia, probenecid was just becoming available. A follow-up of 19 gouty families over an 18-year period was published in 1964[25] and this study demonstrated that the prevalence of gout and asymptomatic hyperuricemia was increased among relatives of gouty patients. They demonstrated that, once hyperuricemia became manifest in a relative of a gouty subject, it tended to persist and increased the risk of the development of gout in that person. They also established again that hyperuricemia tended to become manifest in males after adolescence and that hyperuricemia rarely developed in female subjects until after the menopause.

Gutman had extensive experience of gout prior to the availability of urate-lowering drugs, which he described in a memorial lecture in 1965[26]. He showed that the frequency of attacks was relatively constant in one-third of subjects but that it increased progressively year after year in up to half. In the remainder, the periodicity of acute attacks was quite irregular. In half the patients, the severity of the attacks was relatively constant but in 30% the severity of the attack increased from year to year. He again emphasized the value of colchicine as a prophylactic agent against acute attacks of gout[27]. Many of his patients had taken colchicine prophylactically for up to 10 years without adverse effects. He noted, however, that half of his patients had tophi prior to the start of prophylaxis with colchicine and that one-third of the remainder became tophaceous on colchicine prophylaxis alone. Most of these observations would have referred to the period when there was no effective control of hyperuricemia. However, he did note that treatment with the recently available uricosuric agents both prevented the development of tophi and caused the existing tophi to become smaller. He found that between 10% and 20% of subjects with normal urate excretion developed uric acid calculi and that this doubled in overexcretors of uric acid. It is perhaps notable that Gutman at this time viewed gout as a distinctive disease state with a relatively homogeneous etiology which he believed was principally due to endogenous overproduction of urate.

Now that we appreciate the various factors that can modify the serum urate concentration it is more generally recognized that gout can be a sequel to sustained hyperuricemia whatever the cause, although hyperuricemia alone is not a sufficient cause for the development of gout. This has been well emphasized particularly in a long-term population study of the epidemiology of gout and hyperuricemia[29]. This study found clear evidence that the occurrence of gouty arthritis increased progressively with increasing serum urate concentrations, reaching a prevalence of 36% in those with serum urate concentrations above 8 mg% (0.48 mmol/l). They also found that, by the age of 58 years, 1.5% of the population had suffered at least one attack of gouty arthritis, with an increasing incidence of new attacks up to the age of 48 years. They reported a peak incidence at the age of 48 years with about 1 new case each year per 1000 subjects. However, of the patients they saw, only 1 in 4 had experienced more than 1 attack with the average number being 5. Of the subjects studied, 84% had suffered podagra on at least one occasion. They found urinary calculi in 11% of hyperuricemic subjects and 15% of those with gout. They also commented that subjects with gout tended to be overweight but that they were no more overweight than subjects with hyperuricemia who did not suffer from gout.

Later descriptions of gout inevitably reflect some alteration in the pattern because of the availability of therapy that would lower the serum urate concentration. A study of 354 patients with gout in London in 1970[29] showed some changes in the pattern from those described, but these were such as could be attributed to a different population being studied. In their group, 30% of the patients were regular alcohol drinkers and again the lower limb tended to be involved most frequently. One in 10 of their patients was female and their group included more members of higher social classes. Half of their patients were more than 50% above ideal weight and over one-third were regular drinkers. Twenty percent of patients had tophi. Half displayed hypertension, with about 10% having severe hypertension. Although one quarter showed nitrogen retention, they noted that the incidence of renal failure did not rise until gout had been present for over 40 years. However, they commented upon an apparently different group of young subjects in whom severe hypertension and renal failure were relatively common.

Gutman, again in 1971, commented on the picture of gout as seen at that time and noted a significant association with obesity, arteriosclerotic vascular disease, and essential hypertension[30]. They were so frequently associated with gout and their complications were often so much more serious than those of gout that their association could complicate and/or make difficult the interpretation of the natural history of gout. However, it is important that their significance should not be overlooked. Thus, the advent of drugs that will control hypertension and hyperlipidemia will also have had an effect upon the pattern of untreated gout, and this pattern will be modified not only by drugs that affect urate metabolism but by therapeutic maneuvers that can control hypertension and hyperlipidemia.

Hyperlipidemia and gout

The association between hyperuricemia, gouty arthritis, and other disease states is difficult if one is attempting to determine whether there is an etiologic relationship and the mechanism of any such association. Early examination of the relationship[31] concluded that male subjects with gouty arthritis had higher levels of blood pressure than usual and twice the usual risk of developing coronary heart disease. They also noted that they were more overweight and consumed more alcohol than usual.

The mechanism of the apparent increased risk of developing coronary heart disease in gouty subjects is still not fully defined. However, it has been well established that the common association of primary gout is with hypertriglyceridemia, with between half and three-quarters of gouty subjects showing this abnormality[32]. Hypercholesterolemia is present on occasion but not as consistently[33]. Since hyperlipidemia is also a feature of obesity, it is tempting to attribute the hyperuricemia and the hypertriglyceridemia to a common factor such as the obesity[34]. Different studies have yielded conflicting results. Even when gouty subjects and controls were matched for weight and height, a greater degree of hyperlipidemia was found in gouty subjects[35]. Yet further studies[36,37], however, have confirmed the link between hyperuricemia and hypertriglyceridemia as being mediated through the association with obesity and alcohol excess. The studies of Fessel[38], by contrast, suggested the association with cardiovascular disease was independent of body weight. Family studies of lipid and purine levels in gouty patients revealed the expected increased prevalence of hyperuricemia but no increase in prevalence of hyperlipoproteinemia in the first-degree relatives[39].

However, study of the association of gout with coronary heart disease in the Framingham survey[40] looked at the relationship between gout not associated with the use of diuretics and the development of coronary heart disease in over 5000 subjects. They showed that, in men who had never received diuretics, those who developed gout experienced a 60% excess of coronary heart disease in comparison with those without gout. In men, they showed that correction for systolic blood pressure, cholesterol, alcohol intake, and body mass index failed to alter this association and they reached the conclusion that gout unrelated to the intake of diuretics did impart an additional risk of coronary heart disease in men that was unexplained by the risk factors that had been measured. In addition, studies from Japan[41] concerning abnormalities of lipoprotein metabolism in gout (type 2A in 13% and type 4 in 69%) revealed that the two major associations of hypertriglyceridemia were alcohol intake and hyperuricemia but that the influence of alcohol intake was relatively small. They also showed another group of patients who did not exhibit either obesity or a history of alcohol intake but whose hyperlipidemia was greater than in control subjects. They too concluded that the hyperlipidemia of primary gout is unlikely to be secondary either to alcohol or obesity or both and invoked an additional genetic factor.

Thus, there is no doubt of the continued association of obesity, alcohol consumption, and hypertriglyceridemia in patients with gout and this may lead to the increased prevalence of coronary artery disease in such subjects. Certainly it is unlikely that there is a single answer to this problem so that, in some patients, obesity and alcoholism both independently lead to both hyperuricemia and hypertriglyceridemia, whereas in others different factors may cause one and not the other, and in yet other patients there may be some close association by a mechanism that is not yet fully defined.

Summary of the natural history of untreated gout

Untreated gout usually presented with a distinctive clinical pattern of recurrent severe arthritis with remissions that, in 80% of patients, affected the first metatarsophalangeal joint on at least one occasion. In half of the patients these attacks increased in frequency and severity with the passage of time, whereas in approximately one-third, the recurrent attacks occurred irregularly and with varying severity. After a variable period, usually of at least 10 years, remissions became infrequent and the patient developed a state of chronic gouty arthritis. In the majority of patients, this progressed to produce severe discomfort and disability. At least one-fifth of patients with gout developed tophi. Classically, males were affected much more commonly than females, with males being most affected in the fifth decade and females in the sixth decade of life.

Many other conditions were commonly associated with gouty arthritis, but their frequency depended very much upon the individual case. Several factors often contributed to the underlying hyperuricemia. Obesity was a very common association of gout, being present in over 50% of cases. Alcohol was consumed regularly in at least 30% of cases and hyperlipidemia was also very common. Hypertension was found in over a quarter of gouty patients and this was often associated with arteriosclerotic vascular disease. Ischemic heart disease was a frequent cause of death. Renal colic occurred at some time in 10% of patients but renal insufficiency was less common, being seen consistently in only 5% of patients and this usually only after 10 or more years of recurrent gouty arthritis. This pattern as described here varies widely in individual patients, the variability depending upon the particular factors contributing to gout in any particular individual.

Factors altering natural history over the last 25 years

(a) During this period, and particularly in Western civilizations, there has been a much greater *awareness of the diagnosis of gout*, which has generally led to its earlier recognition. This has presented the opportunity for instituting treatment both to settle the acute attacks and to correct the urate abnormality. With recognition of the role of urate crystals in the development of acute attacks of gout, the possibility of determining a specific diagnosis has increased greatly. Thus, advances in medical care and in early diagnosis and treatment have contributed significantly to changes in the natural history.

(b) This period saw the discovery and ready *availability of effective urate-lowering drugs*. These had the potential to correct the urate abnormality and essentially cure the patient as long as the drugs were taken. The first group of drugs that could normalize serum urate concentrations were the uricosuric drugs, particularly probenecid[42]. This agent is still used and is particularly effective in the commonest form of hyperuricemia due to urate underexcretion. Since that time, the more potent uricosuric agent sulfinpyrazone[43] has been developed as well as the more recent salicylate-like agent diflunisal. However, allopurinol became the most widely used agent to lower the serum urate during this period and proved to be generally effective[44,45]. It could restore in most patients the serum urate to a normal level, this resulting in resolution of tophi and the subsidence of acute attacks of gout. Complications were relatively few but when they occurred, particularly in patients with renal insufficiency or who were receiving diuretics, a severe hypersensitivity phenomenon with exfoliative dermatitis, fever, eosinophilia, hepatitis, and an acute interstitial nephritis could occur and be life-threatening in some patients[46]. Nonetheless, it has been the availability of drugs that, if taken regularly, can restore the serum urate to normal, that has been the dominant effect upon change in the natural history of gout.

(c) *Other drugs.* This period has seen not only the development of drugs that lower urate concentrations but also the development of the benzothiadiazine diuretics, which all reduce renal excretion of urate and cause hyperuricemia[47]. These drugs induce hyperuricemia even when used in low doses as antihypertensive agents and can contribute to further elevation of serum urate concentration and thereby contribute to the development of gout[48]. In addition, the development of nonsteroidal anti-inflammatory drugs (NSAIDs) has proved dramatically effective in the treatment of acute attacks of gout[49], but has often seemed to prevent acute inflammatory reactions at the expense of allowing the formation of urate deposits in the absence of any acute attack. These drugs have been dramatic for symptomatic control, but their side-effects have caused concern.

(d) *The recognition of correctable factors.* During this period, it was gradually recognized that the serum urate concentration was the result of many factors that contribute in a variety of ways either towards raising or towards lowering the serum urate concentrations[50]. Particularly in opulent societies, high-purine and high-protein foods are readily available and frequently consumed. Similarly, obesity is a common problem, and the consumption of beer and other alcohol products is widespread. Thus, the general affluence of Western societies has contributed to higher mean serum urate concentrations in the general population. With higher basal urate levels in the community, it is easier for additional exogenous factors to cause the development of critical hyperuricemia. If this is sufficiently sustained, it will result in a higher incidence of gout. Thus, the common clinical subgroups of gout presently seen are usually those with either (i) underexcretion gout, (ii) underexcretion gout plus exogenous overconsumption of purines, or (iii) overproduction of urate due to genetic mutations or excessive nucleoprotein degradation.

(e) The more serious risk factors relating to gout in relation to longevity are cardiovascular[38,40]. Hyperuricemia has been regularly demonstrated to be an associate of cardiovascular disease, with some studies suggesting that it is independent of obesity and others attributing it to obesity plus hyperlipidemia. Nonetheless, the more widespread recognition of the importance of correcting risk factors for cardiovascular disease has inevitably altered the prognosis for vascular disease in patients with gout. Thus, in a patient who presents with an initial acute attack of gout, it may be more important so far as future health is concerned to correct obesity, hyperlipidemia, hypertension, and smoking than it is to direct attention principally to controlling hyperuricemia.

The factors already mentioned reflect only some of the great changes in medical practice that have developed in the period under study and that have contributed in no small way to changes in the natural history of gout since the early 1960s.

Current clinical presentations of gout

The only acceptable therapeutic result in a patient with gout is a normal serum urate and no acute attacks of gouty arthritis. If this can be achieved, is the prognosis thereafter normal? In seeking an answer to the question, one would comment first that the evidence is not yet completely documented. However, most physicians managing patients with gout act on the basis that a patient with gout whose serum urate has been normalized with drugs should have as normal a prognosis as if he had never suffered from gout, except insofar as that prognosis may be altered by complications of drug treatment.

Gout now presents clinically mostly in the following ways:

Atypical gout

Classical gout is usually of considerable severity, monoarticular, and associated with complete remissions in the early phases. Variations in any of these aspects may be regarded as being atypical and such atypical gout is now recognized more frequently[50]. Our ability to confirm the diagnosis by arthrocentesis and demonstrating urate crystals has provided an objective criterion for diagnosis that was previously lacking. Sometimes this atypical presentation is due to poor compliance with therapy or the use of anti-inflammatory agents that can prevent the symptoms and signs of acute gout but are unable to prevent the crystal deposition. Occasionally, gout may affect the axial skeleton, where it may destroy vertebral bone and cause a radiculopathy[51].

Pauciarticular gout is also seen much more commonly. In one series[52], 40% of 106 consecutive patients had inflammation of at least two joints. As a group, their gout often seemed to be the result of inadequate compliance and understanding of their management, with resulting inadequate control of hyperuricemia. Such patients with polyarticular gout tended to be in the "chronic gouty arthritis" category, with joint involvement starting peripherally in the lower limbs and extending proximally in an asymmetrical fashion to involve finally the upper limb joints, which were sometimes involved at the same time as joints of the lower limb.

Gout in the female

Gout still affects fewer women before the menopause, with 90% of female gout being postmenopausal[53,54]. The onset is thus much later than in the male and the patients are often 70 years of age or more. Clinical features can vary widely. Up to 70% are said to present with a subacute pauciarticular polyarthritis, and in most of these there has been no preceding monoarthritis[55]. In many others, gout may present initially with polyarticular involvement — women are much less likely than men to present with a classical monoarticular pattern[56]. Underlying osteoarthritis is particularly common and tophi are present in between 30% and 40% of patients. In general, the duration of the disease before tophi appear is shorter than in males. Associated factors that may be important etiologically include diuretic therapy (present in up to 80%), renal impairment, and/or hypertension[54]. It is therefore in women that the clinical pattern of acute gouty arthritis appears to have changed most away from the classical description.

Gout in the elderly

With the tendency for people to live longer, more elderly people will be seen to develop renal insufficiency. In addition, modern drug treatment can prevent many of the unpleasant complications of heart failure and prolong life. However, this is often at the cost of hyperuricemia due in part to the modest renal insufficiency frequent in the elderly and in part to diuretic therapy[57,58]. Gout in the elderly is more often atypical, sometimes affecting the hand before the foot[57]. As mentioned, it is particularly common in elderly women[59] who are prone to develop tophi[60].

Diuretic-induced gout

Within a few years of the widespread use of thiazide diuretics, reports appeared of their association with gout[61-63]. There has been much controversy about the mechanism of diuretic-induced hyperuricemia. There is good evidence[64] that the principal cause of this hyperuricemia is plasma volume contraction resulting in excessive proximal tubular reabsorption of many compounds, including urate. There have also been suggestions that there is a specific effect on tubular secretion of urate but this has not been established. However, most of our knowledge about intrarenal handling of urate is indirect and it is difficult to exclude other factors additional to plasma volume contraction[65].

Just how frequently diuretic therapy contributes sufficiently to cause acute gouty arthritis in someone not otherwise likely to develop gout is difficult to determine. Most physicians will have seen patients in whom there were major reductions in the serum urate concentrations with the withdrawal of thiazide diuretics and in some patients it is impossible to control hyperuricemia while they are still receiving these drugs. However, a study of large numbers of hypertensive patients[66] showed relatively few episodes of gout in over 3000 patients treated for hypertension in the Hypertension Detection and Follow-up Program (HDFP). It seems most likely that the increase in serum urate induced by diuretics is relatively slight in the presence of normal renal function but that it can become quite significant when larger doses of diuretics are used in patients with hypertension or in patients with preexisting renal disease. Thus diuretics are an important contributory factor in hyperuricemia and gout, although the extent of their contribution alone is not well defined.

Gout in osteoarthritic joints

In keeping with the atypical nature of gout in the elderly, gout may sometimes present principally as what appears to be an acutely inflamed Heberden's node[67]. Degenerative joint disease has long been recognized as forming a nidus for urate crystal deposition and gout often developed severely in joints affected by osteoarthritis. Similarly, calcium pyrophosphate and urate crystals are sometimes together in a single joint fluid, implying that chondrocalcinosis articularis and gout may coexist.

Tophus formation without acute gouty arthritis

Deposition of urate crystals in soft tissues without the development of an acute inflammatory response, such as usually occurs in joints, can occur in some patients with hyperuricemia. This has been referred to as nonarticular gout[68]. In these patients, no history of acute gouty arthritis can be obtained but silent tophi may develop. This brings up the question of why no inflammatory response is occurring. A similar situation must apply during tophus formation in the ear. However, it has generally been considered to be unusual for tophi to develop in the absence of articular gout. One of the important factors in allowing this to happen more frequently may be the concurrent use of anti-inflammatory drugs and these may so inhibit the inflammatory response to urate crystal formation that any acute gouty arthritis is aborted at a very early stage. Another factor that would minimize the polymorph response to urate crystals would be renal insufficiency. Whether these constitute the true explanation of the development of tophi in skin, cartilage, and other tissues and organs cannot be determined, but certainly the presentation of urate crystal deposition as tophi without gouty arthritis is now an important type of clinical presentation of gout. It seems to be particularly common in women.

Renal gout

The kidney is normally responsible for the elimination of two-thirds of the urate that is produced. Accordingly, any interference with renal elimination of urate will result in hyperuricemia unless compensatory processes either reduce the production of urate or facilitate alternative methods of elimination. Thus, there are two principal mechanisms by which the kidney can cause hyperuricemia due to impairment of renal elimination. Such renal underexcretion of urate can occur either (i) in the absence of any renal disease or renal damage, or (ii) as a component of renal disease.

(i) Renal underexcretion of urate has been postulated as an important cause of hyperuricemia in gouty patients for well over thirty years. In the 1950s, there was intense controversy about whether gout was caused by underexcretion of urate or by overproduction of urate, with active proponents for each view. This was finally resolved by the acceptance that both factors may contribute in different patients. However, in some patients the renal factor is dominant but it occurs as a graded characteristic. Thus, in 1959, Nugent and Tyler[69] provided evidence of defective renal excretion of urate in patients with gout; in 1970 Reiselbach et al.[70] provided data to demonstrate diminished renal excretion of urate per nephron as the basis for primary gout. More recently, impaired tubular transport of urate has been demonstrated in gouty subjects that is unrelated to the serum urate concentration[71]. In all of these patients, renal glomerular function was normal.

(ii) *Renal underexcretion with renal disease.* In most varieties of chronic renal disease, there is reduced renal excretion of many nitrogenous compounds, including uric acid. This results in a decreased urate clearance and hyperuricemia. However, as the GFR falls, renal excretion of urate per nephron rises, which minimizes further progression of hyperuricemia as the renal disease advances[72]. Gout is not a common feature of most varieties of chronic renal disease, and it seems that certain adaptive mechanisms prevent progressive rises in the serum urate concentrations in uncomplicated cases. Moreover, altered leukocyte reactivity occurs in chronic renal insufficiency, and this may reduce the body's response to hyperuricemia and the formation of urate crystals.

However, disproportionate hyperuricemia and a significant association with gout is seen in patients with some specific varieties of renal disease, and there is now good evidence that certain types of chronic renal disease, particularly those that can be broadly classified as being tubulointerstitial, have an increased association with gout. The first of these to be established was chronic lead nephropathy, where half of the patients affected develop gouty arthritis. Such patients have usually had renal disease for about 10 years before developing gout and the gout they developed was less severe than usual, both in the number of attacks and the number of joints involved.[73] This type of gout is rarely as disabling as the chronic tophaceous gout that was reported in the nineteenth century. Other varieties of tubulointerstitial renal disease that may result in the development of gout include several varieties of toxic nephropathy and probably also analgesic nephropathy. Chronic pyelonephritis and hypertensive nephrosclerosis have also been incriminated.[74]

Both polycystic kidney disease and medullary cystic kidney disease (nephronophthisis) are associated with an increased incidence of gout. Up to one-third of patients with polycystic kidney disease suffer from gout and hyperuricemia is even more common[75,76]. The familial occurrence of hyperuricemia and gout in families with medullary cystic disease is also well documented[77,78]. In addition, there are often varieties of kidney disease that present as an insidious nephropathy with a clear inheritance pattern, often dominant, which have a clear association with hyperuricemia and gout[79].

Allopurinol sensitivity

With the widespread use of allopurinol in the community, sometimes for dubious indications such as the presence of asymptomatic hyperuricemia, there is a steady increase in the number of patients who have demonstrated sensitivity to allopurinol. These are most commonly patients with moderate renal insufficiency, often apparently due to aging, who have been on treatment with diuretics, either for heart failure or for hypertension, and who have been receiving allopurinol in a dose that is inappropriately high for the level of their renal function. Thus, allopurinol sensitivity is now a not uncommon finding in patients with severe gout[46]. Such patients may have severe ulcerating tophaceous gout and their management may be rendered difficult if there is associated renal insufficiency or a continuing need for diuretics. The uricosuric response becomes blunted once the GFR has fallen to approximately 60 ml/min, although there is considerable individual difference in the magnitude of the response to uricosuric drugs at different levels of renal function. The necessity to use diuretics concurrently makes it extremely difficult to lower the serum urate and alternative agents to the diuretics need to be tried. Desensitization to allopurinol by steadily increasing doses has rarely proved effective in our hands, although there are several reports of a satisfactory response.[80,81]

It seems likely that the pathogenesis of allopurinol sensitivity does not involve a single homogeneous mechanism. Certainly in some patients, abnormal lymphocyte reactivity to oxypurinol has been demonstrated, suggesting that some of these adverse reactions may represent delayed hypersensitivity to the metabolite.[82] In persistent sensitivity to allopurinol, the only drug that can be used effectively is one of the uricosuric group, usually sulfinpyrazone or diflunisal.

KIDNEY DISEASE DUE TO GOUT

As has already been emphasized, gout is a many-faceted syndrome and not a disease with a homogeneous etiology. Likewise, there are many mechanisms by which the kidney can be damaged. It is therefore not surprising that the relationship between gout and the kidney is varied rather than constant. The type of gout that occurs secondary to primary renal disease has already been emphasized and its distinctive characteristics have been described. What remains to be examined is the renal disease that is sometimes seen in patients with chronic gouty arthritis.

The frequency of renal stones in patients with gout was first noted in 1683 by Sydenham[83] and the association of gout and proteinuria was recorded by Scudamore in 1823[84]. By 1843, Castelnau had described uric acid deposits in the kidney of gouty patients as well as in their joints[85]. Todd in 1857[86] described "a contracted state of the kidney which was particularly apt to be developed in the inveterate gouty diathesis." Garrod in 1876 considered the specific renal lesion of gout as being distinctive crystalline deposits of uric acid that he observed in "all cases of chronic chalk gout where the opportunity of making the examination was afforded[87]." Schnitker and Richter in 1936 could clearly distinguish gout that was secondary to renal disease but still identified an incidence of renal disease in one-third of their patients with primary gout[88]. Brochner-Mortensen in 1940 also recorded renal disease in a quarter of his patients with gout[23]. Brown and Mallory[89] commented on the presence of tubular obstruction that they attributed to intratubular uric acid deposits that occurred together with medullary urate deposits, both of which were complicated by pyelonephritic scarring and vascular disease, which they attributed to hypertension and arteriosclerosis.

However, the most definitive study was that of Talbot and Terplan in 1960[90]. They undertook an extensive autopsy study of almost 300 patients with gout and found a wide variety of lesions. They concluded that the distinctive pathologic feature of the gouty kidney was the presence of urate crystals and that these induced a surrounding giant cell reaction. Most workers subsequently have accepted this definition of the gouty kidney as one in which the primary pathology results from the formation of urate and uric acid crystals.

More recent studies[29] have confirmed the presence of renal insufficiency in 25% of large groups of patients with gout and recorded a positive correlation between impairment of renal function and the presence of tophi. However, renal insufficiency of critical degree was rarely seen until late middle age.

Mechanisms by which uric acid and urate can cause renal damage

Deposition of uric acid within the renal tubules can occur whenever the concentration and pH are appropriate. Very high serum urate concentrations will develop in leukemia and during the chemotherapy of malignancy[91,92]. It is also seen in patients with HGPRT deficiency[93], in whom an elevated uric acid-to-creatinine ratio may be found[94]. However, studies by Seegmiller and Frazier[95] demonstrated the presence of urate crystals in the renal interstitium as well as uric acid crystals within the kidneys of patients with gout. It would be expected that interstitial microtophi can develop between the renal tubules whenever conditions are appropriate for this to occur[16]. Conditions within the renal papilla would often be more favorable towards the formation of such microtophi than that in many other bodily tissues[96]. There is, moreover, evidence that the lining epithelium of the collecting duct can react with intraluminal crystals so that the crystals can pass either through the cells or between the tight junctions between the cells into the renal interstitium where they can induce inflammatory changes and a giant-cell response. When to this is added the presence or absence of hypertension, the presence or absence of vascular disease, the presence or absence of urinary tract infection, and the presence or absence of renal calculus disease, it is not difficult to explain why there is such a variable prevalence of renal disease in patients with gout.

It has recently been said that renal disease in patients with gout is now a rare finding[97]. This would not necessarily be surprising now that we have effective therapy for hyperuricemia, for hypertension, for urinary tract infection, and for hyperlipidemia. We now have available therapeutic measures that should be able to normalize all of the factors that have been postulated as contributing to the development of the gouty kidney. Many of these could contribute to renal disease even in the absence of a uric acid abnormality, so that control of the abnormal urate crystal formation by urate-lowering drugs should at least remove the possibility that gout could contribute to the renal disease. Indeed, there are reports indicating that control of hyperuricemia with allopurinol resulted in no change in renal function over a 2-year period, whereas some deterioration was observed in those not so treated. Again this supports the hypothesis that uric acid and urate crystal formation is essential to the formation of gouty renal disease[98].

Thus, in the 1990s most cases of gout, especially if adequately treated, do not lead to the development of renal insufficiency. Such a generalization may not apply to gout in patients with tophi. However, tophi should not develop in an adequately treated patient. Follow-up of patients with serum urate concentrations of 0.7 mmol/l for over 20 years has not necessarily shown any progression of renal damage, unless factors other than the hyperuricemia were able to contribute. Thus, unless hyperuricemia becomes severe or there are other complicating factors, gout should not be looked upon as a factor that commonly contributes to the development of renal damage[99-101].

The subject of the gouty kidney has been reviewed by the author in greater detail in several recent textbooks of nephrology[102,103].

CRITICAL REVIEW OF THE PROGNOSIS LITERATURE CONCERNING GOUT

The prognosis of untreated gout and the risks of development of the various complications have already been outlined, together with the extent to which the prognosis is altered by control of the hyperuricemia that prevents acute gouty arthritis. A recent study of over 2000 men over a 15-year period revealed that the strongest influence determining the risk of developing acute gouty arthritis was the level of the serum urate concentration[104]. At serum urate concentrations below 0.4 mmol/l, the risk of developing gout was less than 0.1% per annum. At values of between 0.42 mmol/l and 0.53 mmol/l the annual incidence of gouty arthritis was 0.5%. However, this increased to a 5% annual incidence in patients with serum urate concentrations greater than 0.54 mmol/l, at which values the cumulative incidence of gouty arthritis after 5 years amounted to 22%. These more recent data confirm previous studies with similar conclusions. They also revealed that the dominant factors that determined the serum urate consisted of age, body mass index, hypertension, serum cholesterol, and alcohol intake. Study of renal function in these patients failed to reveal any evidence of deterioration of renal function that could be attributed to hyperuricemia per se. This study supports the conservative management of asymptomatic hyperuricemia and stresses the importance of preventive reduction of contributing factors, rather than early drug treatment to lower serum urate concentrations[104].

Thus, essentially all the defined complications of gout, the acute attacks, tophus formation, and the renal disease, can be attributed to urate crystal deposition and subsequent pathologic changes. Effective therapy is available and the prognosis should be excellent as far as uric acid complications are concerned.

Renal stones occur with an increased frequency in gouty patients, with between 5% and 10% of patients suffering from renal colic at some time and occasionally prior to the first attack. This prevalence is much greater than in the nongouty population[105]. The stones consist sometimes of uric acid and in other patients of calcium oxalate. However, both can be prevented either by the use of an alkaline diuresis or regular administration of allopurinol. Thus, this potential complication of gout is similarly preventable and should not adversely affect prognosis once the particular problem has been recognized and appropriate therapy instituted.

However, coronary artery disease is the biggest cause of mortality in patients with gout and this has improved with recognition of risk factors and their prevention. Thus, a significant reduction in the death rate from coronary heart disease has been reported from 46% between 1950 and 1967 to 34% between 1968 and 1979[106]. More recent comparisons of the vascular mortality in patients with gout and their families[107] did not reveal any increased risk of death from coronary artery or cerebrovascular disease in the gouty patients or their relatives. Presumably, the mortality was determined more by other factors than by gout. However, a more recent analysis of the Framingham data[40] showed a 60% excess of coronary heart disease in gouty males as compared with those without gout. Although other pathogenic risk factors were present, the study found that control for the systolic blood pressure, the total cholesterol, the body mass index, or alcohol intake did not alter this excess of coronary heart disease in gouty males. No such association was found in women. It reached the conclusion, unlike earlier studies, that gout imparts an additional risk of coronary heart disease in men that was not explained by recognized risk factors. Hyperuricemia without gout, on the other hand, was not associated with any increased risk of coronary vascular disease. This study emphasized the importance of subjects with gout being assessed for vascular, particularly cardiovascular, disease. It was unable to determine whether correction of hyperuricemia made any difference to this increased incidence of coronary heart disease. This problem was previously studied by life insurance companies, and patients with a history of gout had once been loaded with a higher premium if they were accepted for life insurance. However an extensive study of hundreds of thousands of individuals with over 18 000 deaths in the continental United States in 1954 revealed that mortality in men affected by gout was not different from normal[108]. A separate study of longevity in three groups of patients in the United States (Boston and Buffalo) revealed that the mortality rate of patients with gout was no different from that of the general population[109]. A more recent study by Yu and Talbott[106] failed to show that the development of gout altered the risk of mortality from coronary heart disease. Gutman in New York[30] recorded his extensive experience in gouty subjects in whom urate-lowering therapy had been used to only a limited extent. Of 1600 patients, 14% had died at a mean age of 63 years and 60% of these deaths were due to cardiovascular or cerebrovascular disease. Eighteen percent were attributed to renal insufficiency and of these 30% had renal insufficiency attributable to gouty nephropathy, while similar percentages had malignant hypertension and nephrosclerosis or chronic pyelonephritis[110]. Thus, all data to hand, with the exception of the Framingham study, suggest that mortality from gout is essentially no different from patients who do not develop gout. The Framingham study however, is probably the most comprehensive and reliable and urges caution with this interpretation, at least until we have further leads as to possible mechanisms. Further elucidation will probably depend upon unravelling the interrelationships between uric acid and coronary vascular disease.

With effective therapy so readily available, an important complicating factor in gout is the incidence of complications from drug treatment. The problem of sensivitity to allopurinol has already been mentioned and, while individual cases are dramatic, many either settle or respond rapidly to treatment and the risk to life is numerically small. Uricosuric drugs have the theoretical potential problem of inducing renal damage because of the high urinary uric acid concentrations they initially cause. However, specific comparison by Talbott and Yu[111] failed to demonstrate any difference in the cause of death in treated as opposed to untreated patients with gout. It certainly did not demonstrate any increase in mortality from the use of probenecid or allopurinol. It did not, however, demonstrate any improvement in vascular mortality with the use of these agents, but the numbers studied were relatively small.

In summary, therefore, we now have available a therapeutic armamentarium that should enable the uric acid abnormality associated with gout to be corrected in the great majority of patients. If correction of the associated hyperuricemia can be achieved, the risk of subsequent complications affecting the joints, the kidney, or soft tissue i.e., tophus formation can be regarded as minimal, especially if other risk factors for coronary artery disease can be controlled. A treated gouty patient with a normal serum urate has essentially a similar risk of mortality to that of a nongouty person and this risk is largely dependent upon the asociated risk factors for cardiovascular disease.

PYROPHOSPHATE CPPD CRYSTAL-DEPOSITION DISEASE

In this condition, rhomboidal crystals of calcium pyrophosphate dihydrate (CPPD) or pyrophosphate are found within joint fluid, often associated with calcification in articular cartilage and an inflammatory response, usually involving an accumulation of polymorphs. This condition was not recognized until the early 1960s when the clinical associations of the radiologic appearance, chondrocalcinosis articularis, were first described[112]. This showed up as calcification within joint cartilage. Working independently, McCarty, in extending his studies of arthritis due to urate crystals, found crystals in joint fluid that were not urate but that were associated with acute joint inflammation[113]. These crystals were eventually shown to be pyrophosphate. Injection of these crystals into the normal joints of experimental animals was shown to cause an acute arthritis, so that an etiologic relationship seemed to be established between the presence of the crystals and the associated arthritis. Although the syndrome was originally referred to as pseudogout, the more varied clinical presentations of CPPD crystal deposition disease have generally been elucidated[113,114]. McCarty originally defined pseudogout as "a clinical syndrome of acute, usually recurrent, synovitis of large joints in elderly persons associated with intraleukocytic calcium pyrophosphate dihydrate crystals in the aspirate from the affected joint." However, some patients show symptoms only of degenerative arthritis and synovial fluid from these patients usually shows large numbers of extraleukocytic crystals[115]. Roentgenograms often show characteristic articular calcifications; these calcifications are composed of microcrystals identical to those found in joint fluid. Other early reports indicated that the joints most involved were the knees and that the acute phase was sometimes associated with a fever and leukocytosis. Articular calcification was particularly common in the menisci and other areas of the knee, the wrist, the hip, the symphysis pubis, and the shoulder[114]. Linear calcification in the menisci was particularly common, as was polyarticular involvement.

Diagnosis was greatly assisted by the recognition that CPPD crystals could be identified by polarized-light microscopy, in which the crystals were often seen to be rhomboidal in shape (rather than acicular as with urate) and were positively birefringent (as opposed to the negative birefringence of urate crystsls).

Pathogenesis

Both calcium and pyrophosphate are ubiquitous. Pyrophosphate is the product of many biosynthetic reactions and is readily hydrolyzed to orthophosphate. An increased pyrophosphate concentration has been described in synovial fluid in CPPD deposition disease but not within the plasma. Moreover, collections of crystals have been demonstrated within cartilage and periarticular tissues and this observation has suggested that an acute arthropathy may be precipitated either by shedding of preexisting crystals or by their acute crystallization[116]. It has been shown that CPPD crystals may be taken up by synovial cells and that this can cause release of collagenase, which can then induce further release of deposited crystals. It is also thought that ionic imbalances and localized metabolic disorders or abnormalities within the cartilage matrix can promote deposition of CPPD crystals. However, the precise factors that promote deposition and crystallization are as yet ill-defined. One might also comment that, in regard to urate crystal deposition disease, which is generally a better-understood entity, the factors that precipitate urate crystal formation are also relatively poorly understood. Histologically, CPPD crystal collections have been detected at the border of the articular and subarticular cartilage as well as large agglomerations of randomly arranged crystals, some of which replace chondrocytes[117].

Varieties of CPPD-associated arthritis

Heredofamilial

Chondrocalcinosis is often familial and up to 10% of cases of CPPD-induced arthritis are of familial origin. Pedigree follow-up has enabled mild cases to be defined in whom the arthropathy was not severe but in whom the clinical and radiologic features were otherwise distinctive[118]. In general, these patients are usually of Caucasian origin, are of a younger age group and often show marked radiologic changes. Current evidence suggests an autosomal dominant mode of inheritance in most affected families. Radiologically, the hereditary variety is usually indistinguishable from other types of chondrocalcinosis[119]. An increase in the pyrophosphate content of fibroblasts from affected members of a kindred with hereditary chondrocalcinosis has been reported[120].

Metabolic associated disease

(a) *Hyperparathyroidism.* Chondrocalcinosis has been reported in up to one-third of patients who have had a parathyroidectomy for hyperparathyroidism[121]. This type of patient is usually middle-aged. Pseudogout is a particular risk after parathyroidectomy[122]. It has been postulated that lowering of the ionized calcium after operation tends to dissolve CPPD crystals and that this may loosen them from their deposits and allow them to be shed acutely into a joint.

(b) *Hemochromatosis.* This is a well-established association and needs regularly to be considered[123].

(c) *Hypomagnesemia.* This association is strongly suggested[124]. It has been suggested that, since magnesium promotes solubilization of CPPD, a fall in magnesium concentration can promote the formation of CPPD crystals.

(d) *Hypophosphatasia.* A rare but well-documented association.

(e) *Gout.* Up to 6% of patients with gout show chondrocalcinosis[125].

(f) Other conditions, such as alkaptonuria/ochronosis, hypothyroidism, and Wilson's disease are less definitely associated[123,126].

Sporadic cases

CPPD deposition disease is very common in old age and sporadic cases tend to be especially associated with previously damaged joints. This has been reported in a localized form with unstable joints[127] and in neuropathic joints[128]. CPPD crystal arthropathy has also been associated with osteoarthritis, rheumatoid arthritis, hypermobility, and joint surgery. The condition has also been associated with many other conditions such as hypertension, arteriosclerosis, and diabetes but these are all common in the elderly and it seems more likely that the factor in common in this association is advancing years. Renal insufficiency has been observed as an association in young persons as well, so that there may be some etiologic association between chronic renal failure and CPPD crystal arthropathy in patients with chronic renal failure[129].

Prevalence of chondrocalcinosis in the menisci at autopsy

Extensive studies of knees at autopsy have shown calcification in 5.6%, with 3.3% being composed of CPPD and 2.3% of basic calcium phosphate[130]. More recently, a study of pathologic calcification in menisci in a large group of patients without a history of joint disorder found calcification in 20% of patients, all over 60 years of age[131]. This was much commoner in the female and increased progressively with age. Calcification was in menisci as well as within cartilage and severe damage to articular cartilage was found with an increased frequency in joints showing articular calcification.

Natural history of CPPD deposition disease

The clinical presentations of this condition are diverse. They may be classified as follows.

(1) *Acute arthritis — pseudogout.* The most acute presentation of CPPD crystal arthropathy occurs as an acute arthritis, generally of lesser severity than gouty arthritis. This arthritis tends to be slower to settle but to be ultimately self-limiting. However, it can become recurrent, especially in younger males[132]. Narrowing of the joint space is often seen at an early stage and this has been attributed to concurrence of chondrocalcinosis with osteoarthritis[133]. The knee is the most commonly affected joint in the acute arthritis, followed by involvement of the feet, wrists, or hands[114]. Indeed, involvement of the knees, hands, wrists, and feet is a particularly common feature of CPPD deposition. Pseudogout tends to occur more commonly in persons under the age of 60 years and is a rather more frequent presentation in men than in women. Almost 10% of patients develop acute attacks only[132].

(2) *Subacute arthritis.* This tends to be pauciarticular and presents clinically with features of an acute arthritis that often fails to subside completely. In some it may resemble rheumatoid arthritis.

(3) *Chronic pyrophosphate arthropathy.* Again, this affects particularly the knees but also the ankles and shoulders are frequently involved. It has been referred to as pseudo-osteoarthritis, although it can have superimposed acute episodes. It tends to be bilateral and extraleukocytic crystals are found in the synovial fluid. Effusions are common and may show relatively little evidence of acute inflammation[123]. Radiologic changes are almost invariable. However, it should be noted that acute joint calcification has been observed to clear, suggesting that peripheral shedding of crystal deposits may occur.

This variety is the commonest and may represent over half the patients[134]. The chronic form tends to be polyarticular, although it is rare for the knee not to be involved at some time. Radiologic evidence of osteoarthritis of the hips, back, and hands is often found. Hand disease is particularly common[132], with both the distal and proximal interphalangeal joints being frequently involved. The first carpometacarpal joint is affected in over half of the patients.

Radiologically, the changes are similar to those in osteoarthritis but there are distinctive differences in:

(a) Increased involvement of non-weight-bearing joints such as the wrist, elbow, and shoulder.
(b) An unusual intra-articular distribution.
(c) Prominent subchondral cyst formation.
(d) Progressive bone changes with osteophyte formation being more variable than in osteoarthritis[134]. Linear calcification of cartilage is particularly distinctive and calcification of the fibro-cartilage in the symphysis pubis is highly suggestive. Involvement of hand joints tends to be patchy rather than symmetrical.

(4) *Asymptomatic presentation.* Up to 40% of knees showing meniscal calcification characteristic of CPPD disease are asymptomatic. Thus, the crystal deposition can be silent and the presence of CPPD crystals is insufficient by itself to cause an arthropathy[135]. The precise factors that determine the onset of an inflammatory response to either crystal deposition or release are not well identified.

The clinical features of CPPD arthropathy may be even more varied than implied by the above types of clinical presentation. There are also reports of unusual presentations such as one with acute back pain as the dominant symptom and another with symptoms resembling polymyalgia rheumatica[136] and such deposits have resulted in cervical myelopathy[138]. A most unusual presentation has been with acute inflammation of the temporomandibular joint with severe facial pain[139]. On other occasions, a severe, widespread polyarthritis with severe joint destruction has been recorded[140]. Fever has, at times, been a major feature and this has caused difficulty in diagnosis because the joint symptoms were not particularly dominant[141].

Treatment

Treatment is relevant to prognosis when it can alter the natural history of the disease. The inflammatory component of CPPD-associated arthropathy is usually well-controlled with nonsteroidal anti-inflammatory drugs that inhibit prostaglandin synthetase and have anti-inflammatory effects at higher doses. Aspiration of an affected joint will often promote subsidence of joint inflammation and the addition of intra-articular steroids will often cause subsidence of a joint that is not responding to simpler measures. Intravenous colchicine has been reported to be of value[142] and oral colchicine has also been used. There has been no definitive study of its value vis-à-vis the nonsteroidal anti-inflammatory agents. One would expect that colchicine would demonstrate a beneficial effect principally in the more acute inflammatory varieties. Prophylaxis with colchicine has been shown to be effective in recurrent attacks of pseudogout and has been associated with a reduction of acute episodes by two-thirds. Accordingly, oral colchicine appears to be valuable as a prophylactic agent in recurrent pseudogout[143].

In the absence of knowledge of the basic biochemical abnormality that allows precipitation of the CPPD crystals and the anti-inflammatory response thereto, it is difficult to institute any measures to prevent crystal formation. The judicious use of nonsteroidal anti-inflammatory drugs, aspiration, and intra-articular steroids can usually promote subsidence in any acute inflammation. Even in the subacute to chronic states, these measures, together with physiotherapy, will usually provide symptomatic relief. If joint destruction becomes too severe, joint replacement may be the only measure left. Correction of the associated metabolic disease, while it clearly should be attempted, rarely makes a major difference to the joint symptoms.

Critical review of prognosis

This condition has been known for only a single generation and, since it is principally a condition of the elderly and since knowledge of the basic pathogenesis of the condition is poor, there is little information concerning prognosis in the different varieties of the condition. In the heredofamilial variety, patients often suffered from chronic pain that resulted in earlier retirement from work. Back pain was common but this did not usually cause ankylosis or deformity. Calcification of intervertebral discs was found more commonly in some families than in sporadic cases. They regarded the condition in the familial cases as being severe and incapacitating, much more so than in the sporadic pyrophosphate arthropathy[144].

In most patients with sporadic disease, however, the pattern is one of an initial acute arthritic episode, which may be recurrent. After some years this may pass into a subacute or chronic arthritic state. In the chronic state, pain may be a persistent problem and this may cause considerable disability unless it can be relieved or controlled by anti-inflammatory drugs. Progressive joint damage tends to develop and this may become incapacitating unless it can be corrected. If joint damage is severe, arthroplasty may be needed. There are no reports of prolonged follow-up of large numbers of asymptomatic cases from which to determine their progress.

Future perspectives

Little is known of the factors that result in crystal formation and growth in this condition, although abnormalities of cartilage or pyrophosphate metabolism have been postulated. The increased prevalence in preexisting joint damage is frequently associated with crystal deposition and this suggests that abnormalities in the cartilage are major contributors. Further progress will depend upon an extension of our understanding of the factors that predispose to crystal formation and deposition and the tissue reaction thereto.

BASIC CALCIUM PHOSPHATE (BCP) OR APATITE-ASSOCIATED ARTHROPATHY

The crystals found in this condition consist of a carbonate-substituted hydroxyapatite, together with octacalcium phosphate and tricalcium phosphate, components of most pathological calcifications. The associated arthropathy has been described only since 1976[145,146]. The nature of the crystals can only be confirmed by ultramicroscopy, which is often used with elemental analysis and electron diffraction for definitive diagnosis. Several other simpler procedures, such as the use of alizarin red, merely indicate the presence of calcium phosphate and not the particular salt. With all crystal-associated arthropathies, the question must be asked whether the crystals have induced the joint pathology or whether primary joint damage has predisposed to crystal deposition. In both urate and pyrophosphate crystal arthropathy, while there is good evidence that both situations may apply, it is generally conceded that the usual situation is that the formation of crystals is the primary phenomenon and most of the joint reaction is secondary to this. While some inflammation has been reported following intra-synovial injection of apatite crystals[146], the primary role of these crystals is now considered to be in doubt[123].

Basic calcium phosphate (BCP) or hydroxyapatite is the normal constituent of bone and teeth and has long been recognized as a component of dystrophic and metastatic calcification due to local tissue damage. It is also well-recognized as a feature of acute calcific peri-arthritis, especially that affecting the shoulder; its formation may also be associated with tendonitis and bursitis[147]. Periarticular calcification has been recognized as a common feature of this condition but its involvement in intra-articular pathology has been recognized only more recently.

Natural history of apatite-associated arthropathy

This may be seen in a wide variety of clinical presentations, but usually in one of the following patterns.

Osteoarthritis

Most often, these crystals are found in association with osteoarthritis of the knee and have been reported in 30–60% of synovial fluids from patients who would otherwise be diagnosed as having osteoarthritis of the knee[148]. These patients usually present no distinctive clinical or radiologic feature and, in general, the synovial fluids do not show a leukocytic or inflammatory response and may demonstrate only small numbers of mononuclear cells. These crystals may be found increasingly in association with exacerbations of clinical symptoms. Crystals are found more commonly in patients with the more severe radiologic features of destructive osteoarthritis and in general, the radiologic severity correlates with the concentration of hydroxyapatite crystals in the fluid[149]. This high frequency of association with osteoarthritis has led many to suggest that this type of crystal deposition is an epiphenomenon and does not have etiologic significance. Until its role is more clearly defined, it is not possible to determine its prognostic significance.

Acute arthritis

Occasionally, these crystals have been reported in patients with acute monoarticular arthritis that was otherwise undiagnosable. Radiologic changes were absent but synovial leukocyte counts were increased. There are also a few reports of apatite crystals in association with an erosive arthritis[150]. Considerable radiologic calcification was found and the synovial fluid showed considerable accumulation of crystals. Clinical symptomatology was varied and nonspecific. Some of these crystals were in large, irregular chunks that stained positively for calcium.

Mixed pyrophosphate and apatite crystal disease

This has been associated with advanced destructive disease but otherwise resembles severe osteoarthritis[151].

Apatite-associated destructive arthritis

This symptom was originally described by Dieppe et al.[152]. Shoulders and knees were chiefly affected and features included large, cool effusions, considerable pain, and joint instability with progression of joint damage. There was little inflammatory cell response in the synovial fluid in which calcium hydroxyapatite particles could be readily demonstrated. This was further elaborated in the description of the Milwaukee shoulder by McCarty et al.[153], which further established this entity with its crystal aggregates, its noninflammatory fluid, collagen fragments, and the presence of collagenases and neutral proteases. Most cases had some predisposing condition in the form either of repeated minor trauma with overuse, a neurologic abnormality, recurrent dislocation, or pyrophosphate crystal deposition. It has been reported in association with chronic renal failure. The symptoms, particularly acute symptoms, can often be controlled with nonsteroidal anti-inflammatory drugs.

Periarticular and soft-tissue deposits may clear more rapidly after needling. It is thought that this increases the area of crystals available for contact with reacting cells. Since precipitation of these crystals is regarded more as a local phenomenon than a generalized disorder, there is no reliable method of prevention known. Any prophylaxis will depend, therefore, upon further understanding of the basic process involved.

Problems in determining prognosis

The chief problem in assessing prognosis in this condition is in the fact that it has been described only relatively recently, that the clinical presentations are varied, and that the pathogenic role of the crystals is not clear in all of the various presentations. It seems likely that crystals may be associated with acute exacerbation of arthritis but less likely that crystals, found so frequently in joints that have all the characteristics of osteoarthritis, are actually pathogenetic in inducing the joint damage. Thus, the prognosis depends upon the nature of the clinical manifestation and this will be more severe in joints in which synovial and cartilaginous damage has already occurred. In the osteoarthritic group, it will be that of the underlying disorder.

References

1. Gutman, A. B. (1953). Primary and secondary gout. *Ann. Intern. Med.*, **39**, 1062–1076
2. Brochner-Mortensen, K. (1937). Uric acid in blood and urine. *Acta Med. Scand.*, **84** (suppl.), 1–269
3. Fox, I. H. (1985). Adenosine triphosphate degradation in specific disease. *J. Lab. Clin. Med.*, **106**, 101–110
4. Emmerson, B. T. (1974). Effect of oral fructose on urate production. *Ann. Rheum. Dis.*, **33**, 276–280
5. Sutton, J. R., Toews, C. J., Ward, G. R. and Fox, I. H. (1980). Purine metabolism during strenuous muscular exercise in man. *Metabolism*, **29**, 254–260
6. Emmerson, B. T. (1978). Abnormal urate excretion associated with renal and systemic disorders, drugs and toxins. In Kelley, W. N. and Weiner, I. M. (eds.) *Uric Acid*, pp. 287–315. (Berlin, Heidelberg, New York: Springer-Verlag)
7. Gibson, T., Rodgers, A., Simmonds, H., Court-Brown, F., Todd, E. and Meilton, V. (1983). A controlled study of diet in patients with gout. *Ann. Rheum. Dis.*, **42**, 123–127
8. Tofler, O. B. and Woodings, T. L. (1981). A 13-year follow-up of social drinkers. *Med. J. Aust.*, **2**, 479–481
9. Emmerson, B. T. (1973). Alteration of urate metabolism by weight reduction. *Aust. NZ J. Med.*, **3**, 410–412
10. Yamashita, S., Matsuzawa, Y., Tokunaga, S., Fujioka, S. and Tarui, S. (1986). Studies of the impaired metabolism of uric acid in obese subjects: marked reduction of renal urate excretion and its improvement by a low-calorie diet. *Int. J. Obesity*, **10**, 255–264
11. Yano, K., Rhoads, G. G. and Kagan, A. (1977). Epidemiology of serum uric acid among 8000 Japanese-American men in Hawaii. *J. Chronic Dis.*, **30**, 171–184
12. Spicer, J., McLeod, W. R., O'Brien, K. P. and Scott, P. J. (1979). Distributions and interrelations of coronary risk factors in a community sample of Auckland men. *Aust. NZ J. Med.*, **9**, 158–169
13. Goldbourt, U., Medalie, J. H., Herman, J. B. and Neufeld, H. N. (1980). Serum uric acid: correlation with biochemical anthropometric, clinical and behavioral parameters in 10,000 Israeli men. *J. Chronic Dis.*, **33**, 435–443

14. Gutman, A. B. and Yu, T-F. (1967). Renal function in gout. *Am. J. Med.*, **23**, 600-622
15. Rieselbach, R. E. and Steele, T. H. (1975). Intrinsic renal disease leading to abnormal urate excretion. *Nephron*, **14**, 81-87
16. Emmerson, B. T. and Row, P. G. (1975). An evaluation of the pathogenesis of the gouty kidney. *Kidney Int.*, **8**, 65-71
17. Emmerson, B. T. (1973). Chronic lead nephropathy. *Kidney Int.*, **4**, 1-5
18. Bartels, E. C. (1955). Gout — now amenable to control. *Ann. Intern. Med.*, **42**, 1-10
19. Smyth, C. J. and Frank, L. S. (1962). Treatment of gouty arthritis. *Rheumatism*, **18**, 2-11
20. Adams, F. (transl.) (1886). *The Genuine Works of Hippocrates*. (New York: Wood)
21. Wallace, S. L., Robinson, H. J., Masi, A. T., Decker, J. L., McCarty, D. J. and Yu, T-F. (1977). Preliminary criteria for the classification of the acute arthritis of primary gout. *Arthritis Rheum.*, **20**, 895-900
22. Rodnan, G. P. (1961). A gallery of gout. *Arthritis Rheum.*, **4**, 27-194
23. Brochner-Mortensen, K. (1941). 100 gouty patients. *Acta Med. Scand.*, **106**, 81-107
24. Kuzell, W. C., Schaffarzick, R. W., Naugler, W. E., Koets, P., Mankle, E. A., Brown, B. and Champlin, B. (1955). Some observations on 520 gouty patients. *J. Chronic Dis.*, **2**, 645-669
25. Rakic, M. T., Valkenburg, H. A., Davidson, R. T., Engels, J. P., Mikkelsen, W. M., Neel, J. V. and Duff, I. F. (1964). Observations on the natural history of hyperuricemia and gout. *Am. J. Med.*, **37**, 862-871
26. Gutman, A. B. (1965). Treatment of primary gout: The present status. *Arthritis Rheum.*, **8**, 911-919
27. Yu, T. F. and Gutman, A. B. (1961). Efficacy of colchicine prophylaxis in gout. *Ann. Intern. Med.*, **55**, 179-192
28. Hall, A. P., Barry, P. E., Dawber, T. R. and McNamara, P. M. (1967). Epidemiology of gout and hyperuricemia. *Am. J. Med.*, **42**, 27-37
29. Grahame, R. and Scott, J. T. (1970). Clinical survey of 354 patients with gout. *Ann. Rheum. Dis.*, **29**, 461-468
30. Gutman, A. B. (1971). Views on the pathogenesis and management of primary gout. *J. Bone Joint Surg.*, **54A**, 357-372
31. Hall, A. P. (1965). Correlations among hyperuricemia, hypercholesterolemia, coronary disease and hypertension. *Arthritis Rheum.*, **8**, 846-852
32. Feldman, E. B. and Wallace, S. L. (1964). Hypertriglyceridemia in gout. *Circulation*, **2**, 508-513
33. Barlow, K. A. (1968). Hyperlipidemia in primary gout. *Metabolism*, **3**, 289-299
34. Emmerson, B. T. (1979). Atherosclerosis and urate metabolism. *Aust. NZ J. Med.*, **9**, 451-454
35. Rondier, J., Truffert, J., Go, A. le, Cayla, J., Hila, A., de Gennes, J.-L. and Delbarre, F. (1977). Gout and hyperlipidemia — effect of overweight on the levels of circulating lipids. *Ann. Clin. Res.*, **9**, 239-245
36. Gibson, T. and Grahame, R. (1974). Gout and hyperlipidaemia. *Ann. Rheum. Dis.*, **33**, 298-303
37. Gibson, T., Kilbourn, K., Horner, I. and Simmonds, H. A. (1979). Mechanism and treatment of hypertriglyceridaemia in gout. *Ann. Rheum. Dis.*, **38**, 31-35
38. Fessel, J. (1980). High uric acid as an indicator of cardiovascular disease. *Am. J. Med.*, **68**, 401-404
39. Darlington, L. G., Slack, J. and Scott, J. T. (1982). Family study of lipid and purine levels in gout patients. *Ann. Rheum. Dis.*, **41**, 253-256
40. Abbott, R. D., Brand, F. N., Kannel, W. B. and Castelli, W. P. (1981). Gout and coronary heart disease: The Framingham study. *J. Clin. Epidemiol.*, **3**, 237-242
41. Jiao, S., Kemeda, K., Matsuzawa, Y. and Tarui, S. (1986). Hyperlipoproteinaemia in primary gout: hyperlipoproteinaemic phenotype and influence of alcohol intake and obesity in Japan. *Ann. Rheum. Dis.*, **45**, 308-313
42. Bishop, C., Rand, R. and Talbott, J. H. (1951). Effect of Benemid on uric acid metabolism in one normal and one gouty subject. *J. Clin. Invest.*, **30**, 889-905
43. Kelley, W. N. (1975). Effects of drugs on uric acid in man. In Elliott, H. W., George, R. and Okun, R. (eds.) *Annual Review of Pharmacology*, **15**, 327-350

44. Rundles, R. W., Wyngaarden, J. B., Hitchings, G. H., Elion, G. B. and Silberman, H. R. (1963). Effects of a xanthine oxidase inhibitor on thiopurine metabolism, hyperuricaemia and gout. *Trans. Assoc. Am. Physicians*, **76**, 126
45. Rundles, R. W., Metz, E. N. and Silberman, H. R. (1966). Allopurinol in the treatment of gout. *Ann. Intern. Med.*, **64**, 229-258
46. Hande, K. R., Noone, R. M. and Stone, W. J. (1984). Severe allopurinol toxicity. *Am. J. Med.*, **76**, 47-56
47. Healy, L. A., Magid, G. J. and Decker, J. L. (1959). Uric acid retention due to hydrochlorothiazide. *N. Engl. J. Med.*, **261**, 1358
48. Labeeuw, M., Pozet, N., Hadj Aissa, A., Zech, P. Y., Sassard, J. and Laville, M. (1988). Uric acid renal handling: spontaneous changes and influence of a thiazide alone or associated with triamterene. *Int. J. Clin. Pharmacol.*, **26**, 79-83
49. Emmerson, B. T. (1967). Regimen of indomethacin therapy in acute gouty arthritis. *Br. Med. J.*, **2**, 272-274
50. Emmerson, B. T. (1983). *Hyperuricaemia and Gout in Clinical Practice.* (Syndey: Adis Health Science Press)
51. Arnold, M. H., Brooks, P. M., Savvas, P. and Ruff, S. (1988). Tophaceous gout of the axial skeleton. *Aust. NZ J. Med.*, **18**, 865-867
52. Lawry, II, G. V., Fan, P. T. and Bluestone, R. (1988). Polyarticular versus monoarticular gout: a prospective, comparative analysis of clinical features. *Medicine*, **67**, 335-343
53. Yu, T-F. (1977). Some unusual features of gouty arthritis in females. *Semin. Arthritis Rheum.*, **6**, 247-265
54. Lally, E. V., Ho, G. and Kaplan, S. R. (1986). The clinical spectrum of gouty arthritis in women. *Arch. Intern. Med.*, **146**, 2221-2225
55. Meyers, O. L. and Monteagudo, F. S. E. (1985). Gout in females: an analysis of 92 patients. *Clin. Exp. Rheumatol.*, **3**, 105-109
56. Meyers, O. L. and Monteagudo, F. S. E. (1986). A comparison of gout in men and women — a 10-year experience. *S. Afr. Med. J.*, **70**, 721-723
57. Borg, E. J. T. and Rasker, J. J. (1987). Gout in the elderly, a separate entity? *Ann. Rheum. Dis.*, **46**, 72-76
58. Takala, J., Anttila, S., Gref, C. G. and Isomlaki, H. (1988). Diuretics and hyperuricemia in the elderly. *Scand. J. Rheumatol.*, **17**, 155-160
59. MacFarlane, D. G. and Dieppe, P. A. (1985). Diuretic-induced gout in elderly women. *Br. J. Rheumatol.*, **24**, 155-157
60. Campbell, S. M. (1988). Gout: how presentation, diagnosis, and treatment differ in the elderly. *Geriatrics*, **43**, 71-77
61. Oren, B. G., Rich, M. and Belle, M. S. (1958). Chlorothiazide (diuril) as a hyperuricacidemic agent. *J. Am. Med. Assoc.*, **168**, 2128-2129
62. Aronoff, A. (1960). Acute gouty arthritis precipitated by chlorothiazide. *N. Engl. J. Med.*, **262**, 767-769
63. Bryant, J. M., Yu, T-F, Berger, L., Schvartz, N., Torosdag, S., Fletcher, L., Fertig, H., Schwartz, M. S. and Quan, R. B. F. (1962). Hyperuricemia induced by the administration of chlorthalidone and other sulfonamide diuretics. *Am. J. Med.*, **33**, 408-420
64. Steele, T. H. and Oppenheimer, S. (1969). Factors affecting urate excretion following diuretic administration in man. *Am. J. Med.*, **47**, 564-574
65. Weinman, E. J., Eknoyan, G. and Suki, W. N. (1975). The influence of the extracellular fluid volume on the tubular reabsorption of uric acid. *J. Clin. Invest.*, **55**, 283-291
66. Langford, H. G., Blaufox, M. D., Borhani, N. O., Curb, J. D., Molteni, A., Schneider, K. A. and Pressel, S. (1987). Is thiazide-produced uric acid elevation harmful? *Ann. Intern. Med.*, **147**, 645-649
67. Simkin, P. A., Campbell, P. M. and Larson, E. B. (1983). Gout in Heberden's nodes. *Arthritis Rheum.*, **26**, 94-97
68. Hollingworth, P., Scott, J. T. and Burry, H. C. (1983). Nonarticular gout: hyperuricemia and tophus formation without gouty arthritis. *Arthritis Rheum.*, **26**, 98-101
69. Nugent, C. A. and Tyler, F. H. (1959). The renal excretion of uric acid in patients with gout and in non-gouty subjects. *J. Clin. Invest.*, **38**, 1890-1898

70. Rieselbach, R. E., Sorensen, L. B., Shelp, W. D. and Steele, T. H. (1970). Diminished renal urate secretion per nephron as a basis for primary gout. *Ann. Intern. Med.*, **73**, 359-366
71. Puig, J. G., Anton, F. M., Jimenez, M. L. and Gutierrez, P. C. (1986). Renal handling of uric acid in gout: impaired tubular transport of urate not dependent on serum urate levels. *Metabolism*, **35**, 1147-1153
72. McPhaul, J. J. (1968). Hyperuricemia and urate excretion in chronic renal disease. *Metabolism*, **17**, 430-438
73. Emmerson, B. T., Stride, P. J. and Williams, G. (1980). The clinical differentiation of primary gout from primary renal disease in patients with both gout and renal disease. In Rapado, A., Watts, R. W. E. and De Bruyn, C. H. M. M. (eds.) *Purine Metabolism in Man — III A*, pp. 9-13. (New York: Plenum Press)
74. Sorensen, L. B. (1980). Gout secondary to chronic renal disease: studies on urate metabolism. *Ann. Rheum. Dis.*, **39**, 424-430
75. Newcombe, D. S. (1973). Gouty arthritis and polycystic kidney disease. *Ann. Intern. Med.*, **79**, 605
76. Meijas, E., Navas, J., Lluberes, R. and Martinez-Maldonado, M. (1989). Hyperuricemia, gout and autosomal dominant polycystic kidney disease. *Am. J. Med. Sci.*, **297**, 145-148
77. Thompson, G. R., Weiss, J. J., Goldman, R. T. and Rigg, G. A. (1978). Familial occurrence of hyperuricemia, gout, and medullary cystic disease. *Arch. Intern. Med.*, **138**, 1614-1617
78. Burke, J. R., Inglis, J. A., Craswell, P. W., Mitchell, K. R. and Emmerson, B. T. (1982). Juvenile nephronophthisis and medullary cystic disease — the same disease (report of a large family with medullary cystic disease associated with gout and epilepsy). *Clin. Nephrol.*, **18**, 1-8
79. Leumann, E. P. and Wegmann, W. (1983). Familial nephropathy with hyperuricemia and gout. *Nephron*, **34**, 51-57
80. Meyrier, A. (1976). Desensitization in a patient with chronic renal disease and severe allergy to allopurinol. *Br. Med. J.*, **2**, 458
81. Fam, A. G., Paton, T. W. and Chalton, A. (1980). Reinstitution of allopurinol therapy after cutaneous reactions. *Can. Med. Assoc. J.*, **123**, 128-129
82. Emmerson, B. T., Hazelton, R. A. and Frazer, I. H. (1988). Some adverse reactions to allopurinol may be mediated by lymphocyte reactivity to oxypurinol. *Arthritis Rheum.*, **31**, 436-440
83. Sydenham, T. A. (1788). A treatise of the gout. In *The Works of Thomas Sydenham*, Vol. 2. (London: Robinson, Otridge, Hayes and Newberry)
84. Scudamore, C. (1823). *A Treatise on the Nature and Cure of Gout and Gravel*. (London: Joseph Mallett)
85. Castelnau, N. F. I. (1843). Gouty kidney. *Arch. Gen. Med. J., Comp. de Sci. Med.*, **3**, 285
86. Todd, R. B. (1857). *Clinical Lectures on Certain Diseases of the Urinary Organs, and On Dropsies*. (London: Churchill)
87. Garrod, A. B. (1876). *A Treatise on Gout and Rheumatic Gout*, 3rd edn. (London: Longmans, Green and Co.)
88. Schnitker, M. A. and Richter, A. B. (1936). Nephritis in gout. *Am. J. Med. Sci.*, **192**, 241-251
89. Brown, J. B. and Mallory, G. K. (1950). Renal changes in gout. *N. Engl. J. Med.*, **243**, 325-329
90. Talbott, J. H. and Terplan, K. L. (1960). The kidney in gout. *Medicine (Baltimore)*, **39**, 405-462
91. Barry, K. G., Hunter, R. H., Davis, T. E. and Crosby, W. H. (1963). Acute uric acid nephropathy. *Arch. Intern. Med.*, **3**, 452-459
92. Simmonds, H. A., Cameron, J. S., Morris, G. S. and Davies, P. M. (1986). Allopurinol in renal failure and the tumour lysis syndrome. *Clin. Chim. Acta*, **160**, 189-195
93. Batch, J. A., Riek, R. P., Gordon, R. B., Burke, J. R. and Emmerson, B. T. (1984). Renal failure in infancy due to urate over-production. *Aust. NZ J. Med.*, **14**, 852-854
94. Kelton, J., Kelley, W. N. and Holmes, E. W. (1978). A rapid method for the diagnosis of acute uric acid nephropathy. *Arch. Intern. Med.*, **138**, 612-615

95. Seegmiller, J. E. and Frazier, P. D. (1966). Biochemical considerations of the renal damage of gout. *Ann. Rheum. Dis.*, **25**, 668-672
96. Farebrother, D. A., Pincott, J. R., Simmonds, H. A., Warren, D. J., Dillon, M. J. and Cameron, J. S. (1981). Uric acid crystal induced nephropathy: evidence for a specific renal lesion in a gouty family. *J. Pathol.*, **135**, 159-168
97. Beck, L. H. (1986). Requiem for gouty nephropathy. *Kidney Int.*, **30**, 280-287
98. Gibson, T., Rodgers, V., Potter, C. and Simmonds, H. A. (1982). Allopurinol treatment and its effect on renal function in gout: a controlled study. *Ann. Rheum. Dis.*, **41**, 59-65
99. Fessel, W. J. (1979). Renal outcomes of gout and hyperuricemia. *Am. J. Med.*, **67**, 74-82
100. Berger, L. and Yu, T-F. (1975). Renal function in gout. *Am. J. Med.*, **59**, 605-613
101. Yu, T-F. and Berger, L. (1982). Impaired renal function in gout. *Am. J. Med.*, **72**, 95-100
102. Emmerson, B. T. (1988). Hyperuricemia, gout and the kidney. In Schrier, R. W. and Gottschalk, C. W. (eds.) *Diseases of the Kidney*, 4th edn. pp. 2481-2510. (Boston/Toronto: Little, Brown & Co.)
103. Emmerson, B. T. (1989). Gout and renal disease. In Massry, S. G. and Glassock, R. J. (eds.) *Textbook of Nephrology*, 2nd edn. pp. 756-60. (Baltimore: Williams & Wilkins).
104. Campion, E. W., Glynn, R. J. and DeLabry, L. O. (1987). Asymptomatic hyperuricemia. *Am. J. Med.*, **82**, 421-426
105. Currie, W. J. C. and Turner, P. (1979). The frequency of renal stones within Great Britain in a gouty and non-gouty population. *Br. J. Urol.*, **51**, 337-341
106. Yu, T-F. and Talbott, J. H. (1980). Changing trends of mortality in gout. *Semin. Arthritis Rheum.*, **10**, 1-9
107. Darlington, L. G., Slack, J. and Scott, J. T. (1983). Vascular mortality in patients with gout and in their families. *Ann. Rheum. Dis.*, **42**, 270-273
108. Ungerleider, H. E. (1954). The internist and life insurance. *Ann. Intern. Med.*, **41**, 124-130
109. Talbott, J. H. and Lilienfeld, A. (1959). Longevity in gout. *Geriatrics*, **14**, 409-420
110. Gutman, A. B. (1972). Views on the pathogenesis and management of primary gout. *J. Bone Joint Surg.*, **54A**, 357-372
111. Talbott, J. H. and Yu, T-F. (1976). *Gout and Uric Acid Metabolism*. (New York: Stratton Intercontinental Medical Book Corp.)
112. Zitnan, D. and Sitaj, S. (1963). Chondrocalcinosis articularis, section I, clinical and radiological study. *Ann. Rheum. Dis.*, **22**, 142-152
113. McCarty, D. J., Kohn, N. N. and Faires, J. S. (1962). The significance of calcium phosphate crystals in the synovial fluid of arthritis patients: the "pseudo-gout syndrome". *Ann. Intern. Med.*, **56**, 71-737
114. Moskowitz, R. W. and Katz, D. (1967). Chondrocalcinosis and chrondrocalysynovitis (pseudogout syndrome). *Am. J. Med.*, **43**, 332-334
115. McCarty, D. J. (1963). Crystal-induced inflammation; syndromes of gout and pseudogout. *Geriatrics*, **18**, 467-478
116. Doherty, M. and Dieppe, P. A. (1981). Acute pseudogout: "crystal shedding" or acute crystallization? *Arthritis Rheum.*, **24**, 954-957
117. Pritzker, K. P. H., Cheng, P-T. and Renlund, R. C. (1988). Calcium pyrophosphate crystal deposition in hyaline cartilage. Ultrastructural analysis and implications for pathogenesis. *J. Rheumatol.*, **15**, 828-835
118. Rodriguez-Valverde, V., Zuniga, M., Casanueva, B., Sanchez, S. and Merino, J. (1988). Hereditary articular chondrocalcinosis. *Am. J. Med.*, **84**, 101-106
119. Riestra, J. L., Sanchez, A., Rodriguez-Valverde, V., Alonso, J. L., de la Hera, M. and Merino, J. (1988). Radiographic features of hereditary articular chondrocalcinosis. A comparative study with the sporadic type. *Clin. Exp. Rheumatol.*, **6**, 369-372
120. Lust, G., Faure, G., Netter, P., Gaucher, A. and Seegmiller, J. E. (1981). Evidence of a generalized metabolic defect in patients with hereditary chondrocalcinosis. *Arthritis Rheum.*, **24**, 1517-1527

121. Pritchard, M. H. and Jessop, J. D. (1977). Chondrocalcinosis in primary hyperparathyroidism. *Ann. Rheum. Dis.*, **36**, 146-151
122. Bilezikian, J. P., Connor, T. B., Aptekar, R., Freijanes, J., Aurbach, G. D., Pachas, W. N., Wells, S. A. and Decker, J. L. (1973). Pseudogout after parathyroidectomy. *Lancet*, **1**, 7801-7802
123. Doherty, M. and Dieppe, P. (1986). Crystal deposition disease in the elderly. *Clin. Rheumatol.*, **12**, 97-116
124. Milazzo, S. C., Ahern, M. J., Cleland, L. G. and Henderson, D. R. (1981). Calcium pyrophosphate dihydrate deposition disease and familial hypomagnesemia. *J. Rheumatol.*, **8**, 767-771
125. Hollingworth, P., Williams, P. L. and Scott, J. T. (1982). Frequency of chondrocalcinosis of the knees in asymptomatic hyperuricaemia and rheumatoid arthritis: a controlled study. *Ann. Rheum. Dis.*, **41**, 344-364
126. Alexander, G. M., Dieppe, P. A., Doherty, M. and Scott, D. G. I. (1982). Pyrophosphate arthropathy: a study of metabolic associations and laboratory data. *Ann. Rheum. Dis.*, **41**, 377-381
127. Settas, L., Doherty, M. and Dieppe, P. (1982). Localized chondrocalcinosis in unstable joints. *Br. Med. J.*, **285**, 175-176
128. Jacobelli, S., McCarty, D. J., Silcox, D. C. and Mall, J. C. (1973). Calcium pyrophosphate dihydrate crystal deposition in neuropathic joints. *Ann. Intern. Med.*, **79**, 340-347
129. Ellman, M. H., Brown, N. L. and Katzenberg, C. A. (1979). Acute pseudogout in chronic renal failure. *Arch. Intern. Med.*, **139**, 795-796
130. McCarty, D. J., Hogan, J. M., Gatter, R. A. and Grossman, M. (1966). Studies of pathological calcifications in human cartilage. *Bone Joint Surg. (Am).*, **48**, 309-325
131. Mitrovic, D. R., Stankovic, A., Iriarte-Borda, O., Uzan, M., Quintero, M., Miravet, L. and Kuntz, D. (1988). The prevalence of chondrocalcinosis in the human knee. *J. Rheumatol.*, **15**, 633-641
132. Dieppe, P. A., Alexander, G. J. M., Jones, H. E., Doherty, M., Scott, D. G. I., Manhire, A. and Watt, I. (1982). Pyrophosphate arthropathy: a clinical and radiological study of 105 cases. *Ann. Rheum. Dis.*, **41**, 371-376
133. Ellman, M. H., Brown, N. L. and Levin, B. (1981). Narrowing of knee joint space in patients with pseudogout. *Ann. Rheum. Dis.*, **40**, 34-36
134. Resnick, C. S. and Resnick, D. (1983). Crystal deposition disease. *Semin. Arthritis Rheum.*, **12**, 390-403
135. Gordon, T. P., Smith, M., Ebert, B., McCredie, M. and Brooks, P. M. (1984). Articular chondrocalcinosis in a hospital population: an Australian experience. *Aust. N.Z. J. Med.*, **14**, 655-659
136. Storey, G. O. and Huskisson, E. C. (1977). Unusual presentations of pyrophosphate arthropathy. *Br. Med. J.*, **2**, 21-22
137. Gerster, J-C., Lagier, R. and Boivin, G. (1982). Olecranon bursitis related to calcium pyrophosphate dihydrate crystal deposition disease. *Arthritis Rheum.*, **25**, 989-995
138. Berghausen, E. J., Balough, K., Landis, W. J., Lee, D. D. and Wright, A. M. (1987). Cervical myelopathy attributable to pseudogout. Case report with radiologic, histologic and crystallographic observations. *Clin. Orthop.*, **214**, 217-221
139. Hutton, C. W., Doherty, M. and Dieppe, P. A. (1987). Acute pseudogout of the temporomandibular joint: a report of three cases and review of the literature. *Br. J. Rheumatol.*, **26**, 51-52
140. Webb, J., Deodhar, S. and Lee, P. (1974). Chronic destructive polyarthritis due to pyrophosphate crystal arthritis. *Med. J. Aust.*, **2**, 206-209
141. Bong, D. and Bennett, R. (1981). Pseudogout mimicking systemic disease. *J. Am. Med. Assoc.*, **246**, 1438-1440
142. Spilberg, I., McLain, D., Simchowitz, L. and Berney, S. (1980). Colchicine and pseudogout. *Arthritis Rheum.*, **23**, 1062-1063
143. Alvarellos, A. and Spilberg, I. (1986). Colchicine prophylaxis in pseudogout. *J. Rheumatol.*, **13**, 804-805
144. Bjelle, A., Edvinsson, U. and Hagstam, A. (1982). Pyrophosphate arthropathy in two Swedish families. *Arthritis Rheum.*, **25**, 66-74

145. Dieppe, P. A., Crocker, P., Huskisson, E. C. and Willoughby, D. A. (1976). Apatite deposition diseases: A new arthropathy. *Lancet*, **1**, 266-268
146. Schumacher, H. R., Somlyo, A. P., Tse, R. L. and Maurer, K. (1977). Arthritis associated with apatite crystals. *Ann. Intern. Med.*, **87**, 411-416
147. Thompson, G. R., Ming Ting, Y., Riggs, G. A., Fenn, M. Ellen. and Denning, R. M. (1968). Calcific tendinitis and soft-tissue calcification resembling gout. *J. Am. Med. Assoc.*, **203**, 122-130
148. Dieppe, P. A., Crocker, P. R., Corke, C. F., Doyle, D. V., Huskisson, E. C. and Willoughby, D. A. (1979). Synovial fluid crystals. *Q. J. Med.*, **48**, 533-553
149. Halverson, P. B. and McCarty, D. J. (1986). Patterns of radiographic abnormalities associated with basic calcium phosphate and calcium pyrophosphate dihydrate crystal deposition in the knee. *Ann. Rheum. Dis.*, **45**, 603-605
150. Schumacher, H. R., Miller, J. L., Ludivico, C. and Jessar, R. A. (1981). Erosive arthritis associated with apatite crystal deposition. *Arthritis Rheum.*, **24**, 31-37
151. Gibiliso, P. A., Schumacher, H. R., Hollander, J. L. and Soper, K. A. (1985). Synovial fluid crystals in osteoarthritis. *Arthritis Rheum.*, **28**, 511-515
152. Dieppe, P. A., Doherty, M., MacFarlane, D. G., Hutton, C. W., Bradfield, J. W. and Watt, I. (1984). Apatite associated destructive arthritis. *Br. J. Rheumatol.*, **23**, 84-91
153. McCarty, D. J., Halverson, P. B., Carrera, G. F., Brewer, B. J. and Kozin, F. (1981). "Milwaukee shoulder" — association of microspheroids containing hydroxyapatite crystals, active collagenase, and neutral protease with rotator cuff defects. *Arthritis Rheum.*, **24**, 464-473

6
Ankylosing spondylitis

P. S. HELLIWELL and V. WRIGHT

INTRODUCTION

Ankylosing spondylitis (AS) is a chronic inflammatory condition of the axial skeleton and sacroiliac joints that, untreated, may progress with new bone formation to total bony ankylosis of the spinal column. The origin of the new bone in the axial skeleton occurs at the enthesis, i.e., the point of attachment of ligament to bone. This enthesitis may also occur peripherally, classically at sites such as the insertion of the Achilles tendon and of the plantar aponeurosis into the calcaneum. In addition, a proportion of cases have a seronegative, anodular inflammatory peripheral arthritis.

AS may occur in association with other diseases, notably psoriatic arthritis, Reiter's syndrome, and inflammatory bowel disease. In such cases this may be called secondary AS, although there is evidence to suggest that the spondylitis may be independent of the other diseases.

The arthritis associated with these conditions has been collectively termed seronegative spondarthritis in order to highlight the shared clinical features of these diseases[1]. The recent appreciation of the association between bowel inflammation, enteric bacteria, genetic status, and clinical features in this group of diseases suggests that in the near future we will have a much clearer understanding of the pathogenesis of this group of disorders and will hopefully be able to make an impact on the disease outcome.

This chapter is mainly concerned with primary AS, but secondary AS will be discussed in the context of outcome in different subgroups of the disease. After a short review of the natural history of AS and factors that may have altered the prognosis over the last 20 years, a more detailed discussion and analysis of prognostic factors affecting such outcomes as death, disability, and pain will be presented. Finally, future perspectives with regard to treatment and prognosis in this fascinating group of diseases will be discussed.

NATURAL HISTORY

Some consideration must be given to historical aspects of AS. Up to the mid-1950s and later this disease was often described as rheumatoid spondylitis and it was not until 1961 that the first diagnostic criteria were formulated[2]. In addition to including the disease as a branch of rheumatoid arthritis, many cases were often ascribed to pulmonary tuberculosis, which was prevalent at the time and may have been confused with the nontuberculous apical pulmonary changes known to occur with AS.

Despite these confusions a reasonably homogeneous population seems to have been studied. The general consensus of the early series can be summarized as follows. AS is a disease of insidious onset that progresses with exacerbations and remissions leading to limitation of movement and deformity in the spinal column. Ultimate functional limitation is mild and the disease rarely shortens life but most severe cases occur in those who start with symptoms early in life. Females are less severely affected than males.

This impression of AS had not changed much when the concept of seronegative spondarthritis was introduced by Wright and Moll in 1976[1]. These authors, however, noted that a small percentage of cases followed a particularly unfavorable course leading to permanent invalidity, due to widespread ankylosis, in a relatively short time. The rest of the patient population were described as proceeding with insidiously slow development of ankylosis. In 1977, when the first papers on the association between carriage of *Klebsiella* species and AS were produced, a possible explanation for periods of acute exacerbation and periods of remission was provided[7].

Ankylosing or rheumatoid spondylitis was treated successfully with radiotherapy in the 1940s by Scott[8]. However, it became apparent in the early 1950s that the side-effects of this wide-field X-ray treatment were perhaps more serious than the benefits obtained. Subsequently Court-Brown and Doll reviewed over 14 000 cases of AS treated with radiotherapy between 1935 and 1955. They found that leukemias were increased within 6–8 years of radiation therapy and that carcinomas of other heavily irradiated sites were still increasing up to the end of the 15-year cohort period. They calculated the excess mortality due to radiotherapy of 6 per 1000 patients over 13 years[9]. However, Radford *et al.*, studying a group of patients not treated by X-ray therapy, still found increased mortality in the group as a whole[10]. Increased mortality was associated with the arthritis itself, renal disease, pulmonary disease, cardiovascular disease, and peptic ulcer. It has been suggested that the increase in mortality due to peptic ulceration is a side-effect of treatment with nonsteroidal anti-inflammatory drugs (NSAIDs) and that the increase in deaths attributable to this cause more than offsets that due to the leukemia and other cancers induced by radiotherapy[11].

AS remains, however, a rheumatic disease with a relatively good functional outlook. Patients tend to remain in employment, although modification of their job may be needed[12]. Patients with peripheral arthritis are particularly at risk of functional disability; this may account for up to one-quarter of all patients.

PROBLEMS IN ASSESSING PROGNOSIS IN ANKYLOSING SPONDYLITIS

Nonhomogeneity of disease population

Genetic differences

Approximately 90% of patients with AS carry the HLA-B27 antigen. The 10% of cases who are B27 negative may have a disease different from the B27 positive cases. It has been suggested that B27 negative patients with AS have a later age of onset and possibly milder disease[13,14]. However, American workers have not been able to confirm this finding[15]. Other predisposing genes may occur in B27 negative individuals such as B38 and the B7 Creg group. However, in a disease such as AS where there is a strong genetic marker it would seem sensible to obtain some form of genetic homogeneity in prognostic studies.

Age of onset

Subjects with AS who originally presented in childhood (that is, at less than 16 years of age) may also be a different group prognostically. These subjects more often present with a peripheral arthritis and more frequently suffer with iritis[16,17]. Juvenile spondylitics may have systemic amyloidosis more frequently than patients developing the disease in adulthood[17]. Recently a large anamnestic study of members of the British National Association for AS (NASS), matching subjects for duration of disease, found that subjects with juvenile spondylitis scored better on the social activities scale of the AIMS questionnaire than those with adult-onset disease, and more subjects were in full-time employment[18]. However, 17% had progressed to hip replacement as opposed to 4% in the matched adult-onset population.

Sex differences

Early studies of AS reported a male preponderance. However, more recently it has been suggested that the male-to-female ratio may be closer to unity[19]. Do females have milder disease than males as originally suggested?[20] Overall it was felt that women had less systemic features than men, were likely to have relative sparing of the thoracic spine but were more likely to have hip or shoulder involvement[21].

However, it may be that the higher incidence of peripheral joint involvement produces more severe disability overall[22]. More recently in Leeds, a survey of 62 female and 61 male patients with AS found that the severity of disease in both groups was similar[23].

Primary vs. secondary AS

Is there any difference in severity and prognosis between primary and secondary AS? We have summarized the evidence suggesting that the AS of inflammatory bowel disease may well be independent of and coincidental with the peripheral arthritis[24]. The spondylitis associated with psoriasis and Reiter's syndrome may also follow an independent course, although the radiologic features of spondylitis in these disorders may well differ qualitatively from those in primary AS[25].

It is clear, therefore, that in examining the prognosis of AS an attempt should be made to obtain relatively homogeneous populations classified according to genetic type, sex, age of onset, and associated diseases. The evidence so far presented does not indicate convincingly a difference in the outcome of the spondylitis in any of the subgroups discussed above, but further work needs to be done.

The problem of process assessment in AS

A leading article in the *Lancet* in 1987 identified the difficulties in relating process variables such as ESR to clinical disease activity and outcome in AS[26]. If clinical disease activity in AS is defined as pain and stiffness requiring NSAIDs together with nocturnal pain and prolonged early morning symptoms, then a number of studies have shown that the acute-phase reactants such as ESR, plasma viscosity, and C-reactive protein (CRP) are unrelated to clinical activity[27-30]. What is clear from these studies, however, is that patients with peripheral arthritis have elevated acute-phase proteins and these vary according to the amount of active synovitis present in the peripheral joints. This is the pattern seen in other inflammatory arthritides such as rheumatoid arthritis and presumably occurs because of the different pathologic process involved in peripheral synovitis as opposed to axial enthesitis. Ebringer and colleagues, however, have found a reasonably good association between CRP, ESR, axial disease activity, and *Klebsiella* carriage[31], and have more recently taken this a step further by measuring the reduction in serum IGA levels in relation to improvement in disease activity on a low-starch, high-protein diet[32].

The definition of active disease in axial AS therefore still rests on clinical definitions that vary from study to study. The recently developed Newcastle Enthesis Index may provide some help in assessment of clinical disease activity in a quasi-objective manner but this index awaits further evaluation[33].

Table 1 Causes of death in ankylosing spondylitis

1. Due to arthritis:
    (i) Complete cervical fracture
    (ii) Bronchopneumonia and respiratory failure associated with fused, restricted thoracic cage and severe dorsal kyphosis

2. Due to extra-articular disease:
    (i) Cardiovascular — congestive cardiac failure associated with aortic incompetence, conduction defects, and left ventricular dysfunction
    (ii) Respiratory — apical pulmonary fibrosis with cavitation
    (iii) Renal — amylodosis

Asymptomatic AS

Studies of survival and outcome in AS may be complicated by unidentified apparently healthy people with the disease. Looking at B27 positive blood donors Cohen *et al.* found that 25% of B27 positive cases had a history of low back pain and stiffness, and 54% had limited lumbar flexion compared with 29% of a B27 negative control population. Three out of 24 B27 positive donors had definite AS previously undiagnosed[34]. However, this American study has been challenged by a similar study from Australia where 168 B27 positive apparently normal subjects were screened by questionnaire and X-ray. In the Australian group no cases of AS or sacroiliitis were found. Fifty-two percent of the B27 positive group complained of back pain at some time compared with 49% of the control group[35].

Any study concerned with the natural history and prognosis of a disease must therefore strive to include all cases having the disease. Even in community-based surveys this is not always possible. In hospital-based studies only the worst cases are likely to be seen on a long-term basis and therefore it is likely that we have an unduly pessimistic idea of the prognosis and outcome in AS.

REVIEW OF PROGNOSIS LITERATURE IN DETAIL

Mortality

Mention has already been made of the influence of the iatrogenic factors on mortality, including the effect of radiotherapy and induction of fatal peptic ulceration by NSAIDs. There is little doubt, however, from further studies excluding patients who were treated by radiotherapy, that there is an increased and early mortality in AS[10,38-40] (see Table 1).

Neurologic

Most series that have looked at mortality in AS have included a few cases who have died as a result of a midcervical fracture, often as a result of minor trauma. Cases particularly at risk are those with fused cervical spines. The risk of suffering this complication is not known. AS may cause atlantoaxial subluxation and it has been suggested that this form of cervical instability is more likely to lead to neurologic complications such as tetraplegia and death because of the relative reduction in cervical diameter in AS.

Uncommonly a cauda equina syndrome may occur due to reduction in lumbar canal diameter but this complication is rarely fatal.

Cardiovascular disease

It is well recognized that aortitis at the level of the aortic valve occurs in AS and this can lead to aortic incompetence, cardiac failure, and subsequent death. This is thought to account for between 3% and 14% of all deaths due to AS[36]. In addition conduction defects may occur and contribute to mortality, and recently left ventricular dysfunction has been noted independently of these other cardiac abnormalities[37]. Twenty percent of deaths reviewed by Khan et al. were thought to be due to cardiovascular disease[38]; this figure was 35% in a series from Scandinavia[41].

Pulmonary disease

AS may cause a cystic fibrotic condition of the upper zones of both lungs resembling tuberculosis. Early reports suggested that tuberculosis was more frequently seen in AS[36], but since pulmonary tuberculosis has become uncommon in Western countries, a fibrotic condition specific to AS has been identified. However, 2 out of 30 cases reviewed by Khan in 1981 had pulmonary tuberculosis[38].

Respiratory function is progressively impaired by fusion of the costochondral, costovertebral, and intervertebral joints and death may occur from subsequent pneumonia and respiratory failure. This was the cause of death in 25% of cases (thought to be disease related) that were reviewed by Carette et al.[39]

Amyloidosis

Up to 6% of cases have renal amyloidosis at autopsy[36], but this complication is rarely diagnosed in life. As a cause of death the incidence varies from study to study. None of the cases reviewed by Khan[38] died from amyloidosis and renal amyloid was the cause of death in only a very small percentage of cases in two other series[39,40]. However, a series from Finland found that one-fifth of cases died from uremia due to renal amyloidosis[41]. A subsequent study by the same authors showed that 16% of 76 subjects with AS had a raised creatinine or proteinuria, but none of the subjects had a renal biopsy[42].

Peripheral joint involvement

In some studies there is a hint that extra-articular complications resulting in untimely death may be seen more frequently in subjects with peripheral joint disease and iritis[36,39]. The study by Carette et al. also suggested that patients with iritis and peripheral arthritis had more severe axial changes[39].

Radiographic changes

Despite some scepticism[26], the scintigraphic index of sacroiliac uptake of bone-seeking radioisotopes appears to have greater sensitivity than radiology in the early stages of AS[43]. Moreover, the index appears to be sensitive to changes in pain and stiffness induced by NSAIDs[43,44]. The index is only of use in active sacroiliitis and may be normal where the joints are fused. The presence of sacroiliitis appears to have no prognostic value.

It has been suggested that radiologic changes proceed independently and are a function of the duration of the disease. The apparent improvement that may occur in some cases in spinal mobility would suggest otherwise[39]. As yet we know of no treatment that has been shown to retard the progression of radiologic disease, although this may have been true for radiotherapy[8]. A study by Boersma in 1976 suggested that phenylbutazone had the ability to retard radiologic progression but no allowance was made for the antiphlogistic effect of phenylbutazone in enabling patients to exercise more efficiently. In the next section we will discuss anthropometric changes in response to physical therapy that suggest that active exercise regimes can halt the progressive limitation of movement. It is likely, therefore, that radiologic progression can also be halted by physical methods.

Anthropometric measurements

Early reports suggested that unless the disease was treated aggressively in its early stages progression to complete ankylosis of the spine with deformity was inevitable[8]. The part played by regular exercise therapy in preventing this deterioration was initially emphasized by Hart[46] and further reported by Wynn-Parry[47]. Inevitably some loss of range of movement at presentation is found. Figure 1 depicts the model of gradual deterioration with exacerbations and remissions in a patient with untreated spondylitis. Data to support

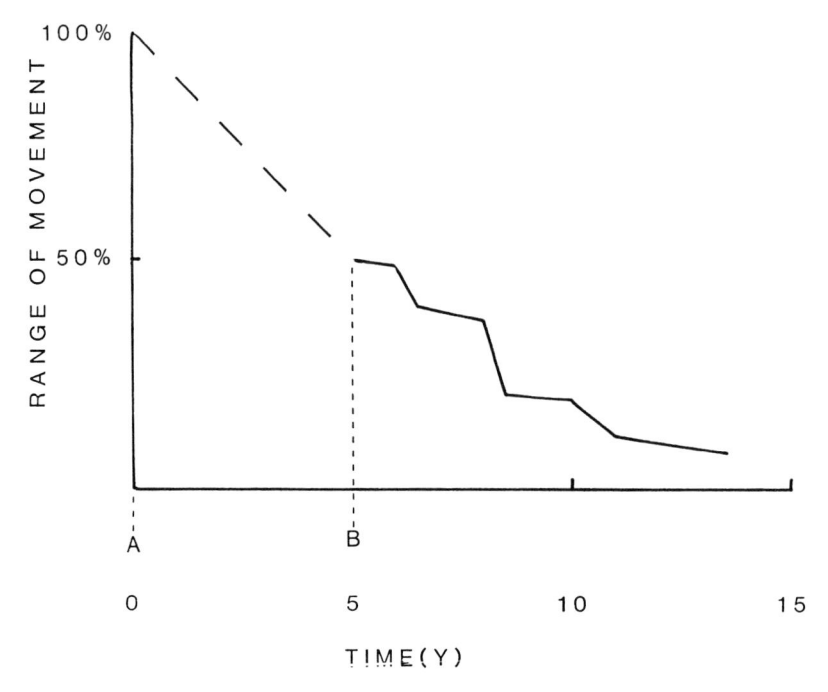

Figure 1 Hypothetical model of anthropometric progression in AS. Point A represents onset of disease (and possibly first symptom). Point B represents time of diagnosis

this hypothetical model are unavailable and are likely to remain so. However, we have information on the effect of treatment on anthropometric measures following presentation.

What are the instruments that have been used to measure spinal mobility and shape? A number of measures have been used over the years, many of which vary from study to study. For example, in the lumbar spine anterior flexion may be measured by the finger-tip to floor distance, by a modified Schöbers test[48], by using the Dunhams spondylometer, or by adapting a flexicurve ruler[49].

The finger to floor distance is a composite movement and may be normal when the lumbar spine is fused providing hip joints are normal and hamstrings are extensible. It is subject to warming-up and diurnal variation (James Smeathers, unpublished data) and is probably age and sex related.

A measure of thoracic spine involvement and costovertebral joint ankylosis is provided by the chest expansion. Unfortunately, this may be measured in a variety of positions from the line of the nipples, the fourth intercostal space, and the xiphisternum. Chest expansion has proved to be one of the more variable measurements between observers. Again this measure is age and sex related. Some measure of the thoracic kyphosis is obtained by recording the occiput to wall or

Table 2 Progression of anthropometric measurements in 51 subjects with ankylosing spondylitis followed from 1947 (average disease duration, 7 years) to 1980 (average disease duration 42 years). Patients categorized according to range of movement in lumbar, thoracic and cervical spine. I – little restriction in movement; II – moderate restriction; III – severe restriction

	1947	1980 I	1980 II	1980 III
I	15	11	1	3
II	14	9	4	1
III	22	1	4	17

Adapted from Carette et al.[39]

tragus to wall distance and recently a new device for measuring this parameter has been developed[50].

Cervical spine measurements were originally made using a tape measure and measuring the distance, for example in cervical flexion, that the chin could be opposed to the sternum. Most studies now measure cervical range of movement using a spirit goniometer.

How reproducible are the anthropometric measurements? Roberts and colleagues showed that warm-up increases the realiability of some of these measures, including finger to floor distance and cervical rotation[51]. Despite this they found intrarater reliability to be good in AS for such measures as Schöbers test, chest expansion, finger to floor distance, and cervical rotation. Stokes et al. noted a large interobserver difference for finger to floor distance and commented that many tape measures made of material are potentially elastic[50]. For all studies involving anthropometric measurements we therefore need to make careful note of the following points: the time of day of the measurements, the observer (preferably the same), a clear statement of the method used, and, in comparative studies, correction of the data for age and sex.

Effects of treatment on anthropometric measures

Carette et al. in a study of 51 long-term survivors with AS seen over a period of 33 years found that improvements in spinal mobility occurred during this time (see Table 2)[39]. No mention of treatment regime was made in this paper but they demonstrated clearly that inevitable deterioration in spinal movements does not occur. Improvement occurred especially in those who presented (after an average of 7 years disease) with reasonably good range of movement.

Centers in the United Kingdom such as Bath and Harrogate are now offering a regular 3-week intensive physiotherapy inpatient regime for

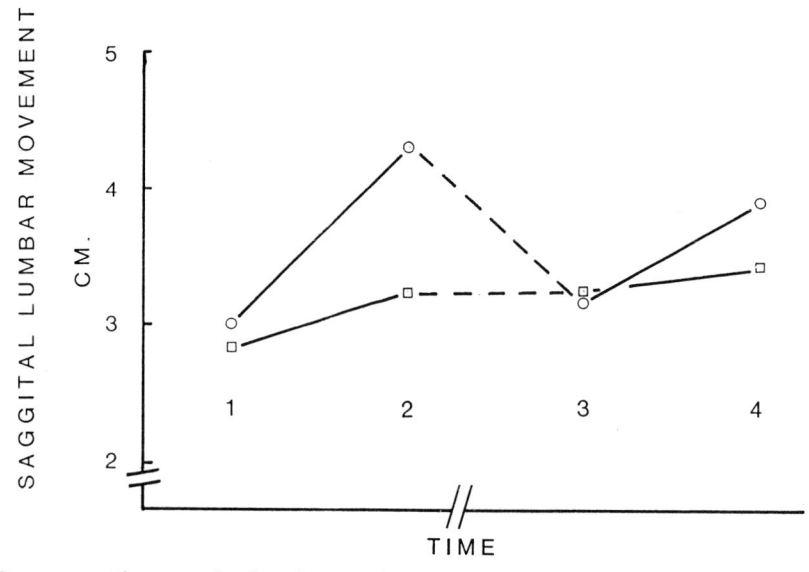

Figure 2a Change in lumbar flexion after two periods of intensive inpatient physiotherapy. *Point 1* = start of first 3-week period. *Point 2* = end of first 3-week period. *Point 3* = start of second 3-week period. *Point 4* = end of second 3-week period. Average interval between points 2 and 3 was 1.5 years for data of Helliwell, Evard, and Wright (circles) and 5.0 years for those of Roberts et al.[53] (squares)

patients with AS. O'Driscoll et al. have demonstrated short-term improvements in cervical mobility in response to such a regime[52]. The effects of these regimes in the long term have recently been evaluated by ourselves (Helliwell, Evard, and Wright, unpublished data) and by Roberts et al[53]. Our own series consisted of 23 patients, all males, with an average age of 42 years and an average duration of disease from first symptom of 15.5 years. Seven had radiologic fusion of the cervical spine, three of the thoracic spine, and five of the lumbar spine and, interestingly, 16 had evidence of peripheral joint involvement. Changes in cervical flexion/extension, lumbar flexion/extension, and chest expansion are presented in Figures 2(a) to (c) together with the results of the study by Roberts et al. In our own series, and that of Roberts et al., chest expansion was measured at the xiphisternum, lumbar flexion/extension by the modified Schöbers method, and cervical movements using a spirit goniometer. Roberts et al. found that the short-term improvements were independent of disease duration in all measures and that improvement on the first visit did not predict improvement on the second.

The improvements in range of movement demonstrated by these studies were only small but may be of functional importance to the already disabled patient. No attempt has yet been made to correlate limited range of movement with functional disability in AS, although

ANKYLOSING SPONDYLITIS

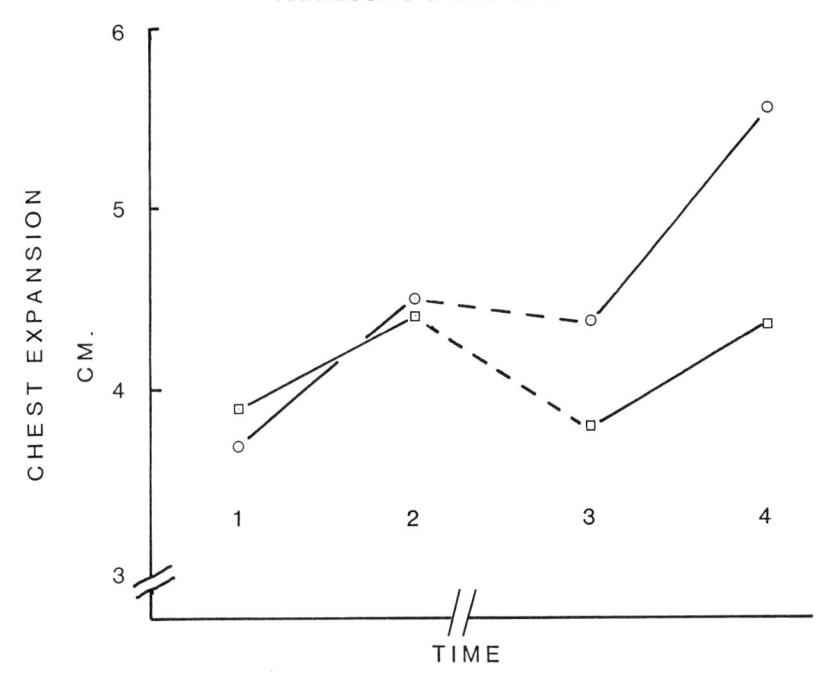

Figure 2b Changes in chest expansion at xiphisternum: same legend as for Figure 2a

this has been done for other rheumatic diseases[54], and we are embarking on a study to examine this question.

These studies have shown that short-term improvement in range of movement can be obtained even in the more severely affected cases of AS. Such improvements may have been due to an increase in ligamentous laxity, or may simply reflect an increase in voluntary effort after 3 weeks of encouraging rest and physiotherapy.

Perhaps a decrease in pain contributed to the small increase in range of movement. Such an effect has been demonstrated in a double blind crossover trial of three NSAIDs in AS[55].

The comparative efficacy of different forms of intensive physiotherapy in this condition has not been compared, although we have just started a study to compare inpatient intensive physiotherapy with outpatient exercises with or without hydrotherapy. A recent study from Nottingham and Peterborough in England casts some doubt on the validity of regular physiotherapy in AS[56]. Comparing a small number of patients from each center, one group received advice only and the other regular physiotherapy during the 2-year period. No difference in spinal shape was seen between patients in the two centers. The only anthropometric improvements obtained were in the intermalleolar distance (for hip involvement) and range of movement of the lumbar spine; both these occurred in the active physiotherapy group.

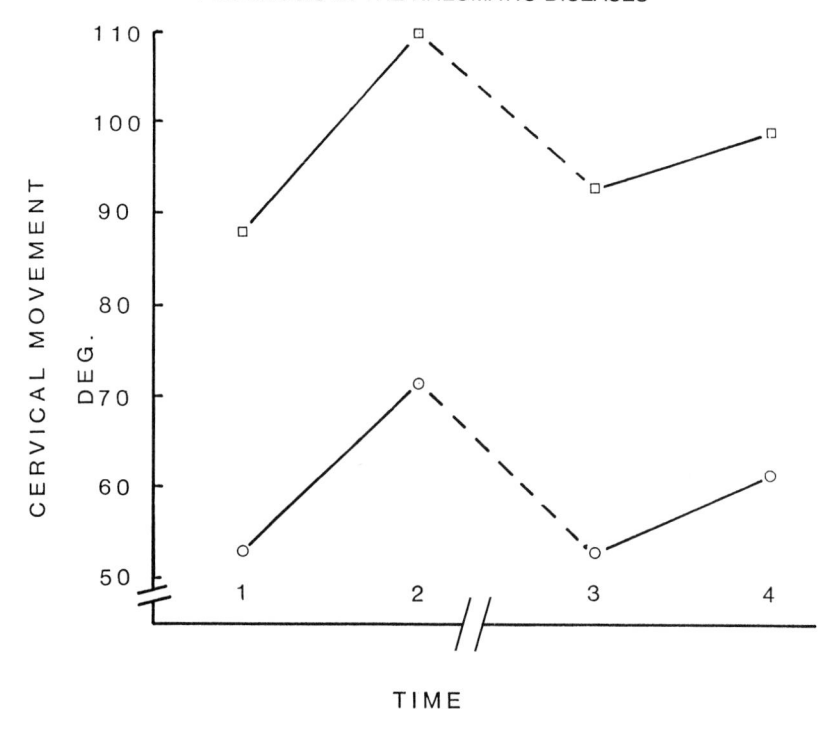

Figure 2c Change in range of movement of cervical spine over same period. Cervical movements were flexion/extension measured by a spirit goniometer for patients of Helliwell, Evard, and Wright (circles) and rotational movement measured with spirit goniometer for those of Roberts et al.[53] (squares)

DISCOMFORT AND PAIN RELIEF

Early studies, such as that of Wilkinson and Bywaters[6] suggested that the first 10 years of the disease were the worst in terms of pain. Hart[36] described a prespondylitic fibrositic stage where pain may be experienced around the chest wall, the pelvis, and the heels. Sometimes there is a systemic illness with anorexia and fever. Weight loss also occurs and may persist throughout the spondylitic's career. However, a recent postal survey of NASS members using both the AIMS and ASAQ questionnaires (see later) found that frequency of NSAID usage and subjective pain and stiffness was identical in subjects divided into cohorts of different disease duration[57]. For all cohorts, females experienced more pain than males. It is difficult to understand how, when the spine is radiologically fused, exacerbations of inflammatory disease persist; most of our patients with fused spines complain of stiffness and deformity rather than pain.

Symptom control in AS is usually readily achieved by treatment with NSAIDs, in particularly phenylbutazone. Despite the risks of agranulocytosis and the withdrawal of this drug from the general market in Britain, phenylbutazone is still prescribable by hospital doctors for AS because of its efficacy in this disease. However, it is probable that other drugs in this class are equally effective. Some NSAIDs are clearly more effective than others: naproxen and indomethacin are superior in clinical trials to azapropazone and aspirin[44,55]. The claim that phenylbutazone was effective in preventing radiologic progression of the disease was probably related to its antiphlogistic effect[45].

Recently an attempt has been made to quantify the extra-articular pain of AS[33]. The Newcastle Enthesis Index (NEI) relies on the response to firm pressure over a number of bony prominences. This group has demonstrated the NEI to be reliable within but not between observers. They also found the NEI to be sensitive to NSAIDs in an "open" trial. Further work needs to be done to determine response of the index to NSAIDs in placebo controlled trials and in relation to other rheumatic diseases such as primary fibromyalgia and rheumatoid arthritis.

Patients with AS who have ankylosed spines often complain bitterly of jarring while traveling in vehicles. In addition we have recently observed that gait in AS can only be described as "cautious." Spondylitics have a decreased stride length and frequency and, weight for weight, produce a smaller heel strike impact than normal[58]. Furthermore, when the spine is ankylosed, the spinal column acts as a rigid strut thus preventing flexion and shock absorption by the spine in response to impact loading. Theoretically this form of discomfort may be alleviated by reducing impact loads at the foot, using appropriate insoles and footwear.

Disability and functional outcome

Spondylitics are customarily regarded as a robust uncomplaining group compared to patients with other rheumatic diseases. Indeed, in comparison to rheumatoid arthritis, functional status after comparable duration of disease is much better in AS, although employment status appears to be related to duration of disease[59]. Unemployment due to illness has been quoted as around 8% after 24 years of disease in New Zealand[60] and 16% after 20 years of disease in Oxford, England[61]. Chamberlain has pointed out that although patients with AS remain in employment they may have to modify their work on account of their disease, which may lead to loss in status and income[12].

Functional outcome and employment status is related to peripheral joint involvement[62,63] and also the severity of spinal involvement[64]. A specific instrument for measuring disability in AS has been developed in Bath, England: the Ankylosing Spondylitis Assessment Questionnaire (ASAQ), which assesses disability, pain, and overall function by a self-administered questionnaire. This has proved reproducible and more appropriate than the commonly used Stanford Health Assessment Questionnaire[64].

Work, leisure, and sexual activity may all be affected by disease severity and extent of peripheral joint involvement. Severe thoracic and rib-cage involvement causes a decease in respiratory tolerance, as measured objectively by a falling vital capacity. Sexual problems are more often admitted by female spondylitics than males: Chamberlain found that 5 out of 6 female spondylitics complained of sexual difficulty, whereas only 8 out of 25 males admitted to this problem[12]. In a later survey it was found that females, who are more likely to have peripheral joint involvement, had more disruption of their social life and had more mobility problems than males[65].

We have commented in an earlier section on the small increase in movement seen in short intensive courses of physiotherapy in this condition; as yet we do not yet know how significant small increases are in terms of function. We have no data on the minimal joint ranges necessary for specific tasks — e.g., cervical extension when shaving. In any case, patients are likely to overcome such disabilities by employing "trick" movements or adaptations.

SUMMARY OF RISK FACTORS IN ANKYLOSING SPONDYLITIS

Mortality

This is clearly related to extra-articular features of the disease such as renal, cardiovascular and respiratory complications. Although extra-articular features are seen more commonly in patients with peripheral arthritis, the data on this are confusing. More juvenile ankylosing spondylitics have peripheral arthritis[18] and a recent survey of patients with AS seen in the outpatient department in Bath found that hip disease was a function of age of onset and was also related to severity of spinal disease[66]. Carette *et al.*[39] also found more peripheral arthritis in the younger spondylitics and found peripheral arthritis to be associated with more severe spinal disease and extra-articular features. However, a postal survey, matching groups of spondylitics for disease duration, showed that those with younger age of onset had a better outcome than adult spondylitics[18]. This contrasts with an earlier survey of the same population comparing those who had joint surgery and those who had not; in the surgical group 51% were found to be unable to work compared with 73% in the nonsurgical group. Surgery in this context was related to age of onset and hip involvement: extra-articular disease was similar in both groups[63]. Indicators of extra-articular disease therefore remain unclear and further study of this question is required.

The other major cause of mortality in this group of patients is cervical fracture, which occurs mainly in patients with a fused cervical spine. Risk factors for cervical fusion are duration of disease and presence of peripheral arthritis.

Table 3 Summary of adverse prognostic factors in AS

Young age onset[39,63,66] (except juvenile spondylitics?[18])

Peripheral arthritis[39]

Iritis[39]

Other extra-articular features (cardiovascular, pulmonary, renal)[36]

Male sex?[20,21]

B27 + ?[14,15]

Range of movement

Radiologic change in the spine that correlates with anthropometric measures is best predicted by duration of disease. There is a suggestion that patients with peripheral arthritis and recurrent iritis are at more risk from progressive ankylosis of the spine. The suggestion that B27 negative patients and females have milder disease has also been discussed in a previous section: again the evidence is conflicting.

Disability

Disability is a function of severity and extent of spinal ankylosis and the presence or absence of peripheral arthritis. These risk factors have been discussed above.

Table 3 summarizes the known risk factors according to mortality, range of movement and disability.

FUTURE PERSPECTIVES

NSAIDs act merely as palliative agents in AS. They are effective in relieving pain and stiffness and allowing the patient to exercise and, therefore, theoretically preventing the progression of spinal disease.

Are there any specific antirheumatic drugs or disease-modifying agents effective in AS? Hill reviewed the use of conventional antirheumatic drugs such as gold, D-penicillamine, and hydroxychloroquine and found no evidence to support the use of these agents in AS[67]. We have attempted to treat severe exacerbations of pain and stiffness with high-dose intravenous pulsed methylprednisolone in a placebo controlled trial in 20 patients with AS (Neumann, Evard, Hopkins, and Wright, unpublished observations). No added benefit was seen in the high-dose steroid group.

Trials with sulfasalazine have been more promising. Initial studies appeared to support a beneficial effect of sulfasalazine on the peripheral arthritis associated with seronegative spondarthritides[68-70]. More recently, sulfasalazine 2 g daily has been shown to have a beneficial effect on subjective and objective indices of spinal involvement[71,72]; the latter study suggested a reduction in radiologic progression. In contrast, a 48-week study published by Corkhill et al. in 1988 failed to show any improvement in either the peripheral or axial arthritis in a group of 62 patients who appeared to have early disease[73].

On balance the evidence supports a beneficial effect of sulfasalazine, although further work needs to be done, in particular on early disease, with studies of progression over a number of years. Why should sulfasalazine work and other conventional antirheumatic drugs not be effective? Recent interest in the etiopathogenesis of AS suggests an interaction between host genetic susceptibility and gut bacteria[32] and may provide the link.

Since *Klebsiella* seems to be frequently implicated in AS, the Leeds group attempted to modify *Klebsiella* carriage by alteration in diet[74]. The carriage of *Klebsiella* was not influenced by the experimental diet, probably because of poor compliance; in addition, the fluctuations in disease activity seen bore no relationship to the carriage of *Klebsiella* organisms. More recently Ebringer and colleagues have attempted to modify *Klebsiella* carriage by giving a low-starch, high-protein diet in a small group of spondylitics[32]. In this open trial there was an overall reduction in pain and stiffness during the 6 months of the diet with corresponding decrease in serum IGA, ESR, and C-reactive protein. However no matching control group was studied; nor were any figures given for the isolation of fecal *Klebsiella*. It is possible that many patients with AS have subclinical bowel inflammation and recent work from Holland has suggested that inflammation of the terminal ileum may be present in seronegative reactive peripheral arthritis and in families having a seronegative spondarthritis[75]. More work on this subject is required and we are in need of a less invasive but reliable test of bowel inflammation. Isotope studies have suggested that iliocecal inflammation and abnormal gut permeability may merely be a side-effect of NSAIDs[76]. It is possible that new developments in molecular biology will lead to further information on the etiopathogenesis of this disease and on further treatment options.

We still do not have a clear idea of which physical regimes are most effective in AS. This sort of information is necessary and may well be used in future for resource planning. We and the team at Bath have shown that a 3-week intensive course of physical therapy prevents progression of anthropometric measurements over a period of some years. However, a study from Nottingham appeared to suggest that such an intensive regime was unnecessary[56]. In order to look further at this question we have just commenced a controlled study of inpatient versus outpatient physiotherapy regimes in AS. An important part of this trial will be an attempt to relate loss of movement in various parts of the spine to functional disability.

Further studies are required to relate changes in anthropometric measures to radiologic changes. We still do not have a system of scoring spinal X-rays that is reliable and reproducible. It is possible that new imaging modalities such as magnetic resonance imaging may help in defining the early changes, although preliminary studies have failed to differentiate early sacroiliitis. An objective quantification of this sort would help with trials of disease-modifying therapy in early disease and reduce our reliance on subjective assessments of disease activity.

References

1. Wright, V. and Moll, J. M. H. (1976). *Seronegative Polyarthritis*, pp. 124-125. (Amsterdam: North Holland)
2. Kellgren, J. H., Jeffrey, M. R. and Ball, J. (eds.) (1963). *The Epidemiology of Chronic Rheumatism*, Vol. 1, pp. 324-327. (Oxford: Blackwell Scientific)
3. Polley, H. F. and Slocumb, C. H. (1947). Rheumatoid spondylitis: a study of 1035 cases. *Ann. Intern. Med.*, **26**, 240-249
4. Hart, F. D. and Maclagan, N. F. (1955). Ankylosing spondylitis: a review of 184 cases. *Ann. Rheum. Dis.*, **14**, 77-83
5. Blumberg, B. and Ragan, C. (1956). The natural history of rheumatoid spondylitis. *Medicine (Baltimore)*, **35**, 1-31
6. Wilkinson, M. and Bywaters, E. G. L. (1958). Clinical features and cause of ankylosing spondylitis. *Ann. Rheum. Dis.*, **17**, 209-228
7. Ebringer, R. W., Cawdell, D. R., Cowling, P. and Ebringer, A. (1978). Sequential studies in ankylosing spondylitis: Association of Klebsiella pneumoniae with active disease. *Ann. Rheum. Dis.*, **37**, 146-151
8. Scott, S. G. (1942). *A Monograph on Adolescent Spondylitis or Ankylosing Spondylitis*. (Oxford: Oxford University Press)
9. Court-Brown, W. M. and Doll, R. (1965). Mortality from cancer and other causes after radiotherapy for ankylosing spondylitis. *Br. Med. J.*, **2**, 1327-1332
10. Radford, E. P., Doll, R. and Smith, P. G. (1977). Mortality among patients with ankylosing spondylitis not given X-ray therapy. *N. Engl. J. Med.*, **297**, 572-576
11. Calman, F. M. B. and Berry, H. (1980). The present position of radiotherapy in ankylosing spondylitis. In Moll, J. M. H. (ed.) *Ankylosing Spondylitis*, pp. 243-248. (Edinburgh: Churchill-Livingstone)
12. Chamberlain, M. A. (1981). Socioeconomic effects of ankylosing spondylitis. *Int. Rehabil. Med.*, **3**, 94-99
13. Van der Berg-Loonen, E. M., Dekker-Saeys, B. J., Meunissen, S. G. M. et al. (1977). Histocompatibility antigens and other genetic markers in ankylosing spondylitis and inflammatory bowel disorders. *J. Immunogenet.*, **4**, 167-175
14. Woodrow, J. C. and Eastmond, C. J. (1978). HLA-B27 and the genetics of ankylosing spondylitis. *Ann. Rheum. Dis.*, **37**, 504-509
15. Khan, M. A., Kushner, I. and Braun, W. W. (1977). Comparison of clinical features in HLA-B27 positive and negative patients with ankylosing spondylitis. *Arthritis Rheum.*, **20**, 909-912
16. Schaller, J. (1977). Ankylosing spondylitis of childhood onset. *Arthritis Rheum.*, **20**, 398-401
17. Ansell, B. M. (1980). Juvenile spondylitis and related disorders. In Moll, J. M. H. (ed.) *Ankylosing Spondylitis*, pp. 120-136. (Edinburgh: Churchill Livingstone)
18. Calin, A. and Elswood, J. (1988). The natural history of juvenile onset ankylosing spondylitis. A 24 year retrospective case-control study. *Br. J. Rheumatol.*, **27**, 91-93
19. Calin, A. and Fries, J. (1975). An extraordinary high prevalence of ankylosing spondylitis in W27 positive males and females. A controlled study. *N. Engl. J. Med.*, **293**, 835-839
20. Tyson, T. L., Thompson, W. A. L. and Ragan, C. (1953). Marie Strumpel spondylitis in women. *Ann. Rheum. Dis.*, **12**, 40-42
21. Hart, F. D. and Robinson, K. C. (1959). Ankylosing spondylitis in women. *Ann. Rheum. Dis.*, **18**, 15-23
22. Marks, S. H., Barnett, M. and Calin, A. (1983). Ankylosing spondylitis in women and men: a case controlled study. *J. Rheumatol.*, **10**, 624-628

23. McKenna, F., Hickling, P., Brophy, T., Taggart, A. and Wright, V. (1986). Ankylosing spondylitis in women and men: a comparative study. *Br. J. Rheumatol.*, **25** (Abstract 69)
24. Helliwell, P. S. and Wright, V. (1987). Seronegative spondarthritides. *Baillière's Clinical Rheumatology*, **1**, 491–523
25. McEwen, C., Di Tata, D., Lingg, C., Porini, A., Good, A. and Rankin, T. (1971). A comparative study of ankylosing spondylitis and spondylitis accompanying ulcerative colitis, regional enteritis, psoriasis and Reiter's disease. *Arthritis Rheum.*, **14**, 291–318
26. Leader (1987). Assessing disease activity in ankylosing spondylitis. *Lancet*, **1**, 1072
27. Kendall, M. J., Lawrence, D. S., Shuttleworth, G. R. and Whitfield, A. G. W. (1973). Haematology and biochemistry of ankylosing spondylitis. *Br. Med. J.*, **2**, 235–237
28. Scott, D. G. I., Ring, E. F. J. and Bacon, P. A. (1981). Problems in the assessment of disease activity in ankylosing spondylitis. *Rheumatol. Rehabil.*, **20**, 74–80
29. Laurent, M. R. and Panayl, G. S. (1983). Acute-phase proteins and serum immunoglobulins in ankylosing spondylitis. *Ann. Rheum. Dis.*, **42**, 524–528
30. Sheehan, N. J., Slavin, B. M., Donovan, M. P., Mount, J. N. and Matthews, J. A. (1986). Lack of correlation between clinical disease activity and erythrocyte sedimentation rate, acute phase proteins or protease inhibitors in ankylosing spondylitis. *Br. J. Rheumatol.*, **25**, 171–174
31. Cowling, P., Ebringer, R., Cawdell, D., Ishll, M. and Ebringer, A. (1980). C-reactive protein, ESR, and klebsiella in ankylosing spondylitis. *Ann. Rheum. Dis.*, **39**, 45–49
32. Ebringer, A., Childerstone, M. and Ptaszynska, T. (1989). Treatment of ankylosing spondylitis using a low starch–high protein diet. *Br. J. Rheumatol.*, **28** (Abstract suppl. 1), 6
33. Mander, M., Simpson, J. M., McLellan, A., Walker, D., Goodacre, J. A. and Carson, Dick, W. (1987). Studies with an enthesis index as a method of clinical assessment in ankylosing spondylitis. *Ann. Rheum. Dis.*, **46**, 197–202
34. Cohen, L., Mittal, K. K., Schmid, F. R. *et al.* (1976). Increased risk for spondylitis stigmata in apparently healthy HLA-BW27 men. *Ann. Intern. Med.*, **84**, 1–7
35. Christiansen, F. T., Hawkins, B. R., Dawkins, R. L., Owen, E. T. and Potter, R. M. (1979). The prevalence of ankylosing spondylitis among B27 positive normal individuals — a reassessment. *J. Rheumatol.*, **6**, 713–718
36. Hart, F. D. (1980). Clinical features and complications. In Moll, J. M. H. (ed.) *Ankylosing Spondylitis*, Chapter 5, pp. 52–68. (Edinburgh: Churchill Livingstone)
37. Sun, J. P., Khan, M. A. and Bahler, R. C. (1987). Impairment of cardiac diastolic function in patients with ankylosing spondylitis as evaluated by Doppler echocardiography. *Br. J. Rheumatol.*, **26** (Abstract suppl. 1), 71
38. Khan, M. A., Khan, M. K. and Kishner, I. (1981). Survival among patients with ankylosing spondylitis: a life-table analysis. *J. Rheumatol.*, **8**, 86–90
39. Carette, S., Graham, D., Little, H., Rubenstein, J. and Rosen, P. (1983). The natural disease course of ankylosing spondylitis. *Arthritis Rheum.*, **26**, 186–190
40. Kaprove, R. E., Little, A. H., Graham, D. C. and Rosen, P. S. (1980). Ankylosing spondylitis: survival in men with and without radiotherapy. *Arthritis Rheum.*, **23**, 57–61
41. Lehtinen, K. (1980). Cause of death in 79 patients with ankylosing spondylitis. *Scand. J. Rheumatol.*, **9**, 145–147
42. Lehtinen, K. (1980). 76 patients with ankylosing spondylitis seen after 30 years of disease. *Scand. J. Rheumatol.*, **12**, 5–11
43. Namey, T. C., McIntyre, J., Buse, M. and Leroy E. C. (1977). Nucleographic studies of axial spondarthritides. *Arthritis Rheum.*, **20**, 1057–1064
44. Dunn, N. A., Mahida, B. H., Merrick, M. V. and Nuki, G. (1984). Quantitative sacroiliac scintiscanning: a sensitive and objective method for assessing efficiency of non-steroidal anti-inflammatory drugs in patients with sacroiliitis. *Ann. Rheum. Dis.*, **43**, 157–159
45. Boersma, J. W. (1976). Retardation of ossification of the lumbar vertebral column in ankylosing spondylitis by means of phenylbutazone. *Scand. J. Rheumatol.*, **5**, 60–64
46. Hart, F. D. (1955). The treatment of ankylosing spondylitis. *Proc. R. Soc. Med.*, **48**, 207–210

47. Wynn-Parry, C. B. (1966). Management of ankylosing spondylitis. *Proc. R. Soc. Med.*, **59**, 619-623
48. Moll, J. M. H. and Wright, V. (1971). Normal range of spinal mobility. *Ann. Rheum. Dis.*, **30**, 381-386
49. Burton, A. K. (1987). The ratio of upper lumbar to lower lumbar sagittal mobility related to age, sex, and low back trouble. *Eng. Med.*, **16**, 233-236
50. Stokes, B. A., Helewa, A., Goldsmith, C. H., Groh, J. D. and Kraag, G. R. (1988). Reliability of spinal mobility measurements in ankylosing spondylitis patients. *Physiotherapy (Canada)*, **40**, 338-344
51. Roberts, W. N., Pallozzi, L., Daltroy, L. and Liang, M. (1986). Warm up increases the reliability of some anthropometric techniques in ankylosing spondylitis. *Br. J. Rheumatol.*, **25**, 123 (Abstract)
52. O'Driscoll, S. L., Jayson, M. I. V. and Baddeley, H. (1978). Neck movements in AS and their responses to physiotheraphy. *Ann. Rheum. Dis.*, **37**, 64-66
53. Roberts, W. N., Larson, M. G., Liang, M. H., Harrison, R. A., Barefoot, J. and Clarke, A. K. (1989). Sensitivity of anthropometric techniques for clinical trials in ankylosing spondylitis. *Br. J. Rheumatol.*, **28**, 40-45
54. Badley, E. M., Wagstaff, S. and Wood, P. H. N. (1984). Measures of functional ability (disability) in arthritis in relation to impairment of range of joint movement. *Ann. Rheum. Dis.*, **43**, 563-569
55. Godfrey, R. G., Calabro, J. J., Mills, D. and Maltz, B. A. (1972). A double blind crossover trial of aspirin, indomethacin, and phenylbutazone in ankylosing spondylitis. *Arthritis Rheum.*, **15**, 110
56. Swannell, A. J. (1988). The case against the value of exercise in the long-term management of ankylosing spondylitis. *Clin. Rehabil.*, **2**, 245-247
57. Will, R., Elswood, J. and Calin, A. (1989). The natural history of ankylosing spondylitis: a cohort study of pain and disability in men and women controlled for disease duration. *Br. J. Rheumatol.*, **28** (Abstract suppl. 1), 20
58. Helliwell, P. S., Smeathers, J. and Wright, V. (1989). Shock absorption by the spinal column in normals and ankylosing spondylitis. Proc. I Mech. Eng, Part H, *Eng. Med.*, **203**, 187-190
59. Lehtinen, K. (1981). Working ability of 76 patients with ankylosing spondylitis. *Scand. J. Rheumatol.*, **10**, 263-265
60. McGuigan, L. E., Hart, H. H., Gow, P. J. *et al.* (1984). Employment in ankylosing spondylitis. *Ann. Rheum. Dis.*, **43**, 604-606
61. Wordsworth, B. P. and Mowat, A. G. (1986). A review of 100 patients with ankylosing spondylitis with particular reference to socio-economic effects. *Br. J. Rheumatol.*, **25**, 175-180
62. Calabro, J. J. and Amante, C. M. (1968). Prognosis in ankylosing spondylitis. *Arthritis Rheum.*, **11**, 471
63. Calin, A. and Elswood, J. (1987). Ankylosing spondylitis: a nationwide analytical review: entry variables determining surgical intervention and outcome. *Br. J. Rheumatol.*, **26** (Abstract suppl. 1), 53
64. Nemeth, R., Smith, F., Elswood, J. and Calin, A. (1987). Ankylosing spondylitis — an approach to measurement of severity and outcome: ankylosing spondylitis assessment questionnaire (ASAQ) — a controlled study. *Br. J. Rheumatol.*, **26** (Abstract suppl. 1), 69-70
65. Chamberlain, M. A. (1983). Socio-economic effects of ankylosing spondylitis in females: a comparison of 25 males with 25 females. *Int. Rehabil. Med.*, **5**, 149-153
66. Calin, A. and Elswood, J. (1987). The relationship between pelvic, spinal and hip involvement in ankylosing spondylitis — one disease process or several? *Br. J. Rheumatol.*, **26** (Abstract suppl. 2), 116
67. Hill, A. G. S. (1980). Drug therapy. In Moll, J. M. H. (ed.) *Ankylosing Spondylitis*. Chapter 14, pp. 163-175. (Edinburgh: Churchill Livingstone)
68. Amor, B., Kahan, A., Dougados, M. and Delriev, F. (1984). Sulphasalazine and AS. *Ann. Intern. Med.*, **101**, 878
69. Dougados, M., Boumier, P. and Amor, B. (1986). Sulphasalazine in ankylosing spondylitis: a double blind controlled study in 60 patients. *Br. Med. J.*, **293**, 911-914

70. Fraser, S. M. and Sturrock, R. D. (1987). An interventional study of sulphasalazine in ankylosing spondylitis with peripheral joint involvement. *Br. J. Rheumatol.*, **26** (Abstract suppl. 2), 117
71. Davis, M. J., Dawes, P. T., Lewin, I. V. and Stanworth, D. R. (1988). The effect of sulphasalazine (SAS) on serum levels of IgA-alpha 1 and the complex of IgA alpha 1 anti-trypsin (IgA/AAT) in ankylosing spondylitis. *Br. J. Rheumatol.*, **27** (Abstract suppl. 1), 57
72. Taylor, H. G., Beswick, E. J., Davis, M. J. and Dawes, P. T. (1989). Sulphasalazine in ankylosing spondylitis: effective in early disease? *Br. J. Rheumatol.*, **28** (Abstract suppl. 1), 6
73. Corkhill, M., Jobanputra, P., Gibson, T. and MacFarlane, D. (1988). Sulphasalazine treatment of ankylosing spondylitis. *Br. J. Rheumatol.*, **27** (Abstract suppl. 2) 81
74. Shinebaum, R., Neumann, V., Hopkins, R., Cooke, E. M. and Wright, V. (1984). Attempt to modify klebsiella carriage in ankylosing spondylitic patients by diet: correlation of klebsiella carriage with disease activity. *Ann. Rheum. Dis.*, **43**, 196–199
75. Mielants, H., Veys, E. M., Joos, R. *et al.* (1986). Familial aggregation in seronegative spondylitis of enteric origin. A family study. 1986. *J. Rheumatol.*, **13**, 126–128
76. Bjarnason, I., So, A., Levi, A. J., Peters, T. J., Williams, P., Zanelli, G. D., Gumpel, J. M. and Ansell, B. (1984). Intestinal permeability and inflammation in rheumatoid arthritis: effects of non-steroidal anti-inflammatory drugs. *Lancet*, **2**, 1171–1173

7
Psoriatic arthritis
D. D. GLADMAN

INTRODUCTION

Psoriasis is a stubborn skin disease affecting up to 3% of the population. Although not life-threatening, it may be associated with important morbidity and disability[1]. Psoriatic arthritis (PSA) has been defined as an inflammatory arthritis, usually seronegative, associated with psoriasis[2]. It has been reported in 10–42% of patients with psoriasis[1-3]. Although the notion of PSA as a separate entity was first proposed by Aliberti in 1822, until some 30 years ago this form of arthritis was considered a variant of rheumatoid arthritis (RA). The concept of PSA as an entity distinct from RA has evolved over the past three to four decades. Epidemiologic studies have shown an increased prevalence of psoriasis among arthritis patients, and conversely, an increased prevalence of arthritis among patients with psoriasis[2-10]. Clinically, it has been noted that, unlike RA, there is no female preponderance in the arthritis associated with psoriasis. The discovery of the rheumatoid factor enabled distinction of RA from PSA, as over 70% of patients with RA have a positive rheumatoid factor, whereas the majority of patients with PSA are seronegative. Thus, PSA has only been studied systematically over the past 30 years.

Most authors have suggested that PSA is a benign arthropathy. However, with the exception of one study[11], the information has been derived from a cross-sectional assessment of patients with PSA at one point in time, and not from prospective follow-up of patients. Thus, it has been difficult to define the prognosis in PSA and to identify the factors that are associated with a benign course or those that lead to severe disease.

NATURAL HISTORY OF PSORIATIC ARTHRITIS

Clinical features

PSA usually begins in the third or fourth decade of life. There is only a slight female preponderance in PSA[2-20]. The arthritis develops after the onset of psoriasis in the majority of patients with a mean interval of 10 years[17]. Some patients note the simultaneous onset of skin and joint disease. However, in each study there is a frequency of about 15% of patients whose arthritis precedes the onset of psoriasis, by as much as 15 years[2-18] (Table 1). The arthritis is inflammatory in nature. It is associated with pain, swelling, and limitation of movement in the affected joints and, unlike rheumatoid arthritis, may be associated with redness or purplish discoloration over the affected joints. At least half of the patients may complain of morning stiffness of more than 30 minutes' duration. In our clinic, 97% of the patients had evidence of actively inflamed joints at their first visit[17]. Any joint may be affected, in a symmetric or asymmetric distribution. The distal interphalangeal joints are involved in half of the patients[17]. Dactylitis, or inflammation of the whole digit, may be seen in a third of the patients, and is more common among patients with distal interphalangeal joint involvement[17]. Our experience suggests that in some patients with PSA, deformity and damage develop quickly after the onset of inflammatory changes in a particular digit. The radiographic features of PSA include erosive changes that are common to inflammatory arthropathies. In some patients these changes may be so advanced as to cause the "pencil and cup" radiologic picture. Tuft resorption may also be seen in patients with PSA. In addition, PSA is associated with periostitis, and other evidence of bony reaction such as enthesopathy, which help differentiate it from RA[2,21]. Spinal involvement occurs in about 35% of the patients[17,18]. Back involvement may be associated with inflammatory back pain and stiffness, as well as limitation of movement, or may be totally asymptomatic[17,20]. Radiographs show changes of sacroiliitis, and evidence of syndesmophytes. The latter may be classical, marginal syndesmophytes in a symmetric fashion, as seen in ankylosing spondylitis, or large, paramarginal syndesmophytes, which are usually asymmetric[2,17-21].

Clinical patterns of psoriatic arthritis

The emergence of the clinical patterns unique to this form of arthritis resulted from the descriptive studies of Wright[3-5] and Moll and Wright[2,7,8], and the radiologic studies of Avilla et al.[9] and Baker[10]. In 1956, Wright studied 42 patients with psoriasis and erosive arthritis, and compared them to patients with classical RA[4]. In addition to the lack of female preponderance in PSA, he concluded that PSA was less often polyarticular at onset and tended to be less severe than RA. However, in a further report by Wright of 118 patients with erosive arthritis and psoriasis[5,6], the majority of patients were found to have an

Table 1 Clinical features of PSA in reported series

Feature	Wright	Little	Roberts	Leonard	Kammer	Scarpa	Gladman
Male/female	18/16	?	57/101	16/14	45/55	33/29	104/116
Age (years)	?	?	?	55	?	54	46
Age onset — skin	35	?	?	35	36	?	29
Age onset — joints	?	?	35–45	44	42	?	36
Family history (%)	35	41	26%	10%	?	?	40
Nail lesions (%)	87	93	?	97	88	?	83
Skin < Joints (%)	64	?	74	?	50	?	68
Simultaneous (%)	13	?	10	?	20	?	15
Joints < skin (%)	23	?	16	?	30	?	17
Asymmetric oligo-arthritis (%)	53	?	?	63	54 (+D)[a]	16.1	11[b]
Symmetric poly-arthritis (%)	31	?	79	23	25 (+D)[a]	39	19[c]
Distal (%)	3	?	28[d]	3	?	7.5	12
Back (%)	10	?	5[d]	7	21	21	2[e]
Mutilans (%)	?	?	5[d]	3	?	2.3	16
Sacroiliitis (%)	87	30	?	30	?	16	27

[a] D=distal joints included.
[b] 14 including symmetric oligoarthritis.
[c] 40 including asymmetric polyarthritis.
[d] Includes more than one category.
[e] 33 including peripheral joint + back involvement.

arthritis indistinguishable from RA, although only 17% of them had a positive rheumatoid factor. In a review paper in 1973, Moll and Wright[8] summarized their concept of PSA, and described five clinical patterns: (1) distal involvement; (2) arthritis mutilans; (3) symmetric polyarthritis, indistinguishable from RA; (4) asymmetric oligoarthritis; and (5) spondyloarthropathy. Despite the fact that in previous papers the majority of patients had an arthritis indistinguishable from RA, the 1973 paper described a "symmetric polyarthritis" in only 15% of the patients, while the "asymmetric" group emerged as the most common form of PSA, occurring in 70% of the patients.

There have been several studies supporting this concept of PSA and its clinical patterns[11-17]. Roberts et al.[11] described 168 patients, the majority of whom had a polyarthritis indistinguishable from RA. Distal joint disease was much less common and did not occur by itself. Axial disease was distinctly uncommon and was associated with severe involvement of peripheral joints. Little et al.[12] and Leonard et al.[13] have stressed the association of arthritis with severe psoriasis. Leonard confirmed the distribution of the five clinical patterns in a population of 30 patients[13]. Kammer et al.[15] reported on 100 patients with PSA. They divided their patients into those with asymmetric oligoarthritis, those with symmetric polyarthritis, and patients with back involvement. The latter group included patients with peripheral joint disease belonging to the other groups. Distal joint disease seemingly did not occur by itself. Scarpa et al.[16] described 62 patients with PSA among 180 patients with psoriasis. They found polyarthritis to be most common among their patients, occurring in 38.7%, followed by back disease in 21%, oligoarthritis in 16%, distal pattern in 7.5%, and arthritis mutilans in 2.3% of the patients. Similarly, polyarthritis was the most common pattern seen among the patient population followed at the PSA clinic at Women's College Hospital in Toronto[17], occurring alone in 40% of the patients, with an additional 21% having polyarthritis and back involvement. Oligoarthritis (fewer than 5 joints involved) occurred in 14% of the patients, and was associated with back disease in another 7%, while the distal pattern occurred in 12% without back disease, and in a further 4% of the patients together with spinal involvement. Thus, a total of 61% of the patients had polyarthritis, 21% had oligoarthritis, and 16% had distal involvement. Back disease alone occurred in 2% of this group of patients. Table 1 compares the clinical features of patients with PSA in the reported series. The frequency of back disease in PSA is difficult to ascertain at times. It appears that back involvement alone is uncommon in PSA. This may be due to the fact that spinal involvement is not always symptomatic, and since not all patients with psoriasis are sent for radiographic evaluation, or even for rheumatological evaluation, many of these patients remain undiagnosed. The reported frequency of back disease in PSA has varied between 2% and 35%. Lambert and Wright[19] reviewed the prevalence of spinal disease in PSA. They evaluated 130 patients with PSA for presence of back disease, based on back pain, and reduction in back and neck mobility. They documented spinal disease in 40% of their patients. Radiographs were available for 103 patients. Radiologic evidence for sacroiliitis was found in 21% of the patients, and syndesmophytes were found in 30%. Patients with and without back disease were compared, and it was found that patients with back disease tended to be older. Patients who had sacroiliitis without peripheral arthritis tended to be males with a shorter duration of psoriasis. Similar observations were described for the Toronto PSA population[17,20].

The description of the clinical patterns of PSA has been helpful in diagnosing the disease and separating it from RA. It is this description that allows the diagnosis of PSA in patients whose psoriasis is not obvious, or even before the onset of skin lesions. However, at times it is difficult to assign a particular pattern to a patient because of overlap of the clinical patterns, especially in the course of follow-up, since the pattern at onset may not necessarily be maintained in the course of the disease. Nonetheless, it is clear that patients with polyarthritis have a more severe disease than patients with oligoarthritis or distal disease. Patients with back disease have a later age of onset of their arthritis. However, the presence of sacroiliitis may be associated with more severe arthritis[6,11].

Associated features of psoriatic arthritis

PSA is defined by the presence of psoriasis. The commonest type of psoriasis associated with PSA is psoriasis vulgaris, which is the most prevalent pattern of psoriasis[1]. Nail lesions appear to be more common among patients with PSA than in patients with psoriasis uncomplicated by arthritis[18,22], but are less common in patients with sacroiliitis without peripheral arthritis[19]. On occasion, the diagnosis of PSA may be confirmed only because of the presence of nail lesions. Some patients with PSA note a strong association between their skin and joint disease, while others do not[11,17]. It has been suggested that joint disease is associated with severe psoriasis[12-14,18]. However, there are patients reported in every study whose arthritis appeared prior to the onset of skin lesions (Table 1). There are also many patients whose arthritis is a major problem, but whose skin lesions are minimal.

Patients with PSA may have other associated extra-articular features. These include features common to all seronegative arthropathies such as iritis, urethritis, colitis, and mucous membrane lesions[2,3,8]. Although Scarpa et al.[16] commented that no extra-articular features were noted in their patients, other series certainly noted these features[15,17]. PSA is also associated with hyperuricemia, and hypergammaglobulinemia[17]. The majority of patients with PSA are seronegative for rheumatoid factor, but there are about 10% who are rheumatoid factor positive and 10% who are antinuclear factor positive[17]. These antibodies are found with the same frequency among patients whose psoriasis is uncomplicated by arthritis, and their relevance to the development of the arthritis is unclear[22]. These antibodies may represent the "normal" occurrence of antibodies in an older population, or may reflect the immunologic phenomena that are present in PSA[23].

HLA antigens as disease markers for psoriatic arthritis

The association between HLA antigens and PSA may be used to identify patients destined to develop psoriasis or PSA[22,24-29]. In addition, HLA antigens may identify patients with a particular pattern of PSA[22,24-27], and thus may be prognostic indicators. In a study of HLA antigen distribution in 158 patients with PSA and 101 patients with uncomplicated psoriasis, HLA antigens B7 and B27 were found more commonly among patients with PSA than patients with psoriasis alone[22]. Among patients with PSA, HLA-B27 was associated with back involvement, while HLA-B38 and B39 occurred more frequently among patients with peripheral polyarthritis. HLA-DR4 was not increased among patients with PSA when compared to controls, however, when patients with RA-like symmetric polyarthritis were analyzed separately, HLA-DR4 was increased compared to controls, in a frequency similar to that seen among RA patients[22]. HLA-DR4 was thought to be more common among patients with more severe PSA[26]. Thus, HLA antigens appeared to be associated with subsets of PSA. However, these studies looked at patients' disease at the time of HLA testing and thus have not related disease course and prognosis to HLA antigens.

Severity of joint disease in psoriatic arthritis

Although studies in the 1950s suggested that PSA was associated with disability[30], more recent studies[11,14,15] have implied that the disease tends to be mild.

In his 1961 study of 118 patients with PSA, Wright[6] noted that deforming arthritis as well as arthritis mutilans was associated with an earlier age of onset of joint disease and with sacroiliitis. Roberts et al.[11] noted the association between back disease and deforming arthritis as well, but felt that in general, PSA tended to be mild. They measured severity by number of admissions to hospital, which were common among their "deforming" group (88%), less common in the "indistinguishable from RA" group (56%) and the "distal" group (44%). Time lost from work was also used as a measure of severity, and was found to be important among patients with deforming arthritis, but less so in the other groups. Molin[14] did not find any patients with mutilating arthritis among his 300 patients. Kammer et al.[15] commented that half of their patients had destructive forms of arthritis. They suggested that although only 25% of the patients with asymmetric oligoarthritis had a destructive form, three-quarters of these patients had a "progressive arthritis." Patients with symmetric arthritis experienced a slowly destructive arthritis. Arthritis mutilans, which is the very deforming form of PSA, was "rarely seen." It was therefore accepted by most rheumatologists that the arthritis associated with psoriasis was of a benign type, and that the synovitis was short-lived and thus did not lead to residual damage in the majority of patients[30].

This concept has recently been challenged, when it was shown that many patients with PSA have deformities and damage, and marked limitation of functional capacity[17]. Eleven percent of the patients had significant disability as measured by the ARA functional class III or IV, and 16% had more than five joints with grade III/IV destructive changes. Stern[18], in a epidemiologic study of patients with psoriasis and arthritis, noted that 50% of patients with PSA reported some limitation in their daily activities as a result of their arthritis. Twice as many patients with PSA were likely to be unemployed than patients with psoriasis who did not have joint complaints, or who had other types of joint disease.

It has been suggested that juvenile-onset PSA may be a more severe disease than adult-onset PSA[31,32]. However, Lambert et al.[33], as well as Hamilton et al.[34] showed that there is no significant difference in juvenile- versus adult-onset PSA, although there may be some differences in genetic predisposition[34].

Course of disease in psoriatic arthritis

In one of his earlier studies, Wright compared patients with psoriasis and erosive arthritis to patients with classic RA, and noted that PSA was less often polyarticular at onset, and tended to be less severe than RA, with fewer affected joints and fewer deformities[4]. In a later study of a larger group of patients, it was noted that deforming arthritis as well as arthritis mulitans were associated with an earlier age of onset of joint disease and with sacroiliitis[5]. A follow-up study of that group of patients concluded that only a small proportion of patients with PSA developed severe arthropathy, in spite of the high prevalence of polyarthritis indistinguishable from RA[11]. A recent longitudinal study of 52 patients with PSA and spondyloarthropathy who had been followed for at least 30 months showed that while there were no important changes in spinal mobility, clinically, there were progressive radiologic changes. There was also significant progression of peripheral joint disease over the mean of 57 months of follow-up in these patients[20]. A 5-year follow-up of 126 patients seen at our PSA clinic revealed that the degree of inflammatory arthritis was decreased, as evidenced by the lower number of patients with inflamed joints and dactylitis at follow-up compared to presentation. However, there was an increased frequency of deformed joints clinically, and progression of damage radiologically[35].

It should be noted that in the course of following patients with PSA we have been impressed with the rapidity with which damage occurs in these patients. We have observed patients with dactylitis who go on to develop ankylosis of a digit within several weeks. We have also observed a number of patients with rapidly progressive deforming arthritis, despite the use of gold therapy.

FACTORS AFFECTING PROGNOSIS

It is unclear whether the prognosis in PSA has changed in the past 20-30 years. As is outlined above, the separation of PSA into its clinical patterns has not always been adhered to, partly because of differences in interpretation of the patterns, and partly because patients do not always fit a pattern clearly. Thus, while PSA has been considered a mild disease by some, it might have been considered more severe by others. In addition, most studies did not include routine radiologic evaluation on all patients, and thus the exact nature of the arthritis, particularly the presence of back disease, was not documented. As a result of this variation, some physicians have tended not to treat patients with PSA with disease-suppressive medications, but would rather prescribe anti-inflammatory or even analgesic medications only for the acute flare of the arthritis.

Treatment modalities used in PSA include nonsteroidal anti-inflammatory medications for mild disease, and disease-modifying drugs for more severe disease[31]. Kammer et al.[15] demonstrated improvement in over 50% of the patients treated with aspirin or other nonsteroidal anti-inflammatory drugs, particularly indocid and phenylbutasone. In our 5-year follow-up study of 126 patients[35], fewer patients displayed inflammatory arthritis at their 5-year follow-up, presumably because of increased use of nonsteroidal anti-inflammatory medications. However, there have been no reports of the long-term outcome of treatment with nonsteroidal medications.

There are several reports suggesting that gold therapy is beneficial in PSA[15,36,37]. A recent double blind study of oral gold (auranofin) in psoriatic arthritis showed only marginal benefit on the number of actively inflamed joints in the treated group[38]. Despite previous concerns, it appears that gold therapy does not exacerbate the psoriasis[15,31]. However, it is unclear what effect gold therapy has on eventual outcome of PSA. Indeed, it has been shown that patients receiving gold therapy were more likely to have erosive disease, but that may have been the reason for the use of this treatment[17]. Antimalarials have also been shown to be beneficial in PSA[15], but there has been persistent concern that these drugs may aggravate the psoriasis[39,40]. D-Penicillamine has also been shown to be effective in psoriatic arthritis[15,41], but its toxic effects, as well as the slow onset of its therapeutic effect, may preclude its use[42]. At present, it is difficult to assess how the use of these "disease-suppressive" medications alters the natural course of PSA, as most of the reported studies describe the therapeutic effect over a 4–6 month period, and there are no follow-up studies describing the long-term effects of these medications.

It has been suggested that the treatment of PSA should include treatment for both psoriasis and arthritis[2,30]. While the majority of patients with psoriasis are treated with topical medications, many are refractory and are therefore treated with systemic therapy[43], including methotrexate[44], PUVA[45], retinoic acid derivatives[46], and more recently cyclosporin[47]. Some of the medications used for PSA have actually been shown to aggravate the psoriasis, such as certain nonsteroidal anti-inflammatory drugs, gold, and chloroquine[39,40,48]. In general, the use of medications that are effective for both skin and joints is preferable for patients with PSA. These medications include methotrexate[49], PUVA[50], and retinoids[51]. Each of these medications has been shown to be effective for PSA, at least in the short term. However, all of these medications are toxic, and their use should be restricted to patients with "severe" disease[30]. Moreover, discontinuation of both methotrexate and retinoic acid derivatives has been associated with severe flares of both the psoriasis and the arthritis. Indeed, we have seen a patient who had previously had minimal joint disease rapidly develop a progressive polyarthritis within 6 weeks of discontinuation of methotrexate. She developed such marked destruction of peripheral joints that she required bilateral hip replacements.

There are no systematic studies of the use of surgery in PSA. The indications for synovectomy and arthroplasty have been the same as those for patients with RA. However, there is disagreement regarding postoperative complications in patients with PSA[2,52,53]. Lambert and Wright reviewed 41 orthopedic procedures in 21 patients with psoriasis and arthritis, 20 of whom had psoriatic arthritis[53]. There were a variety of procedures reported, including synovectomies, arthrodeses, implants, etc. Only one operation was complicated by mild wound infection.

Thus, while there is ample evidence that both nonsteroidal antiinflammatory medications and cytotoxic medications are effective for control of inflammation in psoriatic arthritis, there is no information available as to the effect of treatment on the course and prognosis of PSA.

REVIEW OF PROGNOSIS LITERATURE

Since there is a paucity of long-term studies in PSA, outcome is not always available. From the studies that have been reported, it has been suggested that female sex and early age of onset may be associated with more severe disease. It may also be that severe skin manifestations are associated with more severe joint disease. This may in part be due to the fact that more severe joint disease prevents the patients from looking after their skin disease appropriately. Alternatively, severe skin disease may lead to immobility, and development of contractures. Psoriasis itself rarely causes death, except when there is an exfoliative dermatitis or amyloidosis[1]. Reed and Wright reported 24 deaths, and attributed some of them to corticosteroid therapy, other therapy, or amyloidosis[54]. Roberts et al.[11] provided information on 18 deaths that occurred in the course of follow-up of their 227 patients with psoriasis and arthritis. A major cause of death was ischemic heart disease, but two patients died of infections possibly related to the presence of axial disease, and one patient died of gastrointestinal hemorrhage, possibly related to immunosuppressive therapy. However, only 168 of these 227 patients had psoriatic arthritis, and it is unclear how many of the deaths occurred within this subgroup of their total patient population with psoriasis and arthritis. In our study of PSA patients with a minimum of 5 years' follow-up[35], 12 patients have died. In two of these patients methotrexate side-effects may have been a contributing cause, as both developed liver cirrhosis and its complications.

FUTURE PERSPECTIVES

The exact definition of prognosis in PSA is not clear. There appears to be a group of patients who are particularly destined to develop a more severe disease. These patients usually have a polyarthritis (with or without a spondyloarthropathy) that is rapidly progressive and results in deformity and damage as well as disability. There are other patients with PSA who seem to have a more benign course, and thus a better prognosis, with fewer joints involved, with minimal damage, and who manage to carry on with little or no disability. From the discussion above it appears that the course and prognosis of PSA is variable and may be dependent on sex, age of onset of both psoriasis and PSA, severity of psoriasis, pattern of PSA, HLA antigens, and perhaps other hereditary determinants. Further study is clearly required of patients with PSA with and without spondyloarthropathy in order to assess the factors related to disease severity.

So far, it has been difficult to get a handle on the measurement of prognosis. The term "severe disease" may have different meaning in various reports in the literature. Some authors consider the presence of polyarthritis per se as severe disease. Others refer to the presence of active inflammation as reflecting severe disease. There are investigators who may use the term severe to denote only those patients who have disability. The assessment of disability, deformity, and damage has not been uniform in the literature. Are patients disabled only if they cannot work? Or are patients disabled when they cannot perform every function they would like to? Deformity and damage have not been adequately addressed in many of the reported studies of PSA. This is partly due to the fact that the concept of deformity and damage is not widespread, and partly because of the fact that the measurements themselves are not uniform. It is quite clear that in many studies not all patients have had radiographs, and thus radiologic damage was not uniformly assessed.

In order to study prognosis one must first define the outcome measures, and then assess the prognostic indicators. Damage can be assessed clinically on the basis of the presence of a decreased range of movement of more than 20% of the range that cannot be attributed to active inflammation; the presence of contractures, subluxation, loosening, or ankylosis; or previous surgery. In addition, the change in damage over time can be calculated by dividing the number of clinically damaged joints by the disease duration. Radiologic damage is evidenced by the presence of both erosive changes and joint space narrowing (ARA class III) or when there is complete disorganization or ankylosis of the joint (ARA class IV)[55]. Again, the change of damage over time can be calculated by dividing the number of radiologically damaged joints by the disease duration. The progression of damage may further be studied by defining damage states and analyzing the time for progression between these states.

Measures of disability include functional capacity — as described by the ARA criteria[55], or by other measures of physical activity[56]. The employment status of the patient may further define disability, as well as the number of hospitalizations required for PSA in a defined period of time. Multidimensional health status instruments have been developed[57], and these may be used to assess disability in patients with PSA.

In order to confirm the reliability of the outcome measures to be used in the study of prognostic factors in PSA, we performed a study to evaluate measurements of actively inflamed joints, as well as deformed and damaged joints and radiologically damaged joints in patients with PSA[58]. The Latin square design used in our study allows an improved organizational design, enables examinations during a fixed period of time, and includes specific numbers of observers and patients[58]. This design controls two different sources of variation that may increase the experimental errors: observer variability and order of examination[59,60]. Joint inflammation was documented by the number of joints with stress pain and/or effusions. Clinical damage was documented by the number of deformed joints, and the number of joints with ankylosis, loosening, or limitation of movement of more than 20% of the range. The Latin square design as outlined above was also implemented in reading radiographs of hands and feet of the same patients with PSA. Damage was documented in peripheral joints by the presence of grade III (showing erosions with joint space narrowing) or grade IV (showing ankylosis and/or disorganization of the joint) radiologic change. Five observers examined 5 patients on each of two examination days, for a total of 10 patients. Analysis of variance was used to partition the variance into components, including observer differences, patient differences, and the order of the joint examination. Indeed, for actively inflamed joints and for damaged joints less that 1% of the variance was attributable to observer differences. Similarly, less than 1% was due to order of examination. The major component of the variance was due to patient differences. Indeed, there was a span of patient activity and damage, with the number of actively inflamed joints ranging from 5 to 28 and the number of damaged joints from 2 to 49 among the patients participating in the study. Thus, there was no evidence for systematic observer difference in the measurement of either actively inflamed joints or the damaged joints. Thus, the clinical outcome measures to be used in the prognosis study have been found to be reliable. These may now be used in the study of prognosis in PSA. The results for radiologic assessment were not as good[58], and suggest that further refinement of radiologic evaluation is required.

The extent of disability that occurs among patients with PSA remains to be elucidated. It is clear from the information available that there is a certain proportion of patients with PSA, perhaps more so among those with polyarthritis, who develop significant disability and who are unemployable. With more sophisticated measures of functional outcome more information should become available in the future. We are currently administering the Arthritis Impact Measurement Scales[61] to our patients with PSA.

The study of prognosis in PSA can only be performed by longitudinal follow-up of a large number of patients. Such a study is currently under way at the PSA clinic at the University of Toronto Rheumatic Disease Unit.

References

1. Farber, E. M. and Scott, E. V. (1979). In Fitzpatrick *et al.* (eds.) *Dermatology in General Medicine.* 2nd edn., pp. 233-247. (New York: McGraw-Hill)
2. Wright, V. and Moll, J. M. H. (1976). Psoriatic arthritis. In *Seronegative Polyarthritis*, pp. 169-223. (Amsterdam: North Holland)
3. Wright, V. (1981). Psoriatic arthritis. In Kelly, W. N., Harris, E. D., Ruddy, S. and Sledge, C. B. (eds.) *Textbook of Rheumatology*, pp. 1047-1062. (Philadelphia: Saunders)
4. Wright, V. (1956). Psoriasis and arthritis. *Ann. Rheum. Dis.,* **15**, 348-356
5. Wright, V. (1959). Rheumatism and psoriasis. A Reevaluation. *Am. J. Med.,* **27**, 454-462
6. Wright, V. (1961). Psoriatic arthritis: a comparative study of rheumatoid arthritis and arthritis associated with psoriasis. *Ann. Rheum. Dis.,* **20**, 123-131
7. Wright, V. and Moll, J. M. H. (1971). Psoriatic arthritis. *Bull. Rheum. Dis.,* **21**, 627-632
8. Moll, J. M. H. and Wright, V. (1973). Psoriatic arthritis. *Semin. Arthritis Rheum.,* **3**, 55-78
9. Avila, R., Pugh, D. G., Slocumb, C. H. and Winkelmann, R. K. (1960). Psoriatic arthritis: a roentgenographic study. *Radiology,* **75**, 691-701
10. Baker, H. (1965). The relationship between psoriasis, psoriatic arthritis and rheumatoid arthritis. An epidemiological, clinical and serological study. MD Thesis, University of Leeds
11. Roberts, M. E. T., Wright, V., Hill, A. G. S. and Mehra, A. C. (1976). Psoriatic arthritis. Follow-up study. *Ann. Rheum. Dis.,* **35**, 206-212
12. Little, H., Harvie, J. N. and Lester, R. S. (1975). Psoriatic arthritis in severe psoriasis. *Can. Med. Assoc. J.,* **112**, 317-319
13. Leonard, D. G., O'Duffy, J. D. and Rogers, R. S. (1978). Prospective analysis of psoriatic arthritis in patients hospitalized for psoriasis. *Mayo Clin. Proc.,* **53**, 511-518
14. Molin, J. (1978). Psoriatic arthritis. *Ann. Clin. Res.,* **8**, 305-311
15. Kammer, G. M., Soter, N. A., Gibson, D. J. and Schur, P. H. (1979). Psoriatic arthritis: clinical, immunologic and HLA study of 100 patients. *Semin. Arthritis Rheum.,* **9**, 75-97
16. Scarpa, R., Oriente, P., Pucino, A., Torella, M., Vignone, L., Riccio, A. and Biondi Oriente, C. (1984). Psoriatic arthritis in psoriatic patients. *Br. J. Rheumatol.,* **23**, 246-250
17. Gladman, D. D., Shuckett, R., Russell, M. L., Thorne, J. C. and Schachter, R. K. (1987). Psoriatic arthritis (PSA) — an analysis of 220 patients. *Q. J. Med.,* **62**, 127-141
18. Stern, R. S. (1985). The epidemiology of joint complaints in patients with psoriasis. *J. Rheumatol.,* **12**, 315-120
19. Lambert, J. R. and Wright, V. (1977). Psoriatic spondylitis: A clinical and radiological description of the spine in psoriatic arthritis. *Q. J. Med.,* **56**, 411-425
20. Hanly, G. S., Russell, M. L. and Gladman, D. D. (1988). Psoriatic spondyloarthropathy. A longterm prospective study. *Ann. Rheum. Dis.,* **47**, 386-393
21. Resnick, D. and Niwayama, G. (1981). Psoriatic arthritis. In *Diagnosis of Bone and Joint Disorders*, pp. 1103-1129. (Philadelphia: W. B. Saunders)
22. Gladman, D. D., Anhorn, K. A. B., Schachter, R. K. and Mervart, H. (1986). HLA antigens in psoriatic arthritis. *J. Rheumatol.,* **13**, 586-592
23. Gladman, D. D. (1985). Immunologic factors in the pathogenesis of psoriatic arthritis. In Gerber, L. H. and Espinoza, L. R. (eds.) *Psoriatic Arthritis*, pp. 33-44. (Orlando, Fla.: Grune & Stratton)
24. Espinoza, L. R. (1985). Psoriatic arthritis: Further epidemiologic and genetic considerations. In Gerber, L. H. and Espinoza, L. R. (eds.) *Psoriatic Arthritis*, pp. 9-32. (Orlando, Fla.: Grune & Stratton)
25. Gerber, L. H., Murray, C. L., Perlman, S. G., Barth, W. F., Decker, J. L., Nigra, T. A. and Mann, D. L. (1982). Human lymphocyte antigens characterizing psoriatic arthritis and its subtypes., *J. Rheumatol.,* **9**, 703-707
26. Espinoza, L. R., Vasey, F. B., Gaylord, S. W., Dietz, C., Bergen, L., Brigeford, P. and Germain, B. F. (1982). Histocompatibility typing in the seronegative spondyloarthropathies; A survey. *Semin. Arthritis Rheum.,* **11**, 375-381
27. Kantor, S. M., Hsu, S. H., Bias, W. B. and Arnett, F. C. (1984). Clinical and

immunologic subsets of psoriatic arthritis. *Clin. Exp. Rheumatol.*, **2**, 105-109
28. Beaulieu, A. D., Roy, R., Mathon, G., Morrisette, J., Latulippe, L., Lang, J. Y. et al. (1983). Psoriatic arthritis: Risk for patients with psoriasis — a study based on histocompatibility antigen frequencies. *J. Rheumatol.*, **10**, 633-636
29. McKendry, R. J. R., Sengar, D. P. S., Des Groseilliers, J. P. and Dunne, J. V. (1984). Frequency of HLA antigens in patients with psoriasis or psoriatic arthritis. *Can. Med. Assoc. J.*, **130**, 411-415
30. Fawcitt, J. (1950). Bone and joint changes associated with psoriasis. *Br. J. Radiol.*, **23**, 440-453
31. Bennet, R. M. (1989). Psoriatic arthritis. In McCarthy, D. J. (ed.) *Arthritis and Related Conditions*, 11th edn, pp. 954-971. (Philadelphia: Lea & Febiger)
32. Shore, A. and Ansell, B. M. (1982). Juvenile psoriatic arthritis — an analysis of 60 cases. *J. Pediatr.*, **100**, 529-535
33. Lambert, J. R., Ansell, B. M., Stephenson, E. and Wright, V. (1976). Psoriatic arthritis in childhood. *Clin. Rheum. Dis.*, **2**, 339-352
34. Hamilton, M. L., Gladman, D. and Shore, A. (1990). Juvenile psoriatic arthritis (JPSA) — Clinical analysis and HLA antigens. *Ann. Rheum. Dis.* (in press)
35. Gladman, D. D., Stafford-Brady, F., Chang, C. H., Lewandowski, K. and Russell, M. L. (1989). Longitudinal study of clinical and radiological progression in psoriatic arthritis (PSA). *J. Rheumatol.*, **17**, 809-812
36. Dowart, B. B., Gall, E. P., Schumacher, H. R. and Krauser, R. E. (1978). Chrysotherapy in psoriatic arthritis. Efficacy and toxicity compared to rheumatoid arthritis. *Arthritis Rheum.*, **21**, 513-515
37. Richter, M. B., Kinsella, P. and Corbett, M. (1980). Gold in psoriatic arthritis. *Ann. Rheum. Dis.*, **39**, 279-280
38. Carrett, S. and Calin, A. (1987). Evaluation of auranofin in psoriatic arthritis: a double blind placebo controlled trial. *Arthritis Rheum.*, **30** (suppl.), S25
39. Luzar, M. J. (1982). Hydroxychloroquine in psoriatic arthropathy: exacerbations of psoriatic skin lesions. *J. Rheumatol.*, **9**, 462-464
40. Abel, E. A., DiCicco, L. M., Orenberg, E. K., Fraki, J. E. and Farber, E. M. (1986). Drugs in exacerbation of psoriasis. *J. Am. Acad. Dermatol.*, **15**, 1007-1022
41. Roux, H., Schiano, A., Maestracci, D. and Serratrice, G. (1979). Notre experience du traitement du rheumatisme psoriasique par la D-penicillamine. *Revue de Rheumatisme*, **46**, 631-633
42. Fye, K. H. and Tannenbaum, L. (1982). Penicillamine induced pemphigus vulgaris in psoriatic arthritis. *J. Rheumatol.*, **9**, 331-332
43. Marks, J. M. (1980). Psoriasis: Utilising the treatment options. *Drugs*, **19**, 429-436
44. Roenigk, H. H., Herback, H. I. and Weinstein, G. P. (1973). Methotrexate therapy in psoriasis. *Arch. Dermatol.*, **108**, 35
45. Parish, J. A., Fitzpatrick, T. B., Tanenbaum, L. and Pathak, M. A. (1974). Photochemotherapy of psoriasis with oral methoxsalen and longwave ultraviolet light. *N. Engl. J. Med.*, **291**, 1207-1211
46. Dahl, B., Mollenbach, K. and Reyman, F. (1977). Treatment of psoriasis vulgaris with a new retinoic acid derivative Ro 10-9359. *Dermatologica*, **134**, 261-267
47. Van Joost, T. H., Bos, J. B., Heule, F. and Meinardi, M. M. H. M. (1988). Low-dose cyclosporin A in severe psoriasis. A double-blind study. *Br. J. Dermatol.*, **118**, 183-190
48. Powles, A. V., Griffiths, C. E., Seifert, M. H. and Fry, I. (1987). Exacerbation of psoriasis by indomethacin. *Br. J. Dermatol.*, **117**, 799-800
49. Black, R. L., O'Brien, W. M., Van Scott, E. J., Auerbach, R., Eisen, A. Z. and Bunim, J. J. (1964). Methotrexate therapy in psoriatic arthritis. Double blind study on 21 patients. *J. Am. Med. Assoc.*, **189**, 743-747
50. Perlman, S. G., Gerber, L. H., Roberts, R. M., Nigra, T. P. and Barth, W. F. (1979). Photochemotherapy and psoriatic arthritis. *Ann. Intern. Med.*, **91**, 717-722
51. Klinkhoff, A. V., Gertner, E., Chalmers, A., Gladman, D. D., Stewart, W. D., Schachter, G. D. and Schachter, R. K. (1989). Pilot study of etretinate in psoriatic arthritis. *J. Rheumatol.*, **16**, 779-791
52. Belsky, M. R., Feldow, P., Millender, L. H. et al. (1982). Hand involvement in psoriatic arthritis. *J. Hand Surg.*, **7**, 203-207

53. Lambert, J. R. and Wright, V. (1979). Surgery in patients with psoriasis and arthritis. *Rheumatol. Rehabil.*, **18**, 35-37
54. Read, W. B. and Wright, V. (1966). In *Modern Trends in Rheumatology* (London: Butterworth)
55. Steinbrocker, O., Traeger, C. H. and Battermab, R. C. (1949). Therapeutic criteria for rheumatoid arthritis. *J. Am. Med. Assoc.*, **140**, 659-662
56. The Glossary Committee, American College of Rheumatology. (1988). Physical status instruments. *Dictionary of the Rheumatic Diseases*, Vol. II, *Health Status Measurement*, pp. 7-8. (Bayport, N.Y.: Contact Associates International Ltd.)
57. The Glossary Committee, American College of Rheumatology. (1988). Multi-dimensional health status instruments. *Dictionary of the Rheumatic Diseases*, Vol. III, *Health Status Measurement*, pp. 43-46. (Bayport, N.Y.: Contact Associates International Ltd.)
58. Gladman, D. D., Farewell, V., Buskila, D., Goodman, R., Hamilton, L., Langevitz, P. and Thorne, J. C. (1990). Reliability of measurements of active and damaged joints in psoriatic arthritis. *J. Rheumatol.*, **17**, 62-64
59. Snedecor, G. W. and Cochran, G. W. (1980). *Statistical Methods*, 7th edn. pp. 269-273. (Ames: Iowa State University Press)
60. Cohen, J. (1977). *Statistical Power Analysis for the Behavioral Sciences*, revised edn., p. 323. (New York: Academic Press)
61. Meenan, R. F., German, P. M., Mason, J. H. and Dunalf, R. (1982). The Arthritis Impact Measurement Scales: further investigations of a health status measure. *Arthritis Rheum.*, **25**, 1048-1053

8
Reiter's syndrome

W. F. KEAN and D. W. MACPHERSON

Reiter's syndrome is a postinfectious syndrome characterized by arthritis, conjunctivitis, and urethritis or cervicitis. In 1916 Hans Reiter described the case of a Prussian cavalry officer serving in the Balkans who developed arthritis, urethritis, and conjunctivitis 8 days following a diarrheal illness. Reiter attributed the condition to a spirochetal or syphilitic type of infection, although the patient denied venereal exposure[1]. Reiter was not the first to describe these symptoms. Among others the disease process had already been described by Sir Benjamin Brodie in 1818[2]. A more extensive survey of the historical literature is cited by Paronen[3], Calin[4], and Keat[5]. The eponym, Reiter's syndrome, is now attached to reactive arthritis occurring after such diseases as *Shigella flexneri* dysentery[3,6-13], *Salmonella typhimurium*[7,13-21], *Yersinia enterocolitica*[13,22-30], *Campylobacter jejuni* enterocolitis[31-36], and *Chlamydia trachomatis* urogenital infections[37-46].

There have been several names used to describe the syndrome; these include reactive arthritis, postdysenteric arthritis, sexually acquired reactive arthritis, and others. Our preference is for the term "reactive arthritis" since it best suits the concept of the definition as currently viewed, although we suspect that this will ultimately be changed as is explained in the text. For the purpose of this chapter we shall use the term Reiter's syndrome but reference to the alternative names may be cited where they pertain to their usage by individual authors in the literature.

In 1981 the American Rheumatism Association Sub-Committee on Criteria for Reiter's syndrome accepted that the complete syndrome consists of a seronegative arthritis, urethritis or cervicitis, and conjunctivitis, but acknowledged that the only two necessary abnormalities are an initiating infectious episode, usually dysenteric or urogenital, and the subsequent development of arthritis[47]. Such a definition could therefore support the concept that Lyme disease also may represent a reactive arthritis[48]. The associated features of Reiter's syndrome include inflammatory lesions of the eye, balanitis, oral ulcers, and keratoderma[47]. It is important to establish that gonococcus is not a cause of Reiter's syndrome, but rather causes a septic arthritis. However, "immune-complex" synovitis due to gonococcus could fit the concept of Reiter's syndrome. The organisms implicated as precipitants for Reiter's syndrome should not be cultured from the joint fluid as this would constitute a septic arthritis. Such a definition, however, may have to be challenged if recent work by Keat and colleagues on the identification of *Chlamydia* particles in the synovium and urogenital tract of patients with reactive arthritis confirms the presence of active or latent infectious material[49].

CLINICAL SYMPTOMS AND SIGNS

Musculoskeleton

Patients usually develop arthritis within 3–6 weeks after the infection. The arthritis is usually a very painful asymmetric condition, predominantly affecting the knees, ankles, metatarsal phalangeal joints, and with an associated enthesitis commonly at the base of the calcaneus, or at the insertion of the Achilles tendon into the calcaneus. There is often a plantar fasciitis and Achilles tendonitis. Occasionally upper limb joints are also involved, causing a swelling of the metacarpal phalangeal joints, the wrists, and dactylitis of the fingers. Low back pain due to associated sacroiliitis, or involvement of the lumbar spine, may also occur[3,38].

Urogenital tract

Within 1–15 days after sexual exposure, a nonspecific urethritis may occur[38]. Shreds of mucoid material may be identified in the urine on an early morning specimen of urine, or following prostatic massage. The prostate is frequently exquisitely tender due to associated prostatitis, and in the fluid obtained following prostatic massage there are usually ten or more white cells per high-power field. Cystitis has been identified in 3% of patients, and hemorrhagic cystitis has also been described[38]. Urethritis may follow dysentery and is not necessarily related only to the sexually acquired form but is much less common at less than 1%[3]. If looked for, a cervicitis may be identified in up to 70% of females, but is commonly asymptomatic[38].

Balanitis is a common finding in acute Reiter's syndrome and is characterized by the presence of small, painless ulcers on the glans penis, or in the urethral meatus. The frequency of balanitis is approximately 25% and occurs with similar distribution in both the post-shigella and venereally acquired forms[3,38]. In the uncircumcised patient the lesion is usually a superficial ulcer, which may become scaly, dry, and hyperkeratotic.

Eye

Conjunctivitis of one or both eyes is the most common associated ocular condition and forms part of the classical triad of Reiter's syndrome. It occurs in approximately 40–80% of patients[3,38], and is thought to have a higher incidence in patients with dysentery. Occasionally patients may progress to develop scleritis, keratitis, and corneal ulceration. The most serious abnormality is uveitis and iritis, which may occur in up to 5% of the affected population with as many as 3% having permanently impaired vision[50].

Skin

Nail involvement occurs in approximately 6% of patients with Reiter's[51]. The appearances can be very similar to the nail changes of psoriasis. Frequently there is hyperkeratosis and heaping of cornified material under the nail. There is also dystrophy of the nails and the nail beds. Occasionally patients form pus that collects under the nail bed and can be expressed upon squeezing. The classical rash of Reiter's syndrome, known as keratoderma blennorrhagicum, clinically resembles some of the skin lesions of psoriasis. Keratoderma is a hyperkeratotic lesion that also shares histologic similarity with psoriatic skin lesions. Distribution is predominantly on the soles of the feet, occasionally on the palms and scrotum, but also on the arms, legs, and trunk. It does not necessarily follow a pattern on the extensor surfaces of the elbows, knees, and sacrum as is characteristic of many forms of clinical psoriasis.

Mouth

Stomatitis has been reported in as many as 27% of patients[51]. The lesions are usually, but not always, painless, and occur on the tongue, cheek, inside of the lips, and on the palate[38,51].

Miscellaneous

Following the acute onset of Reiter's syndrome, many patients appear seriously ill with high fever, rigors, rapid heart rate, and exquisitely tender joints that resemble infected joints[3]. Cardiovascular abnormalities in the form of pericarditis, murmur, and conduction abnormalities have been reported in as many as 7% of these patients, and aortic incompetence has also been recognized[52]. The prognosis of aortic disease is theoretically poor and fortunately the incidence appears to be very low. Cardiac conduction defects may be more common than previously suspected and both early and late cases of atrioventricular conduction block have been indentified. Most cases of conduction abnormalities appear to be self-limited but follow-up is necessary to exclude future development of aortic root diseases[52]. Rarely, neurologic abnormalities can occur, such as peripheral neuropathy, meningoencephalitis, individual cranial nerve lesions, and neuropsychiatric manifestations[12].

LABORATORY DIAGNOSIS

Laboratory tests

By definition[47], if there is established clinical evidence of a predisposing preceding infection such as dysentery or nongonococcal venereal infection, the synovial fluid should be negative for any bacterial organism culture. The synovial fluid in Reiter's syndrome commonly has a leukocyte count of 1000 to 8000 cells/mm^3. The erythrocyte sedimentation rate is usually elevated at 68 to 100 mm/h, and the serum white count is commonly elevated. Complement Factor 3 (C3) is usually elevated in both serum and in synovial fluid.

HLA-B27

The most interesting laboratory finding in Reiter's syndrome is the presence of the Class I antigen HLA-B27 in 60–80% of patients with Reiter's syndrome[40]. This antigen occurs in less than 10% of the normal population, and it is stated that an individual who carries HLA-B27 has a 20% chance of developing Reiter's syndrome following infection by one of the specific organisms causing a reactive arthritis. Several hypotheses have been developed to explain the role of the HLA-B27 antigen. The antigen may act as a receptor for components of an arthritis-causing organism. Second, the so-called biologic mimicry theory suggests that bacterial antigenic components mimic the HLA-B27 antigen[53]. This is supported by the fact that a considerable number of patients carry serum antibodies against a synthetic peptide derived from the HLA-B27 heavy chain[54]. Stieglitz and colleagues have reported that there is a bacterial plasmid common to arthritogenic *Shigella* strains that may play a role in triggering reactive arthritis. Their finding that the plasmid encodes an epitope shared with HLA-B27 supports the molecular mimicry hypothesis for the induction of Reiter's syndrome by arthritogenic strains of *Shigella*[55]. The role of HLA-B27 is not absolute since patients who are HLA-B27 negative develop Reiter's syndrome. It is thus postulated that HLA genes on the sixth chromosome, adjacent to, or linked with, HLA-B27, may be responsible for modulating the immune response to infection, which results in the symptom complex we refer to as Reiter's syndrome[56].

Populations such as Polynesians, who lack the histocompatibility tissue antigen HLA-B27, appear to have a low prevalence of Reiter's syndrome[40]. In his World Health Organization investigation of the islands of Java, Darmawan did not find a high incidence of Reiter's syndrome in that population group but suggested it could be due to under-reporting[57].

Urogenital infection

Chlamydia trachomatis is a pathogen associated with trachoma inclusion conjunctivitis, anogenital tract infections, and lymphogranuloma venereum. Only certain serotypes of *Chlamydia trachoma* are associated with ocular and urogenital infections[58]. Chlamydia has been isolated in 36-50% of cases of nongonococcal urethritis[58,59]. Amor and colleagues identified the presence of antibodies to *Chlamydia trachomatis* in 55% and 64% of Reiter's patients in two separate cohort study groups in France[60]. In Amor's study the presence of the HLA-B27 antigen did not appear to influence the susceptibility to *Chlamydia* infection, but patients who were HLA-B27 negative, and had incomplete Reiter's syndrome, had a lower titer of antibody. Antibiotic treatment of *Chlamydia trachomatis* had no direct effect on the arthritis, but it was suggested that it may play a role in prophylaxis[60]. Keat and coworkers identified a significant increase in IgG antibodies to *Chlamydia trachomatis* in sexually acquired reactive arthritis and nongonococcal urethritis compared to healthy male controls[59]. Amor reported that in the 1982 French study, antibodies to *Chlamydia trachomatis* strain D were present in 64% of Reiter's patients compared to 35.6% of rheumatic controls. It was the conclusion of Amor and his colleagues that *Chlamydia trachomatis* may be the initiating agent in about 50% of patients with posturethritic syndrome or sexually acquired reactive arthritis, and possibly even in a few patients with dysenteric Reiter's syndrome, but he held that the evidence that *Chlamydia trachomatis* was a causative agent of Reiter's syndrome was at that date only statistical[60]. In a study of 8 patients with sexually acquired reactive arthritis, Keat and colleagues, using a fluorescein-conjugated monoclonal antibody technique, found chlamydial elementary bodies in synovial membrane preparations, and synovial fluid cell deposits, in 5 of 8 patients they studied, and they also found evidence of *Chlamydia* organisms in the genital tract of 3 of 6 patients[49]. They identified a high serum IgG antibody titer of greater than 64 (reciprocal titer) in 7 of the 8 patients. The identification of chlamydial bodies by a monoclonal technique has significant implications. This may prove to be a faster, cheaper method of detecting the presence of *Chlamydia*. If, as shown by Keat and colleagues, there may be *Chlamydia* organisms within the joint cavity, and if these are viable, there are important implications for treatment. Although oral antibiotic treatment does not appear to influence the course of the disease[61], intravenous and intra-articular antibiotic therapy may influence the disease course. Other routes of application of treatment, such as intraurethral and vaginal antibiotic, may also be required.

We have identified two female patients with the clinical features of Reiter's syndrome who were cervical culture positive for *Ureaplasma urealyticum*. We do not know whether there is a cause and effect relationship but a similar association has been observed by others[62-65].

Dysentery organisms

The dysentery-causing organisms *Campylobacter jejuni, Salmonella typhimurium, Shigella flexneri,* and *Yersinia enterocolitica* are those most commonly associated with the development of Reiter's syndrome. The association of dysentery followed by a Reiter's syndrome is strain-specific. In the case of *Shigella*, the elegant work by Stieglitz and colleagues established that a bacterial plasmid common to arthritogenic strains of *Shigella*, but not to nonarthritogenic strains, encodes an epitope shared with HLA-B27[55]. This finding probably holds true in one form or another for the other species of dysentery-causing bacteria.

The seronegative arthropathy associated with inflammatory bowel disease such as ulcerative colitis and Crohn's disease resembles the arthropathy of Reiter's syndrome and may be an alternative expression of a post-infectious reactive disease, or indeed an expression of the persistence of a chronic antigen trigger as postulated by Keat and colleagues for post-chlamydial disease[8].

NATURAL HISTORY AND PROGNOSIS

The clinical features of Reiter's syndrome develop within 1-6 weeks after two specific types of initiating event — (1) an attack of dysentery or infection with a dysentery-causing agent or (2) a nongonococcal urogenital infection usually due to *Chlamydia trachomatis*.

Reiter's syndrome occurs in approximately 1% of patients following an episode of nongonococcal urethritis[38]. This type typically occurs in young, sexually active males, often with a history of a new partner within the preceding weeks. The high incidence in males has been reported mainly from sexually transmitted disease clinics[38], but probably also reflects referral pattern, diagnostic criteria, and the possibility of asymptomatic cervicitis in females, or a milder disease spectrum in females.

The postdysenteric Reiter's syndrome occurs in approximately 1% of patients following an outbreak of a diarrhea epidemic[3]. This form of Reiter's syndrome has a greater proportion of female patients, and is also seen in sexually inactive children. The majority of cases occur between the ages of 15 and 40 years, with a peak incidence in the early thirties. The range of "sex distribution" is from 9 : 1 to 1 : 1 male to female ratio[3,66]. The diarrhea may be mild, short-lived, and without bloody discharge. Similarly, the associated urethritis is also mild, especially in females, although in males dysuria may be present secondary to prostatitis.

The features of the Reiter's syndrome appear to be a series of symptoms and signs that can be set in motion by a remote but specific group of infectious events, either urogenital or postdysenteric. Presumably there is a common channel through which these unrelated infectious agents trigger the sequences — possibly through a "receptor mechanism" such as a cell-surface mechanism. In our basic understanding of this disease process we know that the presence of the Class I antigen HLA-B27 antigen plays some active or marker role in the commonly held concept of reactive arthritis, which evolves from infection through a latent period to a recognized disease process.

It was originally thought that Reiter's syndrome was a short-lived and self-limiting disease, but many authors in the past 50 years have demonstrated that serious chronic disability and social disability may occur following reactive arthritis[13,38,50-66]. A follow-up report from the original 344 cases identified by Paronen[3] revealed that 40% of those available for study up to 25 years after the onset of disease, had a chronic disability[67]. Reiter's syndrome is described as following three distinct patterns. One is short and self-limiting. The second, which includes the majority of cases, is characterized by recurrent episodes of arthritis. The third form represents a small minority who follow a continuous and unremitting course[3,38,51,67].

Csonka described the clinical course of 185 patients with Reiter's syndrome who attended the Venereal Disease Clinic at St. Mary's Hospital in London between 1942 and 1956[38]. The incidence of Reiter's syndrome in males presenting with urethral infection was 0.8%. Paronen's estimate of Reiter's syndrome occurring postdysentery was 0.2%. Presumably the organism that resulted in the Reiter's syndrome in Csonka's cases was *Chlamydia trachomatis*. In his retrospective analysis, Csonka identified a recurrence rate of 15% of patients per year[68].

Fox and colleagues examined 131 consecutive patients from a university clinic at Stanford, Palo Alto, and from a community clinic at Santa Barbara[51]. They were able to identify 122 patients available for follow-up at a mean of 5.6 years. They found no major difference in the characteristics of the disease between the two centers, but did find that 34% of patients had sustained disease activity, 16% had changed their jobs, and 11% were unemployable. They found no major differences between females and males, or between HLA-B27 positive and negative subjects, except for an increased prevalence of sacroiliitis and chronic uveitis in the HLA-B27 positive group. It is of interest that they identified severe heel involvement as a bad prognostic factor in their patients. Notwithstanding the degree of pain, one can accept that heel pain, by virtue of location alone, might be more of a disability to the average worker than similar pain in an upper limb joint. The same or greater pain in a nondominant wrist or elbow may not be recorded by the patient or by his clinician investigators as a "disability."

In our own experience of Reiter's patients with acute post-chlamydial infection, the majority of patients present with asymmetric arthritis involving the ankles, knees, and occasionally with heel pain, either in the calcaneus or at the insertion of the Achilles tendon. The initial arthritis commonly presents in one ankle, or one knee, but this synovitis may resolve spontaneously within a few days to a few weeks to be followed by the development of acute arthritis in another knee and/or ankle. Involvement of the upper limb joints is uncommon in our experience, although the most commonly involved are the 2nd and 3rd metacarpal phalangeal joints or the wrists. Occasionally there is elbow involvement, and occasionally dactylitis of either the index or middle finger. Dactylitis in one or two toes is a well-recognized accompaniment. The arthritis usually occurs within 3 days to 12 weeks after sexual exposure. It is not known whether the arthritis occurs after the first exposure to the *Chlamydia* organism, or whether some patients may be exposed on several occasions before developing the arthritis. This is similar to the pattern described by Csonka[5] in his follow-up of 30 cases over 10 years. While many patients developed either a mild attack, or full Reiter's syndrome after recurrent episodes of urethritis, some cases of Reiter's syndrome would occur without an apparent precipitating event, and other patients would have episodes of urethritis without the Reiter's syndrome being precipitated. These findings of Csonka and our own experience suggest an alteration in either the resistance of the organism and/or the virulence of the organism and/or the type of exposure that occurred. In the first 2–3 months of arthritis we have found that the joint pain is extremely refractory to management with adequate doses of nonsteroidal anti-inflammatory drugs. The pain is sometimes so severe in joints such as the knees and ankles, or in areas such as the base of the calcaneus, that either intra-articular or oral steroids have been required in order to give the patient pain relief. Investigators who have reported on patients suffering from coexistent acquired immunodeficiency syndrome (AIDS) and Reiter's syndrome have reported on the severity of the joint pain that is refractory to standard doses of nonsteroidal anti-inflammatory drugs[69]. In our experience the majority of patients with newly diagnosed post-*Chlamydia* Reiter's syndrome are unable to continue work, especially if work involves standing or walking. Fox and colleagues reported that heel pain at onset heralded a poor prognosis[51]. The most common complications we have identified in addition to arthritis are enthesitis, urethritis, and cervicitis. Skin rash, nail changes, and ocular lesions have been uncommon in our series. In the majority of our patients with post-chlamydial arthritis the disease process becomes manageable within approximately 6 months to 1 year, allowing the patient to return to meaningful occupation. Many patients will have ongoing disabilities such as pain and swelling in a single joint following the 12-month period, but this is usually not sufficient to restrict them from work except in exceptional circumstances.

In a syndrome with a wide variety of presenting clinical features and

Table 1 Organisms that cause Reiter's syndrome

Urogenital	*Chlamydia trachomatis*
Postdysenteric	*Campylobacter jejuni*
	Salmonella typhimurium
	Shigella flexneri
	Yersinia enterocolitica

several recognized etiologic precipitants it is difficult to identify factors that are predictive for disease occurrence, progression, or severity and duration. Although there appears to be a common association of the presence of HLA Class I antigen HLA-B27 in 60–80% of patients with Reiter's syndrome, those who do not possess this antigen sometimes show a variable expression of signs and symptoms. Reiter's syndrome is triggered by multiple organisms (Table 1). In our experience and that of others[38], the response to treatment of patients infected by *Chlamydia* may be quite different from that of patients suffering from postdystentery Reiter's syndrome, but the clinical presentation, signs, and symptoms are similar[3,5,38,50,51]. We suspect that the virulence of the organism must be taken into account as a factor that might alter the activity of the disease. Most patients who contract Reiter's syndrome are young, in the 20–40 age group, and therefore are likely to be itinerant and follow-up to establish prognosis becomes more difficult. This has been referred to by many authors in the literature as a significant limitation in establishing prognosis[3,38,51]. There is no clinical evidence to date that early diagnosis alters the course of the disease, but early diagnosis of Reiter's syndrome in females may be missed because of the asymptomatic nature of cervicitis. If cervicitis is not diagnosed, it is possible that female patients with inflammatory joint pain could be categorized as having some other disease state, thus ultimately altering prognostic data. In both males and females with Reiter's syndrome there is significant overlap of symptoms and signs with other diseases such as ankylosing spondylitis, psoriatic arthritis, and the arthritis of inflammatory bowel disease. These factors will lead to the possibility of sample contamination when attempting to determine the outcome of a target cohort of Reiter's syndrome sufferers.

SERIES REPORTS

Two of the major series on Reiter's syndrome are the studies by Paronen on postdysenteric syndrome and by Csonka on posturogenital syndrome. Each of the original studies was followed by a subsequent outcome or prognostic report by the same author. In view of the importance of these two series, which examine the two major predisposing infectious types of Reiter's syndrome — postdysenteric and posturogenital — we considered it necessary to review the findings of the authors in detail. The unique *in vivo* experiment of postbacillary dysentery recorded by Commander Noer is also detailed[70]. This is followed by an account of the literature based on the excellent review of Andrew Keat[5].

Paronen's series

In Paronen's original report[3] of 1948, he suggested that the prognosis of Reiter's syndrome was good. He suggested that the disease had not led to death, and that the disease did not cause any permanent or disabling change in affected organs, although he did acknowledge that there had been a few cases of permanent damage to the eye, most likely in relation to iritis. He also acknowledged that some authors had recorded ankylosis of the joints, and one case of urethral stricture had been reported. He stated that recovery was usually spontaneous, and the duration of the disease was usually from 2 to 5 months. However, he did acknowledge that recurrences had been reported in the literature, although these were uncommon. Hollander recorded recurrences in up to 15% of his case studies[71]. In Paronen's original series he noted that none of his cases with marked joint swelling recovered within the first month. The earliest recovery began in the second month. Fifty-three percent of cases recovered during the second to fourth month, although four patients were ill for more than 1 year, with the longest duration being 16 months. In patients who had only arthralgia he observed the start of recovery within the second week. Twenty-four percent recovered from arthralgia in the first month, and 90% were better during the first 3 months, with the longest duration being 8 months. Paronen recorded that 79.4% of all cases with joint involvement recovered completely, although 20.6% had ongoing synovitis characterized by small exudates, swelling, limitation of extension or flexion, or crepitation on palpation. However, he observed that the symptoms were usually mild and caused the patients no appreciable discomfort, except before and during bad weather. He recorded one patient who, after 3 years, continued to have fluid in one knee with associated crepitation in both knees, but stated that the range of motion of the joint resulted in tenderness only on strenuous exertion and in bad weather. He also noted that 1½ years after the onset of disease the patient had returned to agricultural work, and that although his sedimentation rate was high at the onset of disease, it had become normal within 4 months.

Paronen recorded 268 cases of conjunctivitis that lasted from 2 days to 7 months. Eighty percent of cases recovered within 1–4 weeks. He also recorded 17 cases of iritis, 17 cases of keratitis, and 7 cases of keratoiritis, all of which were reported to have recovered within 1–5 months.

He recorded urethritis in 202 cases, the duration of which lasted from 1 day to 9 months. He noted that 87% recovered within 4 weeks. In 60.8% of cases the duration of the urethritis was only 1–2 days, but he stated that in cases that lasted longer, up to several weeks, the symptoms undulated in a pattern similar to the cases of conjunctivitis. He recorded cystitis in 22 cases lasting from 1 week to 9 months, orchitis in 10 cases from 1 week to 2 months, and epididymitis in 4 cases that lasted from 3 to 9 months. Penile eczema or balanitis was recorded in 7 cases and lasted from 1 week to 7 months. In three cases of epididymitis small nodes remained when the treatment had lasted from 3 to 5 months.

Paronen documented that since patients in his series contracted the illness during military service, they were informed that treatment would be at the expense of the state, and that they would receive compensation if their disability was over 10%. He therefore concluded that in view of these economic advantages it would seem reasonable to believe that patients in the event of recurrences would report them. In cases of recurrence that he observed over 3 years he noticed a recurrence of eye manifestations in 50 cases, but 40 of these patients had suffered continuously from arthritis and were still being treated when the eye symptoms recurred. In only 10 cases was there complete freedom from any symptoms for some time before the recurrence of the ocular symptoms. The asymptomatic period varied in duration from 23 days to 20 months. The interval free from eye manifestations while arthritis persisted varied from 2 days to 7 months. Urethritis recurred in 6 cases, 3 of whom had no other symptoms. In one case, urethritis, arthritis, and conjunctivitis reappeared in association with an epididymitis, and in another case urethritis recurred three times during the course of 1 year in association with a mild arthritis, a unilateral orchitis, and an epididymitis. Recurrence of arthritis was noted in 10 cases, and in 4 of them it was preceded by a new episode of diarrhea. In 5 cases the arthritis recurred alone. In the other 5, eye symptoms or urogenital symptoms also occurred. The completely asymptomatic interval of the arthritis was from 3 to 18 months. In one case there were two recurrences with intervals of 7 and 3 months. In 4 cases the recurrence involved only the joints that had been affected the first time, and 5 patients had symptoms both in previously affected and unaffected joints, and in one case the patient's recurrence occurred only in joints that had been unaffected in the original illness. Paronen stated that in his series Flexner dysentery had preceded the Reiter's syndrome in 96.4% of cases[3]. He assumed that the remaining 3.6% of cases also had preceding dysentery. It was his conclusion that nonspecific urethritis was not a precipitant cause of Reiter's syndrome in his series of patients, but indeed a concomitant part of the classical triad, although it is possible that some of the military cases in his series may have been of venereal origin. Paronen was intrigued by the concept of Reiter's syndrome occurring in so few patients, 0.2% of the total affected by the dysentery, and reflected on the predisposition of his patients, either by "allergy or some other constitutional factor, a circumstance which is supported by familial disposition." Paronen concluded that "Reiter's syndrome thus seems to occur only after dysentery, and that dysentery bacillus seems to be the causative factor also in such cases in which no dysenteric infection can be demonstrated by clinical means."

In 1969 Paronen and colleagues reported a follow-up of his original 344 cases[67]. Seventy-five cases were lost to follow-up because of death or travel abroad to ports unknown. One hundred and seventeen patients failed to answer inquiries, but questionnaire responses were achieved from 152. One hundred of these complied by attending for personal examination. It was noted that of the 52 patients who replied,, but did not attend for examination, 22 stated they had no symptoms after the first stage, and the other 30 admitted to symptoms mainly in the joints. The follow-up study group reported by Paronen and his colleagues in 1969 therefore comprised 100 patients, 93 men and 7 women. The average age at the time of follow-up was 50 years, and the average age at the onset of disease was 29 years in the 1940s. In the 100 patients they recorded three separate groups with regard to joint symptoms. The first were patients whose X-ray changes were similar to ankylosing spondylitis. This finding supports our personal opinion, and that of others[5], that ankylosing spondylitis is a form of reactive arthritis of unknown pathogenesis and should be classified as such. The second were those with longstanding joint symptoms, but no changes of ankylosing spondylitis. The third group were those whose joint symptoms had disappeared by 1947 or were only slight and temporary. In the analysis of the group with features similar to ankylosing spondylitis, 31 of 32 had symmetrical sacroilitis and/or ankylosing spondylitis. Thirteen of the 32 had only mild spinal symptoms. Definite limitation of motion occurred in 14 of the 32, and a marked thoracic kyphosis was recorded in 3. The authors concluded that the spinal symptoms were mild compared to those of patients with ankylosing spondylitis. Nineteen of the 32 patients also had peripheral joints involved, most frequently in the hip, knee, and ankle joints, and the metatarsal phalangeal joints. Nine patients had calcaneal spur involvement.

In the second group, namely, patients without changes of ankylosing spondylitis, there were joint changes present in 18 patients. The knee, finger, and toe joints were the most affected. These changes usually involved either one or two joints. There was no morning stiffness in these patients and symptoms had been continuous in only one case. The majority of patients therefore had recurrent symptoms at intervals from 1 to 4 months lasting from 1 week to several months each year. At least 5 of these patients indicated that their joint pains were the result of acute attacks. Erosion was present in only 2 of these patients and calcaneal spur was present in only 2. Rheumatoid factor was positive in one case, but the clinical picture was not that of rheumatoid arthritis.

In the third group there were 30 patients in whom the joint symptoms had disappeared. There was only an occasional patient who had recurrence of mild symptoms, and this was sometimes 20 years after the initial attack. In one such case the patient had developed pain in the left ankle in 1944. The patient had a recurrence of diarrhea in 1966 and developed arthritis, urethritis, and conjunctivitis in association with an increase in temperature and sedimentation rate. The patient reported that he had to use crutches for a few weeks, and then the symptoms disappeared within 1 month. Seven patients had cardiac involvement during the initial illness. Five of these patients were asymptomatic at follow-up. Cardiac insufficiency had developed in one patient, and arrhythmia with total heart block in another. Mitral valve disease was recorded in one patient, but this was thought to be related to rheumatic fever. Nineteen patients reported that they had recurrence of conjunctival irritation, either photophobia, pain, or redness, lasting up to 1-2 weeks. In some cases it occurred once a year, but medication was not usually required. One cannot always assume that recurrent conjunctivitis of an isolated nature is directly related to Reiter's syndrome since it may be due to another infectious cause. However, this pattern of recurrent conjunctivitis has been reported by others[38,51,70]. Iritis, which was usually unilateral, appeared in a total of 7 cases initially. There was recurrence of iritis in all patients except one. One patient developed secondary glaucoma requiring iridectomy, and ultimately severe loss of vision in the right and left eye. Iritis did not appear to be related to the occurrence of joint attacks, but occurred independently. It is of note that in 4 of these cases there were changes resembling ankylosing spondylitis.

Paronen and colleagues recorded that 2 cases had mild psoriasis, but no peripheral joint symptoms. Two other patients showed evidence of dry, scaling eczema, which was stated to have been similar to that which appeared in the original occurrence in the 1940s. In one patient these changes had been present continuously, and in the other they had recurred in 1957 and were persistent until documentation by Paronen in 1969.

Twenty-two patients had symptoms of diarrhea that had lasted for many years without any detectable cause, and one wonders how many of these patients may also have had either Crohn's disease, or ulcerative colitis. Exacerbation of diarrhea caused accentuation of joint symptoms in two of these cases.

The authors noted that one patient, who had encephalitis during the initial stage of Reiter's syndrome in the 1940s, subsequently developed Parkinsonism in 1957. Only one patient had a recurrence of urethritis after 1947. Eight patients had an asymptomatic elevated blood urea, two of whom also had a documented prostatitis. Using a palpation technique, it was found that 24% of Reiter's patients had prostatitis, and 9 of these cases had clinical features resembling ankylosing spondylitis. In a control group of 100 unselected male patients of similar age distribution in the author's medical department, prostatitis diagnosed by this palpation method was present in 31%. Thus, in this series it cannot be proven that prostatitis was a significant finding in relation to the Reiter's syndrome at this late stage in the disease.

Seven of the original 34 women from Paronen's series were available for investigation. Three reported they had been completely cured, two had symptoms of arthralgia or of arthritis in the toe and finger joint, and one reported knee effusion that recurred repeatedly. Iritis had recurred in one patient. Calcaneal spur was found in two of the women, and one of them had ankylosis of the sacroiliac joint that was asymptomatic. There were no cases of inflammation recorded in the genital tract in these patients. The authors also stated that a considerable number (unspecified) of patients had crepitus in the patella area. Subsequent investigations revealed that a considerable number of these patients had chondromalacia. Whether this was secondary to the original disease process was not established.

The hundred follow-up patients were divided into four categories with respect to working capacity: Grade I, fully employable; Grade II, light or part-time work, periodically incapable of working; Grade III, employable, can do light housework; Grade IV, confined to house, but able to care for themselves. The authors established that 58% of patients were in Grade I, with only one in Grade IV, and two in Grade III. It is important to document in the author's review that they found that the severity of the disease at the initial onset did not seem to be directly related to the long-term prognosis based on their criteria. However, the authors had to conclude that Reiter's syndrome was a disabling disease in approximately 50% of all cases documented or at least caused symptoms from which the patients suffered over a period of decades.

Csonka's series

In a series of 185 patients reported by Csonka in 1958, the age of onset ranged from 15 to 59 years, and 82% of attacks occurred between the ages of 20 and 40[38]. Genital infection consisting of nonspecific urethritis, with or without gonorrhea, acute hemorrhagic cystitis, and chronic prostatitis was present in 97.8% of the cases. One hundred percent of patients had joint and tendon involvement, and 46% of patients had eye lesions comprising conjunctivitis, keratitis, and iritis. There was no report of any neurologic abnormality. Five patients had thrombophlebitis, one patient had pericarditis, and 38 patients had balanitis; and 26 patients had keratoderma blennorrhagica. The mean time of onset from sexual intercourse to the development of nonspecific urethritis was approximately 13 days; similarly, the mean time of onset from the nonspecific urethritis to the development of arthritis was 14 days. The duration of the first attack was approximately 3 weeks to 18 months with a mean of 3.8 months. Approximately 20 of the 185 cases showed no evidence of a clear-cut remission, but rather presented a disease process lasting 3 or more years. In the follow-up of this series of patients 80 were observed for less than 1 year, mainly because of default[68]. Csonka mentioned that the majority of those who defaulted had mild disease; however, it cannot be assumed that all of these were ultimately completely disease free. Between 1 and 3 years, approximately 30 patients suffered from multiple attacks. In the follow-up span of 25 years, 104 of the original patient group were recorded as having had multiple attacks. Csonka was able to follow 30 patients for a period of approximately 10 years, and made the interesting observation in this group that reinfection with venereal urethritis, either gonococcal or nongonococcal, did not inevitably lead to further arthritic attacks. There was no clinical difference in the character of these attacks of urethritis, which in some patients produced an episode of arthritis and in others did not, and similarly some attacks of arthritis were not preceded by a urethral infection although this had been the initiating event in the first attack. It was also stated that there was a marked variability in the intervals between attacks, these being as infrequent as 3 months, or as long as 18 years, similar to the observations of Paronen in his postdysenteric Reiter's syndrome study[3]. Forty-eight patients stated that one or more of their later episodes of Reiter's syndrome were "unprovoked" by sexual intercourse in the preceding 2-3 months[68]. In 22 of these attacks urethritis was absent, and in two instances nonspecific urethritis appeared only after the onset of arthritis. The work of Keat and colleagues[49], which has identified the presence of *Chlamydia* particles in the synovial cells and genital tract by a monoclonal antibody technique, may support the clinical observations of Csonka and suggests the possibility of latent infection and the presence of actively infectious *Chlamydia* or *Chlamydia* particles within diseased tissue that have the potential for reactivation without exogenous injections of new organisms such as from a sexual contact. Csonka noted that iritis and sacroiliitis had a high incidence in the patients who suffered multiple attacks[68]. There were 21 cases with iritis, and 9 cases with sacroiliitis. It is important to document that 7 cases of sacroiliitis were also observed in patients with only a single attack of Reiter's syndrome. It is often difficult to separate the problem of disease persistence from reinfection, but it is important to note that Csonka observed that repeated attacks were associated with less-complete recovery. As a further argument to support the concept of activation of a latent infection, Csonka observed four of his original patients with previous sexually acquired Reiter's syndrome in whom diarrhea occurred as a result of food poisoning (2 cases) or antibiotic therapy for unrelated reasons (2 cases) and was followed within 1-5 days by a new attack of arthritis. In another 3 patients second attacks of Reiter's syndrome occurred within 2-7 days after urogenital surgery or instrumentation, and in 6 cases one attack was preceded by tonsillitis. In all of these cases the first attack followed venereal urethritis. Are these examples of reactivation of latent infection? Is the term reactive arthritis incorrect and are we dealing with a special form of septic arthritis syndrome?

Csonka reported that 14 of 109 of his cases gave a positive family history of rheumatic disease in close relatives compared to only 9 of 400 control patients with uncomplicated nonspecific urethritis or gonorrhea. He therefore made the observation in his 1958 report that a hereditary predisposition to the arthritic manifestations of Reiter's syndrome was possible. He commented on the development of Reiter's syndrome occurring in two brothers, who lived in different parts of England, and who developed severe attacks of Reiter's syndrome within 3 months of each other. They denied having a common sexual source. Csonka drew the analogy of recurrence of Reiter's syndrome, and predisposition to the disease of rheumatic fever, which results from a specific organism and can be prevented with early treatment of the hemolytic streptococci. He questioned whether a similar policy of early antimicrobial treatment would be beneficial in the management of patients with a history of previous attacks of Reiter's syndrome.

Csonka reported that although many patients show a rapid development of the classical features of Reiter's syndrome within a matter of days to weeks, many patients present with incomplete manifestations or variations in symptoms. He described one patient who had nonspecific urethritis and arthritis, and 9 years later had a similar attack, but in addition had conjunctivitis. One patient, who had recurrent episodes of urethritis and circinate balanitis over 2 years, later developed severe arthritis and conjunctivitis. One patient had urethritis and arthritis on three occasions and developed iritis after the fourth attack, which was years after the first. This then became the dominant feature in future recurrent attacks. Csonka reported that iritis would usually occur as a late manifestation. Similarly, keratoderma blennorrhagica was a late development. He mentions one patient with an attack of urethritis and arthritis followed by a symptom-free interval of 18 years. The patient then developed arthritis and conjunctivitis after contracting venereal urethritis. He also identified a difference in expression of the disease in the host with regard to the same infectious source. Two patients gave the same female contact as the source of their urethritis. One developed arthritis only, and the other had the full triad. Csonka did not identify any deaths in his series; however, he recorded that some measure of permanent damage was observed in 28 patients. Twenty-one of these had recurrent iritis. Twenty-three had foot deformities including pes valgus, pes cavus, subluxation of the toes, and periostitis of the heel. Eight patients had anklyosis of the peripheral joints, and 16 had sacroiliitis, one with spinal involvement. He also described a further 6 patients who were handicapped by a mild to moderate activity in various joints for up to 2–3 years but who did not show residual joint damage[38].

"*In vivo* experiment" — Noer

In 1966 Commander H. Rolf Noer, a physician in the United States Navy, had the unique experience of being able to observe and document the development of 9 cases of Reiter's syndrome out of 602 cases of bacillary dysentery aboard a United States naval vessel[70]. The ship was visiting a locale that was endemic for shigellosis. A picnic had been arranged for the crew (no officers invited) and all unconsumed food was offered in the mess hall in the evening. Acute dysentery occurred after the picnic and within 12–72 hours more than 90% of those afflicted with diarrhea presented to sick bay. Within 11 days to 1 month, 9 of these patients presented with clinical features of Reiter's syndrome. Commander Noer recorded that there was a strong similarity between the clinical presentation of his patients and those of Paronen[3]. He stated that the 9 patients usually had a single joint that was their worst in terms of severity and duration although other joints were involved. He also recorded that half of the patients had previous joint or tendon disorders and the Reiter's syndrome seemed to select these joints. Two patients had balanitis associated with prolonged urethritis and this was especially worse in the noncircumcised patient. Poor prognosis was associated with prolonged or recurrent conjunctivitis, which in turn was associated with severe, prolonged, and/or recurrent arthritis. Deep bone pain unrelated to a joint was present in three men, but only one man had a calcaneal spur periostitis.

The erythrocyte sedimentation rate (ESR) remained high for an average of 2 months after discharge from the sick list and rose markedly 1 or 2 weeks before relapse.

Immobilization of affected joints in plaster did not appear to shorten the course of morbidity of these joints compared to nonimmobilized joints in the same patient.

Six months after the onset of the Reiter's, all 9 men had returned to some form of duty. In a final follow-up prior to publication of his data, Commander Noer recorded that 4 of the 9 men had no recurrence and were on full duty; 3 of the 9 with recurrent symptoms were found to be disease free and returned to active duty; but the remaining 2 sailors were invalided out of the navy because of continuing disability from Reiter's disease[70]. It was Commander Noer's opinion that severe and prolonged symptoms from the start of the disease identified those men with the poor prognosis who ultimately had to leave the service, but he did record that the severity of the initial dysentery was not related to the severity of the subsequent Reiter's syndrome[70].

Keat's review

One of the most informative dissertations in the Reiter's literature is the review by Keat in the *New England Journal of Medicine* in 1983[5]. He used the now popular meta-analysis approach in comparing *Shigella, Salmonella, Campylobacter, Yersinia,* and sexually acquired Reiter's syndrome. For each group he compiled the data from six or more literature reports. From these data Keat reported that 72–84% of patients were HLA-B27 positive and that the incidence of arthritis in Reiter's syndrome following these infections was in the order of 1–3% except for *Yersinia* infection, which brought an unusually high incidence of 33%. Such a figure, however, may be a product of the problems inherent in meta-analysis and should be viewed in this context. The mean age for the five groups was remarkably similar at approximately 30 years of age, with more young children under 15 years identified in the postdysenteric types. The male-to-female ratio was 28 : 1 in the sexually acquired form. As previously stated this may reflect a true lower incidence in females, lack of symptoms of cervicitis in females, or merely the referral pattern to so-called sexually acquired disease clinics (women may be more likely to be treated by family doctors or by gynecologists than in clinics specifically for sexually acquired disease). The male-to-female ratio for post *Salmonella, Campylobacter,* and *Yersinia* Reiter's syndrome was approximately 1 : 1. The high 9 : 1 male-to-female ratio for post *Shigella* Reiter's, reflects the inclusion of Paronen's military cases in the analysis[3]. The appearance of the Reiter's triad of urethritis, arthritis, and conjunctivitis was more likely to occur after *Shigella* infection (84% incidence) or after the sexually acquired form (35% incidence) than after *Salmonella, Campylobacter* or *Yersinia* 12%, 9.5%, 10% incidence, respectively. The mean period from the onset of infection to the onset of the Reiter's syndrome was 10 days to 3 weeks with more than 80–90% of cases of Reiter's appearing within 30 days of infection. The mean duration of the Reiter's episode was approximately 19 weeks with 60–90% of episodes being less than 6 months. The data showed that many Reiter's patients had multiple episodes — *Yersinia* group 15%, *Salmonella* group 17%, *Campylobacter* group 33%, and sexually acquired group 48% (data for *Shigella* group not available). Many patients had disease beyond 1 year — *Campylobacter* group 5%, *Yersinia* group 10%, sexually acquired group 16.5%, *Shigella* group 18% (data for *Salmonella* group not available).

Most cases in Keat's analysis had approximately three affected joints, usually knee, ankle, and wrist or metatarsal phalangeal. Monoarthritis was present in approximately 19% of the *Salmonella* and *Campylobacter* groups and 15% of the *Yersinia* group, but only 9% of the sexually acquired group and 4% of the *Shigella* group. Sacroiliitis was found in 7–10% of cases, but accurate data analysis was not available for the *Shigella* group. Tendonitis, dactylitis, fasciitis, and enthesitis collectively, occurred in 5–22% of all groups.

Keat's analysis of the extra-articular lesions showed that the majority, but not all of the postdysenteric patients had diarrhea, 89–100%. As expected, the incidence of diarrhea in the sexually acquired form was low at 0.17% but the presence of urethritis occurred in both postdysenteric (13–70%) and sexually acquired (100%) forms. Erythema nodosum (5%) and myositis (27%) were unique to the *Yersinia* form and amyloidosis (0.2%) was unique to the sexually acquired form. Aortic valve disease was recorded only in the *Yersinia* (1.1%) and sexually acquired forms (1.6%), and circinate balanitis was noted only in the *Shigella* (24%) and sexually acquired forms (23%). Keratoderma blennorraghia was noted only in the sexually acquired form (12%).

Keat's data analysis based on more than 40 literature reports provides useful information on the similarity of disease patterns in all forms of Reiter's disease. Perhaps the most useful information is that we can tell patients with Reiter's syndrome derived from any infectious sources that the mean duration of disease is approximately 19 weeks, but that 15-50% of patients have recurrent episodes and 5-18% of patients have symptoms greater than 1 year. The disadvantages of Keat's analysis are the pitfalls of meta-analysis itself, namely, different types of trials and analysis, different patient groups, different or no predetermined diagnostic or laboratory criteria, no predetermined analytical intent, etc.

The unexpected nature of an epidemic of dysentery does not lend itself to the structure required for a carefully planned cohort analysis of signs and symptoms or a double blind controlled trial of a therapeutic agent, but such a network could remain in place in a unit with a special interest in documenting the outcome of Reiter's disease in a prospective fashion. Prognosis of long-term outcome would also depend on careful tracking of the original cohort and matching them by age, sex, and other "environmental" factors to appropriate controls.

A prospective cohort analysis or randomized double blind controlled trial of the sexually acquired form of Reiter's syndrome may prove easier to design based in an established infectious disease unit, especially one that has a sexually acquired disease clinic. However, the very nature and historical significance of such a clinic may induce a referral bias, with fewer women presenting to such a clinic by preferring to be treated by a family physician or by a gynecologist. In addition, the purported less-symptomatic cervicitis of females may result in nonreporting by the patient or misdiagnosis by the health professional.

Cohort analyses of patients who are HLA-B27 positive are of little value since they miss the 20-40% of Reiter's patients who are HLA-B27 negative.

The best opportunity to establish a prognostic clinical and therapeutic index will come from the extension of the monoclonal antibody work of Keat and colleagues, once the presence and exact identification of an infectious agent or part thereof is established in the tissue[49]. This will narrow the diagnostic criteria to the specific offending organism without contamination from other types of Reiter's syndrome. Prognosis can then be charted based on the presence or absence of persistent antigen and therapeutic outcome can be charted both clinically and against the presence of antigen. Until this can be established, prognostic evaluation of Reiter's syndrome, except in broad terms, will be unsatisfactory, as is currently the case. At present even the best series in the literature are contaminated with cases of ankylosing spondylitis, psoriatic arthritis, and the arthritis of inflammatory bowel disease. While these are most likely types of "reactive disease" the presumed differences in the initiating infectious agent preclude their inclusion into a cohort analysis where a tight diagnostic criterion is sought.

REITER'S SYNDROME IN CHILDHOOD

Reiter's syndrome in childhood has a reported male predominance of approximately 10 : 1 with a mean age of 10 years[72]. Rosenberg and Petty describe Reiter's syndrome in childhood in three boys aged 11, 12, and 14 years in a series of 39 children with seronegative enthesopathy and arthropathy[73]. Two of the children who were HLA-B27 negative had persistent arthritis and enthesopathy associated with *Yersinia* infection, and one who was HLA-B27 positive had *Chlamydia* infection with conjunctivitis, urethritis, enthesopathy, and arthritis that included bilateral sacroiliac sclerosis with erosion. It was reported that the boy with the Reiter's syndrome secondary to *Chlamydia* had become entirely asymptomatic, but the time frame was not given. Enthesopathy in children has previously been reported in three of seven children by Singsen[74] and in one of three children reported by Rosenberg and Petty[72]. Sheerin and colleagues reported a long-term clinical and diagnostic follow-up study of HLA-B27 associated arthropathy in 85 children[75]. At a mean follow-up time of 8.9 years (range 5.5 to 22 years), 54 were able to be contacted by telephone and 36 were available for follow-up by examination. At the time of initial diagnosis, and at the time of follow-up, none of these children was categorized as having Reiter's syndrome, although one of two with psoriatic skin lesions without nail pitting had urethritis and subsequently developed what the authors termed incomplete Reiter's syndrome. The absence of Reiter's syndrome in this cohort of 36 could be selection bias reflecting the low incidence of arthritogenic organism infection in children in that particular catchment area at the time of initial diagnosis. It could also reflect diagnostic and investigative criteria that missed the diagnosis of Reiter's syndrome. Furthermore, the study did not include HLA-B27 negative children with arthritis and would thus result in failure to include those Reiter's syndrome patients who were HLA-B27 negative, but who have some or all of the clinical features resembling those who are HLA-B27 positive.

Uveitis in Reiter's syndrome of childhood occurs in about 1% of juvenile rheumatoid disease[72]. It is commonly acute and symptomatic in association with the presence of HLA-B27. The occurrence of blindness can be as high as 15–30%, with visual impairment occurring in a further 30%[76].

ACQUIRED IMMUNODEFICIENCY SYNDROME (AIDS) AND REITER'S SYNDROME

In 1987 Winchester and colleagues reported on 14 patients with arthritis and AIDS[69]. One patient had a 10-year history of spondyloarthropathy and developed psoriasis in conjunction with the onset of AIDS, and 13 patients had a diagnosis of Reiter's syndrome and AIDS. Two of the 13 with Reiter's syndrome had a *Shigella flexneri* enteric infection, and one of 13 had a *Campylobacter fetus* septicemia with septic arthritis preceding the reactive arthritis. Seven patients had a diarrheal illness, and three had a urethral infection at, or preceding, the onset of the Reiter's syndrome. Five patients had a progressive course with a severe proliferative synovitis with joint destruction and erosions. Four of the five had a preceding diarrheal illness of unknown cause. Eight patients had an intermittent course. The attacks generally affected the same joints and were about 6 months apart. Only two of the eight patients had erosions. All patients had oligo- or polyarthritis. The most common joint problem was enthesopathy of the Achilles tendon in eleven of thirteen patients. Posterior tibial tendonitis was present in two. Dactylitis was present in six. The use of nonsteroidal anti-inflammatory drugs was largely ineffective for pain relief. Sulfasalazine was of benefit to the joint disease in two, and the colitis in one, but was without effect in two others. High-dose prednisone was effective in the multiple joint complaints of one patient with progressive disease, but was ineffective in another. When the immune deficiency was diagnosed, the prednisone treatment was stopped. In two patients, methotrexate was used to treat the Reiter's syndrome and both developed Kaposi's sarcoma and pneumocystis carinii as the first manifestation of AIDS. Another patient with AIDS-related complex and severe Reiter's syndrome was treated with azathioprine. The patient developed severe fatigue and weight loss. Winchester and colleagues stated that the concomitant occurrence of Reiter's syndrome and AIDS suggests that the CD4 positive inducer-helper T cell is not a causative factor of Reiter's syndrome. In contrast they suggest that Reiter's syndrome may occur during episodes of immune deficiency such as the presence of high levels of CD8 positive suppressor cytotoxic T cell activity. The authors also suggested that the immune-deficient state could predispose to the increased opportunistic activity of arthritogenic organisms by altering the frequency and site of presentation, such as in the bowel. It was also stated that immune activation by the Reiter's syndrome could activate latent HIV infection. The authors also acknowledge that the coexistence of Reiter's and AIDS may merely represent cooccurrence of two diseases spread by the same host cohort.

Several other authors concur with Winchester and colleagues that complete or incomplete Reiter's syndrome may coexist or predate the diagnosis of AIDS[77-80]. These workers also emphasize the markedly increased severity and degree of joint pain of the Reiter's syndrome concomitant with AIDS compared to that which is not associated. They support the findings of others that use of even high doses of NSAIDs can be without benefit for pain relief[77-80].

SUMMARY

In summary, there appears to be a higher incidence of Reiter's syndrome in males than in females, but this incidence is skewed largely by the male predominance in the sexually acquired form[38]. There is a definite positive association with the presence of the Class I antigen HLA-B27. The pattern of the disease process does not appear to differ much between postdysentery and urogenital infection based on the large series reported by Paronen[3] and Csonka[38], respectively, except for those issues discussed above. Symptoms can last from 20 weeks to longer than 1 year, with 20–50% of patients having recurrent disease. Although death is not a common feature of Reiter's syndrome, acute morbidity can be significant in patients who develop high fever, cardiac involvement, neurologic involvement, iritis, and severe joint pain. Such presentations have been reported with increased severity in patients with coexistent Reiter's syndrome and AIDS. Based on information derived from the larger series, factors that reflect a poor long-term prognosis are involvement of the Achilles tendon, the heel, or the plantar aponeurosis. It should be noted that a similar degree of pain in the upper limbs may not be reported by the patient or recorded by the investigator as causing significant disability, but since almost all daily activities involve walking or standing, the presence of any persistent inflammatory lesion in the feet will result in a perceived poor clinical and social outcome. The presence of iritis, especially a recurrent iritis, obviously augurs a poor prognosis with subsequent development of severe visual impairment and possibly blindness. Patients with recurrent arthritis, and those with persistent arthritis, are obviously at serious prognostic risk. Severe joint pain unresponsive to standard therapy with nonsteroidal anti-inflammatory drugs is characteristic of Reiter's syndrome that coexists in patients with AIDS. In many of our own patients we have noted that Reiter's syndrome, secondary to *Chlamydia*, can also be extremely refractory in response to standard doses of nonsteroidal anti-inflammatory drugs. In patients who suffer from AIDS and Reiter's syndrome the prognosis of the Reiter's is bad, but the long-term prognosis is obviously based on the outcome of the AIDS and not the Reiter's syndrome. It is also recommended that immunosuppressant drugs, such as methotrexate and azathioprine, as well as prednisone, should not be used in the treatment of Reiter's syndrome if concomitant AIDS syndrome is suspected, and should definitely not be given to any AIDS patient with Reiter's syndrome. The consequences of the added immunosuppressant drug are acceleration of the AIDS syndrome[69].

Approximately 5–50% of patients who develop Reiter's syndrome not associated with AIDS may be said to have a poor prognosis. Severe disease at onset, persistence of symptoms, recurrence of symptoms, duration of symptoms beyond 1 year, and the presence of individual disease sites such as the heel, the eye, and the heart augur the worst prognosis. More accurate methods of identifying the cause of Reiter's syndrome such as monoclonal antibody techniques may not only improve diagnostic skills but radically change therapeutic techniques[49]. As discussed in the text, the identification of infectious organism component parts, either active or latent, may lead to a reevaluation of terminology, disease categorization, and ultimately establishment of an accurate prognostic index. At present no clear statement on prognosis can be given because of existing imperfections in diagnostic techniques.

References

1. Reiter, A. (1916). Uber ein bisher uner kannte spirochaeten infektion (spirochaetosis arthritica).
2. Brodie, B. C. (1818). *Pathologic and Surgical Observations on Diseases and Joints*. (London: Longman)
3. Paronen, I. (1948). Reiter's disease: a study of 344 cases observed in Finland. *Acta Med. Scand.* **212** (suppl.), 1-114
4. Calin, A. (1985). Reiter's syndrome. In Kelley, W. N., Harris, E. D., Ruddy, S. and Sledge, C. B. (eds). *Textbook of Rheumatology*, 2nd edn., p. 1007. (Philadelphia: W. B. Saunders)
5. Keat, A. (1983). Reiter's syndrome and reactive arthritis perspective. *N. Engl. J. Med.*, **309**, 1606-1615
6. Davies, N. E., Haverty, J. R. and Boatwright, M. (1969). Reiter's disease associated with shigellosis. *South. Med. J.*, **62**, 1011-1014
7. Berglöf, F. E. (1963). Arthritis and intestinal infection. *Acta Rheum. Scand.*, **9**, 141-149
8. Sairanen, E. and Tiilikainen, A. (1974). HLA-27 in Reiter's disease following shigellosis. *Scand. J. Rheumatol.* 8 (suppl.) abstract no. 30-11
9. Singsen, B. H., Bernstein, B. H., Koster-King, K. G., Glovsky, M. M. and Hanson, V. (1977). Reiter's syndrome in childhood. *Arthritis Rheum.*, **20**, 402-407
10. Good, A. E. and Schultz, J. S. (1977). Reiter's syndrome following Shigella flexneri 2a: a sequel to traveler's diarrhea: report of a case with hepatitis. *Arthritis Rheum.*, **20**, 100-104
11. Calin, A. and Fries, J. F. (1976). An "experimental" epidemic of Reiter's syndrome revisited: follow-up evidence on genetic and environmental factors. *Ann. Intern. Med.*, **84**, 564-565
12. Young, R. H. and McEwen, E. G. (1947). Bacillary dysentery as the cause of Reiter's syndrome (arthritis with nonspecific unrethritis and conjunctivitis). *J. Am. Med. Assoc.*, **134**, 1456-1459.
13. Aho, K., Ahvonen, P., Alkio, P. et al. (1975). HL-A27 and reactive arthritis following infection. *Ann. Rheum. Dis.*, **34** (suppl.), 29-30
14. Vartiainen, J. and Hurri, L. (1964). Arthritis due to Salmonella typhimurium: report of 12 cases of migratory arthritis in association with Salmonella typhimurium infection. *Acta Med. Scand.*, **175**, 771-776
15. Warren, C. P. W. (1970). Arthritis associated with Salmonella infections. *Ann. Rheum. Dis.*, **29**, 483-487
16. Fries, J. and Svejgaard, A. (1974). Salmonella arthritis and HL-A27. *Lancet*, **1**, 1350
17. Hakansson, U., Löw, B., Eitram, R. and Winblad, S. (1975). HL-A27 and reactive arthritis in an outbreak of salmonellosis. *Tissue Antigens*, **6**, 366-367
18. Jones, R. A. K. (1977). Reiter's disease after Salmonella typhimurium enteritis. *Br. Med. J.*, **1**, 1391
19. Jones, M. B., Smith, P. W. and Olhnausen, R. W. (1979). Reiter's syndrome after salmonella infection: occurrence in HLA-B27 positive brothers. *Arthritis Rheum.*, **22**, 1141-1142
20. Lemaire, V. and Ryckewaert, A. (1978). Rheumatisme post-salmonellien: un cas. *Nouv. Presse Med.*, **7**, 2239-2240
21. Stein, H. B., Abdullah, A., Robinson, H. S. and Ford, D. K. (1980). Salmonella reactive arthritis in British Columbia. *Arthritis Rheum.*, **23**, 206-10
22. Winblad, S. (1975). Arthritis associated with Yersinia enterocolitica infections. *Scand. J. Infect. Dis.*, **3**: 83-85
23. Aho, K., Ahvonen, P., Lassus, A., Sievers, K. and Tiilikainen, A. (1974). HL-A27 in reactive arthritis: a study of yersinia arthritis and Reiter's disease. *Arthritis Rheum.*, **17**, 521-526

24. Laitinen, O., Leirisalo, M. and Skylv, G. (1977). Relation between HLA-B27 and clinical features in patients with yersinia arthritis. *Arthritis Rheum.*, **20**, 1121-1124
25. Leirisalo, M., Skylv, G., Kousa, M. *et al.* (1982). Followup study on patients with Reiter's disease and reactive arthritis with special reference to HLA-B27. *Arthritis Rheum.*, **25**, 249-259
26. Marsal, L., Winblad, S. and Wollheim, F. A. (1981). Yersinia enterocolitica arthritis in southern Sweden: a four-year follow-up study. *Br. Med. J.*, **283**, 101-3
27. Laitinen, O., Tuuhea, J. and Ahvonen, P. (1972). Polyarthritis associated with Yersinia enterocolitica infection: clinical features and laboratory findings in nine cases with severe joint symptoms. *Ann. Rheum. Dis.*, **31**, 34-39
28. Caroit, M. (1976). Les manifestations articulaires des infections a Yersinia enterocolitica. *Rev. Rheum. Mal Osteoartica.* **43**, 583-588
29. Jacobs, J. C. (1975). Yersinia enterocolitica arthritis. *Pediatrics*, **55**, 236-238
30. Ahvonen, P. (1972). Human Yersiniosis in Finland. II. Clinical features. *Ann. Clin. Res.*, **4**, 39-48
31. Weir, W., Keat, A. C., Welsby, P. D. and Brear, G. (1979). Reactive arthritis associated with Campylobacter infection of the bowel. *J. Infect.*, **1**, 281-284
32. Gumpel, J. M., Martin, C. and Sanderson, P. J. (1981). Reactive arthritis associated with campylobacter enteritis. *Ann. Rheum. Dis.*, **40**, 64-65
33. Van de Putte, L. B. A., Berden, J. H. M., Boerbooms, A. M. T. *et al.* (1980). Reactive arthritis after Campylobacter jejuni enteritis. *J. Rheumatol.*, **7**, 531-535
34. Kosunen, T. U., Kauranen, O., Martio, J. *et al.* (1980). Reactive arthritis after Campylobacter jejuni enteritis in patients with HLA-B27. *Lancet*, **1**, 1312-1313
35. Leung, G. Y.-K., Littlejohn, G. O. and Bombardier, C. (1980). Reiter's syndrome after Camplylobacter jejuni enteritis. *Arthritis Rheum.*, **23**, 948-950
36. Pönkä, A., Martio, J. and Kosunen, T. U. (1981). Reiter's syndrome in association with enteritis due to Campylobacter fetus ssp. jejuni. *Ann. Rheum. Dis.*, **40**, 414-415
37. Wright, V. (1963). Arthritis associated with venereal disease: a comparative study of gonococcal arthritis and Reiter's syndrome. *Ann. Rheum. Dis.*, **2**, 77-89
38. Csonka, G. W. (1958). The course of Reiter's syndrome. *Br. Med. J.*, **1**, 1088-1090
39. Keat, A. C., Maini, R. N., Pegrum, G. D. and Scott, J. T. (1979). The clinical features and HLA associations of reactive arthritis associated with non-gonococcal urethritis. *Q. J. Med.*, **48**, 323-342
40. Brewerton, D. A., Caffrey, M., Nicholls, A., Walters, D., Oates, J. K. and James, D. C. O. (1973). Reiter's disease and HLA-A27. *Lancet*, **2**, 996-998
41. Morris, R., Metzger, A. L., Bluestone, R. and Terasaki, P. I. (1974). HL-AW27 — a clue to the diagnosis and pathogenesis of Reiter's syndrome. *N. Engl. J. Med.*, **290**, 554-556
42. Oates, J. K. and Young, A. C. (1959). Sacroiliitis in Reiter's disease. *Br. Med. J.*, **1**, 1013-1015
43. Laird, S. M. (1958). Figures and fancies. *Br. J. Vener. Dis.*, **34**, 137-152
44. Hawkes, J. G. (1973). Clinical and diagnostic features of Reiter's disease: a follow-up study of 39 patients. *N.Z. Med. J.*, **78**, 347-353
45. Csonka, G. W. (1979). Clinical aspects of Reiter's syndrome. *Ann. Rheum. Dis.*, **38**, (suppl.), 4-7
46. Kousa, M. J. (1978). Clinical observations on Reiter's disease with special reference to the venereal and non-venereal aetiology. *Acta Dermatol. Venereol. (Stockh.)*, **58** (suppl.), 81
47. Wilkins, R. F., Arnett, F. C., Bitter, T. *et al.* (1981). Reiter's syndrome: Evaluation of preliminary criteria for definitive disease. *Arthritis Rheum.*, **24**, 844-849
48. Weyand, C. M. and Goronzy, J. J. (1989). Immune responses to borrelia burgdorferi in patients with reactive arthritis. *Arthritis Rheum.*, **32**, 1057-1064
49. Keat, A., Dixie, J., Sonex, C., Thomas, B., Osborne, M. and Taylor-Robinson, D. (1987). Chlamydia trachomatis and reactive arthritis: the missing link. *Lancet*, **1**, 72-74
50. Lerisalo, M., Skylv, G. and Kousa, M. (1985). Follow up study on patients with Reiter's disease and reactive arthritis with special reference to HLA B27. *Arthritis Rheum.*, **20**, 249-259
51. Fox, R., Calin, A., Gerber, R. C. and Gibson, D. (1979). The chronicity of symptoms

and disability in Reiter's syndrome: an analysis of 131 consecutive patients. *Ann. Int. Med.*, **91**, 190-193

52. Good, A. E. (1974). Reiter's disease: a review with special attention to cardiovascular and neurological sequelae. *Semin. Arthritis Rheum.*, **3**, 253-286
53. Van Bohemen, C. G., Grumet, F. C. and Zanin, H. C. (1984). Identification of HLA-B27 M1 and M2 cross reactive antigens in Klebsiella, Shigella, and Yersinia. *Immunology*, **52**, 607-610
54. Schwimmbeck, T., Yu, D. T. Y. and Oldstone, M. B. A. (1987). Auto-antibodies to HLA B27 in the sera of HLA B27 patients with ankylosing spondylitis and Reiter's syndrome: molecular mimicry with Klebsiella pneumoniae as potential mechanism of autoimmune disease. *J. Exp. Med.*, **66**, 173-181
55. Stieglitz, H., Fosmire, F. and Lipskie, T. (1989). Identification of a 2-Md plasmid from Shigella Flexneri associated with reactive arthritis. *Arthritis Rheum.*, **32**, 937-946
56. Ford, D. K., da Roza, D. M. and Shulzer, M. (1982). The specificity of synovial mononuclear cell responses to microbiological antigens in Reiter's syndrome. *J. Rheumatol.*, **9**, 561-567
57. Darmarwan, J. (1988). *Rheumatic conditions in the northern port of Central Java. An epidemiological survey*, p. 165. (Indonesia, Kenrose)
58. Taylor-Robinson, D. and Thomas, B. J. (1980). The role of Chlamydia trachomatis in genital tract and associated diseases. *J. Clin. Pathol.*, **33**, 205-233
59. Keat, A. D., Thomas, B. J., Taylor-Robinson, D., Pegrum, G., Maini, R. S. and Scott, J. T. (1980). Evidence of Chlamydia trachomatis infection in sexually acquired reactive arthritis. *Ann. Rheum. Dis.*, **39**, 431-437
60. Amor, B. (1983). Chlamydia and Reiter's syndrome. *Br. J. Rheumatol.*, **22** (suppl. 2), 156-160
61. Popert, A. J., Gill, A. J. and Laird, S. F. (1964). A prospective study of Reiter's syndrome: an interim report on the first 82 cases. *Br. J. Vener. Dis.*, **40**, 160-165
62. Ford, D. K. (1967). Relationships between mycoplasma and the etiology of non-gonococcal urethitis and Reiter's syndrome. *Ann. N.Y. Acad. Sci.*, **143**, 501-504
63. Ford, D. K. (1968). Non-gonococcal urethritis and Reiter's syndrome: personal experience with etiological studies during 15 years. *Can. Med. Assoc. J.*, **99**, 900-910
64. Taylor-Robinson, D., Csonka, G. W. and Prentice, M. J. (1977). Human intraurethral inoculation of ureaplasmas. *Q. J. Med.*, **46**, 309-326
65. Taylor-Robinson, D. and McCormack, W. M. (1980). The genital mycoplasmas. *N. Engl. J. Med.*, **302**, 1003-1010, 1063-1067
66. Neuwelt, C. M., Borenstein, D. G. and Jacobs, R. P. (1982). Reiter's syndrome, a male and female disease. *J. Rheumatol.*, **9**, 268-272
67. Sairanen, E., Paronen, I. and Mahonen, A. (1969). Reiter's syndrome: a follow up study. *Acta Med. Scand.*, **18**, 57-63
68. Csonka, G. W. (1960). Recurrent attacks in Reiter's disease *Arthritis Rheum.*, **4**, 164-169
69. Winchester, R., Bernstein, D. A., Fischer, H., Enlow, R. and Solomon, G., (1987). The co-occurrence of Reiter's syndrome and acquired immuno-deficiency. *Ann. Intern. Med.*, **106**, 19-26
70. Noer, H. R. (1966). An experimental epidemic of Reiter's syndrome. *J. Am. Med. Soc.*, **198**, 693-698
71. Hollander, J. L. (1946). The diagnosis and treatment of Reiter's syndrome. *Med. Clin. N. Am.*, 716-723
72. Rosenberg, A. S. and Petty, R. E. (1979). Reiter's disease in children. *Am. J. Dis. Child.*, **133**, 394-398
73. Rosenberg, A. S. and Petty, R. E. (1982). Syndrome of seronegative enthisopathy and arthropathy in children. *Arthritis Rheum.*, **25**, 1041-1047
74. Singsen, B. A., Bernstein, B. A., Kostar-King, K. G., Glovsky, M. M. and Hansen, V. (1977). Reiter's syndrome in childhood. *Arthritis Rheum.* **20**, (suppl.), 404-407
75. Sheerin, K. A., Giannini, E. A., Brewer, E. J. and Barron, K. S. (1988). HLA B27 associated arthropathy in childhood: long term clinical and diagnostic outcome. *Arthritis Rheum.*, **31**, 1165-1170

76. Petty, R. E. (1987). Current knowledge of the etiology and pathogenesis of chronic uveitis accompanying juvenile rheumatoid arthritis. *Rheum. Dis. Clin. N. Am.*, **13**, 19-36
77. Rynes, R. I., Goldenberg, D. L., Digiacomo, R., Olson, R., Hussain, M. and Veazey, J. (1988). Acquired immunodeficiency syndrome — associated arthritis. *Am. J. Med.*, **84**, 810-816
78. Berman, A., Espinoza, L. R., Diaz, J. D., Aguilar, J. L., Rolando, T., Vasey, F., Germain, B. F. and Lockey, R. F. (1988). Rheumatic manifestation of human immunodeficiency virus infection. *Am. J. Med.*, **85**, 59-64
79. Forster, S. M., Seifert, M. H., Keat, A. C., Rowe, I. F., Thomas, B. J., Taylor-Robinson, D., Pinching, A. J. and Harris, J. R. W. (1988). Inflammatory joint disease and human immunodeficiency virus infection. *Br. Med. J.*, **296**, 1625-1627
80. Davis, P., Stein, M., Latif, A. and Emmanuel, J. (1988). HIV and polyarthritis. *Lancet*, **1**, 936

9
Systemic lupus erythematosus

R. ROUBENOFF and M. C. HOCHBERG

Like many of the rheumatic diseases, systemic lupus erythematosus (SLE) is a disease of unknown etiology. This alone makes prognostication in SLE difficult. In addition, the spectrum of systemic lupus is so wide that many observers consider it to be a syndrome comprising a group of diseases sharing common features, rather than one single entity. Clearly, some patients with systemic lupus erythematosus have a mild disease involving only skin and joints, while others have a life-threatening disease leading to multiple organ failure and death. How do we distinguish these subtypes of systemic lupus prospectively? What do we tell patients about their potential course? What should we follow as clinically relevant parameters that allow us to assess prognosis? This chapter will attempt to answer these questions.

THE NATURAL HISTORY OF SYSTEMIC LUPUS ERYTHEMATOSUS

Given the above remarks, a single "natural history" of systemic lupus is obviously impossible to outline. Nonetheless, a review of the evolution of our understanding of the course of systemic lupus is useful in assessing the present state of our knowledge.

Although Kaposi[1] described visceral involvement in what we now recognize as SLE as early as 1872, lupus was not commonly diagnosed until the beginning of this century, when Osler[2] in Baltimore and Jadassohn[3] in Vienna established the disease as a separate entity. It should be noted that both of the women Osler described, who we would clearly identify today as having systemic lupus, died of renal failure.

During the period 1900 to 1948, much of the progress in understanding systemic lupus was made by pathologists at autopsy[4]. This no doubt reinforced the perception of poor prognosis associated with systemic

Table 1 Cumulative survival (%) in systemic lupus erythematosus by study, 1955-1982[a]

Study	Location/year	Cumulative survival (%) 5-year	10-year
Merrell and Shulman[8]	Baltimore, 1955	51[b]	—[c]
Kellum and Hasericke[83]	Cleveland, 1964	70	53
Estes and Christian[28]	New York, 1971	77	59
Fries et al.[84]	Stanford, 1974	95	92
Lee et al.[64]	Toronto, 1977	91	—[c]
Grigor et al.[85]	England, 1978	98	89
Hochberg et al.[61]	Baltimore, 1981	97	90
Wallace et al.[30]	Los Angeles, 1981	88	79
Ginzler et al.[29]	United States, 1982	77	71
Michet et al.[9]	Minnesota, 1985	75	63

[a]Modified from Hochberg, M.C., Systemic lupus erythematosus VIII: prognosis. *Md. State Med. J.*, **33**, 114-116. Note that date refers to date of publication, not dates of patient accrual.
[b]Four-year survival rate.
[c]Not calculated.

lupus, a disease that often required florid clinical features to be diagnosed *ante mortem*. It was not until Hargreaves et al.[5] described the LE cell in 1948 that the spectrum of clinical manifestations of lupus began to change, with profound impact on our understanding of the disease's prognosis. Shortly thereafter, the introduction of corticosteroid therapy provided the first useful therapy for systemic lupus[6]. McCombs and Patterson[7] reported results of a before-after study assessing the effects of corticosteroid therapy on mortality; 18 of 20 patients (90%) considered to have serious disease died prior to the advent of corticosteroids. In contrast, the case fatality rate among 50 comparable patients treated with corticosteroids was only 36%. When Merrell and Shulman[8] reported the first life-table analysis of lupus survival in 1955, they found the 4-year survival at Johns Hopkins Hospital to be 51%.

The survival rate of systemic lupus has steadily improved over the past 30 years (Table 1). Chronic renal failure is no longer intrinsically fatal. New treatments have led to 10-year survival rates in the 80-90% range. In comparing survival rates from different series, one should note the difference between cumulative survival rates established by life-table techniques (shown in Table 1), mortality rates, and case fatality rates. Life tables allow statistical analysis of the survival of a population over time, and permit correction for duration of follow-up, differences in calendar time, and loss to follow-up. Mortality rates, on the other hand, are simply the number of people who die of a disease divided by the total number of people in the population at a given time. Case fatality ratios are the number of people who die of a disease divided by the total number of people with the disease. By any measure, however, the prognosis of systemic lupus can no longer be considered uniformly bleak. Instead, the specific types of lupus must be considered in evaluating prognosis in this disease.

Table 2 Prevalence of systemic lupus erythematosus by country. Rates are for entire population, unless specified by gender

Study	Year[a]	Prevalence per 100 000 population[b]
United States		
Siegal[11]	1965	14.0(F) 1.8(M)
Fessel[10]	1974	51.0(F,M)
Serdual[11]	1979	15.3(F,M)
Michet[9]	1985	53.8(F) 19.0(M)
United Kingdom[13]	1987	12.5(F) —
New Zealand[12]	1980	23.2(F) 14.7(M)
Japan[14]	1987	19.1(F,M)
Finland[15]	1985	28.0(F,M)

[a] Year of publication, not of data accrual.
[b] (F) = female; (M) = male; (F,M) = both female and male.

THE CHANGING PROGNOSIS OF SYSTEMIC LUPUS ERYTHEMATOSUS

Descriptive epidemiology of SLE

Prevalence

The prevalence of systemic lupus varies from country to country (Table 2). In Rochester, Minnesota, the prevalence of SLE as of January, 1980 was 53.8 cases per 100 000 population for women and 19.0 per 100 000 for men[9]. In San Francisco, Fessel found a prevalence of SLE as of July, 1973 of 51.0 per 100 000 for both men and women[10]. Based on these and other data[11-15], a task force of the National Institute of Arthritis and Musculoskeletal and Skin Diseases recently concluded that at least 100 000–150 000 women with lupus currently reside in the United States (Hochberg, M. C., personal communication).

Incidence

Although prevalence is an important measure of disease, with important implications for health policy, it does not measure the risk of developing disease. The latter is the value of incidence, the rate of development of new cases. Understanding the risk of developing disease is the first step in prognostication. The incidence of systemic lupus erythematosus has been rising for the past thirty years, as case recognition has improved, and a consensus on case definition has developed (Table 3). The incidence of SLE in Rochester, Minnesota, for example, tripled between 1950 and 1979, to 2.1 cases per 100 000 population per year[9]. In San Francisco between 1965 and 1973 the

Table 3 Incidence of systemic lupus erythematosus in the United States, 1965–1985

Study	Year[a]	Incidence per 100 000 population
United States		
Siegal	1965	2.5
Fessel[10]	1974	7.6
Mitchet[9]	1985	2.1
Hochberg[16]	1985	4.6

[a]Year of publication, not of data accrual.

annual incidence of SLE was 7.6 cases per 100 000 population per year[10]. The incidence of SLE in Baltimore between 1970 and 1977 was 4.6 cases per 100 000 population per year[16]. Hochberg[16] found that the incidence of systemic lupus in Baltimore in the 1970s peaked in the 4th decade for black women, was steady but high from age 20 to 50 in white women, while for black men the incidence rose steadily with increasing age.

Mortality

Kaslow and Masi[17] and Gordon et al.[18], using United States mortality statistics, showed that the age- and sex-specific risk of dying of SLE mirror the incidence of the disease. Both gender and race play an important role in affecting mortality. In the United States, mortality rates are higher for women than men at every age group[17]. Combining US death certificate data for SLE and DLE (discoid lupus), Lopez-Acuna et al.[19] found a significant interaction between female gender and nonwhite race in producing increased mortality. In the United Kingdom, age-specific annual mortality rates increase steadily in males, but level off after age 50 in females[20]. United States mortality rates are higher for blacks than for whites in nearly all age and gender categories[17]. Kaslow[21] found that Americans of Asian descent (Chinese, Japanese, and Filipinos) had a significantly higher annual mortality rate than US whites (6.8/million vs. 2.8/million, respectively). Similar results were reported from Hawaii by Serdula and Rhoads, who found the highest prevalence and mortality rates from SLE in Hawaiians of oriental descent[22].

It is heartening to note, however, that mortality rates from SLE have been declining for all age groups for the past 15 years. Gordon et al.[18] found that the most precipitous drop occurred in black women. Significant declines also occurred in both white women and men, while the trends in black men were the least impressive. In the UK, Hochberg[20] found a similar decrease, also more impressive in women than men.

Conclusion

When faced with an increasing incidence of SLE and declining mortality attributed to SLE, we must consider whether there has truly been an increase in the disease of the 1950s, or whether the lupus of the 1970s and 1980s is somehow different. In other words, is there a systematic difference in the criteria by which patients are diagnosed as having systemic lupus? As noted above, in the 1930s and 1940s only the most severe cases of systemic lupus erythematosus were diagnosed as such. In the absence of treatment, many of these patients died. In the 1970s and 1980s, however, with better recognition of the spectrum of lupus and more sensitive serologic tests, many patients are being diagnosed as systemic lupus who have mild, non-life-threatening disease, and who may do well regardless of therapy, or even in the absence of treatment. This is reflected in the rising incidence of systemic lupus. Thus, it may seem that the prognosis of systemic lupus has improved over time due to improved medical care, when part of the change may be due to a dilution of the severe cases by milder cases that can now be diagnosed. A much more pertinent issue, then, is the change in prognosis among comparable subgroups of patients — ones who have the same severity of illness, presence of important risk factors, etc.

CURRENT PROGNOSIS IN SYSTEMIC LUPUS

In developing a prognosis for a patient with systemic lupus, we must consider potential markers of increased risk that are attributes of the patient themselves, as well as features of the disease that may bode ill. Host factors that may affect outcome in systemic lupus include age, gender, race, education, and socioeconomic status (SES). In addition, individual factors such as patient motivation and compliance no doubt play a role. Disease factors of importance include the presence of renal disease, central nervous system (CNS) disease, and the presence of certain serologic markers. In the following sections, these will be discussed with respect to specific outcome measurements.

Prognosis in systemic lupus: host factors

Age

Of all the outcome measures considered in disease, death has traditionally been the best studied. Aside from its obvious importance, death is the most easily ascertained (i.e., "hardest") of all end-points. Although mortality rates from systemic lupus erythematosus generally increase with increasing age (except in black women), there is evidence that "late-onset SLE," beginning after age 50, generally has a good prognosis, with less renal disease, higher serum complement values, and a milder clinical course featuring mainly skin, joint, and serous membrane involvement[23,24,25]. Ballou et al.[26] showed that 5-year survival was similar among the two age groups. When compared to expected survival by age, the older patients actually had a better relative survival rate than patients under age 50.

How do we reconcile the apparent discrepancy between the rising mortality rates with age and the milder disease in older patients? First, mortality rates are derived from death-certificate information. The diagnosis of lupus may appear on the death certificate because the certifying physician knows the patient has systemic lupus, but active disease may not have been the direct cause of death. Second, the age at death (attributed to systemic lupus) does not indicate that the disease began shortly before death. Those dying of lupus at an advanced age may not necessarily have had late-onset SLE.

Gender

Studies generally agree that mortality rates for women are higher than for men[17-20,27]. Using mortality rates, these studies show a synergistic interaction between gender and race, with black women having the highest mortality, and white males the lowest. However, mortality data reflect patterns of incidence, and may be misleading in terms of prognosis. When survival rates are examined, most studies show comparable gender-specific survival rates: Estes and Christian[28] found no significant difference in survival rates by gender. In the multicenter study of outcome in SLE conducted by the Lupus Survival Study Group[29], males had a somewhat more favorable prognosis, as did older patients. On the other hand, Wallace et al.[30] reported worse survival rates in men than in women, although these were not adjusted for age.

Race

A nagging consideration when faced with race as a prognostic risk factor is whether one is actually seeing differences in SES, with race acting as a marker for higher or lower SES. For example, the Survival Study[29] found no racial difference in survival after adjusting for method of payment for medical care (public vs. private), a surrogate for SES. Similarly, Reveille and Alarcon[31] found that privately insured black and white patients had similar cumulative survival rates (93% and 86% for whites vs. 89% and 84% for blacks at 5 and 10 years, respectively), while publicly funded black patients had lower survival rates (81% and 78% at 5 and 10 years, respectively). On the other hand, a second recent study, based on 411 patients seen at Duke University between 1969 and 1983, suggests that these effects are independent, with nonwhite race and low SES contributing independently to decreased survival[32]. These conclusions are indirectly supported by other data from the Survival Study and from Hochberg et al.[33] that demonstrate that blacks have more severe disease than whites. Thus, although blacks seem to have a poorer prognosis than whites, it is not clear whether this is due to an intrinsic difference leading to more severe disease in blacks, or socioeconomic factors resulting in lower compliance and less access to medical care, or a combination of the two.

Prognosis in systemic lupus: disease factors

In a series of articles, Urowitz and colleagues[34-36] proposed that SLE mortality follows a bimodal distribution. In their experience, deaths within the first 2 years after diagnosis were generally due to active disease, while deaths occurring over 5 years after diagnosis were often due to cardiovascular disease, infections, or reappearance of active disease after a prolonged remission.

Renal disease

The largest study of disease-associated risk factors in systemic lupus was the Survival Study mentioned above. This study followed 1103 patients at nine university rheumatology clinics in the United States over 43.5 ± 35.2 months (mean ± standard deviation), and applied life-table techniques to derive survival rates[29]. Not unexpectedly, renal disease was the worst prognostic feature of the disease itself. Thus, several markers of renal function, such as serum creatinine at entry and level of proteinuria at entry were highly correlated with survival. For example, the 10-year survival for patients with serum creatinine greater than 3 mg/dl was only 12%, compared with over 80% in patients with normal serum creatinine. Renal disease accounted for 18% of all deaths in the study. Interestingly, although hemodialysis was available at all nine centers during the second half of the study, this procedure did not alter mortality rates from SLE. Thirty of 57 patients undergoing hemodialysis died, 21 of them with active SLE at the time of death, after having been dialyzed for 3.6 ± 4.5 months (mean ± standard deviation).

In Estes' and Christian's series[25], spanning 1962 to 1970, patients with renal disease had the worst 5-year survival, approximately 50%. In a large series reported by Wallace et al.[30] of patients seen between 1950 and 1979, renal disease was the most common cause of death. Patients with lupus nephritis had a 60% 15-year survival, compared with 85% survival for those without renal disease. In this series, nephrotic syndrome at onset of nephritis was associated with a poor prognosis (45% 15-year survival, vs. 75% in patients without nephrotic syndrome at the onset of nephritis). However, development of nephrotic syndrome after developing nephritis was not associated with a poorer survival. Correia et al.[37] suggested that a rapid deterioration in renal function was associated with worse survival than a gradual decline. These investigators also observed that death within 2 years of diagnosis was associated with active disease in 12 of 13 patients, compared to only 8 of 19 later deaths. Tareyeva et al.[38] found that men with lupus nephritis had a worse survival than women (41% vs. 60% at 10 years).

Many studies have investigated the prognostic usefulness of the renal biopsy in systemic lupus. The issue is confused by the realization that, in some patients at least, renal histology changes over time[39]. Thus, a biopsy that initially shows mild changes can "transition" into more severe disease on a subsequent biopsy. A corollary problem is that of "silent lupus nephritis," in which the urinalysis and serum creatinine are normal, but the biopsy indicates active disease, which can include diffuse proliferative lupus nephritis[40].

Estes and Christian[25] found that patients with diffuse proliferative or membranous glomerulonephritis had a 5-year survival rate of only 22%, compared with better than 60% 5-year survival in patients with focal proliferative glomerulonephritis. In the past 15 years, investigators have attempted to standardize interpretation of the renal biopsy using the World Health Organization criteria[41], which distinguish five categories of lupus nephritis (Table 4). There is general agreement that diffuse proliferative lupus nephritis is associated with a much poorer outcome than other WHO classes, and mild mesangial lesions have the best outcome[38,42-46].

In addition, specific histologic features have been assembled into two prognostic indices: an activity index and a chronicity index (Table 4)[47]. Austin et al.[47] analyzed the prognostic contribution of renal biopsy data in 102 patients with lupus nephritis who had been entered into a series of treatment trials at the National Institutes of Health (USA). They found that age under 24 years, male sex, and serum creatinine greater than 1.35 mg/dl were the most important clinical prognostic indicators. In addition, chronicity index and activity index both significantly enhanced their prognostic model; age and chronicity index alone were as useful as all five factors together. These authors concluded that the renal biopsy does add significantly to prognostic accuracy in lupus nephritis. In another analysis, the NIH group showed that chronicity index rose despite prednisone therapy, but not after cytotoxic therapy[48]. Using multiple linear regression analysis, Whiting-O'Keefe et al.[49] showed that the renal biopsy added significantly to the predictive power of clinical variables, although the amount of variability explained by the model (R^2) rose only from 0.25 to 0.33.

Other investigators have found the renal biopsy to be of only limited prognostic significance. Fries et al.[50] found the renal biopsy did not add

Table 4 World Health Organization classification of lupus renal lesions, and National Institutes of Health activity and chronicity index scoring systems

WHO Class[a]	Description
I	Mesangial lesions only
II	Focal proliferative GN
III	Diffuse proliferative GN
IV	Membranoproliferative GN
V	Membranous GN

Activity Index[b] Maximum score 24 points

Glomerular changes	Tubulointerstitial changes
Cellular proliferation	Mononuclear cell infiltrate
Fibrinoid necrosis (×2)	
Cellular crescents (×2)	
Hyaline thrombi, wire loops	
Leukocyte infiltration	

Chronicity Index[b] Maximum score 12 points

Glomerular changes	Tubulointerstitial changes
Glomerular sclerosis	Interstitial fibrosis
Fibrous crescents	Tubular atrophy

[a]Modified from Ref. 41. GN = glomerulonephritis.
[b]Modified from Ref. 47. Each feature is graded 0, 1, 2, or 3 (absent, mild, moderate, or severe). Fibrinoid necrosis and cellular crescents are weighted by a factor of 2.

significantly to prognosis. Esdaile et al.[51] also found the additional value of the biopsy limited beyond clinical predictors. However, they emphasized that the extent of tubulointerstitial involvement was the strongest biopsy predictor of outcome. Appel et al.[52] applied the chronicity and activity indices to their New York lupus population, and found that neither index significantly predicted renal survival. However, they also found that WHO class was important: patients with mesangial lesions had the best prognosis. Readers should note, however, that the mean chronicity and activity indices in Appel's patients were both low (75% had an activity index less than 5 [out of a possible 24], and 77% had a chronicity index less than 2 [out of a possible 12]), whereas Austin's series included patients with much higher scores. Thus, these indices may be of less prognostic value when restricted to a narrower range.

A related question is the prognosis of patients with systemic lupus once they develop end-stage renal disease. In general, disease activity tends to diminish at this stage, perhaps due to the immunosuppressive effect of uremia, or perhaps due to the salutary effect of thrice-weekly hemodialysis, a form of plasmapheresis[53,54]. Although Jarrett et al.[54] described problems with infection and vascular access in their hemodialysis patients with SLE, Hellerstedt et al.[55] found lupus patients to have a generally favorable outcome. This discrepancy may be due to other factors, such as a differential prevalence of lupus anticoagulant activity in the two populations, difference in age, etc.

Central nervous system disease

Lupus cerebritis has been associated with decreased survival, albeit not as strongly as renal disease has been. Estes and Christian[25] found that the 5-year survival rate in their patients with neuropsychiatric symptoms was 58%, compared to 78% for the series as a whole. They further examined prognosis by type of CNS symptom. Grand mal seizures, in the absence of uremia, were not associated with increased mortality. Neither were "functional psychoses." However, focal neurologic signs, such as cranial nerve abnormalities, tremor, and hemiparesis, or the presence of "organic mental syndromes" were associated with an increased mortality. These findings were independent of renal disease.

The Lupus Survival Study Group[29] also found decreased survival in patients with central nervous system lupus, especially during the first year after entering the study. Both seizures and "organic psychosis" were associated with decreased survival, although neither was an independent predictor of survival in a linear regression model. Seizures in the setting of uremia were associated with a far worse prognosis than seizures in the face of normal renal function. Feinglass et al.[56] found that 10 of 52 (19%) patients with neuropsychiatric features of SLE died over 4.5 years of follow-up, compared to 9 of 88 (10%) patients without such features. Of note, 4 of the 10 neuropsychiatric deaths were due to infection in the setting of high-dose cortiscosteroid therapy for the CNS manifestations of the disease. Similarly, Sergent et al.[57] found that 7 of their 28 patients with CNS lupus died, 5 from infections.

Transverse myelopathy has also been described as a complication of systemic lupus[58]. This condition has been associated with a very poor prognosis. Andrianakos et al.[58] found that 8 of 13 patients with lupus-associated transverse myelitis died, over a range of 4 days to 3 years after onset of symptoms. In contrast, peripheral neuropathy due to systemic lupus erythematosus-associated mononeuritis multiplex is not associated with increased mortality[59,60].

Serology

The presence of antibodies to double-stranded DNA and low complement levels are both associated with active disease, especially nephritis. In addition, hypocomplementemia is more common in black patients[33] and those with a younger age of onset[24]. Since these demographic subgroups are themselves associated with decreased survival, it is hard to know whether these serologic abnormalities are independently associated with poor outcome. Because of this confounding issue, one may best say that serologic markers of active diseases herald a more dangerous situation, one associated with poorer prognosis. In contrast, antibodies to "extractable nuclear antigens" such as anti-RNP and anti-Sm are not associated with increased mortality[61].

Prognosis in systemic lupus: other factors

Infection

Although infections were found to be a frequent problem in patients with systemic lupus erythematosus even in the presteroid era, much of the infectious complication rate of this disease has been attributed to the immunosuppression of corticosteroids and cytotoxic agents[62]. The Lupus Survival Study Group found that infection was the underlying cause of 33% of all deaths, a proportion greater than that due to active disease (31%)[63]. Rubin et al.[36] found that infection was more common in patients with active disease who were also being treated with higher doses of corticosteroids. In another publication[64], this group described major infections (those producing systemic symptoms and requiring parenteral antibiotics) in 10% of their patients with SLE; one-third of these patients died.

When investigating fatal infections in systemic lupus, Hellmann et al.[62] found that opportunistic infections occurred as commonly as bacterial infections but were much less likely to be diagnosed *ante mortem*. Four-fifths of fatal bacterial infections were diagnosed before autopsy, compared to only one-fifth of fatal opportunistic infections. No measure of lupus activity correlated with fatal opportunistic infection, but prednisone and cytotoxic use in the 3 months preceding death were strongly associated with such infections. Thus, infectious complications of SLE continue to be a major cause of mortality, and may be associated with intensive treatment of active disease, rather than with the disease itself.

Coronary artery disease

In recent years, several reports of premature coronary artery disease (CAD) in SLE have appeared. Rubin et al.[36] found that 9 of 30 patients who died 2 or more years after the diagnosis of SLE died of CAD. In the Lupus Survival Study Group experience[64], CAD accounted for 9 deaths (4.5% of all deaths) when myocardial infarction and sudden death were combined. In contrast, the expected number of cardiac deaths in their population was only 2, based on rates provided by the National Center for Health Statistics[63]. Correia et al.[37] found that CAD accounted for 25% (7 of 28) of deaths among their 138 patients with lupus nephritis.

Autopsy data also indicate that there may be an increased prevalence of premature CAD in patients dying of lupus[65]. CAD was associated with prednisone therapy, elevated blood cholesterol levels, and hypertension. In an angiographic series of 100 consecutive women with SLE, ischemic heart disease was found in sixteen[66]. Furthermore, patients with SLE are known to have higher levels of serum cholesterol and triglycerides than do normal controls. Patients taking prednisone have higher levels than patients not taking prednisone, but even the latter group of SLE patients have higher lipid levels than age- and sex-matched normal controls[67]. Thus, as survival of patients with systemic lupus erythematosus improves, coronary artery disease has emerged as an issue of growing importance. Whether this is due to prolonged corticosteroid treatment, as some have suggested[63], or due to other factors, remains to be decided.

PHYSICAL DISABILITY AND PSYCHOSOCIAL ADJUSTMENT IN SYSTEMIC LUPUS

Unlike the extensive literature on mortality, nonfatal outcomes in systemic lupus have not enjoyed the same interest until recently. The World Health Organization[68] has classified the impact of disease on the patient in three categories: impairment, disability, and handicap. Impairment refers to "loss or abnormality of psychological, physiological, or anatomical structure or function." Impairment may then lead to development of disability — "any restriction or lack (resulting from an impairment) of ability to perform an activity in the manner or within the range considered normal for a human being." Finally, a handicap is the inability to fulfill a normal social role, as a result of a disability.

Obviously, a disease with such protean manifestations as systemic lupus often has an explosive impact on a patient's ability to perform normal social functions at work, at home, and at leisure. Depending on the target organ involved in any individual person's disease, the degree of disability may be greater or less. For example, severe photosensitivity and arthralgias could render a farmworker unemployable, but have little effect on a computer programmer. Conversely, mild central nervous system manifestations such as memory or calculation deficits could have severe consequences for the programmer, but pose fewer problems for the agricultural worker. Of course, severe cerebritis or nephritis, or an infectious complication, could disable either one.

Liang et al.[69] interviewed 75 lupus patients and 23 controls with rheumatoid arthritis. They found that nearly half of the SLE patients had difficulty keeping a job, compared to 35% of controls. Two-thirds reported a decrease in their independence since contracting the disease, and 70% admitted to depression ("lowered spirits"). Using the

Minnesota Multiphasic Personality Interview (MMPI), these investigators found that patients with SLE had marked elevations on three scales — hypochondriasis, depression, and hysteria. Similar findings were noted in the rheumatoid arthritis patients. However, nearly a quarter of the SLE patients reported fear of death, compared to none of the rheumatoid arthritis patients.

Stein et al.[70] studied the psychosocial impact of SLE in 120 patients followed at the University of British Columbia. They found that 12.5% were divorced after their diagnosis; this figure is not significantly different from the general population in their area. SLE was not a barrier to completing their education (33% did so after their diagnosis), to getting married (40% were married after diagnosis), or to being employed. Sixty-three percent of patients who had a work history were still working at the time of their survey. In those employed in professional, managerial, or skilled jobs, 95% were working full time (more than 35 hours per week), compared to only 40% of semiskilled workers and 50% of laborers. Sixteen percent of patients with a work history had to retire due to lupus. Overall, 20 patients, including 11 work retirees, had severely affected lifestyles due to lupus while another 62 patients had moderately affected lifestyles. Thus, only one-third of the entire group noted little or no effect of lupus upon their lifestyle.

Hochberg and Sutton[71] administered the Stanford Health Assessment Questionnaire (HAQ) and the Psychosocial Adjustment to Illness Scale (PAIS) to 106 outpatients with SLE in an attempt to characterize the type and extent of physical disability in SLE. In this group of outpatients, only a mild degree of functional limitation was found: the mean disability index score was 0.66 out of a maximum score of 3.0, compared to 1.2 in patients with rheumatoid arthritis. More than 25% of patients had no difficulty with any basic or instrumental activities of daily living, and less than 10% needed assistance with at least one of these activities. The four patients who reported being disabled from work had significantly higher scores than 45 currently working patients (1.25 vs. 0.40, $p<0.05$).

Psychosocial adjustment was measured using the PAIS, an instrument that assesses the impact of chronic illness on 7 domains: health care orientation, vocational environment, domestic environment, social environment, extended family relationships, sexual relationships, and psychological distress[72]. Analysis of these data showed highly significant correlations between self-reported physical disability and poor psychosocial adjustment across all categories except health care orientation[71]. Several sociodemographic factors, including age, race, gender, source of patient care, educational level, and marital status, were analyzed for their association with disability and psychosocial outcomes. In multivariate models, only educational level was inversely associated with disability; the other sociodemographic variables were not associated with disability.

The longitudinal course of physical disability and psychosocial dysfunction was studied in this cohort by Hochberg et al.[73]. Over a 12-month follow-up, 84 (83%) of 102 survivors remained under evaluation. Although there were no overall changes in level of physical disability or psychosocial adjustment for the entire group, there was considerable variation within individual patients, with 34 patients noting increased disability and 29 noting decreased disability (improved function). A highly significant correlation was noted between changes in disability index and psychosocial adjustment among these patients. Furthermore, the only baseline clinicolaboratory variable that predicted increasing disability was therapy with prednisone: 32 (94%) of 34 cases with increased disability index were taking prednisone, compared to 20 (69%) of 29 cases with decreased disability index. In addition, the mean prednisone dose was 19.4 mg/day in the former, vs. 11.5 mg/day in the latter. These data imply that increase in disability might reflect the results of active/severe disease and/or the development of corticosteroid complications.

Patients with systemic lupus erythematosus are at increased risk of developing corticosteroid-induced avascular necrosis of bone (AVN), a major cause of pain and disability. Zizic et al.[74] followed 54 patients with SLE prospectively. Twenty-eight of these patients developed AVN at 93 sites. The development of AVN was correlated with mean prednisone dose at various times in the course of illness. Other corticosteroid-induced complications that might impact on physical disability include osteoporosis with resultant fracture, steroid myopathy, and obesity accompanied by Cushingoid habitus[75].

Because systemic lupus erythematosus is a disease of young women of child-bearing age, any analysis of psychosocial adjustment must consider the impact of the disease on reproductive capacity. Stein et al.[70] found that 47 women had had 124 pregnancies prior to the diagnosis of SLE, resulting in 78% live births. After the diagnosis of lupus, 61 women had 76 pregnancies, resulting in 45% live births. Four births after diagnosis resulted in infants with birth defects, compared to none in the group before diagnosis. Nonetheless, these data should be interpreted with caution. The effect of various medications[76], the age of the mothers, the effect of varying presence of anti-Ro and anti-phospholipid antibodies[77], and the possibility of selection bias cannot be excluded. Readers are referred to a comprehensive review of pregnancy in SLE by Petri for further discussion of this area[78].

SUMMARY AND FUTURE PERSPECTIVES

Of all the rheumatic diseases, systemic lupus erythematosus is the most far-ranging and variable, affecting multiple organ systems in different patients at different times. Like most of its rheumatic counterparts, its etiology remains a matter for speculation. As a result, prognostication in systemic lupus is a difficult problem. In this chapter, we have reviewed the basic tenets that determine outcome in this disease. As summarized in Table 5, we have divided prognostic factors

Table 5 Summary of factors indicating a poorer prognosis in systemic lupus erythematosus. Factors are presented in generally descending order of strength of their association with a poor outcome, both in terms of mortality and of disability

Host factors
Younger age at diagnosis (under 24 years)
Race (black, oriental)
Low socioeconomic status
    Public funding of medical care (US medicaid)

Disease factors
Active nephritis
    Serum creatinine elevation
    Biopsy evidence of diffuse proliferative GN
    Chronicity index, especially interstitial disease
    Active urinary sediment
Active central nervous system disease
    Focal neurologic findings
    Diffuse cerebritis ("organic brain syndrome")

Other factors
Infection
    Dose of corticosteroids
    Use of cytotoxic agents
Coronary artery disease
    Duration and amount of corticosteroid use
Ischemic necrosis of bone
    Duration and amount of corticosteroid use

between host-related factors, disease-related factors, and treatment-related factors.

When considering the impact of systemic lupus on the patient, one must review a hierarchy of potential dangers to the patients. Are they in danger of dying prematurely from renal or CNS involvement? If so, treatment of these severe manifestations must be the first priority. It is here that diagnosis, prognosis, and treatment become inextricably linked. Once the danger of death recedes, however, less dramatic but often more intractable prognostic issues must be grappled with. Will the patient be able to return to work? Will he or she suffer from intractable pain or fatigue? Will she be able to have children if she so desires? Will he or she develop infection or ischemic necrosis of bone? The same considerations — host factors, disease factors, and treatment choices — will to a large degree determine the answers to these questions as well.

Recently, observational cohort studies have been developed to estimate the long-term prognosis of morbidity outcomes, including physical disability and psychosocial adjustment in SLE[71,73,79]. These studies utilize validated indices for measuring disease activity[80-82]. Such indices will greatly assist in standardizing the measurement of this variable and the classification of disease flare as an important outcome. A subcommittee of the American College of Rheumatology Diagnostic and Therapeutic Criteria Committee is currently developing guidelines for use of these measures in clinical research.

When a physician tells a patient a prognosis, he or she is, in essence, attempting to forecast or prophesy the future. Such a task is inherently uncertain at best. Although there is now a large literature regarding fatal outcomes in SLE, research into nonfatal outcomes is sorely needed. As noted above, we do not have reliable data on the financial impact of this disease, nor have we quantified the degree of social and personal suffering it causes. If, to paraphrase Lord Kelvin, science requires the ability to measure outcomes, we are only at the beginning of this task with regard to systemic lupus erythematosus.

References

1. Kaposi, M. K. (1872). Neue Beitrage zur Keantiss des lupus erythematosus. *Arch. Dermatol. Syphilol.*, **4**, 36-78
2. Osler, W. (1904). On the visceral manifestations of the erythema group of skin diseases. *Am. J. Med. Sci.*, **127**, 1-23
3. Talbott, J. H. (1987). Historical background of discoid and systemic lupus erythematosus. In Wallace, D. J. and Dubois, E. L. (eds.) *Dubois' Lupus Erythematosus*, pp. 3-11. (Philadelphia: Lea & Febiger)
4. Blotzer, J. W. (1983). Systemic lupus erythematosus I: Historical aspects. *Md. State Med. J.*, **32**, 439-441
5. Hargraves, M. M., Richmond, H. and Morton, R. (1948). Presentation of two bone marrow elements: the Tart cell and the L. E. cell. *Proc. Staff Meet. Mayo Clin.*, **23**, 25-28
6. Harvey, A. M., Howard, J. E., Wilkenwerder, W. L., Bordley, J. E., Carey, R. A. and Kattus, A. (1950). Observations on effect of adrenocorticotropic hormone (ACTH) on disseminated lupus erythematosus, drug hypersensitivity, and chronic bronchial asthma. *Trans. Am. Clin. Climat. Assoc.*, **61**, 221-234
7. McCombs, R. P. and Patterson, J. F. (1959). Factors influencing the course and prognosis of systemic lupus erythematosus. *N. Engl. J. Med.*, **260**, 1195-1204
8. Merrell, M. and Shulman, L. E. (1955). Determination of prognosis in chronic disease, illustrated by systemic lupus erythematosus. *J. Chronic Dis.*, **1**, 12-32
9. Michet, C. J., McKenna, C. H., Elveback, L. R., Kaslow, R. A. and Kurland, L. T. (1985). Epidemiology of systemic lupus erythematosus and other connective tissue diseases in Rochester, Minnesota, 1950 to 1979. *Mayo Clin. Proc.*, **60**, 105-113
10. Fessel, W. J. (1974). Systemic lupus erythematosus in the community. Incidence, prevalence, outcome, and first symptoms; the high prevalence in black women. *Arch. Intern. Med.*, **134**, 1027-1035
11. Siegel, M. and Lee, S. L. (1973). The epidemiology of systemic lupus erythematosus. *Semin Arthritis Rheum.*, **3**, 1-54
12. Meddings, J. and Grennan, D. M. (1980). The prevalence of systemic lupus erythematosus (SLE) in Dunedin. *N.Z. Med. J.*, **91**, 205-206
13. Hochberg, M. C. (1987). Prevalence of systemic lupus erythematosus in England and Wales, 1981-1982. *Ann. Rheum. Dis.*, **46**, 664-666
14. Nakal, K., Furusawa, F., Kasukawa, R., Tojo, T., Homma, M. and Aoki, K. (1987). A national epidemiological survey of diffuse collagen diseases: estimation of prevalence rate in Japan. In Kasukaw, R. and Sharp, G. C. (eds.) *Mixed Connective Tissue Disease and Anti-Nuclear Antibodies*, pp. 9-13. (Amsterdam: Elsevier Scientific Publishers)
15. Helve, T. (1985). Prevalence and mortality rates of systemic lupus erythematosus and causes of death in SLE patients in Finland. *Scand. J. Rheumatol.*, **14**, 43-46
16. Hochberg, M. C. (1985). The incidence of systemic lupus erythematosus in Baltimore, Maryland, 1970-1977. *Arthritis Rheum.*, **28**, 80-86
17. Kaslow, R. A. and Masi, A. T. (1978). Age, sex, and race effects on mortality from systemic lupus erythematosus in the United States. *Arthritis Rheum.*, **21**, 473-479
18. Gordon, M. F., Stolley, P. D. and Schinnar, R. (1981). Trends in recent systemic lupus erythematosus mortality rates. *Arthritis Rheum.*, **24**, 762-769

19. Lopez-Acuna, D., Hochberg, M. C. and Gittelsohn, A. M. (1982). Mortality from discoid (DLE) and systemic lupus erythematosus (SLE) in the United States, 1968-1978. *Arthritis Rheum.*, **25**, S80 Abstract
20. Hochberg, M. C. (1987). Mortality from systemic lupus erythematosus in England and Wales, 1974-1983. *Br. J. Rheumatol.*, **26**, 437-441
21. Kaslow, R. A. (1982). High rate of death caused by systemic lupus erythematosus among U.S. residents of Asian descent. *Arthritis Rheum.*, **25**, 414-418
22. Serdula, M. K. and Rhoads, G. G. (1979). Frequency of systemic lupus erythematosus in different ethnic groups in Hawaii. *Arthritis Rheum.*, **22**, 328-333
23. Baker, S. H., Rovira, G. H., Campion, E. W. and Mills, J. A. (1979). Late onset systemic lupus erythematosus. *Am. J. Med.*, **66**, 727-732
24. Dimant, J., Ginzler, E. M., Schlesinger, M., Diamond, D. S. and Kaplan, D. (1979). Systemic lupus erythematosus in the older age group: computer analysis. *J. Am. Geriatr. Soc.*, **27**, 58-61
25. Wilson, H. A., Hamilton, M. E., Spyker, D. A., Brunner, C. M., O'Brien, W. M., Davis, J. S. and Winfield, J. B. (1981). Age influences the clinical and serologic expression of systemic lupus erythematosus. *Arthritis Rheum.*, **24**, 1230-1234
26. Ballou, S. P., Khan, M. H. and Kushner, I. (1982). Clinical features of systemic lupus erythematosus. Differences related to race and age of onset. *Arthritis Rheum.*, **25**, 55-59
27. Masi, A. T. and Kaslow, R. A. (1978). Sex effects in systemic lupus erythematosus. A clue to pathogenesis. *Arthritis Rheum.*, **21**, 480-484
28. Estes, D. and Christian, C. I. (1971). The natural history of systemic lupus erythematosus by prospective analysis. *Medicine (Baltimore)*, **50**, 85-95
29. Ginzler, E. M., Diamond, H. S., Weiner, M., Schlesinger, M., Fries, J. F., Wasner, C., Medsger, T. A., Ziegler, G., Klippel, J. H., Hadler, N. M., Albert, D. A., Hess, E. V., Spencer-Green, G., Grayzel, A., Worth, D., Hahn, B. A. and Barnett, E. V. (1982). A multicenter study of outcome in systemic lupus erythematosus. I. Entry variables as predictors of prognosis. *Arthritis Rheum.*, **25**, 601-611
30. Wallace, D. J., Podell, T., Klinenberg, J. R., Forouzesh, S. and Dubois, E. L. (1981). Systemic lupus erythematosus — survival patterns. *J. Am. Med. Assoc.*, **245**, 934-938
31. Reveille, J. D. and Alarcon, G. S. (1986). Survival in systemic lupus erythematosus: demographic, socioeconomic, clinical factors, and causes of death. *Arthritis Rheum.*, **29** (suppl. 4), S27 (Abstract)
32. Studenski, S., Allen, N. B., Caldwell, D. S., Rice, J. R. and Polisson, R. P. (1987). Survival in systemic lupus erythematosus. A multivariate analysis of demographic factors. *Arthritis Rheum.*, **30**, 1326-1332
33. Hochberg, M. C., Boyd, R. E., Ahearn, J. M., Arnett, F. C., Bias, W. B., Provost, T. T. and Stevens, M. B. (1985). Systemic lupus erythematosus: a review of clinico-laboratory features and immunogenetic markers in 150 patients with emphasis on demographic subsets. *Medicine (Baltimore)*, **64**, 285-295
34. Urowitz, M. B., Bookman, A. M., Koehler, B. E., Gordon, D. A., Smythe, H. A. and Ogryzlo, M. A. (1976). The bimodal mortality pattern of systemic lupus erythematosus. *Am. J. Med.*, **60**, 221-225
35. Urowitz, M. B. and Gladman, D. D. (1980). Late morality in SLE — "the price we pay for control". *J. Rheumatol.*, **7**, 412-416
36. Rubin, L. A., Urowitz, M. B. and Gladman, D. D. (1985). Mortality in systemic lupus erythematosus: the bimodal pattern revisited. *Q. J. Med.*, **55**, 87-98
37. Correia, P., Cameron, J. S., Lian, J. D., Hicks, J., Ogg, C. S., Williams, D. G., Chantler, C. and Haycock, D. G. (1985). Why do patients with lupus nephritis die? *Br. Med. J.*, **290**, 126-131
38. Tareyeva, I. E., Janushkevitch, T. N. and Tuganbekova, S. K. (1984). Lupus nephritis in males and females. *Proc. Eur. Dial. Transp. Assoc. — Eur. Renal Assoc.*, **21**, 712-714
39. Ginzler, E. M., Nicastri, A. D., Chen, C-K., Friedman, E. A., Diamond, H. S. and Kaplan, D. (1974). Progression of mesangial and focal to diffuse lupus nephritis. *N. Engl. J. Med.*, **291**, 693-696
40. Stemankovic, I., Favre, H., Donath, A., Assimacopoulos, A. and Chatelanat, F. (1986).

Renal biopsy in SLE irrespective of clinical findings: long-term follow-up. *Clin. Nephrol.*, **26**, 109-115
41. McCluskey, R. T. (1975). Lupus nephritis. In Sommers, S. C. (ed.) *Pathology Decennial*, pp. 435-460. (New York: Appleton-Century-Crofts)
42. Ponticelli, C., Zucchelli, P., Moroni, G., Cagnoli, L., Banfi, G. and Pasquali, S. (1987). Long-term prognosis of diffuse lupus nephritis. *Clin. Nephrol.*, **28**, 263-271
43. Leaker, B., Fairley, K. F., Dowing, J. and Kincaid-Smith, P. Lupus nephritis: clinical and pathological correlation. *Q. J. Med.*, **62**, 163-179
44. Walker, R. J., Bailey, R. R., Swainson, C. P. and Lynn, K. L. (1986). Lupus nephritis: a 13-year experience. *N.Z. Med. J.*, **99**, 894-896
45. Schwartz, M. M., Kawala, K. S., Corwin, H. L. and Lewis, E. J. (1987). The prognosis of segmental glomerulonephritis in systemic lupus erythematosus. *Kidney Int.*, **32**, 274-279
46. Magil, A. B., Ballon, H. S., Chan, V., Lirenman, D. S., Rae, A. and Sutton, R. A. L. (1984). Diffuse proliferative lupus glomerulonephritis. Determination of prognostic significance of clinical, laboratory, and pathologic factors. *Medicine (Baltimore)*, **63**, 210-220
47. Austin, H. A., Muenz, L. R., Joyce, K. M., Antonovych, T. A., Kullick, M. E., Klippel, J. H., Decker, J. L. and Balow, J. E. (1983). Prognostic factors in lupus nephritis. Contribution of renal histologic data. *Am. J. Med.*, **75**, 382-391
48. Balow, J. E., Austin, H. A., Muenz, L. R., Joyce, K. M., Anonovych, T. T., Klippel, J. H., Steinberg, A. D., Plotz, P. H. and Decker, J. L. (1984). Effect of treatment on the evolution of renal abnormalities in lupus nephritis. *N. Engl. J. Med.*, **311**, 491-495
49. Whiting-O'Keefe, Q., Henke, J. E., Shearn, M. A., Hopper, J., Biava, C. G. and Epstein, W. V. (1982). The information content from renal biopsy in systemic lupus erythematosus. *Ann. Intern. Med.*, **96**, 718-723
50. Fries, J. F., Porta, J. and Liang, M. H. (1978). Marginal benefit of renal biopsy in systemic lupus erythematosus. *Arch. Intern. Med.*, **138**, 1386-1390
51. Esdaile, J. M., Federgreen, W., Levinton, C., Hayslett, J. P. and Kashgarian, M. (1988). Biopsy predictors in SLE nephritis: import of interstital disease. *Arthritis Rheum.*, **31**, S37 (Abstract)
52. Appel, G. B., Cohen, D., Pirani, C. L., Meltzer, J. L. and Estes, D. (1987). Long-term follow-up of patients with lupus nephritis. A study based on the classification of the World Health Organization. *Am. J. Med.*, **83**, 877-885
53. Coplon, N. S., Diskin, C. J., Petersen, J. and Swenson, R. S. (1983). The long-term clinical course of systemic lupus erythematosus in end-stage renal disease. *N. Engl. J. Med.*, **308**, 186-190
54. Jarrett, M. P., Santhanam, S. and Del Greco, F. (1983). The clinical course of end-stage renal disease in systemic lupus erythematosus. *Arch. Intern. Med.*, **143**, 1353-1356
55. Hellerstedt, W. L., Johnson, W. J., Ascher, N., Kjellstrand, C. M., Knutson, R., Shapiro, F. L. and Sterioff, S. (1984). Survival rates in 2728 patients with end-stage renal disease. *Mayo Clin. Proc.*, **59**, 776-783
56. Feinglass, E. J., Arnett, F. C., Dorsch, C. A., Zizic, T. M. and Stevens, M. B. (1976). Neuropsychiatric manifestations of systemic lupus erythematosus: diagnosis, clinical spectrum, and relationship to other features of the disease. *Medicine (Baltimore)*, **55**, 323-339
57. Sergent, J. E., Lockshin, M. D., Klempner, M. S. and Lipsky, B. A. (1975). Central nervous system disease in systemic lupus erythematosus. Therapy and prognosis. *Am. J. Med.*, **58**, 644-654
58. Andrianakos, A. A., Duffy, J., Suzuki, M. and Sharp, J. T. (1975). Transverse myelopathy in systemic lupus erythematosus. Report of three cases and review of the literature. *Ann. Intern. Med.*, **83**, 616-624
59. McCombe, P. A., McLeod, J. G., Pollard, J. D., Guo, Y-P. and Ingall, T. J. (1987). Peripheral sensorimotor and autonomic neuropathy associated with systemic lupus erythematosus. Clinical, pathological, and immunological features. *Brain*, **110**, 533-549
60. Hellmann, D. B., Laing, T. J., Petri, M., Whiting-O'Keefe, Q. and Parry, G. J. (1988).

Mononeuritis multiplex: the yield of the evaluation for occult rheumatic diseases. *Medicine (Baltimore)*, **67**, 145-153
61. Hochberg, M. C., Dorsch, C. A., Feinglass, E. J. and Stevens, M. B. (1981). Survivorship in systemic lupus erythematosus. Effect of antibody to extractable nuclear antigen. *Arthritis Rheum.*, **24**, 54-59
62. Hellmann, D. B., Petri, M. and Whiting-O'Keefe, Q. (1987). Fatal infections in systemic lupus erythematosus: the role of opportunistic infections. *Medicine (Baltimore)*, **66**, 341-348
63. Rosner, S., Ginzler, E. M., Diamond, H. S., Weiner, M., Schlesinger, M., Fries, J. F., Wasner, C., Medsger, T. A., Ziegler, G., Klippel, J. H., Hadler, N. M., Albert, D. A., Hess, E. V., Spencer-Green, G., Grayzel, A., Worth, D., Hahn, B. A. and Barnett, E. V. (1982). A multicenter study of outcome in systemic lupus erythematosus. II. Causes of death. *Arthritis Rheum.*, **25**, 612-617
64. Lee, P., Urowitz, M. B., Bookman, A. A. M., Koehler, B. E., Smythe, H. A., Gordon, D. A. and Ogryzlo, M. A. (1977). Systemic lupus erythematosus. Review of 110 cases with reference to nephritis, the nervous system, infections, aseptic necrosis, and prognosis. *Q. J. Med.*, **181**, 1-32
65. Bulkley, B. H. and Roberts, W. C. (1975). The heart in systemic lupus erythematosus and the changes induced in it by corticosteroid therapy: a study of 36 necropsy patients. *Am. J. Med.*, **58**, 243-264
66. Badui, E., Garcia-Rubi, D., Robles, E., Jimenez, J., Juan, L., Deleze, M., Diaz, A. and Mintz, G. (1985). Cardiovascular manifestations in systemic lupus erythematosus. Prospective study of 100 patients. *Angiology*, **36**, 431-448
67. Ettinger, W. H., Goldberg, A. P., Applebaum-Bowden, D. and Hazzard, W. R. (1987). Dyslipoproteinemia in systemic lupus erythematosus. Effect of corticosteroids. *Am. J. Med.*, **83**, 503-509.
68. Wood, P. H. N. (1980). Appreciating the consequences of disease: the international classification of impairments, disabilities, and handicaps. *WHO Chronicle*, **34**, 476-380
69. Liang, M. H., Rogers, M., Larson, M., Eaton, H. M., Murawski, B. J., Taylor, J. E., Swafford, J. and Schur, P. F. (1984). The psychosocial impact of systemic lupus erythematosus and rheumatoid arthritis. *Arthritis Rheum.*, **27**, 13-19
70. Stein, H., Walters, K., Dillon, A. and Schulzer, M. (1986). Systemic lupus erythematosus — a medical and social profile. *J. Rheumatol.*, **13**, 570-576
71. Hochberg, M. C. and Sutton, J. D. (1988). Physical disability and psychosocial dysfunction in systemic lupus erythematosus. *J. Rheumatol.*, **15**, 959-964
72. Derogatis, L. R. and Lopez, M. C. (1983). *The Psychosocial Adjustment of Illness Scale: Administration, Scoring, and Procedures Manual*. (Baltimore: Clinical Psychometric Research)
73. Hochberg, M. C., Sutton, J. D. and Engle, E. W. (1988). Longitudinal course of physical disability and psychosocial dysfunction in systemic lupus erythematosus. *Arthritis Rheum.*, **31**, S94 (Abstract)
74. Zizic, T. M., Hungerford, D. S. and Stevens, M. B. (1980). Ischemic necrosis of bone in systemic lupus erythematosus. The early diagnosis of ischemic necrosis of bone. *Medicine (Baltimore)*, **59**, 134-142
75. Hochberg, M. C. (1985). Collagen-vascular disease and disability. In Hadler, N. M. and Gillings, D. B. (eds.) *Arthritis and Society. The Impact of Musculoskeletal Diseases*, pp. 17-35. (London: Butterworth)
76. Roubenoff, R., Hoyt, J., Petri, M., Hochberg, M. C. and Hellmann, D. B. (1988). Effects of antiinflammatory and immunosuppressive drugs on pregnancy and fertility. *Semin. Arthritis Rheum.*, **18**, 88-110
77. Petri, M., Watson, R. and Hochberg, M. C. (1990). Anti-Ro antibodies and neonatal lupus. *Rheum. Dis. Clin. N. Am.*, **15**, 355-360
78. Petri, M. (1988). Outcomes encouraging in mothers with lupus. *Contemp. Obstet. Gynecol.*, 103-115
79. Engle, E. W., Callahan, L. F., Pincus, T. and Hochberg, M. C. (1990). Validation of the rheumatology attitudes index (RAI) in systemic lupus erythematosus (SLE). *Arthritis Rheum.*, **34**, 281-286
80. Committee on Prognosis Studies in SLE. (1986). Prognosis studies in SLE: an activity index. *Arthritis Rheum.*, **29**, S93 (Abstract)

81. Liang, M. H., Socher, S. A., Roberts., W. N. and Esdaile, J. M. (1988). Measurement of systemic lupus erythematosus activity in clinical research. *Arthritis Rheum.*, **31**, 817–825
82. Petri, M., Hellmann, D. B. and Hochberg, M. C. (1989). Validity and reliability of the lupus activity index: comparison with the Toronto activity index (SLEDAI) and systemic lupus erythematosus activity measure (SLAM) (Abstract). *Arthritis Rheum.*, **32** (4, Suppl.), 530
83. Kellum, R. E. and Hasericke, J. R. (1964). Systemic lupus erythematosus. A statistical evaluation of mortality based on a consecutive series of 299 patients. *Arch. Intern. Med.*, **113**, 200–202
84. Fries, J. F., Weyl, S. and Holman, H. R. (1974). Estimating prognosis in systemic lupus erythematosus. *Am. J. Med.*, **57**, 561–565
85. Grigor, R., Edmond, J., Lewkon, A. R., Bresnihan, B. and Hughes, G. R. V. (1978). Systemic lupus erythematosus: a prospective analysis. *Ann. Rheum. Dis.*, **37**, 121–128

10
Systemic sclerosis (scleroderma)

V. D. STEEN and T. A. MEDSGER

PROBLEMS IN DETERMINING PROGNOSIS

Estimating prognosis in systemic sclerosis is particularly difficult for a number of reasons. First, it is a disorder of remarkable clinical heterogeneity. Patients may be classified as having diffuse (widespread) or limited (restricted) cutaneous involvement. Additional variants not yet described are likely to exist. Although most rheumatologists are well aware of the differences between disease subsets, many earlier treatment studies[1-4] included patients with different variants and different stages of the disease without stratification. It was thus very difficult or impossible to interpret results. The natural history of these variants is quite different, having important implications for prognosis, patient and family education, anticipation of future complications, and monitoring and treatment of patients.

Second, there is a lack of standardized terminology. We must define terms and organ system involvement. Lung involvement may be defined by some as pleural thickening on chest roentgenogram, reduced vital capacity, reduced diffusing capacity for carbon monoxide (DLCO), or bibasilar rales on physical examination. Others may require pulmonary symptoms together with pulmonary fibrosis on roentgenogram. These issues need to be resolved. In the difficult areas where symptoms are evaluated, such as the frequency and severity of Raynaud's phenomenon, more objective methods of measurement are needed. The psychological status of the patient and the placebo effect in therapy trials must be considered. Most importantly, we need to be precise in defining all outcome and prognosis terms.

A third problem is that there are no standardized, widely accepted methods to measure disease stage or activity. Clear definitions of disease stage and activity will allow investigators to study patients most likely to have the abnormality that is being studied. Prognostic information based on this type of system would be more meaningful. Basic research to identify pathogenetic mechanisms of scleroderma would be assisted by clarification of which patients are in early active stages of disease.

Fourth, studies in systemic sclerosis must be of adequate size and duration to answer the important outcome questions. Cross-sectional reports are inferior to those of longitudinal design, but the latter require many years of observation. Multicenter efforts are often necessary to locate adequate numbers of patients with the desired variants and stages of disease.

NATURAL HISTORY OF DISEASE

The natural history of systemic sclerosis is best understood by reviewing the two major variants and their early and late stages.

Early diffuse disease

Patients with early diffuse scleroderma are sometimes difficult to diagnose. They often have fatigue, arthralgias, carpal tunnel syndrome, puffy fingers, swollen legs, and a positive serum antinuclear antibody test prior to developing Raynaud's phenomenon or characteristic skin changes (Table 1). Helpful clues at this point, when the diagnosis is not clear, include capillary dropout on nail-fold microscopy[5], the presence of palpable tendon friction rubs and serum anti-Scl 70 antibody[6]. After this prodromal phase, there is most often a rapid progression of diffuse cutaneous scleroderma. Skin thickening begins in the fingers, but within 6–12 months progresses proximally up the arms and legs to include the trunk. Tendon rubs (due to fibrous tenosynovitis), which may be painful or asymptomatic, are most commonly found in the palms, wrists, and ankles. Arthralgias, alone or with true synovitis in a rheumatoid distribution, are common in early diffuse scleroderma. The combination of accelerated skin thickening and tendon and joint involvement often leads to severe contractures with marked decrease in function. Raynaud's phenomenon may result in finger-tip ulcerations, while ulcers found over the dorsal surface of the proximal interphalangeal joints are more likely due to a combination of skin stretching, trauma, and circulatory insufficiency. Muscle involvement, either inflammatory or noninflammatory, can cause proximal muscle atrophy and weakness.

Visceral changes are frequent in early diffuse scleroderma. Gastrointestinal involvement, particularly esophageal dysmotility, is present in half of the patients at the time of initial evaluation. More severe small-intestinal hypomotility may develop subsequently but is uncommon. Figure 1 graphically displays the onset of visceral disease in

Table 1 Clinical characteristics of patients with diffuse cutaneous scleroderma with early disease (less than 3 years of symptoms) and late disease (more than 6 years of symptoms)

	Early (less than 3 years) (n=425)		Late (more than 6 years) (n=319)
Symptoms duration (years)	2.2	$p < 0.001$	12
Fatigue	83%	$p < 0.01$	71%
Arthralgias	52%		49%
Puffy fingers	58%	$p < 0.0001$	35%
Tendon rubs	67%	$p < 0.0001$	27%
Carpal tunnel	27%	$p < 0.01$	10%
Contractures	88%		93%
Muscle weakness	39%	$p < 0.01$	50%
Raynaud's phenomenon	89%		94%
Digital ulcers	22%	$p < 0.0001$	47%
Total skin score	40	$p < 0.001$	28
Calcinosis	10%	$p < 0.0001$	53%
Telangiectasia	51%	$p < 0.0001$	82%

relation to the time after disease onset. Pulmonary interstitial changes are also frequent in early diffuse disease (approximately 50%). In some patients, a mononuclear cell inflammatory component has been identified by bronchoalveolar lavage[7,8] and these individuals may respond to corticosteroids or combined steroid and immunosuppressive regimens. Subclinical evidence of heart disease (from electrocardiogram, echocardiogram, or thallium perfusion scan) is more common than symptomatic heart disease[9]; the latter occurs in only 10% of patients. The most dramatic complication is renal involvement with malignant hypertension (renal crisis). Eighty percent of patients with renal crisis develop it during the first 4 years of the illness[10]. This problem was almost uniformly fatal until the advent of new, potent antihypertensive agents, especially angiotensin-converting enzyme inhibitors. Today with these drugs and better physician and dialysis management, survival is the rule rather than the exception.

Late diffuse disease

We consider the change from early to late diffuse disease to occur when skin thickening has passed its peak extent and severity and has begun to lessen. Cutaneous improvement almost always begins in areas that have been affected last, i.e., usually the anterior chest, abdomen, and upper arms. Once this regression is obvious[11], puffiness, arthralgias, and tendon rubs also decrease, allowing a patient to be more functional, depending on the severity of the joint contractures that occurred early in disease (Table 1). Systemic features such as fatigue often subside, and renewed energy and sense of well-being return. Although the

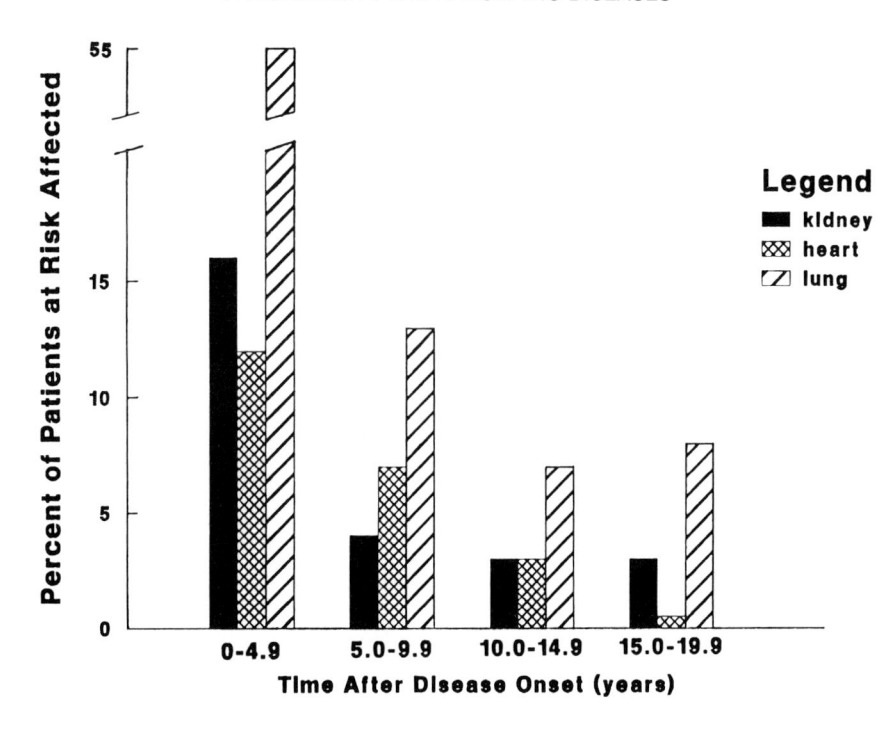

Figure 1 The timing of internal organ involvement in systemic sclerosis with diffuse cutaneous scleroderma

fibrotic process in internal organs may continue to progress slowly, it is distinctly unusual for there to be rapid worsening of skin thickening in the late stage of diffuse scleroderma. After many years, telangiectasias and calcinosis may appear similar to patients with limited scleroderma. Considering the simultaneous regression of cutaneous changes, late-stage diffuse disease can be misdiagnosed as limited disease. The presence of severe hand contractures suggests that such patients initially had diffuse cutaneous scleroderma. In this late stage, complications result from fibrotic and atrophic changes rather than inflammatory events. The gastrointestinal problems include a flaccid, atonic esophagus, esophageal stricture, or small intestinal hypomotility that may result in malabsorption. Symptoms can usually be managed with various medications for reflux, obstipation, pseudoobstruction, hypomotility, or bacterial overgrowth. In the unusual circumstance of complete gastrointestinal failure, permanent hyperalimentation may be required.

Anti-Scl 70 antibody is associated with an increased frequency and severity of pulmonary fibrosis[6,14]. In most cases, pulmonary fibrosis is benign, producing few symptoms except mild dyspnea on exertion. Pulmonary function usually does not deteriorate rapidly, although smokers may experience more accelerated functional loss[12,13]. In a few cases, rapid worsening of pulmonary function occurs, resulting in respiratory failure. Secondary pulmonary hypertension with cor pulmonale supervenes and death due to bacterial pneumonia or hypoxia or arrhythmia is the rule.

Heart disease is the least predictable of the visceral involvements during late-stage diffuse scleroderma. Conduction disturbances, electrocardiographic abnormalities, echocardiographic evidence of pericardial effusion, thallium perfusion scan defects, or decreased left ventricular function can be seen in patients with early or late disease[15-17]. The abnormalities found during early disease may persist asymptomatically without progression or evolve to serious left ventricular dysfunction, life-threatening arrhythmia, or rarely pericardial tamponade. Both ventricular ectopy and supraventricular tachycardia are strongly associated with increased mortality[18].

As noted above, the small minority of instances of renal crises occur in late disease. Some investigators believe that mild hypertension, proteinuria, or azotemia developing during the course of scleroderma represent evidence of "scleroderma kidney"[16,19,20]. Our experience suggests that these findings are often nonspecific and due to nonsclerodermatous or nonrenal causes.

Early limited disease

Detailed information on early limited scleroderma is relatively unavailable because these patients often do not seek medical attention. Patients with limited scleroderma most often have Raynaud's phenomenon for years (often one or more decades) before other clinical manifestations of systemic sclerosis appear. In early disease, arbitrarily defined here as the first 5 years after onset of Raynaud's, patients may next experience mild digital puffiness, occasional digital tip ulcers, or heartburn (Table 2). Excessive fatigue and severe arthralgias are unusual, and true synovitis and tendon friction rubs are rare. Calcinosis and telangiectasias, which are considered classic markers of disease (often termed CREST syndrome), can take years to develop and thus are less common in this early stage. The presence of skin thickening restricted to distal extremities (fingers, hands, distal forearms) for several years and the presence of serum anticentromere antibody are strong clues to classification as limited cutaneous scleroderma. Gastrointestinal and pulmonary interstitial findings are frequent, and indistinguishable from these same manifestations in diffuse disease, but myocardial and renal scleroderma are rare.

Late limited disease

In late-stage limited scleroderma, cutaneous changes remain stable. The most remarkable finding is the presence of numerous matlike

Table 2 Clinical characteristics of patients with limited cutaneous scleroderma with early disease (less than 5 years of symptoms) and late disease (more than 10 years of symptoms)

	Early (less than 5 years) (n=175)		Late (more than 10 years) (n=417)
Symptoms duration (years)	3.7	$p < 0.001$	22.0
Fatigue	69%		74%
Arthralgias	32%		40%
Puffy fingers	69%		63%
Tendon rubs	5%		8%
Carpal tunnel	19%		16%
Contractures	47%	$p < 0.01$	60%
Muscle weakness	23%	$p < 0.0001$	44%
Raynaud's phenomenon	91%	$p < 0.01$	98%
Digital ulcers	24%	$p < 0.0001$	43%
Total skin score	6		9
Calcinosis	28%	$p < 0.001$	59%
Telangiectasias	75%	$p < 0.001$	93%

telangiectasias (93%), especially on the fingers, lips, and face, and the appearance of subcutaneous calcinosis affecting fingers, forearms (elbows), and knees (55%). Digital tip ischemia may lead to ulcerations or gangrene with secondary bacterial infection. The occurrence of inflammatory ulcerative calcinosis, digital ischemic ulcers, or secondary bacterial infection in these sites may lead to significant disability.

In this late stage, esophageal reflux and stricture are frequently severe and small-bowel malabsorption with recurrent episodes of pseudoobstruction may progress and become life-threatening. Pulmonary interstitial fibrosis may be present and may be progressive, but this complication is less frequent in patients with the anticentromere antibody[21]. As noted above, clinically meaningful myocardial and/or renal involvement are rare in this variant.

The most serious problem in late-stage limited scleroderma is the development of pulmonary arterial hypertension, which is uniformly fatal. This complication occurs many years after the onset of Raynaud's phenomenon, most often in patients who have had few other scleroderma problems[22]. Rapid progression of dyspnea (over months) is the most frequent initial symptom. Once hypoxemia and/or secondary right heart failure develop, the mean survival is less than 2 years. No known pharmacologic intervention has proven successful. At autopsy there is noninflammatory subintimal proliferation of small- and medium-sized pulmonary arteries without significant interstitial fibrosis[23].

Another problem that can occur in late limited disease is cutaneous vasculitis with mononeuritis multiplex. This complication is believed to be most strongly linked to associated Sjögren's syndrome[24]. Pulmonary fibrosis, pulmonary hypertension, and severe gastrointestinal disease account for most of the disease-related deaths in limited scleroderma.

HISTORICAL REVIEW OF PROGNOSIS

There have been numerous studies of survival in different groups of systemic sclerosis patients; these have been reviewed in detail recently and are summarized in Table 3[25]. Using the above definitions of diffuse and limited disease we have found marked differences in survival between these groups[6,26]. From onset of first symptom, early diffuse scleroderma patients who have had symptoms less than 3 years have a 70% survival at 5 years compared to 90% in the early limited groups who have had symptoms less than 5 years (Figure 2) ($p < 0.001$). Similar results are observed if the starting point is first physician diagnosis of systemic sclerosis or first evaluation at our center. This difference remains constant after the third year, suggesting that the excess mortality in diffuse scleroderma is within the first 3 years of disease.

Scleroderma-specific serum autoantibodies predict survival because of their association with the above-described clinical variants[6,27,28]. Anticentromere antibody, which is found in limited cutaneous scleroderma, is thus associated with a better prognosis than anti-Scl 70 antibody, which is associated with diffuse cutaneous disease[6]. Attempts have been made to describe a variant that is "intermediate" with regard to skin thickening[29-31] but there are no distinctive clinical, laboratory, or autoantibody findings in that group of patients. In our opinion the two-way classification system should be used until other clear-cut subsets are described.

In two recent studies the 10-year survivals from first diagnosis of diffuse scleroderma in Italy and Australia were 26% and 22%, respectively[29,30]. Our Pittsburgh diffuse scleroderma patients with truncal involvement seen during a similar period (1972-1983) had a 10-year cumulative survival rate from first diagnosis of 55%. The reasons for this difference are unknown but may reflect, in part, improved prognosis in US patients with renal crisis, or possibly the use of D-penicillamine therapy[59].

Male sex, nonwhite race, older age, and early visceral involvement have been found to be associated with decreased survival[25] (Table 3). Our more recent experience has been similar, although we have not found a significantly reduced survival in black patients. In nearly all studies, visceral involvement is associated with a higher mortality. This is particularly true for restrictive lung disease[13], severely depressed pulmonary diffusing capacity[22,23], congestive heart failure[33], pericardial involvement[34], and renal disease[35].

Survival is not the only end-point for evaluation of outcome. Morbidity and disability from visceral disease as well as from cutaneous, joint, and tendon involvement are equally important. Functional

Table 3 Selected survival studies in systemic sclerosis

Reference	Number of patients	Cumulative survival (life-table method) 5 year	10 year	Demographic	Clinical	Laboratory
Farmer (1960)	236		51[b]	Age > 40	Heart Kidney Trunk skin	ESR > 50 mm/h (Westergren) Anemia
Tuffanelli (1962) Bennett (1971)	727 67	70+ 73	40	Age > 40	Lung Trunk skin	BUN > 40 mg/dl ECG abnormal
Medsger (1971)	309	60	35	Age > 45 Males Blacks	Lung Heart Kidney	
Medsger (1973)	358	44		Age > 50 Blacks Heavy alcohol and cigarette use		
Barnett (1978)	113	70	55	Age > 40 Males	Lung Heart Kidney Trunk skin	ESR > 32 mm/h Anemia Proteinuria
Eason (1981)	47	60	42	Lung Heart Kidney Non-CRST		
Wynn (1985)	64	69	51	Age > 50	S3 gallop corticosteroid use	
Giordano (1986)	90	72	32		Trunk skin	

[b]Percentage of patients alive (years of follow-up).
[a]Modified from Masi, 1988[25] and reprinted by permission of the publisher.

PROGNOSIS IN SYSTEMIC SCLEROSIS (SCLERODERMA)

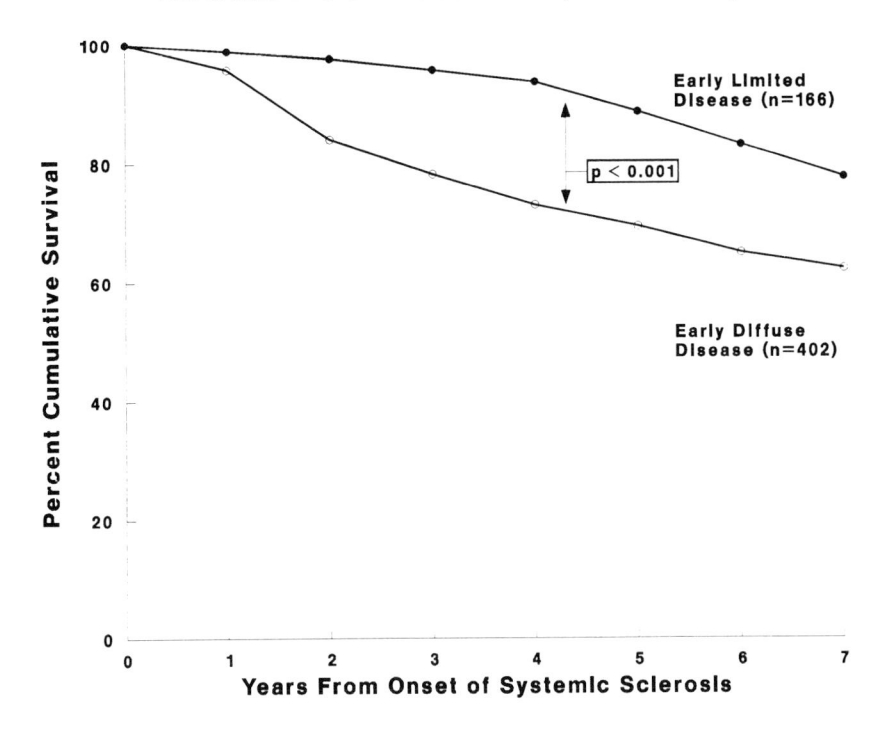

Figure 2 The percent cumulative survival in patients with early limited cutaneous and diffuse cutaneous scleroderma

assessments have documented marked deficits in the ability to perform activities of daily living[36,37]. Using the Health Assessment Questionnaire (HAQ), we found a mean disability index of 1.02 for patients with diffuse scleroderma and 0.67 for those with limited scleroderma[38]. Comparable figures are 0.82 for rheumatoid arthritis patients and 0.67 for systemic lupus erythematosus[86,87]. The scleroderma HAQ disability index scores correlated well with the extent of skin thickening, loss of fist closure, proximal muscle weakness, and tendon friction rubs but not with the presence of digital ulcers. The latter finding points out the need for additional scleroderma-specific questions to assess the impact of such manifestations as Raynaud's phenomenon, cardiopulmonary, gastrointestinal, and renal disease on the quality of life. The HAQ pain scale may not be as accurate in scleroderma as in rheumatoid arthritis since scleroderma-related functional limitations, especially those due to visceral disease, are not necessarily painful. We therefore used an overall "disease difficulty" visual analog scale. In the same patients, this measure of disease activity had a higher mean value (0.96) than did the pain index (0.85, $p < 0.05$). Additional visual analog scales relating to these organ systems may prove useful in quantifying important subjective symptoms of visceral disease.

Hand involvement from Raynaud's phenomenon, skin thickening, arthritis, or tenosynovitis is common and often severe. Several investigators have recommended special procedures for evaluating the scleroderma hand, including a scleroderma goniometer[39], measurement of finger-tip to palm distance in full flexion[40], and a carefully developed but complicated hand function score[41]. Physical therapy using paraffin[42] and an aggressive exercise program[41] were considered helpful. However, dynamic splinting did not improve digital flexibility[43].

Patient and iatrogenic factors may play an important role in scleroderma outcomes, both fatal and nonfatal. Cigarette smoking is recognized to be a potent adverse influence on Raynaud's phenomenon and also a deleterious factor in the progression of pulmonary interstitial fibrosis[13]. Nonsteroidal anti-inflammatory drugs (NSAIDs), intended to ameliorate joint and tendon discomfort, may exacerbate reflux esophagitis and cause gastritis. Calcium channel blocking agents, commonly used in the management of Raynaud's phenomenon, also reduce lower esophageal sphincter pressure and thus may aggravate reflux esophagitis. Both of these types of drugs can cause peripheral edema, which may already be present due to scleroderma. Corticosteroids are sometimes used to treat the inflammatory phase of early diffuse scleroderma, but it is in these patients that steroids may be implicated in the precipitation of renal crisis, particularly of the normotensive variety[44]. Agents intended to induce remissions of early diffuse disease may themselves have serious adverse effects. D-Penicillamine, one of the more popular drugs, cannot be tolerated by close to 25% of scleroderma patients[45]. Fortunately, most of the adverse effects are not life-threatening and are reversible when the drug is discontinued. However, aplastic anemia, pemphigus, nephrotic syndrome, and myasthenia gravis may be debilitating or even fatal. Immunosuppressive drugs, particularly alkylating agents, have been implicated in the later developments of malignancy[46,47], as is the case in other rheumatic diseases[48].

Similar to other chronic diseases, the direct costs (physician visits, medications, laboratory tests, physical and occupational therapy, hospitalizations) and indirect costs (work time lost, help from others) involved for the scleroderma patient are high. No formal studies have been published, but we believe that costs for diffuse disease are similar to or greater than those for rheumatoid arthritis.

SUMMARY OF OUTCOME RISK FACTORS

Outcome in patients with systemic sclerosis is extremely variable. As described above, male sex, black race, and older age are host factors associated with reduced survival[25]. The primary disease feature predicting a poor prognosis is classification as diffuse scleroderma. This distinction is best made using the extent and pace of skin thickening, as

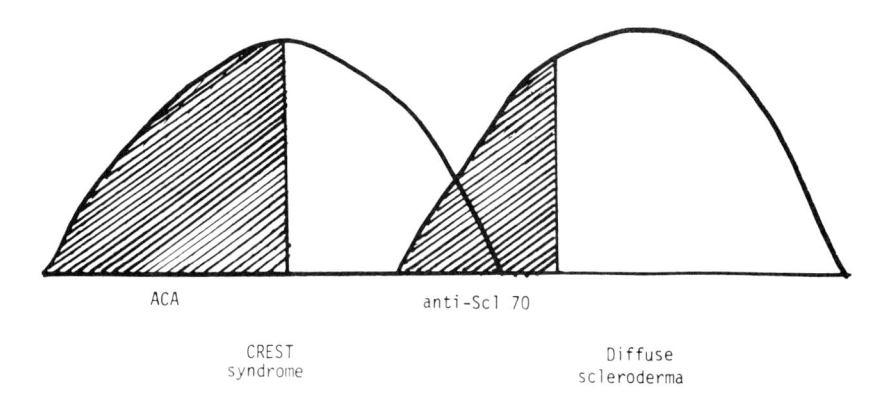

Figure 3 The frequency of scleroderma-specific antibodies in subsets of scleroderma

described earlier, but cutaneous changes in the absence of Raynaud's phenomenon[49], palpable tendon friction rubs[50], and capillary loop dropout[5] are also frequent precursors of diffuse scleroderma.

The scleroderma-specific autoantibodies have been very useful in predicting the variant of disease, but within variants these serum antibodies do not correlate with survival. Certain clinical features are autoantibody linked, however, including anticentromere with telangiectasias and calcinosis in limited disease, and anti-Scl 70 with pulmonary interstitial fibrosis and peripheral vascular disease among diffuse-disease patients[6]. Figure 3 graphically depicts the frequency of these antibodies in these scleroderma variants.

Different HLA markers have been found to correlate with systemic sclerosis in reports from several centers. Whether these discrepancies represent ethnic variations or result from the study of small populations is not clear. In our large series we found a small but significant increase of HLA-DR5 in patients with anti-Scl 70 antibodies and of HLA-DR1 in patients with anticentromere antibodies[6].

Certain manifestations appear with equal frequency in both disease variants and are therefore not prognostically useful, including Raynaud's phenomenon, gastrointestinal disease, and pulmonary interstitial fibrosis. Several studies have identified a markedly decreased diffusing capacity for carbon monoxide (DLCO), smoking, and severe Raynaud's phenomenon as risk factors for reduced survival in patients with severe lung disease[13,32].

Heart and kidney involvement are seen far more commonly in patients with diffuse scleroderma than in those with limited scleroderma. The electrocardiogram and newer methods of evaluation of cardiac function including Holter monitor, echocardiogram, thallium, and MUGA scans may identify abnormalities including arrythmias[51], pericardial effusions[20], and ventricular ectopy[18] that are poor prognostic signs. The outcome implications of the common conduction defects[15,16], asymptomatic pericardial effusions, and thallium defects are not known.

Until recently, scleroderma renal crisis almost always resulted in death. Patients with early diffuse scleroderma and rapidly increasing skin thickening are those at greatest risk to develop this complication[10]. Although elevated plasma renin levels, malignant hypertension, and proteinuria are a part of renal crisis, they do not antedate it by weeks or months and thus are not useful in predicting its future development. Microangiopathic hemolytic anemia, seizures, and cardiac dysfunction may herald the onset of renal disease[10,20].

Modification of prognosis

Established systemic sclerosis is remarkably recalcitrant to intervention with medication or other forms of therapy. However, several recent advances have improved prognosis and reduced morbidity in certain disease subsets. The new family of calcium channel blockers can symptomatically and plethysmographically reduce the frequency and severity of Raynaud's phenomenon and enhance healing of digital ulcers[52]. Other drugs including serotonin antagonists[53], and prostaglandin derivatives[54] hold some promise. Digital sympathectomy and microsurgical revascularization of hand arteries are newer surgical methods to improve blood flow[55].

Potassium *para*-aminobenzoate (Potaba)[56], colchicine[2], dimethyl sulfoxide (DMSO)[57], azathioprine[58], and chlorambucil[1,4] have been studied for their ability to alter the natural course of cutaneous and visceral disease, but there is little evidence that they are effective. D-Penicillamine has had broad support because of the belief that, in uncontrolled studies, it is associated with improvement in skin thickening and survival and possibly reduced frequency of new renal disease[59,59a].

The arthropathy and myopathy of scleroderma are frequently resistant to therapy. An aggressive hand and joint exercise program is recommended for most early diffuse scleroderma patients, who are at greatest risk for developing contractures. Wrist and dynamic finger splints have been used but not found to be helpful[43].

Symptomatic esophageal reflux has been improved by the use of histamine receptor blockers. Whether these agents will serve as effective prophylaxis for esophageal stricture is unknown. The prokinetic drugs metoclopramide and cisapride may be useful in enhancing esophageal motility[60], but are not likely to overcome circumstances in which there is severe atrophy and fibrous replacement of esophageal smooth muscle. The bacterial overgrowth that results from small intestinal hypomotility contributes to disabling diarrhea in patients with small-bowel malabsorption. The diarrhea can often be transiently improved but not eliminated by the use of rotating courses of broad-spectrum antibiotics[61].

Pulmonary fibrosis with restrictive lung disease is more severe in scleroderma patients who smoke[13]. Several investigators have used the results of bronchoalveolar lavage to identify a subgroup of pulmonary fibrosis patients with a lymphocytic inflammatory process that might be amenable to treatment[7,8,62]. There are anecdotal reports of improvement with corticosteroids and/or immunosuppressive drugs in such patients[62]. Although D-penicillamine has been shown to improve pulmonary diffusing capacity and perhaps stabilize lung disease[63,64], it does not appear to reverse the fibrotic process. The treatment of isolated pulmonary hypertension, a late consequence of limited cutaneous disease, has been uniformly unsuccessful; numerous vasodilators have failed to alter this inevitably fatal complication. Only a rare patient survives more than 5 years from its first detection[22]. Earlier identification of these patients using echo-doppler or other newer noninvasive techniques may allow the initiation of therapy before the changes are irreversible. However, the dominant histopathologic feature is that of subintimal proliferation of small arteries with luminal occlusion[65] for which no effective therapy is known.

Cardiac abnormalities noted on electrocardiogram, echocardiogram, thallium perfusion scans, and at autopsy are much more frequent than is symptomatic cardiac disease[9]. Although several agents have been shown to improve myocardial perfusion measured by thallium scans[66,67], the significance of this finding for the natural history of cardiac disease is unknown.

The prognosis of renal crisis has been dramatically improved during the past decade by the introduction of angiotensin-converting enzyme (ACE) inhibitors (Figure 4). Survival is now the rule rather than the exception[68]. Patients may maintain or improve when these agents are administered early in the course of renal crisis. In addition, more than half of the patients who have been on dialysis for 3 or more months and continue to take an ACE inhibitor are able to discontinue dialysis after 5–15 months[69].

FUTURE OUTCOMES

One of the most difficult aspects of determining prognosis in systemic sclerosis is the lack of standardized measurements of disease status and activity. Survival is a clear-cut end-point, and the HAQ may be used to monitor functional aspects of the disease, although it was designed for a population with arthritis rather than one in which multisystem involvement is the rule. Scleroderma is such a varied disease that additional and preferably standardized measures of organ involvement are needed.

The severity and extent of skin thickening has received the most attention. Evaluation of skin tethering and palm prints[70] are cumbersome and have not generally been used. Newer objective methods using

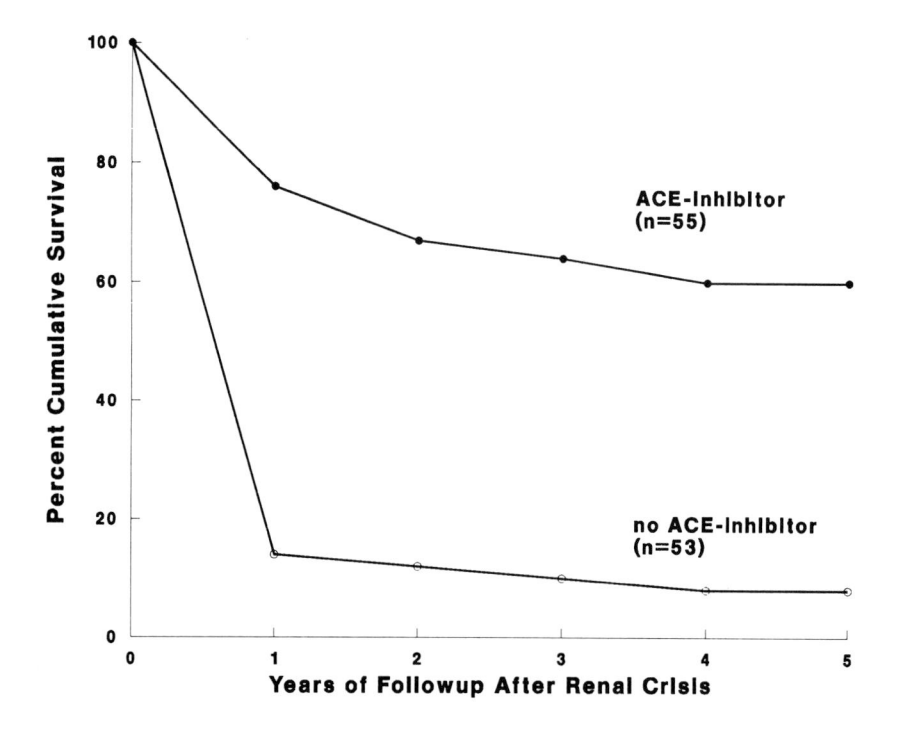

Figure 4 The cumulative survival of patients with scleroderma renal crisis who were treated or not treated with angiotensin-converting enzyme inhibitor

ultrasound[39,71,72] have been reported but are expensive, not generally available, and have not yet been correlated with physical examination. The most popular methods of monitoring skin thickening are those that are performed by physical examination since they are simple, rapid and inexpensive. A skin scoring system has been developed that has been validated with excellent interrater reliability (data not published). A modified scoring system and a method using the percentage of body surface area affected[59a] have also been proposed. A consensus statement will be necessary to gain uniformity.

Muscle strength and hand function can be assessed by quantitative methods of evaluation, but even here standardization would be helpful. Pulmonary function tests are reliable, reproducible, and the best available method to assess lung function; the percent predicted FVC (restrictive disease) and the percent predicted DLCO (vascular disease) are the two most useful measurements. The cine-esophagram is sensitive in identifying dysmotility, but is difficult to quantitate. Newer radionuclide scintigraphic methods are able to quantitate esophageal emptying over time, and have been favorably compared with the cine study and manometry[75]. Renal function can be monitored easily with blood pressure, urinalysis, and serum creatinine and creatinine clearance, although a more sensitive, inexpensive, and reproducible method to estimate renal blood flow would be welcome.

Cardiac abnormalities as seen on electrocardiogram, Holter monitor, echocardiogram, and thallium scan are difficult to interpret because their significance is unknown. The MUGA scan is helpful for evaluating overall cardiac function, and the left ventricular ejection fraction can be quantified. Additional noninvasive ways of monitoring pulmonary arterial pressure and right ventricular function using echo-doppler or even magnetic resonance imaging would be useful.

Another major issue to be addressed is the difficulty in determining the stage or activity of the disease. In contrast to rheumatoid arthritis and lupus, scleroderma is a more fibrotic and less inflammatory disorder. Standard markers of disease activity such as the erythrocyte sedimentation rate are not useful. Our attempt to classify patients into groups as above (early diffuse, late diffuse, etc.) is a crude beginning. Other investigators have tried to quantitate disease severity[4,76,77], but each approach is different and none separates severity from activity. Further work is needed to develop disease scales that are reliable and helpful in determining prognosis.

In the laboratory, attempts to identify evidence of the primary pathophysiologic processes in scleroderma are being made. For example, damage of vascular endothelium may be signalled by elevated plasma levels of factor VIII-von Willebrand factor antigen[76,78,79]. Such elevations do not appear to correlate with acute-phase reactants, but do with disease severity. Serum endothelial cell cytotoxicity activity has been found in some series[80] but not all[81,82]; it may not correlate either with "severe" or "active" disease. Activation of lymphocytes can be measured using serum-soluble interleukin-2 receptor levels, which are increased in early active diffuse disease and decline toward but not to normal later in disease[83,84]. Finally, production of procollagen by fibroblasts can be assayed using a serum radioimmunoassay for procollagen III peptide breakdown products[85]. These fragments were found in increased amounts in diffuse scleroderma patients and in those with evidence of recent disease progression, but not in the circumstance of remission. It is possible that these or related laboratory tests will ultimately describe disease activity and influence therapeutic intervention decisions.

Crucial to any attempt at early intervention in systemic sclerosis is early detection, since therapy must be designed to affect the disease process in its formative stages and prior to the development of irreversible fibrosis. Nevertheless, the outlook for a longer and better quality of life for patients with this disease has importantly improved during the last two decades.

References

1. Steigerwald, J. C. (1979). Progressive systemic sclerosis: management. III. Immunosuppressive agents. *Clin. Rheum. Dis.*, **5**, 289-294

2. Alarcon-Segovia, D. (1979). Progressive systemic sclerosis: management IV. colchicine. *Clin. Rheum. Dis.*, **5**, 294-302
3. Jayson, M. I. V., Lovell, C., Black, C. M. *et al.* (1977). Penicillamine therapy in systemic sclerosis. *Proc. R. Soc. Med.*, **70** (suppl. 3), 82-88
4. Furst, D. E., Clements, P. H., Hillis, S. *et al.* (1989). Immunosuppression with chlorambucil vs placebo for scleroderma. Results of a 3-year parallel, randomized, double-blind study. *Arthritis Rheum.*, **32**, 584-593
5. Maricq, H. R., Spencer-Green, G. and LeRoy, E. C. (1976). Skin capillary abnormalities as indicators of organ involvement in scleroderma (systemic sclerosis). *Am. J. Med.*, **61**, 862-870
6. Steen, V. D., Powell, D. L. and Medsger, T. A., Jr. (1988). Clinical correlations and prognosis based on serum autoantibodies in patients with systemic sclerosis. *Arthritis Rheum.*, **31**, 196-203
7. Owens, G. R., Paradis, I. L., Gryzan, S. *et al.* (1986). The role of inflammation in the lung disease of systemic sclerosis: comparison with idiopathic pulmonary fibrosis. *J. Lab. Clin. Med.*, **107**, 253-262
8. Silver, R. M., Metcalf, J. F., Stanley, J. H. *et al.* (1984). Interstitial lung disease in scleroderma. Analysis by bronchoalveolar lavage. *Arthritis Rheum.*, **27**, 1254-1261
9. Follansbee, W. (1986). The cardiovascular manifestations of systemic sclerosis (scleroderma). *Curr. Probl. Cardiol.*, **11**, 242-298
10. Steen, V. D., Medsger, T. A., Jr., Osial, T. A., Jr. *et al.* (1984). Factors predicting development of renal involvement in progressive systemic sclerosis. *Am. J. Med.*, **76**, 779-786
11. Black, C., Dieppe, P. K., Huskisson, T. *et al.* (1986). Regressive systemic sclerosis. *Ann. Rheum. Dis.*, **45**, 384-388
12. Schneider, P. D., Wise, R. A., Hochberg, M. C. *et al.* (1982). Serial pulmonary function in systemic sclerosis. *Am. J. Med.*, **73**, 385-394
13. Steen, V. D., Owens, G. R., Fino, G. J. *et al.* (1985). Pulmonary involvement in systemic sclerosis (scleroderma). *Arthritis Rheum.*, **28**, 759-767
14. Bernstein, R. M., Steigerwald, J. C. and Tan, E. M. Association of antinuclear and antinucleolar antibodies in progressive systemic sclerosis. *Clin. Exp. Immunol.*, **48**, 43-51
15. Follansbee, W. P., Curtiss, E. I., Rahko, P. S. *et al.* (1985). The electrocardiogram in systemic sclerosis (scleroderma): A study of 102 consecutive cases with functional correlations and a review of the literature. *Am. J. Med.*, **79**, 183-192
16. Smith, J. W., Clements, P. J., Levisman, J. *et al.* (1979). Echocardiographic features of progressive systemic sclerosis (PSS). Correlation with hemodynamic and postmortem studies. *Am. J. Med.*, **66**, 28-33
17. Follansbee, W. P., Curtiss, E. I., Medsger, T. A., Jr. *et al.* (1984). Physiologic abnormalities of cardiac function in progressive systemic sclerosis with diffuse scleroderma. *N. Engl. J. Med.*, **310**, 142-148
18. Kostis, J. B., Seibold, J. R., Turkevich, D. *et al.* (1988). The prognostic importance of cardiac arrhythmias in systemic sclerosis. *Am. J. Med.*, **84**, 1007-1015
19. Cannon, P. J., Hassar, M., Case, D. B. *et al.* (1974). The relationship of hypertension and renal failure in scleroderma (progressive systemic sclerosis) to structural and functional abnormalities of the renal cortical circulation. *Medicine*, **53**, 1-46
20. LeRoy, E. C. and Fleischmann, R. M. (1978). The management of renal scleroderma. Experience with dialysis, nephrectomy and transplantation. *Am. J. Med.*, **64**, 974-978
21. Steen, V. D., Medsger, T. A., Jr., Rodnan, G. P. *et al.* (1984). Clinical associations of anticentromere antibody (ACA) in patients with progressive systemic sclerosis. *Arthritis Rheum.*, **27**, 125-131
22. Stupi, A. M., Steen, V. D., Medsger, T. A., Jr. *et al.* (1986). Pulmonary hypertension (PHT) in the CREST syndrome variant of progressive systemic sclerosis (PSS). *Arthritis Rheum.*, **29**, 515-524
23. Salerni, R., Rodnan, G. P., Leon, D. F. *et al.* (1977). Pulmonary hypertension in the CREST syndrome variant of progressive systemic sclerosis (scleroderma). *Ann. Intern. Med.*, **86**, 394-399
24. Oddis, C. V., Eisenbeis, C. H., Jr., Reidbord, H. E. *et al.* (1987). Vasculitis in systemic

sclerosis: a subset of patients with the CREST variant Sjogren's syndrome and neurologic complications. *J. Rheumatol.*, **14**, 942-948
25. Masi, A. T. (1988). Clinical-epidemiological perspective of systemic sclerosis (scleroderma). In Jayson, M. I. V. and Black, C. M. (eds.) *Systemic Sclerosis: Scleroderma*, pp. 7-31. (Chichester: Wiley)
26. Medsger, T. A., Jr. (1989). Systemic sclerosis (scleroderma), localized scleroderma, eosinophilic fasciitis, and calcinosis. In McCarty, D. J. (ed.) *Arthritis and Allied Conditions*, pp. 1118-1163. (Philadelphia: Lea & Febiger)
27. McCarty, G. A., Rice, J. R., Bembe, M. L. et al. (1983). Anticentromere antibody: clinical correlations and association with favorable prognosis in patients with scleroderma variants. *Arthritis Rheum.*, **26**, 1-7
28. Tramposch, H. D., Smith, C. D., Senecal, J-L. et al. (1984). A long-term longitudinal study of anticentromere antibodies. *Arthritis Rheum.*, **27**, 121-124
29. Giordano, M., Valentini, G., Migliaresi, S. et al. (1986). Different antibody patterns and different prognoses in patients with scleroderma with various extent of skin sclerosis. *J. Rheumatol.*, **13**, 911-916
30. Barnett, A. J., Miller, M. H. and Littlejohn, G. O. (1988). A survival study of patients with scleroderma diagnosed over 30 years (1953-1983): the value of a simple cutaneous classification in the early stages of the disease. *J. Rheumatol.*, **15**, 276-283
31. Masi, A. T. (1988). Classification of systemic sclerosis (scleroderma): relationship of cutaneous subgroups in early disease to outcome and serologic reactivity. *J. Rheumatol.*, **15**, 894-898
32. Peters-Golden, M., Wise, R. A., Hochberg, M. C. et al. (1984). Carbon monoxide diffusing capacity as predictor of outcome in systemic sclerosis. *Am. J. Med.*, **77**, 1027-1034
33. Wynn, J., Fineberg, N., Metzer, L. et al. (1985). Prediction of survival in progressive systemic sclerosis by multivariate analysis of clinical features. *Am. Heart J.*, **110**, 123-127
34. McWhorter, J. E. and LeRoy, E. C. (1974). Pericardial disease in scleroderma (systemic sclerosis). *Am. J. Med.*, **57**, 566-575
35. Traub, Y. M., Shapiro, A. P. and Rodnan, G. P. et al. (1984). Hypertension and renal failure (scleroderma renal crisis) in progressive systemic sclerosis. Report of a 25-year experience with 68 cases. *Medicine*, **62**, 335-352
36. Coppock, J. S. and Bacon, P. A. (1988). Outcome, assessment and activity. In Jayson, M. I. V. and Black, C. M. (eds.) *Systemic Sclerosis: Scleroderma*, pp. 279-288. (Chichester: Wiley)
37. Coppock, J. S., England, S. E., Harris, P. et al. (1985). Clinical measurement of the hand in scleroderma, its relationship to hand function. *Br. J. Rheumatol.*, **24**, 96
38. Poole, J. and Steen, V. D. (1986). The use of the Health Assessment Questionnaire (HAQ) to determine physical disability in systemic sclerosis. *Arthritis Rheum.*, **29**(4), S152
39. Serup, J. (1983). Measurement of contractures of the digits in systemic sclerosis. Development of digit-goniometers and definitions of normal joint mobility of the digits of elderly persons. *Dermatologica*, **167**, 250-255
40. England, S. E., Coppock, J. S. and Bacon, P. A. Objective assessment of hand movements in scleroderma: a pre-requisite to trials of physiotherapy. *Int. J. Rehabil. Res.*, **8**, 399
41. Askew, L. J., Beckett, V. L., Kai-Nan, A. et al. (1983). Objective evaluation of hand function in scleroderma patients to assess effectiveness of physical therapy. *Br. J. Rheumatol.*, **22**, 224-232
42. Coppock, J. S., England, S. E., Harris, P. et al. (1985). Clinical measurement of the hand in scleroderma, its relationship to hand function. *Br. J. Rheumatol.*, **24**, 96
43. Seeger, M. W. and Furst, D. E. (1987). Effects of splinting in the treatment of hand contractures in progressive systemic sclerosis. *Am. J. Occup. Ther.*, **41**, 118-121
44. Helfrich, D. J., Banner, B., Steen, V. D. et al. (1989). Renal failure in normotensive patients with systemic sclerosis. *Arthritis Rheum.*, **32**, 1128-1134
45. Steen, V. D., Blair, S., Medsger, T. A., Jr. (1986). The toxicity of D-penicillamine in systemic sclerosis. *Ann. Intern. Med.*, **104**, 699-705

46. Roumm, A. D. and Medsger, T. A., Jr (1985). Cancer in systemic sclerosis: an epidemiologic study. *Arthritis Rheum.*, **28**, 344-360
47. Medsger, T. A., Jr. (1985). Editorial. Systemic sclerosis and malignancy — are they related? *J. Rheumatol.*, **12**, 1041-1043
48. Baker, G. L., Kahl, L. E., Zee, B. C. et al. (1987). Malignancy following treatment of rheumatoid arthritis with cyclophosphamide: a long-term case-control followup study. *Am. J. Med.*, **83**, 1-96
49. Young, E., Steen, V. D., Medsger, T. A., Jr. (1986). Systemic sclerosis without Raynaud's phenomenon. *Arthritis Rheum.*, **29**, S43
50. Steen, V. and Medsger, T. A., Jr. (1989). Natural history of patients with limited cutaneous systemic sclerosis (lcSSc) and anti-Scl antibody. *Arthritis Rheum.*, **32**(4), S92
51. Clements, P. J., Furst, D. E., Cabeen, W. et al. (1981). The relationship of arrhythmias and conduction disturbances to other manifestations of cardiopulmonary disease in progressive systemic sclerosis (PSS). *Am. J. Med.*, **71**, 38-46
52. Finch, M. B., Dawson, J. and Johnston, G. D. (1986). The peripheral vascular effects of nifedipine in Raynaud's syndrome associated with scleroderma: a double-blind crossover study. *Clin. Rheumatol.*, **5** 493-498
53. Seibold, J. R. and Jageneau, A. H. M. (1984). Treatment of Raynaud's phenomenon with ketanserin, a selective antagonist of the serotonin 2 (5-HT2) receptor. *Arthritis Rheum*, **27**, 139-146
54. Martin, M. F. R. and Tooke, J. E. (1982). Effects of prostaglandin E1 on microvascular haemodynamics in progressive systemic sclerosis. *Br. Med. J.*, **285**, 1688-1690
55. Jones, N. F., Raynor, S. C. and Medsger, T. A., Jr. (1987). Microsurgical revascularisation of the hand in scleroderma. *Br. J. Plastic Surg.*, **40**, 264-269
56. Zarafonetis, C. J. D., Dabich, L., Negri, D. et al. (1988). Retrospective studies in scleroderma: effect of potassium para-aminobenzoate on survival. *J. Clin. Epidemiol.*, **41**(2), 193-205
57. Williams, H. J., Furst, D. E., Dahl, S. L. et al. (1983). Double-blind multicenter controlled trial comparing dimethyl sulfoxide and normal saline in treatment of hand ulcers in patients with scleroderma. *Arthritis Rheum.*, **28**, 308-314
58. Jansen, G. T. et al. (1968). Generalized scleroderma. Treatment with an immunosuppressive agent. *Arch. Dermatol.*, **97**, 690-698
59. Steen, V. D., Medsger, T. A., Jr. and Rodnan, G. P. (1982). D-Penicillamine therapy in progressive systemic sclerosis (scleroderma). *Ann. Intern. Med.*, **97**, 652-659
59a. Jimenez, S. A., Andrews, R. P. and Myers, A. R. (1985). Treatment of rapidly progressive systemic sclerosis with D-penicillamine: A prospective study. In Black, C. M. and Myers, A. R. (eds.) *Current Topics in Rheumatology, Systemic Sclerosis (Scleroderma)*, pp. 387-393. (New York: Gower Medical)
60. Ramirez-Mata, M., Ibanez, G. and Alarcon-Segovia, D. (1977). Stimulatory effect of metaclopramide on the esophagus and lower esophageal sphincter of patients with PSS. *Arthritis Rheum.*, **20**, 30-34
61. Kahn, I. J., Geffries, G. H. and Sleisinger, M. H. (1966). Malabsorption in scleroderma: correction by antibiotics. *N. Engl. J. Med.*, **274**, 1339-1344
62. Kallenberg, C. G. M., Jansen, H. M., Elema, J. D. et al. (1984). Steroid-responsive interstitial pulmonary disease in systemic sclerosis. Monitoring by bronchoalveolar lavage. *Chest*, **86**, 489-492
63. Steen, V. D., Owens, G. R., Redmond, C. et al. (1985). The effect of D-penicillamine on pulmonary findings in progressive systemic sclerosis. *Arthritis Rheum.*, **28**, 882-888
64. deClerck, L. S., Dequeker, J., Francx, L. et al. (1987). D-Penicillamine therapy and interstitial lung disease in scleroderma. A long-term followup study. *Arthritis Rheum.*, **30**, 643-650
65. Al-Sabbagh, M. R., Steen, V. D., Zee, B. C. et al. (1989). Pulmonary arterial histology and morphometry in systemic sclerosis: a case-control autopsy study. *J. Rheumatol.*, **16**, 1038-1042
66. Kahan, A. et al. (1986). Nifedipine and thallium-201 myocardial perfusion in progressive systemic sclerosis. *N. Engl. J. Med.*, **314**, 1397-1402

67. Alexander, E. L. et al. (1986). Reversible cold-induced abnormalities in myocardial perfusion and function in systemic sclerosis. Ann. Intern. Med., 105, 661-668
68. Whitman, H. H., III, Case, D. B., Laragh, J. H. et al. (1982). Variable response to oral angiotensin-converting enzyme blockade in hypertensive scleroderma patients. Arthritis Rheum., 25, 241-248
69. Steen, V. D., Shapiro, A. P., Medsger, T. A., Jr. (1990). Outcome of renal crisis in systemic sclerosis. Ann. Intern. Med., 113, 352-357
70. Bluestone, R., Graham, A., Holloway, V. et al. (1970). Treatment of systemic sclerosis with D-penicillamine: a new method of observing the effects of treatment. Ann. Rheum. Dis., 29, 153-158
71. Akesson, A., Forsberg, L., Hederstrom, E. et al. (1986). Ultrasound examination of skin thickness in patients with progressive systemic sclerosis (scleroderma). Acta Radiol. Diagnosis, 27, 91-94
72. Myers, S. L., Cohen, J. S., Sheets, P. W. et al. (1986). B-mode ultrasound evaluation of skin thickness in progressive systemic sclerosis. J. Rheumatol., 13, 577-580
73. Kahaleh, M. B., Sultany, G. L., Smith, E. A. et al. (1986). A modified scleroderma skin scoring method. Clin. Exp. Rheumatol., 4, 367-369
74. Davidson, A., Russell, C. and Littlejohn, G. O. (1985). Assessment of esophageal abnormalities in progressive systemic sclerosis using radionuclide transit. J. Rheumatol., 12, 472-477
75. Greaves, B. Y. M., Malia, R. G., Ward, A. M. et al. (1988). Elevated von Willebrand factor antigen in systemic sclerosis: relationship to visceral disease. Br. J. Rheumatol., 27, 281-285
76. Furst, D. E., Clements, P. J., Saab, M. et al. (1984). Clinical and serological comparison of 17 chronic progressive systemic sclerosis and 17 CREST syndrome patients matched for sex, age and disease duration. Ann. Rheum. Dis., 43, 794-800
77. Kahaleh, M. B., Osborn, I. and LeRoy, E. C. (1981). Increased factor VIII/von Willebrand factor antigen and von Willebrand factor activity in scleroderma and Raynaud's phenomenon. Ann. Intern. Med., 94, 482-484
78. Lee, P., Conolly, S. N., Sukenik, S. et al. (1985). The clinical significance of coagulation abnormalities in systemic sclerosis (scleroderma). J. Rheumatol., 12, 514-517
79. Kahaleh, M. B., Sherer, G. K. and LeRoy, E. C., (1979). Endothelial injury in scleroderma. J. Exp. Med., 149, 1326-1335
80. Shanahan, W. R., Jr. and Korn, J. H. (1982). Cytotoxic activity of sera from scleroderma and other connective tissue diseases. Lack of cellular and disease specificity. Arthritis Rheum., 25, 1391-1395
81. Drenk, F., Mensing, H., Serbin, A. et al. (1985). Studies on endothelial cell cytotoxic activity in sera of patients with progressive systemic sclerosis, Raynaud's syndrome, rheumatoid arthritis, and systemic lupus erythematosus. Rheumatol. Int., 5, 259-263
82. Engel, E. E., Charley, M. R., Steen, V. D. et al. (1989). Soluble interleukin 2 receptors in systemic sclerosis (scleroderma). Arthritis Rheum., 32, S42
83. Peter, J. B., Agopian, M. S., Clements, P. J. et al. (1989). Elevated serum levels of interleukin-2 receptor (IL-2R) and IL-2 in diffuse (DS) and limited scleroderma (LS). Arthritis Rheum., 32, S77
84. Horslev-Petersen, K., Ammitzboll, T., Engstrom-Laurent, A. et al. (1988). Serum and urinary animoterminal type III procollagen peptide in progressive systemic sclerosis: relationship to sclerodermal involvement, serum hyaluronan and urinary collagen metabolites. J. Rheumatol., 15, 460-467
85. Krieg, T., Langer, I., Gerstmeier, H. et al. (1986). Type III collagen aminopropeptide levels in serum of patients with progressive systemic scleroderma. J. Invest. Dermatol., 87, 788-791
86. Fries, J. F., Spitz, P. W. and Young, D. Y. (1982). The dimensions of health outcomes: The Health Assessment, Disability and Pain Scales. J. Rheumatol., 9, 789-793
87. Hochberg, M. C. and Sutton, J. D. (1988). Physical disability and psychosocial dysfunction in systemic lupus erythematosus. J. Rheumatol., 15, 959-964

11
Polymyositis-dermatomyositis

C. V. ODDIS and T. A. MEDSGER

INTRODUCTION

Polymyositis-dermatomyositis (PM-DM) is a serious, chronic, inflammatory disorder of striated muscle of unknown etiology. It occurs in both children and adults and is characterized by proximal muscle weakness. The generally accepted subtypes of PM-DM include polymyositis, dermatomyositis (when a typical rash is also present), myositis in overlap with another connective-tissue disease, and myositis associated with malignant neoplasm[1]. PM-DM is an uncommon disease but by no means rare; its recognition is increasing, as evidenced by a survey of hospital-diagnosed cases revealing an annual incidence of over 10 new cases per million population during 1978-1982[2].

In addition to causing symmetric muscle weakness, the disease affects numerous other organ systems and has significant morbidity, functional disability, and mortality. This chapter will examine the natural history of treated and untreated polymyositis-dermatomyositis. Emphasis will be on clinical features that predict both good and poor outcomes as well as those interventions that may alter prognosis.

PROBLEMS IN THE DETERMINATION OF PROGNOSIS

Assessment of prognosis in polymyositis-dermatomyositis is difficult. Because of its relative rarity, most studies involve single referral centers reporting retrospectively on small numbers of patients followed for brief periods of time. Such cross-sectional studies have obvious limitations in their ability to accurately describe the natural history of disease and to identify prognostic factors. One prospectively designed study addressed 18 juvenile dermatomyositis patients over a 10-year period (1960–1969) but it is now outdated. Some series have included patients from several different institutions or geographic areas; the retrospective analysis of prognosis in such diverse groups of patients is inherently difficult. Likewise, there is considerable variation in the time from symptom onset to clinical presentation or disease diagnosis from study to study. Patients in late stages of myositis should be grouped and analyzed separately from those examined early in their disease course. Finally, published methods of analysis are highly variable. Long-term prospective follow-up of well-defined incident cohorts of myositis patients is obviously needed.

A second difficulty with the inflammatory myopathies is the lack of a pathophysiologically meaningful classification of disease subsets. No serious attempt has been made to use new clinical, laboratory, immunologic, and pathologic findings to develop an improved classification system. Identifiable disease subsets undoubtedly have unique clinical and prognostic features. Although collective generalizations about PM-DM can certainly be stated, subset analysis maximizes the information gained concerning outcome and methods of improving it.

Objective criteria for improvement (or deterioration) in PM-DM are not well defined. Patients may certainly demonstrate increased muscle strength but this is often subjectively assessed through standard manual muscle strength grading. This traditional method does not permit adequate gradation in the range of weakness where most myositis patients fall. An accurate, reproducible, inexpensive, and convenient means of quantifying muscle strength is needed to test therapeutic interventions. Related issues are the lack of adequate criteria for staging disease severity or determining disease activity. Such criteria would allow critical comparison of patients receiving similar treatment. Finally, prognostic assessment in PM-DM must attempt to distinguish disease-related from treatment-induced factors in the analysis of outcome. Most previously published mortality studies report death rates but fail to clearly elaborate on the contribution of corticosteroids, immunosuppressive agents, or other therapeutic interventions to poor outcome. More importantly the impact of medication-induced side-effects on patient disability, discomfort, and need for additional medical or surgical intervention is poorly documented. Their elucidation may lead to new or innovative approaches in the management of PM-DM patients.

NATURAL HISTORY OF UNTREATED DISEASE

Four published series of untreated PM-DM patients are summarized in Table 1. The earliest report by O'Leary and Waisman in 1940 described 38 dermatomyositis patients[3]. Nineteen (50%) died, six because of bronchopneumonia, after an average disease duration of 2 years. Seven additional patients (18%) had residual but stable disability, and six (16%) had continued deterioration at the time of publication. Only four patients (10%), all with mild disease, were felt to have recovered completely with adequate follow-up of 7-14 years such that a transient remission had been ruled out. More often, untreated patients with acute onset progressed quickly to severe involvement but a more indolent onset was associated with milder illness, less disability, and a more favorable outcome. The course of illness was usually progressive to a certain point, but if one survived, then disease activity thereafter abated and muscle "repair" was thought to have occurred. Intracutaneous or subcutaneous calcification developed in four survivors and if patients lived long enough, both muscle fibrosis and contractures were likely to ensue.

Another group of 25 untreated dermatomyositis patients seen over a 20 year period was reported by Sheard in 1951[4]. Thirteen (52%) died after a mean disease duration of 20 months. The 12 remaining patients were observed for an average of 5 years and had chronic, low-grade myositis. It was felt that the majority of patients who lived beyond 1 year would ultimately survive, but rapidity of disease onset was not correlated with prognosis. Mortality was high in younger patients; 5 of 7 under age 20 died.

Fourteen of 89 patients reported by Rose and Walton[5] were untreated. One followed a progressively severe course and died after 6 years while another continued to deteriorate 3 years after disease onset. Another patient made a spontaneous partial recovery but later relapsed after 2 years. Two recovered but with persistent muscle weakness of moderate degree. Interestingly, three children in this series seen between 1950 and 1952 were not treated and recovered fully. However, in each the disease course was quite protracted and school attendance was erratic owing to muscle weakness or pain. Both untreated patients and patients receiving delayed corticosteroid therapy had more residual disability than those treated with steroids.

The largest reported group of 122 untreated myositis patients comes from a comparative study of untreated and corticosteroid-treated patients from the Mayo Clinic[6]. Neither the death rate nor the remission rate was significantly different in the untreated versus corticosteroid-treated patients. Steroid therapy did, however, appear to accelerate disease remission. Contractures and calcinosis occurred in both groups. Nevertheless, the authors concluded that since one-half of remissions occurred spontaneously, myositis should be viewed as self-limiting, thus distinguishing it from the other connective-tissue diseases.

It is our impression that a high proportion (up to 50%) of untreated PM-DM patients referred to major medical centers died from its complications during the precorticosteroid era. Among the survivors, the course is extremely variable. Some have unexplained cessation of disease activity and a small subset achieves spontaneous, complete remission without treatment. This intriguing group of patients is poorly understood and will undoubtedly remain so since corticosteroids are now universally prescribed.

Table 1 Natural history of non-corticosteroid-treated PM-DM patients

Author (year)	Total patients	Died	Progressive	Stable chronic	Recovered	Comments
O'Leary (1940)[3]	38	19 (50%)	6 (16%)	7 (18%)	4 (10%)	36/38 with dermatomyositis 2/38 with short follow-up precluding outcome determination
Sheard (1951)[4]	25	13 (52%)	12 (48%)	—	0	22/25 with dermatomyositis 12 "chronic, smoldering" 5/7 under age 20 died
Rose (1966)[5]	14	1 (13%)	1 (13%)	3 (38%)	3 (38%)	follow-up available in 8; 3 who recovered all had childhood DM and protracted course
Winkelmann (1968)[6]	122	35 (29%)	14 (12%)	25 (20%)	48 (39%)	

HISTORICAL REVIEW OF FACTORS ALTERING PROGNOSIS

The prognosis of myositis improved in patients having disease onset after 1950, with survival rates ranging from 53% to 86% after mean follow-up periods of 4.3 to 8 years[5-14]. This trend in mortality coincides with the introduction of cortisone and ACTH treatment[15,16]. Winkelmann was the first to retrospectively compare corticosteroid-treated versus untreated patients from the same institution[6]. The 279 patients with PM-DM were diagnosed prior to 1959 and included 122 untreated patients and 157 treated with corticosteroids (118 "high-dose", cortisone 50+ mg per day, and 38 "low-dose", < 50 mg of cortisone daily). Overall 87 (31%) died during follow-up, 80 from myositis and 7 from other causes. Although a lower proportion died in the high-dose group (28/119, 24%) compared to the untreated group (42/122, 34%), an appropriate life-table analysis was not performed. The highest death rate (45%) was in the low-dose group, but was possibly confounded by their older age.

Although nearly all studies over the past 30 years have documented the clinical efficacy of corticosteroids, several have not found significant survival differences[9,11]. In Winkelmann's study, spontaneous remission occurred as often as steroid-induced remission, but the latter occurred earlier with more rapid suppression of constitutional and muscle symptoms and with fewer permanent sequelae[6]. In reality what was termed "high-dose" cortisone in this study is lower than the recommended optimal initial therapy with corticosteroids today, which may have biased against finding any effect of therapy. Considerably higher doses (prednisone 40–60 mg per day, the equivalent of cortisone 160–240 mg) were later advocated by Pearson and Vignos[1,8].

In the corticosteroid treatment era, controlled prospective trials supporting their efficacy in polymyositis are lacking, primarily because they are considered unethical. Several retrospective analyses indicate that muscle weakness is improved and pain is lessened in steroid-treated patients. In one report where detailed documentation of sequential strength was made, 31 patients clearly responded to corticosteroid therapy[7]. The majority of those who improved were treated with 40 mg or more of prednisone daily for at least 3 months, while only a few improved on a dose of 20–39 mg per day. A Scandinavian study[12] assessed the effect of different corticosteroid treatment regimens using a standardized disability scale. In comparing steroid-responsive vs. steroid-resistant patients, the degree of improvement was greatest in those receiving therapy early (< 24 months after onset) and higher mean doses during the first 3 months.

Further support for corticosteroid efficacy came from Rose and Walton, who objectively documented relapses following steroid withdrawal and improvement after its reinstitution[5]. Ten years later, researchers from the same institution demonstrated improved functional ability in all myositis patient subsets receiving initial high-dose corticosteroid and found that only 18% of adequately treated cases were severely disabled[10]. A recent community hospital-based study of 27 steroid-treated adult PM-DM patients revealed that 64% had little or no muscle weakness after 3 months with a number of patients having discontinued all therapy[17]. The experience of referral centers may be skewed to more severe cases.

Immunosuppressive medications, either alone or in combination with corticosteroids, appear to improve prognosis in myositis. A prospective, randomized, controlled trial of prednisone versus a combination of prednisone and azathioprine showed no statistical difference in muscle strength at 3 months[18]; but, at 1 and 3 years, the combination therapy was superior as judged by functional ability and dose of prednisone necessary for disease control[19]. Methotrexate was considered effective in 17 of 22 steroid-resistant patients given 25-35 mg intravenously each week[20]. In addition, a retrospective analysis of 25 patients treated with methotrexate concluded that 16 (64%) had improved by more than one full muscle strength grade[7,21].

The improved prognosis in polymyositis over the last several decades is also attributable to better supportive care, such as optimal management of pneumonitis resulting from dysphagia with aspiration. A recent mortality study of PM-DM in the United States from 1968 to 1978 demonstrated a temporal increase in mean age at death[22]. Although this trend may indicate increased incidence in older persons, it more likely represents improved prognosis.

RELATION OF PROGNOSIS TO SPECIFIC OUTCOMES

Mortality

Mortality rates for polymyositis-dermatomyositis vary significantly among published retrospective studies. The two earliest reported series of non-corticosteroid-treated patients recruited between 1925 and 1947 had mortality rates of about 50% with short follow-up periods[3,4]. In Table 2, we have summarized 10 published studies, dividing them according to the decade in which the average patient was entered. There were four reports including 554 patients studied primarily during the 1950s and followed 2.5-6.1 years[5,6,9,11]. Both corticosteroid-treated and untreated patients were included in these series. The mortality rate was remarkably similar (28-36%). Factors associated with poor survival were older age at onset[5,9]; black race[9]; malignancy[5,6,11]; rapid progression[6] and severe muscle weakness[9,11]; and overlap with other connective tissue diseases[5,11], especially scleroderma[6], dysphagia[9,11], and pulmonary infiltration[9]. Aspiration pneumonia due to pharyngeal muscle dysfunction was the most frequent cause of lung disease[9].

In the 1960s, almost all patients were treated with corticosteroids. Three series described 265 patients followed for 1.8-5.0 years[7,14,23]. The case fatality rate was more variable in this time period, ranging from

Table 2 Mortality statistics and poor prognostic features in several PM-DM series stratified by decade of patient entry

Author (year)	Dates of patient entry	Number of patients	Mean follow-up from entry (years)	Mortality rate	Poor prognostic features
Rose (1966)[5]	1954–1964	89	6.1	30%	Malignancy, other CTD[a], acute course
Winkelmann (1968)[6]	Before 1959	279	3.0	32%	Malignancy, scleroderma, rapid progression
Medsger (1971)[a]	1947–1968	124	2.5[b]	36%	Pulmonary infiltrates, dysphagia, severe weakness, age > 50, black race
Carpenter (1977)[11]	1947–1971	62	NS[c]	45%	Dysphagia, severe weakness
Bohan (1977)[7]	1956–1971	153	4.3	14%	Malignancy, older age, delayed treatment
Benbassat (1985)[14]	1956–1976	92	1.8	32%	Dysphagia, older age, leukocytosis, fever, failure to induce remission, shorter disease duration
Riddoch (1975)[23]	1960–1970	20	5	40%	(Excluded children, cancer, CTD[c])
Henriksson (1982)[12]	1967–1978	107	5	23%	Malignancy, older age, delayed treatment, cardiac involvement
Hochberg (1986)[24]	1970–1981	76	NS	17%	Age > 45, cardiac involvement
Tymms (1985)[25]	1970–1982	105	4	18%	Older age, delayed treatment

[a] CTD = connective-tissue disease.
[b] median.
[c] NS = not stated.

14% in a large medical center referral population[7] to 40% in a small series of 20 patients in which children were excluded and therapy was begun a mean of 2.8 years after onset of symptoms. The latter study may not be representative for the above reasons. Poor prognostic signs continued to be older age[7,14], associated malignancy[7,23], delayed treatment[7,23], and dysphagia[14]. There is some disagreement concerning the effect of another connective-tissue disease on mortality in patients with myositis in overlap[7,23].

Investigators publishing on patients seen during the 1970s have noted improved survival[12,24,25]. Among 288 patients in these three series, 56 (19%) died, and the mortality rate varied from 17% to 23%. As expected, older age[12,24,25], malignancy[12], and delayed therapy[12,25] adversely influenced prognosis, and, for the first time, cardiac involvement[12,24] and complications of corticosteroid and immunosuppressive therapy[25] were implicated.

In contrast to systemic sclerosis[26], where male sex is recognized to be a poor prognostic sign, no such significant differences have been reported in polymyositis. Similarly, no studies have identified dermatomyositis as having a higher mortality rate, with the exception of its closer association with malignancy than polymyositis. The reason for improved survival in recent times is uncertain, but may reflect earlier diagnosis, detection of milder cases, better general medical care, and more judicious use of the required potent therapeutic agents.

A number of studies deal exclusively or separately with mortality in juvenile myositis. Before the introduction of corticosteroids, at least one-third of children with myositis died[27,28]. Over the last 20 years, survival has improved but the prognosis in children continues to be extremely variable and difficult to predict. For example, the combined mortality rate from three published series was 7.2% with only 9 of 125 patients dying[29-31]. Another prospective study of 18 patients seen between 1960 and 1969 and followed for a mean of 5 years had no deaths attributable to dermatomyositis and 17 patients were ambulatory and functionally independent[32]. On the other hand, in a recent study of 28 children with DM, 5 died during treatment[33], while 7 (one suicide) of 66 in another series died of myositis or its complications[34].

While malignancy, cardiac disease, and pulmonary complications such as pneumonia from aspiration are the most common causes of death in adults, children die because of progressive intractable muscle weakness, sepsis, gastrointestinal vasculitis, respiratory failure, or cardiomyopathy[34-37]. A time period during which life-threatening complications are particularly frequent is the initial 12-month period of treatment[34]. Overall, we conclude that the judicious use of corticosteroids and immunosuppressive drugs and other modern clinical management advances have greatly improved the prognosis of juvenile polydermatomyositis during the past two decades. The current expected survival is 90% or more 10 years after diagnosis.

Disability

Factors correlated with disability are quite different from those associated with death. Information on the short- and long-term morbidity and functional disability from PM-DM is limited. Morbidity from myositis results not only from the primary inflammatory process but also from its treatment.

Most survivors of myositis experience considerable improvement in their functional status, with maximum benefit occurring in the 3-5 years after beginning treatment. Reduction in discomfort and objective increase in muscle power in corticosteroid-treated compared with untreated patients has been noted[5]. Early treatment has permitted the introduction of physiotherapy for passive range of motion and more rapid mobilization, which has prevented muscle and tendon shortening with contractures. Untreated patients and those receiving delayed treatment had more residual disability. In a 20-year follow-up study, a 6-level disability grading system was applied to 118 patients[10]. In all clinical subsets of PM-DM the average disability at onset was severe, with gait abnormalities and an inability to climb stairs without arm support in most cases. After 4 years, the average disability grade was slightly less than 3 (6 being the worst), corresponding to minimal atrophy or weakness in one or more muscle groups without functional impairment. Improvement in disability was greatest during the first 3 years and remained relatively constant thereafter. The disability grade at presentation was similar in all myositis subsets, and all showed improvement after treatment, including patients with cancer (until they failed due to malignancy). Late disability was worse in the overlap category (particularly rheumatoid arthritis and systemic sclerosis), and some statistical improvement in this and other groups was spurious due to early death of severely disabled cases who were thus excluded from subsequent analysis. A small group of patients (20%) still had "active" disease during follow-up; however, from the fourth year of follow-up 30%, and from the seventh year 50% of these "active" cases had elevated serum muscle enzymes but a stable clinical picture. It is possible that, in these cases, enzyme leakage from previously damaged myofibrils represents an end-stage, inactive process. At study end, two-thirds of 82 survivors had no functional disability, but the toxicity of treatment was not well described.

In the UCLA series, 40 of 124 patients treated with prednisone had a detailed muscle strength evaluation preceding treatment. On a scale of 1 to 5[21] strength improved an average of one grade or more after a mean of 2.1 months[7]. Forty-six patients received 50 courses of immunosuppressive medications, and in 50% muscle strength improved by an average of one grade. Virtually every patient treated with high-dose corticosteroids (in the range of 40 mg daily) for more than several months developed side-effects. Immunosuppressive medications led to severe side-effects, e.g., bone marrow suppression, gastrointestinal hemorrhage, and hepatic toxicity, in 22% of users.

A favorable functional outcome was reported from Sweden in long-term survivors of PM-DM[12]. Eighty-seven percent of patients who improved with therapy had minimal or no disability at follow-up (mean 5 years), in contrast to only 9% of patients who were treatment failures. Of 18 patients in whom treatment was delayed greater than 24 months after the onset of weakness, 3 improved, and these only temporarily. Side-effects from corticosteroids or immunosuppressive drugs were found in 42% of the patients, but their contribution to long-term disability was not addressed.

In a community-based series of 27 adult myositis patients 64% had little or no weakness and no patients had severe impairment after 3 months of treatment[17]. Eight less severely ill patients received alternate-day prednisone from the outset with excellent clinical results and without subsequent need for daily therapy. More importantly, when toxicity was compared between daily and alternate-day cortico-steroid regimens, Cushing's syndrome, severe infection, compression fractures, and new-onset insulin-dependent diabetes mellitus all occurred more frequently and were more severe in the group treated daily[17]. In another series of 22 adult patients (none with overlap), 14 were followed for a mean of 5.6 years[38]. By life-table analysis, the proportion discontinuing corticosteroids was 42% at 3 years from diagnosis, but corticosteroid complications had occurred in 7 patients (32%). Although mean strength at follow-up rose one grade, 5 of 14 (36%) patients had substantial disability related to the disease or its treatment.

Further support for the frequency of complications of high-dose corticosteroid therapy comes from a 105-patient study in which 8 had osteoporotic vertebral compression fractures, 7 each had osteonecrosis of the femoral head, complicated peptic ulcer, and posterior subcapsular cataracts; and 4 developed diabetes mellitus[25]. Two others died from septicemia associated with cytotoxic drug-induced agranulocytosis while a cyclophosphamide-treated patient later died of acute myeloid leukemia. In our own retrospective series of 30 corticosteroid treated patients, four suffered osteoporotic bone fractures, two had osteo-necrosis (five different joints), and two each had peptic ulcer disease, hypertension requiring treatment, and diabetes mellitus[39]. One patient experienced a recrudescence of a *Mycobacterium tuberculosis* infection[39]. In these two studies combined, significant corticosteroid complications affected 39 of 135 (29%) patients.

The major limitation in properly assessing disability in PM-DM is that all reported data are retrospective. Assessment of iatrogenic factors must be prospective and long-term especially to detect such complications as late malignancy. Also, longitudinal prospective quantitation of disability using validated patient self-report instruments may provide valuable information. Although developed for persons with arthritis, the Health Assessment Questionnaire (HAQ) or Arthritis Impact Measurement Scales (AIMS) may accurately reflect limitations due to other musculoskeletal conditions. Thirty-five of our connective-tissue disease (CTD) patients with myopathy had a mean HAQ disability index of 1.54 compared with 455 nonmyopathy CTD patients, whose mean disability index was 1.19 ($p < 0.01$). Again, prospective studies and separation of disease from therapy-related disability must be addressed.

Three distinct courses for juvenile dermatomyositis (JDMS) have been described, i.e., monocyclic, chronic polycyclic, and chronic continuous[40]. No onset features predicted children who would experience a severe continuous illness. Relapse in a child with an apparent monocyclic course is uncommon, but was observed 8 years after recovery from the initial episode of myositis[41]. There is one report of morbid progression in JDMS, with biopsy evidence of disease activity years after initial successful corticosteroid therapy and intensive physical therapy[30]. Finally, a subgroup of patients with severe generalized vasculitis do poorly despite an optimal therapeutic regimen[42,46].

Of 41 children with JDMS followed 0.5 to 15 years, 25 were functionally normal, 11 were ambulatory and capable of normal activities with residual weakness or contractures, 6 had nonhandicapping calcinosis, 2 had severe disability and were wheelchair dependent, and 3 had died[31]. No patient had progressive muscle weakness or decreased physical function late in the illness (5-15 years after onset). In another study of 47 JDMS patients, the best predictor of functional recovery was prompt, high-dose corticosteroid therapy[42]. Children receiving such treatment had 78% good functional outcomes and less than 20% developed disabling calcinosis. This is in contrast to the British view that low-dose corticosteroids (1 mg kg^{-1} d^{-1}) for a brief period of time produces better outcome and less long-term iatrogenic complications[43,44]. These authors concluded that nearly all of their severely disabled patients had received excessive doses of steroids and/or immunosuppressives[45]. Known side-effects of corticosteroid therapy commonly reported in JDMS patients include growth retardation, changes in bone density, cataract formation and avascular necrosis of the femoral head.

Dermal and subcutaneous calcification (calcinosis) is reported in 20-50% of JDMS patients[32,47,48] and is a major source of chronic disability. In severe cases an exoskeleton-like calcification may result[42]. Calcinosis persists even after active disease remits and causes focal atrophy of muscle and skin, leading to contractures and both deep and superficial cutaneous ulcerations. Lesions tend to progress inexorably, and treatment is generally unsatisfactory.

Other features leading to chronic disability in JDMS include arthritis[49], Raynaud's phenomenon[49], and muscle contractures. Physical therapy is extremely important. In the acutely ill or very weak child, bed rest and passive range of motion exercises are recommended. After clinical improvement, active motion is begun with a goal of early mobilization. Gait retraining and swimming are particularly helpful in rehabilitation. If fixed contractures occur in chronic myositis, functional disability may result, preventing ambulation even though adequate muscle power has been restored[44].

Discomfort

The frequency of pain at the onset of myositis is variable, but in one series was found in 73% of cases[10]. When present, it responds very well to corticosteroid therapy and is not a disabling factor except when it occurs in association with known steroid side-effects, e.g., osteoporotic fractures, osteonecrosis, or complications of the disease, e.g., calcinosis or arthritis.

Economic status

Very little has been reported on the short- or long-term economic impact of myositis. An encouraging study of 18 JDMS patients evaluated an average of 18.5 years after diagnosis found that their educational achievement and employment status was better than both a corresponding group of adults with juvenile rheumatoid arthritis and the general adult population of British Columbia[49]. Fifty percent were married and their annual income was quite good. Residual disability related to calcinosis and flexion contractures were present in only three people.

Economic considerations in the adult would include both immediate and delayed loss of work and decrease in earning capacity. No studies have been reported on this subject. The costs of medical intervention for the consequences of disease and treatment-related complications are unknown. Particular areas of concern would be the need for joint replacement in patients with osteonecrosis and the treatment of opportunistic infections or secondary malignancy after the use of chemotherapeutic agents.

OTHER PROGNOSTIC FACTORS

There is no correlation between the initial serum creatine kinase (CK) level and the grade of disability or degree of weakness at disease presentation[10]. Similarly, chronic low-level CK elevation does not always imply ongoing muscle destruction. In adults, histopathologic changes in muscle are of no value in predicting survival[11] or identifying those who will experience spontaneous remission[6]. However, in children, it has been suggested that a noninflammatory, occlusive vascular lesion of muscular arteries identifies a severe subset of JDMS[46].

Pulmonary involvement

Pulmonary involvement in PM-DM has been long recognized as a serious complication that may be underappreciated[50,51]. In a literature review, lung disease accounted for 58% of all PM-DM deaths, and others have confirmed this diminished survival[52,53]. Most recent studies note the association of the Jo-1 antibody with interstitial lung disease in polymyositis. In a series of 42 patients recently reported, 45% developed clinically evident pulmonary disease (chest radiograph or pulmonary function testing) during a mean follow-up of 35 months, and in 10% it contributed directly to death[54]. Response to corticosteroids has been reported but is inconsistent[51].

Aspiration pneumonia is the most common pulmonary complication of PM-DM and occurred in 14% of patients in one series[54]. It is usually associated with pharyngeal dysfunction and nearly all who aspirate complain of pharyngeal dysphagia, a well-recognized predictor of poor outcome in myositis[9,11]. Ventilatory insufficiency due to weakness of respiratory muscles is present in 4–8% of PM-DM patients[3,5,10,54]. It is associated with severe generalized muscle weakness, but the ultimate prognosis for recovery of respiratory function is good with corticosteroid treatment[54].

Iatrogenic pulmonary complications include opportunistic infection, kyphosis with restrictive lung disease following vertebral compression fractures, and drug-induced interstitial pneumonitis from either methotrexate or cyclophosphamide[55-57].

Cardiac

Cardiac involvement is associated with a poor prognosis in PM-DM[10,23,58,59]. Comparing the course of five patients with cardiac involvement to eight patients without it, one study noted a longer history of persistently active more severe skeletal myositis in those with cardiac disease[60]. In another report, 11 of 16 (69%) cases with well-documented cardiac involvement, and all four with congestive heart failure died[59]. A correlation between EKG changes and death has been noted in JDMS[28].

Abnormalities that may signal cardiac involvement in PM-DM are frequent[58] and include EKG abnormalities[61], conduction disturbances[62,63], arrhythmias[64], congestive heart failure[7,59,65], coronary arteritis[66], and myocarditis[65,67]. Other causes of these common problems must, of course, be excluded. Persistent elevation of the serum CK-MB isoenzyme fraction above 3% of the total CK usually correlates with cardiac involvement and has been associated with fatal congestive heart failure[58,64].

Serology

A number of serum autoantibodies have been found in association with PM-DM. Their correlations with certain clinical features make them important for both diagnosis and prognosis. Anti-nRNP is found in myositis associated with SLE and/or systemic sclerosis. Anti-Mi-2 is detected almost exclusively with DM where its frequency approaches 20%[68]. Anti-Jo-1 is uncommon in DM but is found in 20–40% of adult PM patients[69,70]. It has a strong association with interstitial lung disease, which may dominate the clinical picture[71]. Other clinical features associated with anti-Jo-1 include Raynaud's phenomenon, sicca syndrome, and an arthritis that may become chronic and deforming[72]. Two other rarely encountered anti-cytoplasmic antibodies, anti-PL-7 and anti-PL-12, have similar clinical associations[73]. Anti-PM-Scl is associated with myositis and scleroderma in overlap[74], and anti-SSA has been found in 60% of 55 patients with myositis of whom 69% (23 of 33) had cardiac damage[75]. Not enough is known as yet to predict long-term outcome in these serologic subgroups, but an attempt is being made to determine whether they respond differently to corticosteroid and immunosuppressive therapy[76].

FUTURE PERSPECTIVES

Reliable prognostic information is crucial for the physician in patient and family counseling, anticipating disease complications, and selecting an optimal therapeutic regimen. Unfortunately, the available data in PM-DM are limited and most often derived from short-term retrospective studies, often performed on unrepresentative patients. In the future, it will be necessary to plan careful prospective, longitudinal studies of incident cohorts, including clinical, laboratory, serologic, and functional outcome data. The acquisition of such data may lead to important new concepts of disease classification and prognosis.

References

1. Pearson, C. M. (1963). Patterns of polymyositis and their responses to treatment. *Am. J. Med.*, **59**, 827–838
2. Oddis, C. V., Conte, C. G., Steen, V. D. and Medsger, T. A., Jr. (1990). Incidence of polymyositis-dermatomyositis: a 20-year study of hospital-diagnosed cases in Allegheny County, PA, 1963–1982. *J. Rheumatol.*, **17** (10)
3. O'Leary, P. A. and Waisman, M. (1940). Dermatomyositis. *Arch. Derm. Syph.*, **41**, 1001–1019
4. Sheard, C., Jr. (1951). Dermatomyositis. *Arch. Intern. Med.*, **88**, 640–658
5. Rose, A. L. and Walton, J. N. (1966). Polymyositis: a survey of 89 cases with particular reference to treatment and prognosis. *Brain*, **89**, 747–768
6. Winkelmann, R. K. *et al.* (1968). Course of dermatomyositis-polymyositis: comparison of untreated and cortisone-treated patients. *Mayo Clin. Proc.*, **43**, 545–556
7. Bohan, A., Peter, J. B., Bowman, R. L. and Pearson, C. M. (1977). A computer-assisted analysis of 153 patients with polymyositis and dermatomyositis. *Medicine*, **56**, 255–286
8. Vignos, P. J., Bowling, G. F. and Watkins, M. P. (1964). Polymyositis: effect of corticosteroids on final results. *Arch. Intern. Med.*, **114**, 263–277
9. Medsger, T. A., Jr., Robinson, H. and Masi, A. T. (1971). Factors affecting survivorship in polymyositis: a life-table study of 124 patients. *Arthritis Rheum.*, **14**, 249–258
10. DeVere, R. and Bradley, W. G. (1975). Polymyositis: its presentation, morbidity and mortality. *Brain*, **98**, 637–666

11. Carpenter, J. R., Bunch, T. W., Engel, A. G. and O'Brien, P. C. (1977). Survival in polymyositis: corticosteroids and risk factors. *J. Rheumatol.*, **4**, 207-214
12. Henriksson, K. G. and Sandstedt, P. (1982). Polymyositis — treatment and prognosis: a study of 107 patients. *Acta Neurol. Scand.*, **65**, 280-300
13. Hochberg, M. C., Feldman, P., Zizic, T. M. and Stevens, M. B. (1983). Survival in adult poly (dermato) myositis. *Arthritis Rheum.*, **26**, S9
14. Benbassat, J., Gefel, D., Larholt, K., Sukenik, S., Morgenstern, V. and Zlotnick, A. (1985). Prognostic factors in PM-DM: a computer-assisted analysis of 92 cases. *Arthritis Rheum.*, **28**, 249-255
15. Elkinton, J. R., Hunt, A. D., Jr., Godrey, L., *et al.* (1949). Effects of pituitary adrenocorticotropic hormone (ACTH) therapy. *J. Am. Med. Assoc.*, **141**, 1273-1279
16. Oppel, T. W., Cohen, C. and Milhorat, A. T. (1950). The effect of pituitary ACTH in dermatomyositis. *Ann. Intern. Med.*, **32**, 318-324
17. Hoffman, G. S., Franck, W. A., Raddatz, D. A. *et al.* (1983). Presentation, treatment and prognosis of idiopathic inflammatory muscle disease in a rural hospital. *Am. J. Med.*, **75**, 433-438
18. Bunch, T. W., Worthington, J. W., Combs, J. J. *et al.* (1980). Azathioprine with prednisone for polymyositis: a controlled clinical trial. *Ann. Intern. Med.*, **92**, 365-369
19. Bunch, T. W. (1981). Prednisone and azathioprine for polymyositis: long-term followup. *Arthritis Rheum.*, **24**, 45-48
20. Metzger, A. L., Bohan, A. and Goldberg, L. S. (1974). Polymyositis and dermatomyositis: combined methotrexate and corticosteroid therapy. *Ann. Intern. Med.*, **81**, 182-189
21. British Medical Research Council. (1943). *Aid to the Investigation of Peripheral Nerve Injuries*, 2nd edn. (London: HMSO)
22. Hochberg, M. C., Lopez-Acuna, D. and Gittelsohn, A. M. (1983). Mortality from polymyositis and dermatomyositis in the United States, 1968-1978. *Arthritis Rheum.*, **26**, 1465-1471
23. Riddoch, D. and Morgan-Hughes, J. A. (1975). Prognosis in adult polymyositis. *J. Neurol. Sci.*, **26**, 71-80
24. Hochberg, M. C., Feldman, D. and Stevens, M. B. (1986). Adult onset polymyositis/dermatomyositis: an analysis of clinical and laboratory features and survival in 76 patients with a review of the literature. *Semin. Arthritis Rheum.*, **15**, 168-178
25. Tymms, K. E. and Webb, J. (1985). Dermatopolymyositis and other connective tissue diseases. A review of 105 cases. *J. Rheumatol.*, **12**, 1140-1148
26. Medsger, T. A., Jr., Masi, A. T., Rodnan, G. P., Benedek, T. G. and Robinson, H. (1971). Survival with systemic sclerosis (scleroderma): A life-table analysis of clinical and demographic factors on 309 patients. *Ann. Intern. Med.*, **75**, 369-376
27. Wedgewood, R. J. P., Cook, C. D. and Cohen, J. (1953). Dermatomyositis: report of 26 cases in children with a discussion of endocrine therapy in 13. *Pediatrics*, **12**, 447-466
28. Bitnum, C., Darvschnor, C. W. and Travis, L. B. (1964). Dermatomyositis. *J. Pediatr.*, **64**, 101-131
29. Hanson, V. (1976). Dermatomyositis, scleroderma and polyarteritis nodosa. *Clin. Rheum. Dis.*, **2**, 445-467
30. Miller, J. J. and Koehler, J. P. (1972). Persistence of activity in dermatomyositis of childhood. *Arthritis Rheum.*, **20**, 332-337
31. Sullivan, D. B., Cassidy, J. T. and Petty, R. (1977). Dermatomyositis in the pediatric patient. *Arthritis Rheum.*, **20**, 327-331
2. Sullivan, D. B., Cassidy, J. T., Petty, R. E. and Burt, A. (1972). Prognosis in childhood dermatomyositis. *J. Pediatr.*, **80**, 555-563
33. Bruguier, A., Texier, P., Clement, M. C. *et al.* (1984). Dermatomyositis infantiles. A propos de vingthuit observations. *Arch. Fr. Pediatr.*, **41**, 9-14
34. Spencer, C. H., Hanson, V., Singsen, B. H., Bernstein, B. H., Kornreich, J. H. and King, K. K. (1984). Course of treated juvenile dermatomyositis. *J. Pediatr.*, **105**, 399-408
35. Yoshioka, M., Okuno, T. and Mikawa, H. (1985). Prognosis and treatment of polymyositis with particular reference to steroid resistant patients. *Arch. Dis. Child.*, **60**, 231-244

36. Goel, K. M. and King, M. (1986). Dermatomyositis-polymyositis in children. *Scott. Med. J.*, **31**, 15-19
37. Miller, L. C., Michael, A. F. and Kim, Y. (1987). Childhood dermatomyositis: clinical course and long-term followup. *Clin. Pediatr.*, **26**, 561-566
38. Baron, M. and Small, P. (1985). Polymyositis/dermatomyositis: clinical features and outcome in 22 patients. *J. Rheumatol.*, **12**, 283-286
39. Oddis, C. V. and Medsger, T. A., Jr. (1988). Relationship between serum creatine kinase level and corticosteroid therapy in polymyositis-dermatomyositis. *J. Rheumatol.*, **15**, 807-811
40. Spencer, C., Kornreich, H., Bernstein, B. *et al.* (1979). Three courses of juvenile dermatomyositis. *Arthritis Rheum.*, **22**, 661-665
41. Lovell, H. B. and Lindsley, C. B. (1986). Late recurrence of childhood dermatomyositis. *J. Rheumatol.*, **13**, 821-822
42. Bowyer, S. L., Blane, C. E., Sullivan, D. B. *et al.* (1983). Childhood dermatomyositis: factors predicting functional outcome and development of dystrophic calcification. *J. Pediatr.*, **103**, 882-888
43. Dubowitz, V. (1976). Treatment of dermatomyositis in childhood. *Arch. Dis. Child.*, **51**, 494
44. Miller, G., Heckmatt, J. Z. and Dubowitz, V. (1983). Drug treatment of juvenile dermatomyositis. *Arch. Dis. Child.*, **58**, 445-450
45. Dubowitz, V. (1984). Prognostic factors in dermatomyositis (letter). *J. Pediatr.*, **105**, 336-337
46. Crowe, W. E., Bove, K. E. and Levinson, J. E. (1982). Clinical and pathogenic implications of histopathology in childhood poly-dermatomyositis. *Arthritis Rheum.*, **25**, 126-139
47. Muller, S. A., Winkelmann, R. D. and Brumstring, L. A. (1959). Calcinosis in dermatomyositis. *Arch. Dermatol.*, **95**, 669-673
48. Pachman, L. M. and Cooke, N. (1980). Juvenile dermatomyositis: a clinical and immunologic study. *J. Pediatr.*, **96**, 226-234
49. Chalmers, A., Sayson, R. and Walters, K. (1982). Juvenile dermatomyositis: medical, social and economic status in adulthood. *Can. Med. Assoc. J.*, **126**, 31-33
50. Miller, E. S. and Mathews, W. H. (1956). Interstitial pneumonitis in dermatomyositis. *J. Am. Med. Assoc.*, **160**, 1467-1470
51. Arsura, E. L. and Greenberg, A. S. (1988). Adverse impact of interstitial pulmonary fibrosis on prognosis in polymyositis and dermatomyositis. *Semin. Arthritis Rheum.*, **18**, 29-37
52. Lakhanpal, S., Lie, J. T., Conn, D. L. and Martin, W. J., II (1987). Pulmonary disease in polymyositis-dermatomyositis: a clinico-pathological analysis of 65 autopsy cases. *Ann. Rheum. Dis.*, **46**, 23-29
53. Takizawa, H., Shiga, J., Moroi, Y. *et al.* (1987). Interstitial lung disease in dermatomyositis. Clinicopathologic study. *J. Rheumatol.*, **14**, 102-107
54. Dickey, B. F. and Myers, A. R. (1984). Pulmonary disease in polymyositis/dermatomyositis. *Semin. Arthritis Rheum.*, **14**, 60-76
55. Sastman, H. D., Matthay, R. A., Putman, C. E. *et al.* (1976). Methotrexate-induced pneumonitis. *Medicine (Baltimore)*, **55**, 371-388
56. Gockerman, J. P. (1982). Drug-induced interstitial lung disease. *Clin. Chest Med.* **3**, 521-536
57. Patel, A. R., Shah, P. C., Rhee, H. L. *et al.* (1976). Cyclophosphamide therapy and interstitial pulmonary fibrosis. *Cancer*, **38**, 1542-1549
58. Askari, A. D. (1984). Cardiac abnormalities in inflammatory myopathy. *Clin. Rheum. Dis.*, **10**, 131-149
59. Oka, M. and Raasakka, T. (1978). Cardiac involvement in polymyositis. *Scand. J. Rheumatol.*, **7**, 203-208
60. Sharratt, G. P., Danta, G. and Carson, P. H. (1977). Cardiac abnormality in polymyositis. *Ann. Rheum. Dis.*, **36**, 575-578
61. Stern, R., Godbold, J. H., Chess, Q. and Kagen, L. J. (1984). ECG abnormalities in polymyositis. *Arch. Intern. Med.*, **144**, 2185-2189

62. Schaumberg, H. H., Nielsen, S. L. and Yurchak, P. M. (1971). Heart block in polymyositis. *N. Engl. J. Med.*, **284**, 480-481
63. Kehoe, R. F., Bauerfeind, R., Tommaso, C. *et al.* (1981). Cardiac conduction defects in polymyositis: electrophysiologic studies in four patients. *Ann. Intern. Med.*, **94**, 41-43
64. Askari, A. D. and Huettner, T. L. (1982). Cardiac abnormalities in polymyositis/dermatomyositis. *Semin. Arthritis Rheum.*, **12**, 208-219
65. Denbow, C. E., Lie, J. T., Tancreli, R. G. *et al.* (1979). Cardiac involvement in polymyositis. A clinicopathologic study of 20 autopsied patients. *Arthritis Rheum.*, **22**, 1088-1092
66. Okada, T. and Shiokawa, Y. (1975). Cardiac lesions in collagen disease. *Jpn Circ. J.*, **39**, 479-484
67. Hill, D. L. and Barrows, H. S. (1968). Identical skeletal and cardiac muscle involvement in a case of fatal polymyositis. *Arch. Neurol.*, **19**, 545-551
68. Targoff, I. N. and Reichlin, M. (1985). The association between Mi-2 antibodies and dermatomyositis. *Arthritis Rheum.*, **28**, 796-803
69. Reichlin, M. and Arnett, F. C. (1984). Multiplicity of antibodies in myositis sera. *Arthritis Rheum.*, **27**, 1150-1156
70. Yoshida, S., Akizuki, M. and Mimori, T. (1983). The precipitating antibody to an acidic nuclear protein antigen, the Jo-1, in connective tissue diseases: a marker for a subset of polymyositis with interstitial pulmonary fibrosis. *Arthritis Rheum.*, **26**, 604-611
71. Wasicek, C. A., Reichlin, M., Montes, M. and Raghu, G. (1984). Polymyositis and interstitial lung disease in a patient with anti-Jo-1 prototype. *Am. J. Med.*, **76**, 538-544
72. Oddis, C. V., Medsger, T. A, Jr. and Cooperstein, L. C. (1990). A subluxing arthropathy associated with the anti-Jo-1 antibody in polymyositis dermatomyositis. *Arthritis Rheum.*, **33**
73. Bernstein, R. M. and Mathews, M. B. (1985). Jo-1 and other myositis autoantibodies. In Brooks, P. M. and York, J. R. (eds.) *Rheumatology - 85*, pp. 273-278. Excerpta Med Int. Cong. Ser. Amsterdam: Elsevier Science Publishers
74. Reichlin, M., Maddison, P. J., Targoff, I. *et al.* (1984). Antibodies to a nuclear/nucleolar antigen in patients with PM-DM overlap syndrome. *J. Clin. Immunol.*, **4**, 40-44
75. Behan, W. M., Behan, P. O. and Gairns, J. (1987). Cardiac damage in polymyositis associated with antibodies to tissue ribonucleoprotein. *Br. Heart J.*, **57**, 176-180
76. Miller, F. W., Love, L. A., Leff, R. L., Fraser, D. D. and Plotz, P. H. (1989). Clinical and autoantibody subgroups predict therapeutic responses and prognosis in the idiopathic inflammatory myopathies. *Arthritis Rheum.*, **32**(suppl.), S125

12
Vasculitis

F. J. BARBADO, J. J. VÁZQUEZ, M. KHAMASHTA, and
G. R. V. HUGHES

PROBLEMS IN DETERMINING THE PROGNOSIS OF THE VASCULITIDES

Concept and definition of vasculitis

The label "vasculitis" embraces a large group of diseases that lack a clearly defined etiology and have heterogeneous clinical expressions, their common denominator being an inflammatory process with vascular wall necrosis. Systemic vasculitis can be the principal or sole manifestation, as in polyarteritis nodosa (PAN), Churg-Strauss' allergic and granulomatous angiitis and Wegener's granulomatosis, or it can be a part of other primary disease processes such as connective-tissue disease, infections, or neoplasms[1,2].

Classification of vasculitis and its relation to prognosis

Systemic vasculitis classification is difficult and has been based on: caliber of vessels affected[3]; histologic features of lesions, e.g., granulomatous inflammation[4,5]; clinical manifestations[6,7]; pattern of systemic involvement; causative factors; and immunopathogenic mechanisms implicated[6,7]. No combination of these features is specific[8].

The classification of the vasculitides is of particular importance in the analysis of the prognosis and course of the process[9-11].

Table 1 summarizes the classification of Fauci et al.[1,2], based on clinical, pathologic, and immunopathogenic criteria. This is presently the most widely accepted classification and it is a rational tool for establishing prognosis and therapeutic strategy.

The three main systemic vasculitis categories having important prognostic implications are: (1) Predominantly systemic vasculitis syndromes (e.g., PAN, Wegener's granulomatosis) that lead to irreversible organ dysfunction and fatal outcome if not treated. Acceptance of this

Table 1 Classification of the vasculitis syndromes

Systemic necrotizing vasculitis
  Classic polyarteritis nodosa
  Churg-Strauss' allergic angiitis and granulomatosis
  Polyangiitis overlap syndrome
Hypersensitivity vasculitis
Wegener's granulomatosis
Giant-cell arteritis
Other vasculitis syndromes

---

group, although provisional, is based on proven practical arguments, such as their potentially life-threatening nature and the need for combined corticosteroid and immunosuppressive treatment. (2) Hypersensitivity vasculitides. These are confined mainly to the skin, rarely produce visceral damage, are often self-limiting and have a different therapeutic management and more favorable clinical connotations. (3) Polyangiitis overlap syndrome. Aside from clarifying the similarities and differences between different groups of vasculitides, this category permits a more precise division of systemic and localized forms. Although the overlap syndrome was at first recognized as a distinct entity situated between PAN and Churg-Strauss' angiitis[1,2], the crossover between PAN and hypersensitivity vasculitides was later enlarged[12,13]. At the present it is becoming clear that this overlap includes the principal well-defined vasculitides (PAN, Wegener's granulomatosis, giant-cell arteritis)[14-16]. It is important to recognize the polyangiitis overlap syndrome because of its serious prognosis and the need for aggressive therapy. This entity illustrates the existence of a continuous spectrum of clinicopathologic manifestations in the vasculitis syndromes[12].

In reality, this classification is a tool for prognosis and treatment and does not imply that each syndrome constitutes a distinctive entity. For the moment, as far as our knowledge of systemic vasculitis is concerned, precise labels are less important than the analysis of prognostic variables and therapeutic options.

The prognostic outlook of systemic vasculitis is complex and difficult to predict due to the heterogeneity of the group and its diverse manifestations[17]. There are no prognostic factors that indicate which patients will experience progressive disease with severe visceral involvement[18].

Natural history of untreated systemic vasculitides

The 5-year survival rate in the presteroid era was 10-13%[19-23]. However, this figure probably included patients with cutaneous and muscular forms of disease, who had a more favorable prognosis, so the true survival rate of untreated PAN was probably lower[2].

The prognosis of untreated Churg-Strauss' angiitis is poor, with a 5-

year survival rate of 25%[20,23]. The clinical course and prognosis of untreated polyangiitis overlap syndrome is similar to that of PAN.

In contrast, most hypersensitivity vasculitides resolve spontaneously, although some, like Henoch–Schonlein purpura, may exhibit recurrent intestinal or renal disease and have a worse prognosis[2].

Factors that modify the prognosis of systemic vasculitis

The corticosteroid era

Corticosteroids have been used in the treatment of PAN since 1950[24,25]. Early reports of steroid treatment in PAN were of isolated cases and sometimes showed a moderate effect on the course of the disease[24,26]. In a comparative study of the 5-year survival of patients with PAN who were treated versus not treated with steroids, it was found that the survival rose from 13% to 48% in the treated group[19]. Moreover, a report by the Medical Research Council (1960) cites a 3-year survival rate in treated patients of 62%[27]. These findings are confirmed by a more recent study reporting a 5-year survival rate of 57%[28]. Two findings of this study can be highlighted: (1) arterial hypertension did not invariably carry an unfavorable prognosis, perhaps due to improved antihypertensive treatment, and (2) the first 3 months were the most critical for survival — 78% of deaths occurred in this period. Other authors[18,29,30] report 5-year survival rates of 55–59% in PAN patients treated with steroids.

The era of immunosuppressives

The successful use of cytotoxic regimens in severe systemic vasculitis was first established in Wegener's granulomatosis, a process that until then had a high mortality[31-34]. Later, the use of immunosuppressive treatment was tried in other severe systemic vasculitides including PAN[18,21,34,35]. Most authorities today consider cyclophosphamide as the drug of choice in severe and progressive PAN and in polyangiitis overlap syndrome, particularly steroid-resistant forms with involvement of medium-caliber arteries[36]. Although still not properly evaluated, apparently the early use of cyclophosphamide can notably ameliorate the gravity of the prognosis. Some authors[3,37] still propose azathioprine as the immunosuppressive agent of choice because of its efficacy and limited adverse effects, although in severe vasculitis it clearly lacks the efficacy of cyclophosphamide.

Other factors

The effectiveness of plasmapheresis, used in some patients with systemic vasculitis to eliminate circulating immune complexes, has not been evaluated because it is generally used as an adjunct to conventional treatment. In a prospective randomized study no significant difference was found in the survival rate of patients treated with plasmapheresis and steroids as compared to those treated with plasmapheresis, steroids, and cyclophosphamide[29,38].

Arterial hypertension, often resistant to treatment, is another factor of systemic visceral damage (kidneys, heart, CNS) that probably increases early morbidity and mortality. It is likely that modern antihypertensive regimens (ACE inhibitors, vasodilators, beta-blockers) have modified the less favorable prognosis associated with this disorder, including malignant forms[39].

Hemodialysis of patients with renal vasculitis and oliguria or chronic kidney failure has improved the prognosis of some patients, as has kidney transplantation[29,39].

A CRITICAL REVIEW OF PROGNOSIS IN THE LITERATURE: MORTALITY, IATROGENIC FACTORS, AND ECONOMIC COSTS

Mortality

The cause of death in PAN can be divided into four categories: (1) Death resulting directly from active vasculitis (early death pattern). Death is due to acute kidney failure or to progressive renal insufficiency with arterial hypertension; gastrointestinal complications, particularly perforation, intestinal infarction, or hemorrhage; peritonitis; pancreatitis; coronary arteritis with ischemic heart disease or heart failure; multisystemic vasculitis[18,29,40]. (2) "Late death pattern" with inactive vasculitis, e.g., chronic kidney failure, late complications of arterial hypertension[18,29,40]. (3) Complications of steroid and/or immunosuppressive treatment[21,28,40]. (4) Unrelated or intercurrent causes.

As for the cause of death determined by post-mortem study, kidney damage (vasculitis, glomerulonephritis, hypertensive changes), followed by CNS, and cardiac and gastrointestinal injury (intestinal infarction, gastrointestinal hemorrhage) are notable[2].

The mortality rate of PAN ranges from 26% to 53%[18,21,29,30]. The peak mortality rate occurs within the first 3-6 months after beginning treatment[19,28,40], and most deaths take place in the first 2 years[29,30].

In our own experience with the long-term follow-up of 32 patients with PAN, the survival rate declined in the first two years to 70%; after this initial drop, survival rates remained at 55% and 65% throughout follow-up. The 5-year overall survival rate was 60%[30] (Figure 1). These findings are similar to those of other authors[18,28,29] and, mathematically, reflect the fact that the majority of patients die in the first and second years after diagnosis, the survival rate then tending to level off. This is why classic idiopathic PAN is presently conceived as a "one-shot" disease[41,42]. Patients with PAN associated with hepatitis B virus infec-

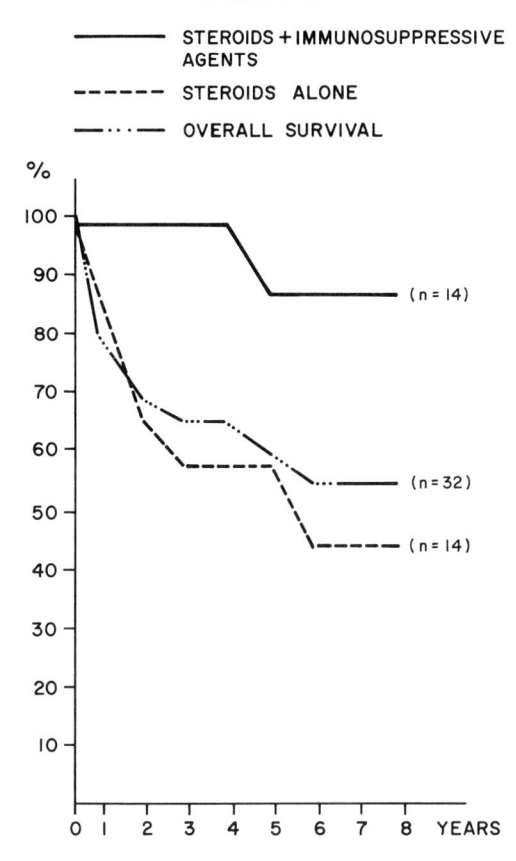

Figure 1 Actuarial probability of survival in 32 patients with systemic necrotizing vasculitis of the polyarteritis nodosa group. Survival by treatment groups

tion suffer a self-limited disease that can last months, and sometimes leaves chronic and consumptive sequelae. Once the initial episode has been overcome, recurrence of vasculitis is rare[35,41], in spite of the persistence of viral replication markers.

Some authors[43,44] consider the prognosis of Churg-Strauss' allergic and granulomatous angiitis to be more benign because hypertensive nephropathy is less common. It is also claimed that the incidence of life-threatening intestinal or abdominal hemorrhage is less because of a lower incidence of microaneurysms. Kidney disease is characteristically discrete, but renal hypertension occasionally can be severe. According to Fauci et al.[2] the clinical course and prognosis are similar to PAN. Likewise Scott et al.[40], studying patients with PAN and lung involvement, particularly asthma or pulmonary infiltrates, found no such favorable outcome and postulated an early mortality similar to that of classic PAN. Nonetheless, in our series of 16 patients with Churg-Strauss' angiitis, only 1 had a fatal course, in more than 10 years of follow-up[30]. Perhaps the most striking difference with respect to classic

PAN is a higher morbidity and mortality from heart disease (congestive heart failure, myocardial infarction) as compared to renal and gastrointestinal disease[45]. The frequency of vasculitis recurrence could also be higher in Churg-Strauss' angiitis[30].

In our experience — 16 patients prospectively followed up for 13 years — polyangiitis overlap syndrome had a 26% mortality rate. The main causes of death were kidney failure, intestinal infarction, and pulmonary vasculitis. The clinical behavior and prognostic indicators were thus similar to those of PAN[16].

Incapacity and physical suffering

In the systemic vasculitides, incapacity results from the residual effects of vasculitic episodes. The organic or visceral sequelae secondary to the acute inflammatory phase have not been described in detail. Many survivors have residual lesions and require continued treatment for the control of hypertension, heart failure, kidney failure, and neurologic alterations.

Peripheral neuropathy is the most common and most important incapacitating sequel of systemic vasculitis. Although at the onset the typical model is polyneuritis or mononeuritis multiplex, systemic vasculitis can also exhibit distal and symmetric polyneuropathy[46]. Peripheral neuropathy is the most intractable complication. CNS involvement is uncommon and late[47], and its clinical manifestations are polymorphic. The cerebral arteries in the carotid and vertebrobasilar systems can be affected. The residual neurologic morbidity is important (stroke, focal ischemic or hemorrhagic manifestations). Although cranial nerve neuropathy is rare, the eighth nerve can be damaged, producing deafness. The oculomotor nerves can also be affected[48].

The kidney is the organ most often affected in PAN[2].

Cardiac involvement in the form of primary vascular disease (coronary arteritis) can lead to chronic ischemic heart disease, sometimes exacerbated by arterial hypertension and disturbances of the cardiac conduction system[49]. Coronary vascular inflammation can mimic occlusive arteriosclerosis and can predispose to early atherosclerosis.

Liver disease, particularly when associated with HB_sAg, can be manifest as chronic active hepatitis that on occasion evolves into hepatic cirrhosis[35].

Travers et al.[41] have called attention to the frequency (41%) of functional respiratory alterations in PAN. In Churg-Strauss' angiitis and in the postvasculitis phase, important limitations can remain, such as chronic bronchial asthma or frequent recurrences of severe bronchospasm that are resistant to conventional treatment and are corticosteroid dependent[45].

Ocular vasculitis can be manifest by alterations in the visual field, loss of visual acuity, and transient or permanent unilateral amaurosis due to retinal ischemia or infarction[28,48,50]. Hypertensive changes are more common than ocular vasculitis and can improve in the long term with effective control of arterial hypertension.

Iatrogenic factors

Complications can appear with short- or long-term steroid and/or immunosuppressive treatment.

Among the many serious and well-known adverse effects of steroids, the most common problems are suppression of the hypothalamic-adrenal axis, which occurs even after modest doses. Cataracts and osteoporosis appear with prolonged daily drug treatments. Induction of hyperlipidemia, possibly complicated by atherosclerosis, and an enhanced propensity to certain infections, particularly bacterial sepsis, mycosis, and tuberculosis, should also be kept in mind. Serious opportunistic infections are frequent — particularly pneumonia and sepsis. Some adverse side-effects of steroid treatment specific to serious systemic vasculitis have been reported.

Cyclophosphamide produces both local and distant complications[36,51]. One must be particularly alert to:

(1) Bone marrow depression.
(2) Increased susceptibility to infection.
(3) Gonadal disorders.
(4) Carcinogenic potential.

Carcinogenesis may occur as a late complication of cyclophosphamide. Critical analysis of other conditions treated with immunosuppressives (e.g., kidney transplant, rheumatoid arthritis[52]) shows that the possibilities of neoplastic development are much higher than in the general population. However, in a 21-year period Fauci et al.[53] encountered only a single neoplasm — diffuse histiocytic lymphoma — in 85 patients with Wegener's granulomatosis. Nevertheless, we have observed solid tumors in three patients with SLE undergoing prolonged immunosuppressive treatment out of a series of 107 cases compiled since 1974[54]. These carcinogenic risks have not been sufficiently evaluated for systemic vasculitis and further studies are required[2].

(5) Lower urinary tract complications, such as hemorrhagic cystitis, telangiectases, and bladder wall fibrosis.
(6) Other possible effects. Alopecia is a minor problem.

At the onset of treatment there can be gastrointestinal symptoms — nausea and vomiting. A rare late complication is pulmonary fibrosis[55].

Economic costs

Albert et al.[56] have demonstrated that an aggressive strategy (repeated invasive procedures until a definite diagnosis is reached or available

%
           20   40   60   80   100

GLOBAL SURVIVAL

PERIPHERAL NEUROPATHY

RENAL

GASTRO INTESTINAL

HYPERTENSION

CARDIAC

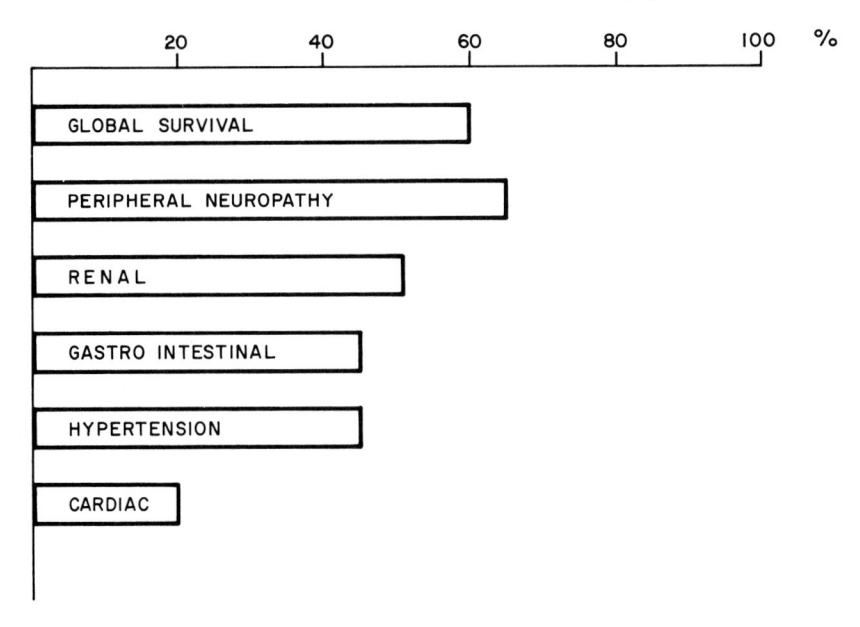

Figure 2 Estimated 5-year survival for five manifestations of systemic necrotizing vasculitis[30]

tests are exhausted) is no more sensitive or specific than a conservative strategy (a single biopsy procedure accompanied by an angiographic evaluation if necessary). The importance of this point is underlined by the fact that the aggressive approach is more expensive ($2986 per patient versus $1961) and has a higher incidence of morbidity (3.8 versus 2.7 days of hospitalization) per patient than the conservative strategy.

PAN also results in other health care and social costs. The mean hospital stay can be prolonged by occasional difficulties in establishing the diagnosis, resulting from overlapping or insidious forms of presentation, toxic syndromes, monomorphic forms, or prolonged fever.

The loss of workdays of active middle-aged adults over prolonged or repeated intervals, or sometimes permanently, carries a high social cost. With the exception of infrequent measures like plasmapheresis or hemodialysis, treatment with steroids or immunosuppressives, and complementary symptomatic medication, is not very expensive. Formal studies of the economic impact of the vasculitides are lacking.

CLINICAL MARKERS OF PROGNOSIS (FIGURE 2)

Age

Sack et al.[28] reported a higher mortality in older patients with PAN and Leib et al.[21] cited an age-dependent decline within the average survival of patients treated with either steroids or immunosuppressives. Guillevin et al.[29] noted that mortality was significantly higher in patients over 50 years than in younger patients; at 6 years the actuarial survival rates were 24% and 60% respectively.

Nephropathy

Up to 70% of PAN cases show functional renal disturbance. Nephropathy (renal vasculitis, hypertensive changes, glomerulonephritis) is an important marker of prognosis, and kidney failure is responsible for almost half of the deaths[2]. Rapidly progressive necrotizing glomerulonephritis can present with hypertension and kidney failure. Spontaneous rupture of aneurysms of the renal vessels can produce peritoneal hemorrhage or perirenal hematoma. In our PAN series without nephropathy the 5-year survival was 100% versus 51% when nephropathy was present. Similar results have been obtained by other authors[19,29,57]. On the other hand, it has been noted that the initial presence of alterations in the urinary sediment or proteinuria without raised serum creatinine are not predictive of a poorer prognosis[18]. Renal damage, particularly when accompanied by uremia, is thus an important clinical indicator of poor prognosis.

The predictive value of renal histologic findings in the evolution of PAN is little known. In our experience, poor prognosis was associated more often with the gross intrarenal vascular alterations (thrombosis, stenosis, luminal irregularities, aneurysms) of PAN.

While necrotizing glomerulonephritis has traditionally been considered a severe form of kidney disease with progressive clinical course, microscopic polyarteritis and focal necrotizing glomerulonephritis have had better prognosis with survival rates of up to 65% at 5 years[57,59]. In the study of Furlong et al.[60] although early treatment reduced mortality rate, there was still a 30% mortality at 2 years of follow-up. While crescentic glomerulonephritis (extracapillary proliferation with crescent formation) is usually idiopathic, several authors have associated it with systemic vasculitis. However, it has not been established whether these two entities are distinct subgroups requiring different treatments and having a different prognosis[61].

Arterial hypertension

Hypertension, present in more than half of the cases (54%), can persist after active vascular inflammation and contribute to chronic deterioration of kidney function. Diffuse renal vasculitis is a well-known cause of hypertension but its effect on survival studies is uncertain[18,28]. Control of hypertension has improved and older data probably need revising.

CNS involvement

CNS vasculitis occurs in 20-40% of cases of PAN. It has been described as the second cause (after kidney disease) of fatal complications, particularly late mortality from stroke[2]. In our experience, CNS involvement — with focal and diffuse defects in cerebral function — was an indicator of poor prognosis, being present significantly more often in the group of patients who died. However, in other studies[28,29] clinical CNS involvement did not significantly influence survival.

Peripheral nervous system

Involvement of peripheral nerves, while common and often a cause of severe disability, is not a major contributor to mortality[18-20].

Liver disease

In our experience, liver involvement (hepatic arteritis, chronic active hepatitis, liver cirrhosis) was more frequent among patients who died than among survivors[21]. These findings have not been recognized in other systemic vasculitis follow-up studies[28,29,62].

Heart disease

Cardiac involvement (coronary vasculitis, ischemic heart disease, congestive heart failure, arrhythmias, nonvalvular and nonatherosclerotic cardiomyopathy, pericarditis) is clinically apparent in a third of patients. However, in post-mortem studies the heart is damaged in up to two-thirds of cases[2]. This finding suggests that the presence of heart disease in systemic vasculitis indicates a poorer prognosis, as has been recognized in PAN. Heart disease is the second cause, after nephropathy, of fatal outcome[29,40,43]. We have found that mortality from cardiac damage secondary to vasculitis declines progressively from the first (60%) to the fifth year of survival (20%)[30].

Gastrointestinal involvement

PAN affects the gastrointestinal system in 44% of patients[2]. The clinical spectrum is varied, ranging from nonthreatening symptoms (nausea, vomiting, diarrhea, nonspecific abdominal pain) to potentially catastrophic manifestations, such as hemorrhage, obstruction, perforation, intestinal infarction, and ruptured mesenteric aneurysms with retroperitoneal hemorrhage and hypovolemic shock[18,29,63].

Clinical markers of prognosis in the polyangiitis overlap syndrome

The course and prognostic markers of polyangiitis overlap syndrome are similar to those of PAN. As in classic systemic vasculitis, nephropathy with uremia, intestinal infarction, and stroke are clinical markers of a poor prognosis[16]. Since skin involvement (hypersensitivity vasculitis) is frequent in polyangiitis overlap syndrome (63% in our experience, higher than that of nephropathy; 93% in the series of Leavitt and Fauci[14]), it is important to recognize it as a distinct entity. It has different prognostic connotations (potentially irreversible organ damage or death) from isolated to localized cutaneous vasculitis[14-16].

Clinical markers of prognosis in Churg-Strauss' angiitis

Churg-Strauss' allergic and granulomatous angiitis usually responds quickly, and sometimes dramatically, to steroids and immunosuppressives. It has been considered more benign than other systemic vasculitides, with a more discrete renal involvement than classic PAN[43,44]. Perhaps the most striking difference from other systemic vasculitides is the prominence of heart disease[45]. Cardiopulmonary complications account for more than half of the deaths, unlike the case of classic PAN, in which kidney disease predominates[45]. Many authors[2,29,40,45] consider that Churg-Strauss' angiitis belongs to the PAN group with a clinical course and global prognosis similar to that of classic PAN.

Biologic and immunologic indicators of prognosis

Biologic parameters

A poorer prognosis has been associated with the presence of anemia and azotemia[30,40], functional liver disorders[40], rheumatoid factor[28], and acute-phase reactants[30]. However, in other studies[39,62] laboratory findings did not affect any aspect of prognosis or influence survival.

Immunologic parameters

Disturbances in the immunologic profile (hyperimmunoglobulinemia, decreased complement factors, presence of circulating immune complexes) in the acute phase of disease are of no value as modulators or indicators of prognosis[3,18,30]. As for serologic markers of HBV, the clinical course and response to treatment of patients with HB_sAg positive PAN do not differ from those who are HB_sAg negative[35]. No significant difference has been found in the 5-year survival of HB_sAg negative PAN patients[17,29,30]. In the series of Sergent et al.[35] of 9 patients with HB_sAg positive PAN, none of the 6 who achieved a prolonged remission had recurrence of vasculitis, in spite of discontinuing treatment.

Although the presence of HBV does not clearly identify a specific clinical profile in this population of patients, we have noted a higher frequency of hepatic involvement, heart disease, joint disease, peripheral neuropathy, and hypertension, and a lower frequency of pleuropulmonary involvement[65].

The long-term prognosis of patients with PAN associated with HBV is unknown. There are no data on the frequency of chronic active hepatitis or evolution of liver cirrhosis in the postvasculitic phase[29].

Antineutrophil cytoplasmic antibody has been found to be a specific and sensitive test for Wegener's granulomatosis but its value as a prognostic marker is still to be defined.

Angiographic alterations as prognostic markers

Visceral angiography can identify PAN patients with a potentially more severe form of disease and poorer prognosis, by demonstrating multiple aneurysms, which carry the risk of mortality from rupture. However, the presence or absence of aneurysms per se is not a predictor of poor prognosis[30]. It has been suggested that regression of aneurysms with treatment is a favorable prognostic development (Figure 3). In several studies[30,66,67], improvement of the angiographic picture paralleled clinical improvement. Some authors[68,69] consider that aneurysmal regression lacks clinical importance and merely represents the natural histologic evolution of the disease to thrombosis or sclerosis.

TYPE OF TREATMENT AND COURSE

Leib et al.[21] and Scott et al.[40] found a significant difference in the pattern of survival in patients with PAN who were treated with corticosteroids and immunosuppressives versus those treated with steroids alone. We found that the combination of steroids and cyclophosphamide produced a 5-year survival of 100% with a later survival of 85%. In contrast, patients treated with corticosteroids alone had a high mortality in the first 2 years, after which survival declined to 65%, reaching 57% at 5 years (Figure 1). In both groups the presence or absence of nephropathy, hypertension, nervous system alterations, gastrointestinal manifestations, and heart disease were randomly distributed[30]. However, Cohen et al.[18], in an actuarial analysis of a patient population (36 cases) treated with corticosteroids alone and another treated with steroids and immunosuppressives, found no significant difference.

All these studies have the drawback of being retrospective. Guillevin et al.[29] studied the random addition of cyclophosphamide in the group of patients with PAN treated with prednisone or plasmapheresis. In order to compare survival curves, 87 cases were treated with one of two regimens: corticosteroids alone (65 patients), or cyclophosphamide and

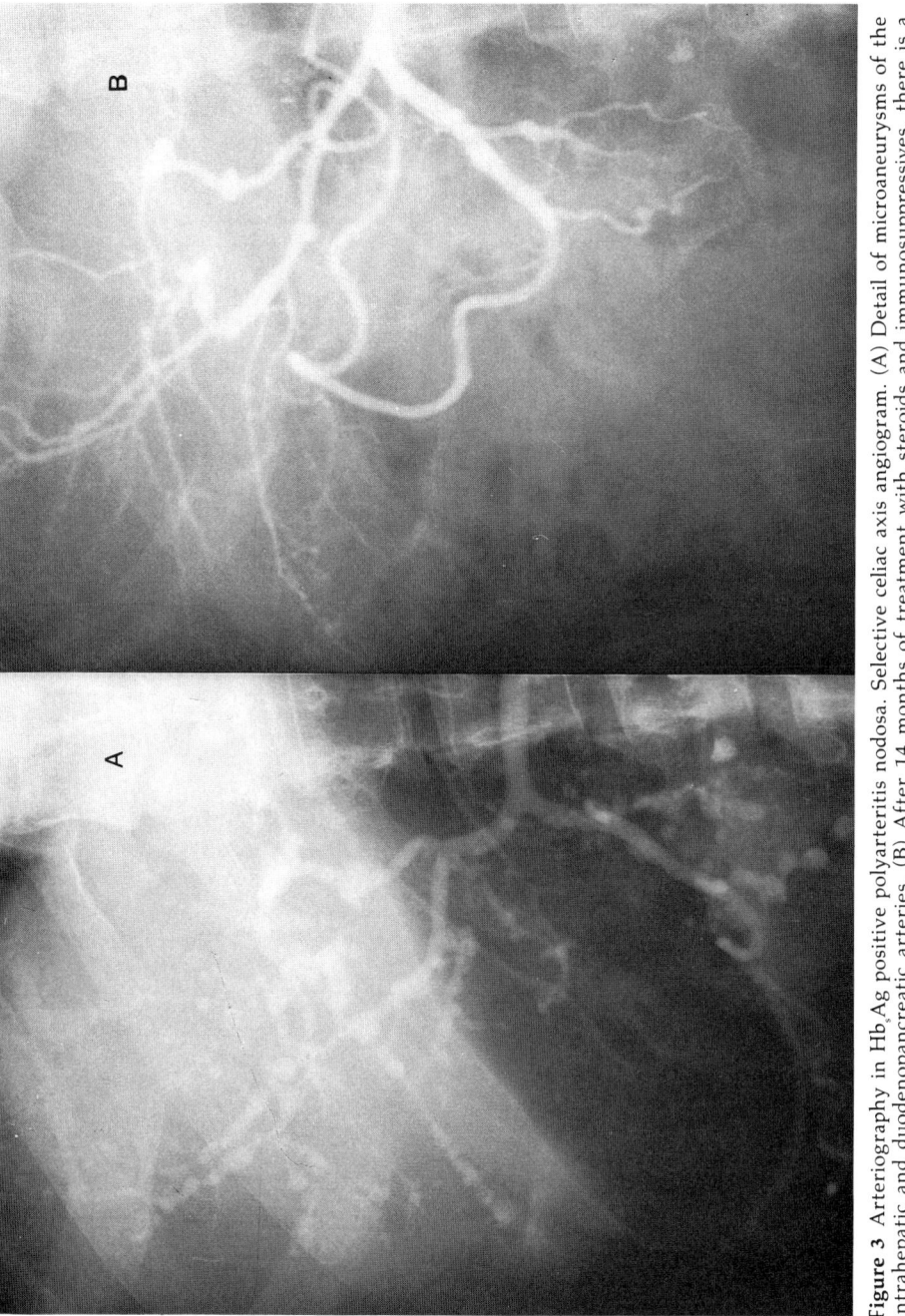

Figure 3 Arteriography in Hb$_s$Ag positive polyarteritis nodosa. Selective celiac axis angiogram. (A) Detail of microaneurysms of the intrahepatic and duodenopancreatic arteries. (B) After 14 months of treatment with steroids and immunosuppressives, there is a notable reduction in the number and size of microaneurysms.

corticosteroids (22 patients). At 5 years there was no statistically significant difference between the two groups of patients. The addition of plasmapheresis produced no difference in mortality.

Most clinicians now recommend combined treatment with methylprednisolone and cyclophosphamide, in the form of either oral administration or an intravenous bolus[42].

FUTURE PERSPECTIVE

In spite of the value of cyclophosphamide, less-toxic alternatives would be welcome. It is likely that some vasculitides might respond similarly to less-toxic agents. Only randomized studies will resolve this question[72].

Recently, the existence of circulating antineutrophil antibodies has been recognized in systemic vasculitis (Wegener's granulomatosis and polyarteritis nodosa). It is not clear whether these antibodies are causative, or a consequence of an as yet unknown epiphenomenon of vascular injury, but a cross-reaction has been observed with endothelial cell determinant antigens and a direct attack on the endothelial cell has been postulated[72].

As long as the etiopathogenesis of systemic vasculitis remains unknown, research programs cannot overlook nonimmunologic mechanisms such as the effects of free oxygen radicals or cellular factors on the probable target organ, the endothelial cell. Together with viral infections, these are alternatives that could be important in the vasculitides[73].

New findings could lead to new treatments that might modify the evolution of the vasculitides. For example, monoclonal antibodies could be used eventually to modulate the role of the endothelial cell in the pathogenesis of vasculitis[74].

References

1. Fauci, A. S., Haynes, B. F. and Kayz, P. (1978). The spectrum of vasculitis. Clinical, pathologic, and therapeutic considerations. *Ann. Intern. Med.*, **89**, 660–676
2. Cupps, T. R. and Fauci, A. S. (1981). Systemic necrotizing vasculitis of the polyarteritis nodosa group. In Smith, L. H. (ed.) *The Vasculitides*, pp. 26–49. (Philadelphia: W. B. Saunders)
3. Fan, P. T., Davis, J. A., Somer, T., Kaplan, L. and Bluestone, R. (1980). A clinical approach to systemic vasculitis. *Semin. Arthritis Rheum.*, **9**, 248–304
4. Paronetto, F. (1976). Systemic nonsuppurative necrotizing angiitis. In Miescher, P. A. and Müller-Eberhard, H. J. (eds.) *Textbook of Immunopathology*, pp. 1012–1024. (New York: Grune & Stratton)
5. Zvaifler, N. J. (1978). Vasculitides: classification and pathogenesis. *Aust. N.Z. J. Med.*, **8**(suppl. 1), 134–8
6. Christian, C. L. and Sergent, S. S. (1976). Vasculitis syndromes: clinical and experimental models. *Am. J. Med.*, **61**, 385–392
7. Duffy, J., Lidsky, M. D., Sharp, J. T., Davis, J. S., Person, D. A., Hollinger, F. B. and Min, K. (1976). Polyarthritis, polyarteritis and hepatitis B. *Medicine*, **55**, 19–37
8. Christian, C. L. (1984). Vasculitis: genus and species. *Ann. Intern. Med.*, **101**, 862–3

9. Alarcón-Segovia, D. (1977). The necrotizing vasculitides. A new pathogenetic classification. *Med. Clin. North Am.*, **61**, 241-259
10. Lockshin, M. D. (1979). Vasculitis. *Bull. N.Y. Acad. Med.*, **55**, 867-73
11. Fauci, A. S. (1979). Vasculitis. *Am. J. Med.*, **67**, 916
12. Cupps, T. R. and Fauci, A. S. (1982). The vasculitis syndrome. *Adv. Intern. Med.*, **27**, 315-344
13. Fauci, A. S. (1983). Vasculitis. *Allergy Clin. Immunol.*, **72**, 211-228
14. Leavitt, R. Y. and Fauci, A. S. (1986). Polyangiitis overlap syndrome. Classification and prospective clinical experience. *Am. J. Med.*, **81**, 79-85
15. Leavitt, R. Y. and Fauci, A. S. (1986). Pulmonary vasculitis. *Am. Rev. Respir. Dis.*, **134**, 149-166
16. Barbado, F. J., Vázquez, J. J., Mostaza, J. M., Fernández-Martín, J., Peña, J. M., Gil, A., Picazo, M. L., Gutiérrez, M. and Ortiz-Vázquez, J. (1988). Síndrome poliangeítico de solapamiento: un nuevo síndrome o más confusión? *An. Med. Intern. (Madrid)*, **5**, 603-10
17. Godeau, P. and Guillevin, L. (1982). Périartérite noueuse systémique. In Khan, M. F. and Peltier, A. P. (eds.) *Maladies Dites Systémiques*, pp. 414-445. (Paris: Flammarion Médecin-Sciences)
18. Cohen, R. D., Conn, D. L. and Ilstrup, D. M. (1980). Clinical features, prognosis, and response to treatment in polyarteritis. *Mayo Clin. Proc.*, **55**, 146-155
19. Frohnert, P. P. and Sheps, S. G. (1967). Long-term follow-up of periarteritis. *Am. J. Med.*, **43**, 8-14
20. Fauci, A. S. (1987). The vasculitis syndromes. In *Harrison's Principles of Internal Medicine*, 11th edn, pp. 1438-1445. (New York: McGraw-Hill)
21. Leib, E. S., Restivo, C. and Paulus, H. E. (1979). Immunosuppressive and corticosteroid therapy of polyarteritis nodosa. *Am. J. Med.*, **67**, 941-947
22. Rose, G. A. (1957). The natural history of polyarteritis. *Br. Med. J.*, **2**, 1148-1152
23. Rose, G. A. and Spencer, H. (1957). Polyarteritis nodosa. *Q. J. Med.*, **26**, 43-81
24. Baggenstoss, A. H., Schick, R. M. and Polley, H. F. (1951). The effect of cortisone on the lesions of periarteritis nodosa. *Am. J. Pathol.*, **27**, 537-559
25. Goldman, R., Adams, W. S. and Back, W. S. (1950). The effect of ACTH on one case of polyarteritis nodosa. *Proceedings of the 1st Clinical ACTH Conference*, p. 467. (Philadelphia: Balckiston)
26. Mundy, W. L., Walker, W. G., Bickerman, H. A. and Beck, G. J. (1951). Periarteritis nodosa: report of a case treated with ACTH and cortisone. *Am. J. Med.*, **11**, 630-637
27. Medical Research Council (1960). Treatment of polyarteritis nodosa with cortisone: results after three years. *Br. Med. J.*, **1**, 1399-1400
28. Sack, M., Cassidy, J. T. and Bole, G. G. (1975). Prognostic factors in polyarteritis. *J. Rheumatol.*, **2**, 4111-4120
29. Guillevin, L., Le Thi Huong Du, P., Godeau, P., Jaiis, P. and Wechsler, B. (1988). Clinical findings and prognosis of polyarteritis nodosa and Churg-Strauss angiitis: a study in 165 patients. *Br. J. Rheumatol.*, **27**, 258-264
30. Barbado, F. J. (1984). Vasculitis necrotizante sistémica tipo poliarteritis nodosa. Esturdio de los marcadores de pronóstico. Doctoral thesis, Universidad Autónoma de Madrid
31. Melam, H. and Patterson, R. (1971). Periarteritis nodosa: a remission achieved with combined prednisone and azathioprine therapy. *Am. J. Dis. Child.*, **121**, 424-427
32. Turpin, J., Loussounarn, J. and Vivien, P. (1971). Sur un cas de périartérite noueuse traiteé pendant trois ans par immunodépresseurs. *Therapie*, **26**, 149
33. Fauci, A. S. and Wolff, S. M. (1973). Wegener's granulomatosis: studies in eighteen patients and a review of the literature. *Medicine*, **52**, 535-561
34. Fauci, A. S., Katz, P., Haynes, B. F. and Wolff, S. H. (1979). Cyclophosphamide therapy of severe systemic necrotizing vasculitis. *N. Engl. J. Med.*, **301**, 235-238
35. Sergent, J. S., Lockshin, M. L., Christian, C. L. and Gocke, D. T. (1976). Vasculitis with hepatitis B antigenemia. Long-term observations in nine patients. *Medicine*, **55**, 1-18
36. Kovarsky, J. (1983). Clinical pharmacology and toxicology of cyclophosphamide: emphasis on use in rheumatic diseases. *Semin. Arthritis Rheum.*, **12**, 359-371

37. Pirofsky, B. and Bardana, E. J. (1977). Immunosuppressive therapy in rheumatic diseases. *Med. Clin. North Am.*, **61**, 419–437
38. Guillevin, L., Le Thi Huong D, P., Bussel, A., Leon, A., Raviart, M., Gie, S. Ang, K. S., Hubert, D., Quaranta, J. F. and Godeau, P. (1985). Treatment of polyarteritis nodosa with plasma exchange: a randomized trial in 69 patients. *Plasma Ther. Transfus. Technol.*, **6**, 483–485
39. Cohen, L., Guillevin, L., Meyrier, A., Bironne, P., Blétry, O, and Godeau, P. (1986). L'hypertension artérielle maligne de la périartérite noueuse. *Arch. Mal. Coeur*, **6**, 773–778
40. Scott, D. G.-I., Bacon, P. A., Elliot, P. J., Tribe, C. P. and Wallington, T. B. (1982). Systemic vasculitis in a District General Hospital 1972–1980: clinical and laboratory features. Classification and prognosis of 80 cases. *Q. J. Med.*, **203**, 292–311
41. Travers, R. L., Allison, D. J., Brettle, R. P. and Hughes, G. R. V. (1979). Polyarteritis nodosa: a clinical and angiographic analysis of 17 cases. *Semin. Arthritis Rheum.*, **8**, 184–199
42. Hughes, G. R. V. (1987). Polyarteritis. In Hughes, G. R. V. (ed.) *Connective Tissue Diseases*, 3rd edn., pp. 200–218. (Oxford: Blackwell Scientific Publications)
43. Vertztman, L. (1980). Polyarteritis nodosa. In Alarcón-Segovia, D. A. (ed.) *Clinics in Rheumatic Disease. Necrotizing Vasculitides*, pp. 279–317. (Philadelphia: W. B. Saunders)
44. Chumbley, L. C., Harrison, E. G. and De Remee, R. A. (1977). Allergic granulomatosis and angiitis (Churg-Strauss). Report and analysis of 30 cases. *Mayo Clin. Proc.*, **52**, 447–484
45. Lanham, J. G., Keith, B. E., Pusey, C. D. and Hughes, G. R. V. (1984). Systemic vasculitis with asthma and eosinophilia: a clinical approach to the Churg-Strauss syndrome. *Medicine*, **63**, 65–81
46. Cruz Martínez, A., Barbado, F. J., Ferrer, M. T., Vázquez, J. J., Pérez Conde, M. C. and Gil, A. (1988). Electrophysiological study in systemic necrotizing vasculitis of the polyarteritis nodosa group. *Electromyogr. Clin. Neurophysiol.*, **28**, 167–173
47. Moore, P. M. and Fauci, A. S. (1981). Neurologic manifestations of systemic vasculitis. A retrospective and prospective study of the clinicopathologic features and responses to therapy in 25 patients. *Am. J. Med.*, **71**, 515–524
48. Ford, R. G. and Siekert, R. G. (1965). Central nervous system manifestations of periarteritis nodosa. *Neurology*, **15**, 114–122
49. Parrillo, J. E. and Fauci, A. S. (1980). Necrotizing vasculitis, coronary angiitis and cardiologist. *Am. Heart J.*, **99**, 547–554
50. Manjiani, M. R. (1967). Ocular manifestations of polyarteritis nodosa. *Br. J. Ophthalmol*, **51**, 696–701
51. Clements, P. J. and Davis, J. (1986). Cytotoxic drugs: their clinical application to the rheumatic diseases. *Semin. Arthritis Rheum.*, **4**, 231–254
52. Baker, G. L., Kahl, L. E., Zee, B. E., Stolzer, B. L., Agarwal, A. K. and Medsger, T. A. (1987). Malignancy following treatment of rheumatoid arthritis with cyclophosphamide. Long-term case-control follow-up study. *Am. J. Med.*, **83**, 1–9
53. Fauci, A. S., Haynes, B. F., Katz, P. and Wolff, S. M. (1983). Wegener's granulomatosis: prospective clinical and therapeutic experience with 85 patients for 21 years. *Ann. Intern. Med.*, **98**, 76–85
54. López, J. M., Sendino, A., Barbado, F. J., Gil, A., Valencia, M. E., Mostaza, J. M., Lavilla, P., Pintado, V. and Vázquez, J. J. (1988). Tumores sólidos en pacientes con lupus eritematoso en tratamiento inmunosupresor prolongado. *An. Med. Intern. (Madrid)* (Suppl. 3), 88
55. Weiss, R. B. and Muggia, F. M. (1980). Cytotoxic drug-induced pulmonary disease: update 1980. *Am. J. Med.*, **68**, 259–266
56. Albert, D. A., Rimon, D. and Silverstein, M. D. (1988). The diagnosis of polyarteritis nodosa. I. A literature based decision analysis approach. *Arthritis Rheum.*, **31**, 1117–1127
57. Serra, A., Cameron, J. S., Turner, D. R., Hartley, B., Ogg, C. S., Neild, G. H, Williams, D. G., Taube, D., Brown, C. B. and Hicks, J. A. (1984). Vasculitis affecting the kidney: presentation, histopathology and long-term outcome. *Q. J. Med.*, **210**, 181–207

58. Savage, C. O. S., Winearls, C. G., Evans, D. J., Rees, A. J. and Lockwood, C. M. (1985). Microscopic polyarteritis: presentation, pathology and prognosis. *Q. J. Med.*, **220**, 467-483
59. Coward, R. A., Hamdy, N. A. T., Shortland, J. S. and Brown, C. B. (1986). Renal micropolyarteritis, a treatable condition. *Nephrol. Dial. Transplant.*, **1**, 31-37
60. Furlong, T. J., Ibels, L. S. and Eckstein, R. P. (1987). The clinical spectrum of necrotizing glomerulonephritis. *Medicine*, **66**, 192-201
61. Velosa, J. A. (1987). Idiopathic crescentic glomerulonephritis or systemic vasculitis? *Mayo Clin. Proc.*, **62**, 145-147
62. Le Thi Huong, D., Guillevin, L., Godeau, P., Jais, J., Wechsler, B., Bletry, O., Piete, J. C. and Herson, S. (1985). Facteurs pronostiques de la périartérite nouese et de lángéite de Churg et Strauss. *Presse Médicale*, **14**, 1341
63. Camilleri, M., Pusey, C. D., Chadwick, V. S. and Res, A. J. (1983). Gastrointestinal manifestations of systemic vasculitis. *Q. J. Med.*, **206**, 141-149
64. Cupps, T. R. and Fauci, A. S. (1982). The vasculitis syndromes. *Adv. Intern. Med.*, **27**, 315-344
65. Ferrer, J., Barbado, F. J., Seone, G. J. and Vázquez, J. J. (1981). Vasculitis associated with hepatitis Bs antigen. *Mayo Clin. Proc.*, **56**, 136
66. Fauci, A. S., Doppman, J. L. and Wolff, S. M. (1978). Cyclophosphamide-induced remissions in advanced polyarteritis nodosa. *Am. J. Med.*, **64**, 890-894
67. Vázquez, J. J., San Martín, P., Barbado, F. J., Gil, A., Guerra, J., Arnalich, F., García Puig, J. and Sánchez Mejías, F. (1981). Angiographic findings in systemic necrotizing vasculitis. *Angiology*, **32**, 773-779
68. Robins, J. M. and Bookstein, J. J. (1972). Regressing aneurysms in periarteritis nodosa. *Radiology*, **104**, 39-42
69. Leonhardt, E. T. G., Jakobson, H. and Ringqvist, O. T. A. (1972). Angiographic and clinico-physiologic investigation of a case of polyarteritis nodosa. *Am. J. Med.*, **53**, 246-256
70. Guillevin, L. (1982). Utilización de la terapeútica inmunosupresora en el tratamiento de la periarteritis nodosa. *Nouv. Presse Med.* (Spanish edn.), **1**, 587
71. Steinberg, A. D. (1984). Cyclophosphamide: should it be used daily, monthly, or never? *N. Engl. J. Med.*, **310**, 458-459
72. Lockwood, C. M., Jones, S., Moss, D. W., Bakes, D., Whitaker, K. B. and Savage, C. O. (1987). Association of alkaline phosphatase with an autoantigen recognised by circulating antineutrophil antibodies in systemic vasculitis. *Lancet*, **1**, 716-720
73. Anonymous (1985). Vasculitis sistémica. *Lancet* (Spanish edn.), **7**, 263-264
74. Bacon, P. A. (1985). Evolving concepts in vasculitis. *Q. J. Med.*, **222**, 609-610

13
Polymyalgia rheumatica and giant cell arteritis

L. A. HEALEY

The prognosis of polymyalgia rheumatica can be described as excellent. Patients respond promptly to prednisone and, with rare exceptions, the disease can be suppressed with a small, safe dose of 5 mg a day. While it may be necessary to continue this medication for years, the natural history is one of eventual remission without residual joint damage.

Since most reported series of polymyalgia date from the steroid era, there is little information on the course of untreated disease. In one of the early papers, Bagratuni in 1963 reported 50 patients with "anarthritic rheumatoid disease" who were treated with aspirin from 1945 to 1961. They ranged in age from 19 to 78 so not all of them could be considered to represent polymyalgia. Remission occurred in 15, and 31 improved greatly. The mean duration of symptoms was 7 years[1].

While polymyalgia rheumatica itself is a benign self-limited illness, its possible association with other diagnoses bears on the question of eventual prognosis. The most obvious is the appearance of giant cell arteritis. How frequently does it occur? Is polymyalgia always a manifestation of giant cell arthritis? In addition, there have been speculations that polymyalgia might be a manifestation of an occult malignancy, or that it may be the prodrome of rheumatoid arthritis. A number of long-term reports are now available to provide answers to these questions and will be cited. My own observations on patients with polymyalgia rheumatica followed for as long as 18 years have not yet been published but will also be referred to. The prognosis will be considered in three respects: polymyalgia rheumatica alone; its possible association with rheumatoid arthritis; and, finally, its relation to giant cell arteritis.

POLYMYALGIA RHEUMATICA

Polymyalgia rheumatica has been defined as a syndrome of pain and stiffness of the neck, shoulders, and pelvic girdle in older patients who show little in the way of physical findings. It was initially identified by a very rapid sedimentation rate. Experience soon showed that the rapid response to prednisone was so invariable that this became a helpful aid in confirming the diagnosis. The cause of symptoms was not initially evident but synovitis has been demonstrated by arthroscopy and biopsy of shoulder joints[2,3]. This finding has several important consequences. It explains why patients with polymyalgia have pronounced morning stiffness as a characteristic symptom. It helps to separate polymyalgia from the diffuse pains associated with occult malignancy that are not due to synovial inflammation and lack this characteristic symptom of stiffness. It confirms that polymyalgia can exist without an elevated sedimentation rate. In fact, there are a significant number of such patients who have pain, stiffness, and characteristic response to steroid in the face of normal sedimentation rates. Finally, as will be discussed, it helps to explain the possible relation to rheumatoid arthritis.

The question of polymyalgia as a symptom of an occult malignancy can be dismissed. Von Knorring and Somer[4] followed 45 patients of their own and reviewed nine reported series for a total of 568 patients. There were 20 patients with malignant neoplasms, a number that is not greater than that to be anticipated in this age group. Subsequent experiences by others have confirmed the conclusion that polymyalgia is not associated with cancer[5,6]. The suspicion of this association arose from initial misdiagnosis of the malaise, musculoskeletal pain, and elevated sedimentation rate associated with the malignant disease as symptoms of polymyalgia rheumatica. Such patients with cancer can be distinguished from those with polymyalgia since they do not have the profound morning stiffness and they also do not show the prompt steroid response.

Most of the early reports suggested that polymyalgia was a self-limited disease requiring steroid treatment for perhaps 1-2 years before remitting[7]. Subsequent studies with longer follow-up reflected the more chronic nature of the synovial inflammation, the need for longer steroid treatment, and the frequency of relapse[8,9].

Kyle and Hazelman have reviewed the published reports[10]. While recognizing the difficulty in interpretation because of varying length of follow-up, the limits of retrospective studies and the different percentages of patients with and without giant cell arteritis, they concluded that patients should expect treatment for at least 2 years and that most can be off steroid after 5 years, although a few may need to continue it indefinitely. Von Knorring followed 53 patients for 10 years[11]. Steroid treatment was stopped in 19 patients after 1-4 years (mean 16 months) and continued in 34 for up to 9 years (mean 3 years). Of these 34 patients, 20 experienced relapses when trying to stop prednisone.

A report from the Mayo Clinic[5] described 96 patients who were followed for a mean duration of 4.5 years. During the period of observation, 83 achieved remission. Recurrences were uncommon, being noted only in four patients after intervals of 3 months to 4 years. Thirty-nine patients were treated with aspirin or nonsteroidal anti-inflammatory drugs (NSAIDs); 54 received steroid, 37 of them having initially received NSAIDs. Steroid-treated patients responded more rapidly but the duration of illness was shorter in the NSAID-treated patients (a median of 8 months versus 17 months). However, the authors decided that, based on lower initial sedimentation rates and clinical picture, this difference was probably more a reflection of milder disease than of a drug effect.

Of 246 of my own patients with polymyalgia followed for as long as 16 years (mean follow-up 5.2 years), only 76 (30%) were able to stop the prednisone within 2 years[6]. Additional patients were able to discontinue prednisone each subsequent year, although a few found it necessary to continue for at least 15 years. Most patients preferred not to continue prednisone because of the well-known risks and made repeated attempts to stop, experiencing a recurrence of pain and stiffness as frequently as on four different occasions. Even if prolonged treatment was required, low doses of prednisone continued to suppress inflammation and relieve symptoms. There was no evidence of joint damage. Neither the initial sedimentation rate, severity of symptoms, nor presence of temporal arteritis were predictors of the duration of disease.

Ayoub and co-workers treated 75 patients with an initially favorable response[12]. Prednisone was continued for 1-2 years in 59 patients, for 2-3 years in 35, for longer than 3 years in 20, and for 4 or more years in 12. Relapses were frequent as the dose was tapered but patients responded when it was raised again. Thirteen of 37 had a recurrence when prednisone was stopped. The authors interpret their findings as suggesting a bimodal distribution indicating two separate patient populations, one with self-limited and one with persistent disease. They found a similar distribution in two other reports[5,11] with a duration of 14-16 months for self-limited disease and 36-40 months for prolonged disease.

This concept of bimodal distribution may not be correct, since the frequency of recurrence increases with the duration of follow-up. For example, in my unpublished study of patients followed for as long as 18 years, 39 of 98 patients with polymyalgia experienced a recurrence. The interval during which patients remained free of symptoms and off prednisone could be as long as 7 years. Most reported studies have a shorter period of observation and such patients might erroneously be included in the first half of a bimodal curve. Recurrences tended to be less severe than the original episode, often were not accompanied by an elevated sedimentation rate, and once again responded very well to small doses of prednisone.

Symptoms in a recurrence were often similar to the initial episode, with pain and stiffness of shoulders and hips. However, at times, the relapse was not like the original episode but involved joints such as wrists, hands, or knees and resembled rheumatoid arthritis. Of 39 patients with polymyalgia who relapsed, 24 again had polymyalgia, whereas 15 had an episode suggestive of rheumatoid arthritis. Four patients, who saw a different rheumatologist for each episode, were diagnosed as polymyalgia on one occasion and as seronegative rheumatoid arthritis on another. Nonsteroidal drugs given for the diagnosis of rheumatoid arthritis were minimally effective and prednisone again produced an excellent result. Patients such as these lead to a discussion of the second category — polymyalgia as a possible prodrome of rheumatoid arthritis.

POLYMYALGIA RHEUMATICA AND RHEUMATOID ARTHRITIS

Most reports with a long follow-up period include a number of patients who at some time in their course show peripheral synovitis. Hamrin in Sweden[13] found swelling of the hands in 25 of 98 patients. A polyarthritis was noted by Ayoub[12] in 13 of 76, and in 16 of 42 patients followed for 5 years in an Italian city[14]. Myles followed 84 patients for 7 years and the initial diagnosis of polymyalgia rheumatica was considered to be incorrect in 5 when they developed polyarthritis[15]. In the Mayo Clinic series[5], synovitis was noted in 27 of 96, and 17 of them had symmetric arthritis that met the criteria for rheumatoid arthritis. In six patients, it predated the appearance of the polymyalgia, while in 11 it occurred from 1 month to 9 years later. This frequency suggested to the authors a strong association with a "rheumatoid arthritis-like process" but no association with definite seropositive rheumatoid arthritis which was noted in only three patients, a frequency that would be expected statistically by chance alone.

In my experience, synovitis is encountered frequently, either at the onset or in subsequent recurrences, and was noted in 77 of the 246 patients reported in 1984[6]. Some of my patients have also had a course as described in the Mayo Clinic series, with symmetric synovitis of wrists and hands at the outset and a picture of polymyalgia in a recurrence. Kyle et al. thought synovitis to be uncommon; noting it in 5 of 56 patients but the mean follow-up period was only 16 months[16].

A review of the American Rheumatism Association criteria for the diagnosis of rheumatoid arthritis[17] reveals that a patient with symmetric synovitis of wrists and hands meets the requirements for the diagnosis. A comparative study of patients whose arthritis began after age 60 indicated significant differences between those with seropositive and seronegative disease[18]. Both had frequent involvement of wrists and metacarpophalangeal joints as might be expected, since these are essential for the diagnosis, but the seronegative group had more frequent involvement of the shoulders, rare involvement of the metatarsal phalangeal joints, and an excellent response to prednisone. The two groups also had differing immune-response gene frequency patterns[19].

Thus, there appears to be a benign synovitis in older patients that might present as polymyalgia rheumatica if shoulders and hips are involved or as rheumatoid arthritis if there is swelling of wrists and metacarpophalangeal joints. This would provide an explanation for the earlier observations that polymyalgia is a precursor of rheumatoid arthritis. Both types respond well to prednisone and, although the duration of disease might be prolonged or recurrent, there is no joint destruction. The similarity in clinical course and the frequent concurrence of the two syndromes suggest they might be manifestations of the same disease. Conversely, the coincidence of polymyalgia rheumatica and seropositive erosive rheumatoid arthritis is infrequent[20].

POLYMYALGIA RHEUMATICA WITH GIANT CELL ARTERITIS

Some patients with polymyalgia rheumatica also have giant cell arteritis (temporal arteritis, cranial arteritis), but exactly how many is difficult to determine since the biopsy sample may fail to show inflammation in patients with an unquestioned clinical presentation of headache and blindness. Conversely, a biopsy may be positive in a patient with only polymyalgia and no cranial artery symptoms. In Scandinavia, the coincidence of the two syndromes is so frequent (35–45%) that polymyalgia is considered an expression of an underlying giant cell arteritis[21]. In the United States[5], the percentage of polymyalgia patients who develop arteritis is closer to 15%. The majority of patients with polymyalgia never show evidence of arteritis and about 35% of arteritis patients do not have polymyalgia. This suggests that the two are separate syndromes that may appear in the same population of patients who share a predisposition of unknown type.

When giant cell arteritis occurs, it is often coincident with or closely related in time to the onset of polymyalgia, but it may either precede or follow at a considerable interval. Of 45 patients who had both polymyalgia and biopsy-proven temporal arteritis, the syndromes appeared simultaneously or within 1 year in 29. However in 16, the interval between the two was from 1 to 6 years. Polymyalgia was the initial manifestation in 7 and the arteritis appeared first and the polymyalgia later when steroids had been tapered and stopped in the remaining 9[22]. Subsequent to this report, I have seen a patient in whom the arteritis appeared 10 years after the polymyalgia was diagnosed and treated. Similar intervals have been noted by others[5,23]. These findings suggest that polymyalgia is a chronic or recurrent synovitis and that giant cell arteritis is more likely to be a single episode of vasculitis, which can occur at various times in relation to it.

While giant cell arteritis may involve any medium or large artery, there is a predilection for extracranial arteries of the head and neck, and the clinical manifestations of headache, jaw claudication, diplopia and vision loss reflect this distribution. In contrast to polyarteritis, giant cell arteritis rarely involves the pulmonary or renal vessels, so that lung or kidney failure is not seen. Aortic aneurysm, myocardial infarction due to arteritic occlusion of a coronary artery, and stroke have been documented but are not common. Only 5 patients in a series of 166 suffered a stroke, which does not exceed the expected frequency for the age[24]. Wilkinson and Russell have suggested that the infrequency of stroke may be due to the fact that the cranial arteries lose much of their elastic tissue when they penetrate the dura, and propose this as a possible reason why arteritis of intracranial arteries is relatively rare[25]. Inflammation is often found in vertebral arteries examined at autopsy, but clinical manifestations such as lateral medullary syndrome are infrequent and, when seen, have been attributed to extension of a thrombus from the site of vertebral arteritis leading to brain-stem damage.

Save-Soderbergh et al.[26] have described 9 patients in whom giant cell arteritis was the cause of death. Two patients died of myocardial infarction with giant cell arteritis demonstrated in coronary arteries; 2 of dissecting aneurysm of the aorta; and 5 of stroke. These 9 cases were among 208 patients with giant cell arteritis in the Goteborg area. Based on this sample and an additional group of 90 patients followed for 9–16 years[27], the authors conclude that fatalities due to giant cell arteritis are so rare that they do not influence the statistical survival rate for patients in this age group. This was also the conclusion reached at the Mayo Clinic in a study of 42 patients[28]. However, on reviewing a larger series of 284 patients from Goteborg, the Swedish investigators suspected an increased number of deaths from cardiovascular causes during the first 4 months after starting treatment. Thereafter, the death rate was as anticipated for age[29].

Patients may have systemic symptoms with giant cell arteritis, such as fever, anemia, weight loss, and malaise. At times, there are no local cranial symptoms and the systemic features are the predominant or only manifestations of what has been called occult giant cell arteritis[30]. These respond well to steroid treatment.

Peripheral neuropathy was described in 23 (14%) of 166 patients. Histologic examination suggested that this was the result of arteritis of larger nutrient arteries rather than inflammation of the smaller vasa nervosum supplying the nerves. Most neuropathic symptoms improved with steroid treatment[31].

The most serious complication of giant cell arteritis is sudden irreversible blindness. While this is occasionally the first sign of the disease, it is more often preceded by other symptoms indicative of cranial arteritis. These include headache, either in the temporal or occipital area or generalized; diplopia; and jaw claudication. Less common manifestations are ear pain, deafness, pain or burning in the tongue, sore throat and cough. Recognition at this stage and treatment with high-dose prednisone, 50 mg a day for 1 month, will usually control the inflammation and prevent loss of vision.

Blindness in 90% of cases is due to ischemic optic neuropathy from blockage of the posterior ciliary branches of the ophthalmic artery. Central retinal artery occlusion accounts for the remainder. It is difficult to know the exact incidence of blindness because the mix of patients in each report depends on referral patterns and the specialty involved. Early papers and those originating in ophthalmologic clinics suggested that patients with temporal arteritis had as much as a 60% risk of sustaining some permanent loss of vision. Later studies show much lower figures, perhaps because of greater awareness of the disease, earlier recognition before visual symptoms appear and prompt treatment with high doses of prednisone. The series of reports from the Mayo Clinic shows both an increased frequency of diagnosis and decreased incidence of vision loss over time. In 42 patients seen between 1950 and 1974, 7 (17%) sustained permanent loss of vision[28]. Of 100 patients seen from 1976 to 1978, 14 (14%) lost vision[32]. In a more recent report[24] of 166 patients seen from 1980 to 1983, the figure was 14 (8%). In our own patients, reported in 1977[30], the figure for permanent loss of vision was 6% and in our recent experience, it is less than 5%. No patient of the 90 reported from Goteborg lost vision[33].

Visual loss occurs early in the course of the arteritis, within the first 3 months after the onset of cranial symptoms. Transient blindness or blurring are sometimes seen but often the loss is permanent. Treatment with prednisone in the range of 60 mg/day relieves the headache and other symptoms but usually does not restore vision. Treatment is primarily to prevent further loss of vision. A report of one patient suggests that 1 g of methylprednisolone intravenously every 12 hours may restore vision but this has not been confirmed[34].

Giant cell arteritis responds well to high-dose prednisone but even in the presteroid days Horton reported that if blindness did not occur the outlook was good and the episode subsided spontaneously. Headache cleared when the temporal artery was biopsied for diagnosis[35]. The great majority of cases (over 95%) of giant cell arteritis involve a single episode. Documented recurrences are extremely rare. Most reports of persistent or recurrent disease describe an elevated sedimentation rate and either polymyalgia or nonspecific symptoms such as tension headache. The sedimentation rate may rise late in the course of the disease without representing a flare in the arteritis. While the reason for this is not known, patients often do not develop symptoms or complications. Attempts to treat the sedimentation rate by increasing the steroid dose are the main cause of osteoporosis and other steroid toxicity.

Unlike polymyalgia rheumatica, which may be persistent or recurrent, giant cell arteritis almost always represents a single episode which either is controlled by steroid or subsides spontaneously.

References

1. Bagratuni, L. (1963). Prognosis in the anarthritic rheumatoid syndrome *Br. Med. J.*, **1**, 513-18
2. Douglas, W. A. C., Martin, B. A. and Morris, J. H. (1983). Polymyalgia rheumatica: an arthroscopic study of the shoulder joint. *Ann. Rheum. Dis.*, **42**, 311-16

3. Chou, C. T. and Schumacher, H. R. (1984). Clinical and pathologic studies of synovitis in polymyalgia rheumatica. *Arthritis Rheum.*, **27**, 1107–18
4. Von Knorring, J. and Somer, T. (1974). Malignancy in association with polymyalgia rheumatica and temporal arteritis. *Scand. J. Rheumatol.*, **3**, 129–135
5. Chuang, T. Y., Hunder, G. G., Ilstrup, D. M. and Kurland, L. T. (1982). Polymyalgia rheumatica. A 10-year epidemiologic and clinical study. *Ann. Intern. Med.*, **97**, 672–80
6. Haley, L. A. (1984). Long-term follow-up of polymyalgia rheumatica: evidence for synovitis. *Semin. Arthritis Rheum.*, **13**, 322–8
7. Plotz, C. M. and Spiera, H. (1969). Polymyalgia rheumatica. *Bull. Rheum. Dis.*, **20**, 578–81
8. Coomes, E. N., Ellis, R. M. and Kay, A. G. (1976). A prospective study of 102 patients with polymyalgia rheumatica syndrome. *Rheumatol. Rehabil.*, **15**, 270–6
9. Behn, A. R., Perera, T. and Myles, A. B. (1983). Polymyalgia rheumatica and corticosteroids: How much for how long? *Ann. Rheum. Dis.*, **42**, 374–8
10. Kyle, V. and Hazelman, B. L. (1990). Stopping steroids in polymyalgia rheumatica and giant cell arteritis. *Br. Med. J.*, **300**, 344–5
11. Von Knorring, J. (1979). Treatment and prognosis in polymyalgia rheumatica and giant cell arteritis. A ten-year survey of 53 patients. *Acta Med. Scand.*, **205**, 429–35
12. Ayoub, W. T., Franklin, C. M. and Torretti, D. (1985). Polymyalgia rheumatica. Duration of therapy and long-term outcome. *Am. J. Med.*, **79**, 309–15
13. Hamrin, B. (1972). Polymyalgia arteritica. *Acta Med. Scand.*, Suppl. 533, 1–164
14. Salvarani, C. *et al.* (1987). Synovitis in polymyalgia rheumatica: A 5-year follow up study in Reggio Emilia, Italy. (Letter.) *J. Rheumatol.*, **14**, 1209–10
15. Myles, A. B. (1975). Polymyalgia rheumatica and giant cell arteritis: A seven-year survey. *Rheumatol. Rehabil.*, **14**, 231–5
16. Kyle, V., Tudor, J., Wraight, E. P., Gresham, G. A. and Hazelman, B. L. (1990). Rarity of synovitis in polymyalgia rheumatica. *Ann. Rheum. Dis.*, **49**, 155–7
17. Arnett, F. C. *et al.* (1988). The American Rheumatism Association 1987 revised criteria for the classification of rheumatoid arthritis. *Arthritis Rheum.*, **31**, 315–24
18. Healey, L. A. and Sheets, P. K. (1988). The relation of polymyalgia rheumatica to rheumatoid arthritis. *J. Rheumatol.*, **15**, 750–2
19. Nepom, G. T. *et al.* (1989). HLA genes associated with rheumatoid arthritis. *Arthritis Rheum.*, **32**, 15–21
20. Hall, S. B., Ginsburg, W. W., Vollersten, R. S. and Hunder, G. G. (1983). The coexistence of rheumatoid arthritis and giant cell arteritis. *J. Rheumatol.*, **10**, 995–7
21. Bengtsson, B. A. (1990). Giant cell arteritis. *Curr. Opinion Rheum.*, **2**, 60–5
22. Healey, L. A. (1986). The relationship of polymyalgia rheumatica to giant cell arteritis — single or separate syndromes? (Letter.) *J. Rheumatol.*, **13**, 1190
23. Jones, J. G. and Hazelman, B. L. (1981). Prognosis and management of polymyalgia rheumatica. *Ann. Rheum. Dis.*, **40**, 1–5
24. Caselli, R. J., Hunder, G. G. and Whisnant, J. P. (1988). Neurologic disease in biopsy-proven giant cell (temporal) arteritis. *Neurology*, **38**, 352–9
25. Wilkinson, I. M. S. and Russell, R. W. R. (1972). Arteries of the head and neck in giant cell arteritis. *Arch. Neurol.*, **27**, 378–91
26. Save-Soderbergh, J., Malmvall, B. E., Andersson, R. and Bengtsson, B. A. (1986). Giant cell arteritis as a cause of death. *J. Am. Med. Assoc.*, **255**, 493–6
27. Andersson, R., Malmvall, B. E. and Bengtsson, B. A. (1986). Long-term survival in giant cell arteritis including temporal arteritis and polymyalgia rheumatica. *Acta Med. Scand.*, **220**, 361–4
28. Huston, K. A., Hunder, G. G., Lie, J. T., Kennedy, R. H. and Elveback, L. R. (1978). Temporal arteritis: A 25 year epidemiologic, clinical and pathologic study. *Ann. Intern. Med.*, **88**, 162–7
29. Nordborg, E. and Bengtsson, B. A. (1989). Death rates and causes of death in 284 consecutive patients with giant cell arteritis confirmed by biopsy. *Br. Med. J.*, **299**, 549–50
30. Healey, L. A. and Wilske, K. R. (1977). Manifestations of giant cell arteritis. *Med. Clin. North Am.*, **61**, 261–70

31. Caselli, R. J., Daube, J. R., Hunder, G. G. and Whisnant, J. P. (1988). Peripheral neuropathic syndromes in giant cell (temporal) arteritis. *Neurology*, **38**, 685-9
32. Calamia, K. T. and Hunder, G. G. (1980). Clinical manifestations of giant cell (temporal) arteritis. *Clin. Rheum. Dis.*, **6**, 389-403
33. Andersson, R., Malmvall, B. E. and Bengtsson, B. A. (1986). Long-term treatment in giant cell arteritis. *Acta Med. Scand.*, **220**, 465-9
34. Rosenfeld, S. J., Kosmorsky, G. S., Klingele, T. G., Burde, R. M. and Cohn, E. M. (1986). Treatment of temporal arteritis with ocular involvement. *Am. J. Med.*, **80**, 143-5
35. Horton, B. T. and Magath, T. B. (1937). Arteritis of the temporal vessels: Report of seven cases. *Proc. Staff Meet. Mayo Clin.*, **12**, 548-53

14
Arthritis in pregnancy

N. BELLAMY, R. R. GRIGOR, and R. P. NADEN

The issues that pertain to arthritis in pregnancy differ from those of the other chapters in this book by virtue of the finite duration of the gestational period. The key issues relate to the effects of pregnancy on the musculoskeletal condition and the effects of the musculoskeletal condition on pregnancy. This broader categorization is preferred to that which limits the discussion to the interaction between pregnancy and the articular condition, since in some disorders, e.g., SLE, the severity and progression of major organ involvement outweighs any articular effects. In addition to discussing gestational effects in the major musculoskeletal conditions, this chapter also examines, where relevant, issues relating to fertility, the post-partum period and drug effects in pregnancy and lactation. Although an attempt will be made to discuss the outcomes according to the paradigm advanced by Fries[1], it is of note that economic outcomes (dollar costs) are poorly delineated, most investigators exploring the incidence of maternal and fetal fatality (death), the fluctuating severity of pain (discomfort) and suffering (disability), and the effects of pharmacologic therapy (iatrogenic effects).

RHEUMATOID ARTHRITIS

Possibly one of the most outstanding clinical events in rheumatology is the ameliorating effect of pregnancy on rheumatoid arthritis (RA). Indeed, this effect is so striking that it led the late Nobel Laureate, Dr. Philip S. Hench[2], to the discovery of cortisone. In spite of this observation, it has not been proven possible to date to replicate the clinical condition outwith the gestational state. Indeed, for many years the literature was relatively fallow and it is only in the last 10 years, with the availability of additional technologies, that a concerted attempt has been made to unravel this enigma. The early literature is limited not only by a relative paucity of sophisticated biochemical and immunologic probes, but also by difficulty in defining the articular condition itself[3]. Thus, while Sir Alfred Baring Garrod (1819-1907) was apparently the first person to use the term "rheumatoid arthritis", it was not until 1959 that the American Rheumatism Association established a revised set of diagnostic criteria for the condition[4]. It is possible that some patients reported prior to 1959 may have had an alternative diagnosis. Even as recently as 1986, Mitchell et al. noted an ongoing difficulty in making a correct diagnosis of RA[5]. In spite of these reservations, it is possible to provide a reasonable overview given the consistency with which some, but not all, of the phenomena have been reported.

Fertility

The effects of RA on fertility are uncertain, there being few relevant published data. It has been reported that the pain and disability of RA may adversely effect sexuality[6] by reducing sexual desire and, in particular, the frequency of sexual intercourse[7]. Yoshino and Uchida noted that married females with RA were concerned about pregnancy and had difficulty with some sexual intercourse positions if hips or knees were affected[7]. Those with unsatisfactory sexual relationships reported a decreased frequency of orgasms and a decreased demand for intercourse from their spouses. The etiology of these problems falls into two broad categories, physical and emotional. It is of note that over 50% of patients report arthralgia during intercourse, 4% experiencing an invariable exacerbation, and 18% only occasional exacerbation of symptoms the day after intercourse. Less is known about sexual disorders in the RA male.

An early study of subfertility by Kay and Bach[8] was initiated following the casual clinical observation that RA females attending a rheumatology clinic had few, if any, children. Indeed, Hargreaves[9] had made a similar observation 7 years previously. Considering that in their series abortion rates were not different between RA and control populations, it is of note that RA women, whether they were premenopausal or postmenopausal at the time of onset, had fewer children than controls. This apparent subfertility in RA women was further underscored by differences in family size between controls and those RA patients who were married (and presumably sexually active) before the onset of disease. Even when corrected for number of years at risk of pregnancy, the number of births per 100 years at risk was still less for RA patients (10.8) than controls (16.8).

The study of Kay and Bach supports the contention that women with RA, as well as those destined to develop RA, are subfertile and have reduced menstrual spans. Unfortunately, the two studies[7,8] are both somewhat restricted. That of Yoshino and Uchida is limited to a Japanese population based on survey data and lacks a control group, while that of Kay and Bach utilizes an English population and lacks data on sexuality. It is not surprising, therefore, that other investigators have failed to find evidence of subfertility[10]. In contrast, there is some suggestion that multiparity itself may be associated with the age-adjusted prevalence of RA[10]. In a recent review[11] it has been postulated that the link between RA and pregnancy may be mediated immunologically. Repeated fetal stimulation of the maternal immune system might account for both the increased risk of disease[10] and the increased spontaneous abortion rate seen in seropositive RA patients[8]. Such inconclusive data clearly necessitate a more rigorous and comprehensive evaluation of the relationship between RA and fertility. At present, the relationship remains uncertain.

The rheumatoid pregnancy: methodologic considerations

Observations on the ameliorating effects of RA on pregnancy span just over a half a century from 1938 to 1989[2,12-27]. In order to avoid confusion, the use of the term "amelioration" will include those patients noting a partial or complete improvement (syn: remission) in their condition. Such improvement may be recognized by any of the following: (a) a reduction in the symptoms of RA, e.g., pain, stiffness and disability; (b) a reduction in the signs of inflammation, e.g., soft-tissue swelling (synovial fluid or membrane), heat, and tenderness; or (c) reduced requirements for simple analgesics, antirheumatic drugs or other therapeutic modalities. Frequently such effects are summarized in the patient's or physician's global assessment of the activity or severity of disease. In the early literature, the exact measures selected and the methods of application employed (i.e., blinded versus unblinded) often are not specified, neither is there any indication given of the bounds of the clinical state described as unchanged (syn: same), nor is the clinical importance of any improvement or deterioration defined. Finally, interpretation of the literature is made more difficult by the disparity between the number of patients studied and the number of pregnancies. This is an important potential source of interpretative error since the proportion of primipara versus multiparous women and those showing consistent versus inconsistent responses in serial pregnancies may account for some of the apparent differences between studies.

Relationship between onset of RA and pregnancy

There are several reports of the first symptoms of RA occurring either during pregnancy[12,15,18,19,22], after cesarean section[12], following spontaneous abortion[12], or in the first 6 months following delivery[12]. When considered as a percentage of the number of RA women followed, it appears that 2–13% may experience initial onset during pregnancy. It is of note that pregnancy-associated onset does not always occur with the very first pregnancy. Thus, in Oka's series[12] of 90 cases onsetting in pregnancy, 31% related to the first, 38% to the second, 13% to the third, 8% to the fourth, and 10% to the fifth or later pregnancy. When onset occurs in pregnancy, it may occur in any of the three trimesters, the relative frequency in each trimester differing between studies[12,15,19,22]. Cecere and Persellin[20] analyzed 308 pregnancies in RA patients and found that the onset of RA occurred in 2% in the second trimester of pregnancy, 3% in the third, with first-trimester onset being less frequent. It is debatable, given the age at which RA usually onsets and the general prevalence of the disease, whether a single pregnancy (cf. multiparity) represents an etiologic risk factor for RA.

The experience with disease onset following cesarean section and spontaneous abortion is limited to a few individual cases and no firm conclusion can be drawn from the data[12]. Certainly no etiologic association has been demonstrated to date and the events are likely coincidental. In contrast, there are data suggesting an increased risk of RA within 6 months of delivery[12]. Oka reported that in 90 cases temporally related to pregnancy, 70 onset within 0-6 months of delivery. This phenomenon accounted for 10% of the 732 female RA patients followed by Oka, and is thought to be more frequent than can be accounted for by chance alone[16]. The risk of developing RA following pregnancy is also greatest in the first month postpartum and declines progressively thereafter[12,16]. The onset of RA is frequently acute or subacute if it arises *de novo* within 1 month of delivery[12].

Course of RA during pregnancy

Pregnancy generally has a beneficial effect on RA[2,12,15-23] and, with few exceptions, patients conceiving while their disease is in remission are likely to remain in that state during the gestational period[22]. While many studies focus on global effects[12,15-18,20], only a few have reported on specific aspects of disease, i.e., activity scores or joint counts[19,21-23]. It is estimated that 62-91% of patients will improve (partial or complete remission) during pregnancy[2,12,15,16,18,19,21], many requiring little or no drug therapy[15,16,20,22]. Improvement often occurs in the first trimester (50-100%)[15,16,18-20,22] and may continue to evolve in the latter two-thirds of the pregnancy[18,19], being maximal in the last trimester[16]. In some cases, however, remission does not develop until the second (14-34%)[16,18-20] or even third trimester (6-9%)[16,18-20]. With rare exception, any improvement achieved is thereafter maintained throughout the pregnancy[20,22]. Cecere and Persellin noted that there often appears to be complete amelioration during pregnancy, allowing complete discontinuation of medication, but that partial improvement is probably as likely as total subsistence[20]. Most reviews have estimated the probability of at least some degree of improvement at approximately 75%[10,18,24,25]. Furthermore, a remission in one pregnancy tends to be predictive of remission in future pregnancies and a failure to remit is equally predictive[20,22,27]. Even those who experience improvement, however, may note continued fluctuation in their disease activity[20,23]. In addition to a reduction in the activity of articular disease, a reduction in the size and/or number of rheumatoid nodules has also been observed[23]. A similar phenomenon has been reported in two patients with rheumatoid nodulosis[26]. In contrast, no effects on the extra-articular features of RA were noted by Ostensen et al.[22] A minority of patients either fail to notice any change in their disease during pregnancy (24–38%)[12,15-21], or experience a worsening of their condition (14–23%)[12,15-21]. When it occurs, deterioration may develop in any of the three trimesters, but may be more frequent in the second and third trimesters[17,19]. Progressive erosion may accompany persistent activity throughout pregnancy as evidenced by comparative radiographs taken prior to conception and following delivery[23].

Most of the preceding discussion has dealt with the level of musculoskeletal morbidity rather than other medical complications of pregnancy or maternal mortality. In the aforementioned studies and reviews, there is little mention of obstetric comorbidity and no mention of any maternal deaths[12-26]. In a small series reported by Morris[17], specific note was made that all patients survived and none appeared in danger during the course of the pregnancy. Ostensen et al. also reported a similar favorable experience[22,23]. Even a patient with pelvic encroachment from a diseased hip (prior central dislocation arthrodesis surgery) had a spontaneous vaginal delivery[17]. Rheumatoid involvement of the hip, if severe, may make delivery more complex and possibly more painful, although in general, birth complications have not been reported[22]. There is no evidence that hypertension, preeclampsia, eclampsia, or other medical complications of pregnancy are any more or less common than in the general obstetric population[19,20]. It seems likely, from current data, that women with RA (and who are otherwise healthy) are at no increased personal risk from undertaking a pregnancy. The greater consideration relates to the severity of any permanent joint damage, major organ involvement, and the patient's capacity to cope physically and socioemotionally with her offspring.

Course of RA following pregnancy

In spite of the major improvements frequently noted, amelioration is not curative, symptoms generally recurring (62–100%) within 4–8 weeks after delivery[12,15,16,18-20,22]. On occasion the remission is more prolonged and may last several months (35%)[12,15,16,18,20] or rarely even years[19]. Relapse may occur in the same joints[12,15] or in previously unaffected joints[12,15]. It may result in disease that, in the short term, is similar in severity[12,15] to, or more severe than that existing prior to conception[12,15]. By the end of 1 year postpartum, however, it is estimated that disease activity is the same as prior to conception[22]. The tendency for RA to relapse following pregnancy has been underscored by Felbo and Snorrason[14] in a study of disease activity before and after therapeutic abortion. There may be a tendency for some improvement immediately following abortion, but two-thirds subsequently note an exacerbation of their disease. The modulating effects of lactation and return of menses on arthritis has received little attention. It would seem that lactation neither delays nor facilitates any relapse[16,22].

Effects of RA on pregnancy

Effects of RA on pregnancy have to be viewed in the context, not only of the patient's disease, but also with respect to the patient's premorbid obstetric history, any comorbidity or concomitant medication, and the "natural" occurrence rates of fetal abnormality and wastage in the general population. Most of the series reported are small and uncontrolled. It is difficult, therefore, to draw inferences regarding the relative risk of fetal events. The major considerations are those of abortion, perinatal mortality and fetal abnormality. Discussion on antirheumatic drugs in pregnancy and lactation will be deferred until the end of this chapter, as many antirheumatic drugs are used to treat several of the conditions under review.

Abortion

The termination of a pregnancy may occur deliberately or spontaneously. The landmark study of Felbo and Snorrason on RA and therapeutic abortion[14] was undertaken to address observed differences between the rate of granting permission for abortion, by a Danish agency, to RA patients (permission rate = 80%) versus applicants in general (permission rate = 40%). This study was undertaken some years ago in a country whose practice does not necessarily reflect that elsewhere. These restrictions notwithstanding, a few patients with RA apply for therapeutic abortion either because they feel physically or emotionally unable to cope with the baby or fear the potential teratogenicity of one of the DMARDs. Clearly, therapeutic abortion does not solve any articular problems relating to the disease, since joint activity either remains the same or in two-thirds of cases worsens following termination, just as it does following the normal delivery of a term pregnancy[14,22]. Felbo and Snorrason felt that "other things being equal, this does not speak for granting permission to induce abortion in cases of rheumatoid arthritis". It is of note that although their numbers were small, clinical progression of disease was most pronounced in 39 patients with "early disease" (ARA stages 1-3) who had induced or spontaneous abortions.

It is controversial whether RA patients are at more risk of spontaneous abortion. Kay and Bach noted an increased risk in seropositive but not seronegative RA patients, but no overall difference between premenopausal-onset RA patients and their controls[8]. Likewise, Felbo and Snorrason noted no differences in spontaneous abortion rates in patients prior to, versus following, the onset of RA. In a comparative study of RA versus OA patients, Kaplan[28] demonstrated a statistically significant increase in abortion rates in RA subjects (p = 0.005), this being evident even before the onset of RA (p = 0.007). This difference could not be explained on the basis of any subgroup with a high frequency of abortion but appeared to be a characteristic of the group as a whole. Given that the estimated figure for spontaneous abortion in the general population is 10-20% and the rate for the OA group was 16.5%, an abortion rate of 25.1% in the RA group appears to represent a clinically important increase in risk. In contrast, Silman et al. were unable to detect any difference in spontaneous abortion rate between RA patients and their unaffected female relatives (relative risk = 1.2, 95% CI 0.5-2.9), the spontaneous abortion rates being in the "normal range" for both groups (11% and 8%, respectively)[29]. However, two recent studies, one from Greece[30] and the other from England[31], observed a tendency for spontaneous abortion rates to be greater after disease onset (27% and 28%, respectively) than before (16% and 15%, respectively). The fetal loss rates in the control populations in these studies were 12% and 16%, respectively. Taken together with spontaneous abortion rates noted in other studies[12,17,22], this experience suggests that spontaneous abortion may be more likely in RA patients once they have established disease. Whether spontaneous abortion is more frequent among those destined to develop rheumatoid disease is far more controversial.

Perinatal mortality

Early reports suggested that stillbirth rates in RA were not apparently increased, although some cases were reported and occasional autopsies have been performed[8,17,19]. More recent evaluations have been conflicting. Silman et al. reported an increased frequency (72.9/1000 vs. 6.2/1000) and risk (relative risk = 12.4) of stillbirth in RA patients compared with their unaffected female relatives, albeit with a large 95% confidence interval (1.6-91.1) and in a small group of patients[29]. In contrast, a study by Siamopoulou-Mavridou et al. showed no such increase (stillbirth rates: RA = < 2%, control = 3%)[30]. Although not the principal focus of these studies, no differences were observed between patients and controls with respect to fertility rates[28,30,31].

Fetal abnormality

RA does not apparently increase the risk of any type of fetal abnormality, although a certain level of fetal morbidity can be anticipated just as in the general population. Single cases of intrauterine growth retardation[17,32], neonatal jaundice[19], and subtle reductions in birth weights[32] have been reported. Most patients, however, have been delivered normally, data being scarce on the timing and duration of labor but not suggesting any deviation from experience in the general population[20]. Likewise, lactation and resumption of menses do not appear to be affected[20]. In general, reviewers have rated pregnancy in RA patients as an event with short-term but no long-term benefits, being attended by low maternal and fetal risk similar to that seen in the general population[10,16,20,24,25,27,33-35].

Predicting the response

Although many years passed between Hench's original discovery and further elucidation of potential mechanisms underlying the ameliorating effects of pregnancy (Table 1), there is now a body of information that might offer some prognostic opportunity[20]. Circulating factors in pregnancy sera that may have immunoregularity or anti-inflammatory activity are of particular interest (Table 2). One of the most promising areas of research has been into pregnancy associated alpha-2-glycoprotein (PAG) formerly termed pregnancy zone protein (PZP). This glycoprotein, arising from the maternal decidua, has a molecular weight of 364 000 daltons and is normally present in the serum but increases during gestation. Both Persellin[36] and Unger[37] have noted an inverse association between PAG levels and the activity of arthritis in pregnant RA patients. However, Ostensen et al.[38], using a different technique, were unable to confirm this association and found no correlation. It was, doubtless, the concept of a potential therapeutic agent circulating in gestational plasma that led to the evaluation of plasma transfusion as a treatment modality. After some initial enthusiasm, it was noted that the benefits could not be duplicated[18], and even in a recent report in juvenile rheumatoid arthritis no benefit was derived from the infusion of autologous third-trimester plasma[39]. Currently there is no method of predicting which patients will have a favorable course during pregnancy, which will deteriorate, which will experience early postpartum relapse, and which will experience a more sustained remission. In particular, rheumatoid factor status, type of joint involvement, disease duration, parity, sex of fetus, and placental weight do not appear to influence the activity of RA in pregnancy[23]. At the present time it is only possible to reassure patients that a remission, partial or complete, during pregnancy is likely in 75% of cases, and that a remission in one pregnancy will likely predict a remission in future pregnancies, deteriorations being equally predictive.

Considering the predominant female involvement of RA and the frequent onset of disease prior to the menopause, it is disappointing that relatively few data have been gathered on RA in pregnancy. However, these studies are difficult to conduct, particularly with respect to patient accrual, and therefore relatively few investigators have pursued this problem. Success may lie in a co-ordinated multidisciplinary approach to investigation bringing together pregnant patients, clinical investigators, and basic scientists. To date only a few

Table 1 Potential factors in the amelioration of rheumatoid arthritis during pregnancy

Humoral factors
　Immunomodulation by circulating trophoblast–anti-trophoblast immune complexes
　Removal of circulating aggregated immunoglobulins by the placental "sponge"
　Alteration in immunoglobulin carbohydrate side-chain composition leading to decreased "stickiness"
　Decreased IgG levels (mild)

Fetal suppression of the maternal immune system
　Soluble factors including alpha-fetoprotein
　Fetal suppressor cells in maternal circulation

Depression of cell-mediated immunity
　Depression of delayed hypersensitivity by skin testing
　Delayed rejection of skin allografts
　Increased virulence or recurrence of intracellular pathogens
　Decreased lymphocyte counts
　Decreased helper T-cells with decreased helper/suppressor ratio
　Depressed *in vitro* lymphocyte responses
　Decreased NK activity (killing)
　Circulating suppressors of cell-mediated immunity including blocking antibodies

Suppression of inflammatory reactions
　Impaired chemotaxis, adherence, phagocytosis, NBT reduction
　Decreased cathepsin B activity
　Suppressive serum factor(s)

From ref. 10 with permission of the author and W. B. Saunders Co.

Table 2 Circulating factors with immunoregulatory or anti-inflammatory activity in pregnancy sera

Fetal factors
　Alpha-fetoprotein
　Other factors in maternal sera

Trophoblast hormones
　Estrogens
　Progesterone
　Human chorionic gonadotropin (hCG)
　Human placental lactogen (hPL)

Maternal factors
　Corticosteroids
　Blocking antibodies including anti-trophoblastic antibodies

Trophoblastic-decidual placental proteins
　Pregnancy-associated plasma protein A (PAPP-A)
　Pregnancy-associated alpha-2 globulin (PAG)
　Placental protein 14 (PP-14)
　Pregnancy-specific beta-1 glycoprotein (SP1)
　Other pregnancy serum proteins

From ref. 10 with permission of the authors and W. B. Saunders Co.

centers have achieved the necessary patient numbers and logistic support, but in doing so have made an invaluable contribution to the literature.

Adult-onset Still's disease (AOSD)

Although a relatively infrequent variant of rheumatoid disease, cases of AOSD have been reported increasingly in the last decade. During that time there have been case reports of AOSD arising *de novo* during pregnancy[40], as well as one recurring after each of two pregnancies[41]. In addition, there has been one observed occurrence of juvenile-onset Still's disease in a pregnancy following 12 years of partial remission[42]. Little etiologic significance can be drawn from these reports, although they serve to alert other investigators that arthritis onsetting in pregnancy or in the puerperium may be AOSD and that further data on this disorder are required.

SERONEGATIVE SPONDYLOARTHRITIS

Ankylosing spondylitis

Ankylosing spondylitis frequently has its onset during the childbearing years[43]. Clinical descriptions of ankylosing spondylitis in women generally suggest that the disease is milder and often atypical compared with men but comprehensive community-based surveys have yet to be done[44-47]. Practically all of the pregnant ankylosing spondylitis patients described in the literature have been seen at rheumatology clinics, implying a bias towards the more serious cases[47]. It is likely that many pregnancies occur in undiagnosed disease. The most significant studies have been those of Ostensen and Husby in Norway, who have also recently reviewed the literature[23, 47-49].

Effect of ankylosing spondylitis on pregnancy

There are no reports of reduced fertility in ankylosing spondylitis. In the absence of severe hip or pelvic joint involvement, which appears to be uncommon during child-bearing years, ankylosing spondylitis women have uncomplicated deliveries of healthy children. There is no increased frequency of spontaneous abortion, premature labor, or stillbirth[23,47,48,50].

The long-term prognosis of the offspring of an ankylosing spondylitis mother is strongly influenced by genetic factors. The offspring of an HLA-B27 positive patient will have a 50% chance of inheriting the HLA-B27 antigen. Several studies have demonstrated a considerably increased risk of ankylosing spondylitis in HLA-B27 positive first-degree relatives of HLA-B27 positive patients compared with unselected HLA-B27 positive subjects in the population[51-54]. Van der Linden found that about one in five HLA-B27 positive first-degree relatives will eventually develop ankylosing spondylitis[51]. Thus, 10% of all children born to an HLA-B27 positive ankylosing spondylitis mother will ultimately get ankylosing spondylitis, but, if the HLA-B27 status of the child is known, 20% of the HLA-B27 positive ones are likely to develop ankylosing spondylitis, whereas the HLA-B27 negative ones virtually never develop the disease[52].

Effect of pregnancy on ankylosing spondylitis

Assessment of spondylitis activity during gestation is difficult because nonspecific low back pain and elevated ESR are both associated with otherwise normal pregnancies[20]. Ostensen and Husby analyzed 9 case reports of 28 pregnancies and found the symptoms of ankylosing spondylitis improved in 46%, remained unchanged in 46%, and worsened in 7%[47]. In their own retrospective series of 87 pregnancies, 20% improved, 55% remained unchanged, and 24% worsened[48]. Being an uncontrolled study, it is uncertain whether the observed changes in disease activity might have been naturally occurring relapses or remissions. Remissions were more likely to occur in patients with accompanying small-joint arthritis. In a further prospective study of 27 pregnancies[23], disease activity was unchanged in 10 patients, and aggravation of spinal symptoms occurred in 11. Only the 6 patients who had accompanying ulcerative colitis or psoriasis experienced marked improvement in their disease symptoms (including back pain and stiffness) when pregnant, and this became apparent between the fifth and tenth weeks of gestation. A need for NSAIDs at some stage of pregnancy was felt in 21 cases though only 16 patients actually took their medication. Postpartum, there was a flare of spinal and extraspinal symptoms unrelated to the return to menses and the period of lactation in 23 pregnancies[23]. This has also been observed in retrospective studies, where, with few exceptions, most patients returned to their prepregnancy disease course[47,48].

It is not known whether pregnancy and childbirth alter the long-term prognosis of ankylosing spondylitis. There are isolated reports of worsening of radiologic changes during pregnancy, but there has been no controlled study to date[47].

Psoriatic arthritis

There are few studies of pregnancy in psoriatic arthritis[50,55]. Ostensen prospectively studied 12 pregnancies in 10 women with psoriatic arthritis. Fetal outcome did not seem influenced by psoriatic arthritis, even when anti-inflammatory drug therapy was necessary. Maternal outcome resembled that in rheumatoid arthritis, with a tendency to gradual amelioration both of peripheral and axial symptoms. The return of the prepregnancy disease pattern was delayed by several months after delivery. Psoriatic skin lesions remained unchanged[47,50].

McHugh and Laurent reported three pregnancies during established arthritis, noting no change in arthritis activity. Psoriatic arthritis appeared to begin in another two patients during the third trimester and in five in the postpartum period[55]. However, such cases most likely represent the coincidental onset of disease in women of child-bearing age. Even in ankylosing spondylitis, an 8% incidence of onset in pregnancy is thought to be explained by chance alone[47].

SYSTEMIC LUPUS ERYTHEMATOSUS

The effect of pregnancy on systemic lupus erythematosus

For the patient contemplating pregnancy the key questions in relation to her systemic lupus erythematosus (SLE) are: what is the likelihood of the disease being active during pregnancy and is the pregnancy itself likely to aggravate the disease? What will be the effect on the disease, of limitations on treatment imposed by the necessity to consider potential iatrogenic effects on the fetus? What is the risk to the fetus?

In answering these questions, there are a number of difficulties in interpreting much of the published data. To date there has been no generally agreed-upon definition of SLE activity, although several authors have recently addressed this problem[56-58]. Manifestations of normal pregnancy that may be mistaken for active lupus include increased facial blushing and palmar erythema, knee effusions, and postpartum hair loss. Flares in some single organ systems may be virtually impossible to distinguish from pregnancy complications, particularly preeclampsia, and phospholipid antibody syndrome[59,60]. Many older studies were either uncontrolled or used historical or self-controls, which did not allow for the fact that SLE may show fewer manifestations with increasing time from diagnosis[61]. Furthermore, recent studies may include more patients with milder disease. Other biases may include self-selection of well women to plan pregnancies (particularly those with previous success), and referral patterns to reporting institutions. Pregnancy and concern for fetal welfare may require modification of the usual treatment. This may in itself lead to flares in disease activity (e.g., Lockshin observed exacerbation of cutaneous lupus in two patients following withdrawal of hydroxychloroquine therapy)[59]. Flares in other organ systems may have more serious significance (e.g., renal failure, hypertension, cerebritis) and be more difficult to treat, particularly when therapeutic options need to be considered in relation to the fetus as well as the mother.

Activity of SLE in pregnancy

Cecere and Persellin reviewed the medical literature in decades during the period 1950-1980. Overall, among 688 pregnancies in women with SLE, 360 (52%) were associated with lupus activity, a proportion remaining constant throughout that time period despite the incidence of maternal deaths falling from 17% to 1%[20]. Two recent prospective studies have provided more precise information. Lockshin reported a frequency of 26% (21/80) for patients displaying disease activity during pregnancy in a group in which 25% (20/80) were active at conception[59]. Urowitz reported a more severely affected group, of whom 70% (43/61) showed activity during pregnancy and 72% (44/61) were active at conception[62]. These data indicate that the likelihood of SLE being active during pregnancy is closely related to the activity of the disease at conception.

Risk of exacerbation in pregnancy

The likelihood of a flare of SLE also appears to be related to disease activity before pregnancy. Ramsey-Goldman further analyzed the data of Cecere and Persellin along with her own and that of Mintz[64] and estimated that women with inactive lupus at conception can expect approximately a 10-30% chance of disease exacerbation during the course of pregnancy or the first few months postpartum[63]. When lupus is active at the time of conception, the overall frequency of exacerbation appears to be twofold to threefold higher, particularly during the second and third trimesters and also postpartum. In two recent studies in which the criteria for flares superimposed on active disease have been carefully defined, this trend has been confirmed. Lockshin reported a prospective evaluation of 80 pregnant women. Disease activity was scored in terms of global assessment, prednisone therapy, cumulative number of organ systems with abnormalities and display of abnormalities in each organ system. Most abnormalities detected were attributable to pregnancy-related complications of preeclampsia or phospholipid antibody syndrome rather than to SLE activity. If only SLE-specific abnormalities were counted, disease exacerbation occurred in 9 of 20 (2%) patients whose disease was quiescent[59]. Urowitz reported a more severely affected group in which many of the patients were on steroid therapy. In this group flares during pregnancy occurred in 7 of 17 (41%) patients whose disease was inactive at conception, whereas 25 of 44 (57%) patients with active SLE at conception experienced a flare in activity[62]. These studies support the conclusion that an exacerbation of SLE is more likely in pregnancy when the disease is active at conception.

The issue of whether lupus exacerbations are more frequent in the pregnant state or whether they occur with the same frequency as in the nonpregnant lupus patient has been addressed in several studies. The observation that the frequency of active disease was virtually the same during pregnancy as before conception in the studies of Lockshin and Urowitz (approximately 25% and 70%, respectively — see above) suggests that pregnancy has no consistent effect on disease activity[59,62].

In a prospective case control study by Lockshin and colleagues[58], a prospective study by Mintz et al.[64] (with all patients routinely receiving corticosteroids during pregnancy, and control patients on oral contraceptives containing only progestagens), and a retrospective report by

Meehan and Dorsey[65], no differences were found in the frequency of exacerbations between pregnant and nonpregnant matched control patients, either during the pregnancy or in the first postpartum year, raising the possibility that exacerbations of SLE during gestation may in fact not be attributable to the pregnancy. Possibly patients with relatively active disease are more likely to be active at the time of conception and to experience further (coincidental) exacerbations during pregnancy. Conversely, those who are relatively inactive are less likely to be active at the time of conception or to exacerbate during the pregnancy.

Renal lupus in pregnancy

Patients with lupus nephritis during pregnancy may be particularly difficult to evaluate. Proteinuria may increase in pregnancy because of the normal increase in glomerular filtration, or because of superimposed preeclampsia or because of active SLE, and there are few clues permitting differentiation[60]. Burkett summarized the outcome of 242 pregnancies in 156 patients[66]. Renal function deteriorated during 27% of pregnancies but usually returned to the prepregnancy level after delivery. It appears likely that most transient impairment in renal function is due to superimposed preeclampsia.

Effect of pregnancy on long-term prognosis

The long-term prognosis of SLE after pregnancy has received little attention. Siegal found no difference in long-term outcome between women who had been pregnant and those who had not[67]. Burkett noted permanent loss of renal function in 7% of patients with renal lupus. Since no control data were available, it is uncertain whether this observation represented a significant difference from the natural progression that might have been expected[66].

Summary

The available evidence leads to the conclusion that the major factor predicting the course of SLE during pregnancy is the activity of the disease prior to conception. Pregnancy itself does not appear to increase the frequency of exacerbations or to worsen the long-term prognosis.

Effect of systemic lupus erythematosus on pregnancy

Maternal

Fertility. In larger series of women with SLE, overall fertility appears to be similar to the normal population, both in the number of women eventually becoming pregnant (75–80%)[68-70] and the number of pregnancies (2.3) per fertile patient[68]. In individuals, however, SLE may impair fertility at times when the disease is active. Estes and Larsen reported only 4 of 68 pregnancies occurring at times when the activity of SLE was moderate or severe[71]. Amenorrhea is more common when SLE is active[72,73], and decreased frequency of sexual intercourse would be expected. The overall effect of corticosteroid drugs on fertility is unknown; these hormones may impair normal ovulation and post-conceptional physiology, but may improve the chance of conception by ameliorating active disease.

Pregnancy-related complications. The major pregnancy-related complication for the mother is preeclampsia. Distinguishing preeclampsia from a flare of lupus nephritis can be very difficult: edema, weight gain, proteinuria, hypertension, hyperuricemia, convulsions, thrombocytopenia, and even hypocomplementemia may occur in both[59,60]. Nevertheless, the distinction is very important in selecting the appropriate treatment for the mother. The decision whether to terminate the pregnancy or not is critically important to the prognosis of the premature fetus/neonate.

Proteinuria may increase in lupus pregnancy because of active lupus nephritis, preeclampsia, or in the presence of stable membranous glomerulonephritis because of the normal increase in glomerular filtration. Clinical and immunologic signs of active SLE and the appearance of hematuria or erythrocyte casts suggests lupus nephritis[60]. A rapidly progressive increase in proteinuria (e.g., doubling every 10 days and reducing shortly after delivery) is more typical of preeclampsia.

Hypertension and hyperuricemia are common in both preeclampsia and renal lupus. Rapidly increasing blood pressure and plasma urate without significant elevation in plasma creatinine, and spontaneous reduction of the hypertension and plasma urate after the first few days postpartum are more suggestive of preeclampsia.

Convulsions are reported to occur in 3–18% of those with SLE[74]. However, the distinction between eclampsia and lupus cerebritis may be difficult.

Thrombocytopenia occurring late in pregnancy is most often associated with preeclampsia[59]. Active SLE is more likely to be manifest as steroid responsive thrombocytopenia and to occur early in pregnancy.

Complement components tend to increase in normal pregnancy. Thus complement levels may be normal in the presence of active renal lupus in pregnancy. Conversely, reduced complement may occur in both preeclampsia and active SLE. Although very low levels are more suggestive of SLE, this is often not helpful in the individual case. More precise measurements of classical and alternate pathway activation may assist differentiation in some circumstances[75,76].

Major complications of SLE (e.g., renal failure, hypertension, cerebritis) may be more difficult to manage in pregnancy because of the need to consider the effect of treatment on the fetus.

There is a high reported incidence of cesarean section (32–34%)[64,67] an event associated with a desire by clinicians to deliver the fetus early. Urowitz and Gladman noted "this can, in part, perhaps be explained by the fact that these patients are looked after by specialists, usually in university centers, and therefore, any concern for maternal or fetal safety might more likely result in surgical delivery"[25].

Clinically significant hip disease, usually a consequence of avascular necrosis, may occasionally cause mechanical problems during delivery. There is one report suggesting that prosthetic hip joints may be at risk during lupus pregnancies[77].

Fetal

Overall fetal mortality has been noted by many to be increased in women with SLE. Rates vary in different series, but fetal loss of 50% or greater has often been reported[78-80]. This fetal wastage comprises a number of different causes, detailed below. However, in their careful review, Cecere and Persellin noted a remarkably consistent rate of overall fetal wastage, excluding "therapeutic" abortions, of 28% over the three decades 1950–1980, despite advances in therapy and monitoring; and the inclusion in later studies of less severe cases of SLE[20]. The most significant component of this increased fetal loss appears to be the substantial increase in stillbirths.

Early abortions. Earlier authors suggested an increased incidence of spontaneous abortions (28–36%)[72,73,81,82]. In a review of such studies, Chesley reported this outcome in 126 of 613 (21%) uninterrupted pregnancies[83]. Subsequent reports, however, have consistently shown a rate of spontaneous abortion of 17% or less[27,64,78,84,85]. Cecere and Persellin noted a similar rate (approximately 17%) in their detailed review, with no apparent change in the three decades 1950–1980, despite advances in therapy and inclusion of milder cases in more recent series[20]. This rate is not significantly different from the expected rate of spontaneous abortion in the normal population of 15%[86]. A more definite increased incidence of spontaneous abortions is described in the subgroup of women who have antiphospholipid antibodies.

Intermediate and late fetal deaths. In contrast, many reports have noted a marked increase in fetal mortality later in pregnancy. Cecere and Persellin noted a stillbirth rate of 7–10% over the period 1950–1980[20], and later authors have reported a similar phenomenon[27,84]. It now appears likely that much of this increased late fetal risk is also related to antiphospholipid antibodies.

There is a relative paucity of information regarding placental changes in SLE patients, but a reduction in placental size may be the result of a variety of pathologic changes including placental infarction, intraplacental hematoma, deposition of immunoglobulin and complement, thickening of the trophoblast basement membrane, and decidual vasculopathy[87,117]. It seems likely that there are several mechanisms that can lead to placental injury in women with SLE, with the clinical significance of the resulting placental damage being enhanced by reduced placental size. Careful monitoring of the size of the placenta throughout pregnancy may allow more accurate identification of those SLE patients who are at greatest risk of fetal loss. Assessment of uteroplacental blood flow by Doppler flow velocimetry may also be useful in the future.

Prematurity. Premature delivery of the baby (before 36 or 37 weeks gestation) is more common in women with SLE — up to 59% in one series[77,84,88]. Much of this reflects a medical decision to deliver the fetus early (iatrogenic prematurity). The incidence of spontaneous premature labor has not generally been increased, there being only two in Lockshin's series of 67 births[77].

Fetal growth. Birth weight tends to be lower than the population average. This is mainly due to deliberate preterm delivery. Fetal intrauterine growth retardation (small for gestational age) occurs in up to 23% of pregnancies[82,84], particularly in those women with antiphospholipid antibodies, but the precise frequency of this complication is unknown.

Effect of lupus activity on fetal outcome

Fetal outcome appears to be affected by the state of the SLE. When lupus nephritis is present, the prognosis is reported to be worse. Earlier reports were conflicting, but a recent review by Burkett of the literature since 1980 reveals an overall fetal wastage in this group of 31% (64 of 208) when therapeutic abortions are excluded[66]. This is similar to the prognosis in SLE generally (28% see above), as is the rate of spontaneous abortion (37 of 202 = 18%). The later perinatal mortality, however, is substantially increased (13%). Several authors report a greater risk of perinatal death in association with more severe renal disease (e.g., serum creatinine 1.5 mg/dl or more) or active disease[78,80,85,89]. Jungers *et al.* showed that fetal survival (overall 82%) may be nearly normal if disease activity is mild at conception or has been in remission for several months. In contrast, onset of SLE in pregnancy was associated with 43% fetal wastage. Urowitz, however, found no increase in fetal loss in women with active compared with inactive disease[62].

The aforementioned studies have generally not related fetal outcome to the presence of antiphospholipid antibodies. Recent data, however, suggest that the presence of these antibodies may be a major determinant of fetal outcome, possibly more than any other feature of SLE.

In summary, overall fetal mortality is increased in women with SLE. The rates of spontaneous early abortion and premature labor are not apparently different from the normal population. However, there is a significant increase in the risk of stillbirth and intrauterine growth retardation, probably due to placental vascular pathology. Induced premature delivery and cesarean section are much more common. The risk to the fetus is significantly increased in the presence of antiphospholipid antibodies. It is less clear whether there is an increased risk to the fetus from other signs of disease activity.

ANTIPHOSPHOLIPID ANTIBODY SYNDROME

Although the clinical association of antiphospholipid antibodies (APAs) (lupus anticoagulant and anticardiolipin antibodies) was first studied in patients with SLE, it has become apparent that these antibodies also occur in patients with few or none of the criteria for SLE. Thus, they appear to define a syndrome with only partial overlap with SLE. Nevertheless, many of the complications of pregnancy in women with SLE are associated with these antibodies.

Clinical features

Antiphospholipid antibodies have been definitely associated with venous thrombosis, arterial occlusion (especially cerebral and ocular), thrombocytopenia, and increased fetal loss[91-96,101]. Chorea[90], livedo reticularis[97], migraine[101,107], and valvular heart disease[98,100,101] may also be more frequent. Possible mechanisms for these effects have been reviewed recently[102,114].

Laboratory tests

Many of the clinical abnormalities were described initially in the context of abnormal coagulation tests (APTT) i.e., the lupus anticoagulant. Subsequently antibodies to cardiolipin (aCL) were shown to be more sentisive, especially for fetal loss[103-105]. However, concordance is only 76% and both APTT and aCL tests may be better than either one alone[103]. The IgG aCL-isotype appears to be strongly associated with thrombosis, thrombocytopenia, and fetal loss[98]. The IgM aCL isotype is less specific but has been associated with endocardial disease[106]. The IgA aCL-isotype has also been reported to be strongly predictive of thrombosis and fetal loss but these data await confirmation. Combinations of the antibody types may provide the most sensitive prediction of risk[98,106].

Relationship of APAs to SLE

The relationship of the antiphospholipid antibody syndrome to SLE remains uncertain. Certainly the majority of patients with APA have few if any of the criteria of SLE[107]. Reports on the frequency of APAs in patients with SLE are also extremely variable, from 21% to 81%[98]. Since criteria for "positive ACL" tests were set in 1986[108], prevalences of 25%[109] and 42%[98] have been reported. This variability likely represents different selection biases in the groups studied.

Prognosis for the mother in pregnancy

Irrespective of the precise relationship between the two syndromes, the presence of APA is a major predictor of complications in pregnancy for the woman with SLE. For the mother, APA is associated with increased risk of venous thrombosis and arterial occlusion. It has been suggested that the risk of thrombosis is increased further in pregnancy[110] but this has been disputed by others[111]. Thrombocytopenia, however, is frequently aggravated by pregnancy[111]. Other problems associated with APA occur in pregnancy, but it is not clear whether they are more common than outside pregnancy. It also appears that the development of preeclampsia, especially of early onset, is more frequent when APAs are present[77].

Prognosis for the fetus

Antiphospholipid antibodies markedly increase the risk for the fetus. This risk has been somewhat exaggerated in the past in series of patients selected because of previous fetal loss. In a prospective series the frequency of fetal loss has been reported as 36%[98]. Lockshin has suggested that the risk of fetal loss is about 50% for a woman in her first pregnancy or with previous live children[111], although no data were presented.

The nature of the fetal loss is similar to that seen in SLE in general. Most losses are spontaneous first-trimester abortions, but these are a common occurrence in normal women. APAs have been reported in about 6–11% of women with habitual abortion[112,113].

The increase in risk of second- or third-trimester fetal death is more dramatic, with fetal growth retardation and intrauterine death with or without maternal signs of preeclampsia[101].

The risk to the fetus is clearly increased further by the concurrent presence of thrombocytopenia[77]: 78% fetal loss when APA is associated with thrombocytopenia versus 38% when platelets are normal. Premature delivery is extremely common, partly reflecting the high level of concern for the fetus *in utero* and consequent early intervention.

The exact cause of the fetal losses in the second and third trimester is not known. The clear association of IgG idiotypes of aCL with fetal loss suggests a direct effect of transplacental IgG antibodies on fetal tissues, possibly producing vascular and thrombotic damage similar to that seen in adults. There are few data available on fetal tissues except for the placenta. The placenta is usually small[105] and a range of histologic abnormalities have been described[117]. In contrast to earlier suggestions[115,116], infarction is not usually present. Abnormal fetal placental blood flow patterns have been observed by Doppler techniques[119]. Impaired placental function may also be caused by lesions in the maternal uterine circulation. Antiphospholipid antibodies may affect uteroplacental perfusion by direct endothelial damage, by impairment of prostacyclin synthesis, or by causing intravascular thrombosis through various effects on the coagulation and fibrinolytic systems[102].

Effect of treatment

Faced with a high risk of fetal loss, and often a patient who has lost one or more babies already, the clinician is under considerable pressure to use drug treatment. The early reports of successful pregnancies after treatment with aspirin or heparin and high-dose steroids, usually after many earlier losses[115,116], generated considerable enthusiasm for this treatment. In the last 5 years there has been increasing caution, as complications associated with high-dose steroids (osteoporosis, avascular necrosis of the femoral head, miliary tuberculosis) have been encountered. The appropriate level of steroid treatment is difficult to determine since APA levels may not decrease with steroid therapy. A number of women with APA have had successful pregnancies without any therapy, or with aspirin alone[77,112,118,119,121]. Lockshin[77] has even reported a series in which the fetal outcome was worse in the group treated with higher doses of steroids, although these patients were not randomly assigned to treatment groups. There is clearly a need now for a properly randomized controlled trial and this is in progress — the Kingston Antiphospholipid Antibody Study (KAPS)[120]. In the meantime there is no clear evidence that high-dose, or even low-dose, steroids improve the prognosis in pregnancies complicated by APA, although treatment is usually considered if there have been three or more spontaneous first-trimester abortions, or a previous fetal/neonatal loss. In these latter circumstances, there is an increasing trend toward aspirin alone, or aspirin plus low-dose steroids (up to 30 mg/day) while the result of the KAPS is awaited.

Summary

APAs are a major risk factor for the mother and fetus in pregnancy. Indeed it may well be that most of the adverse prognosis associated with SLE in pregnancy can be predicted by the presence or absence of APAs. Although this hypothesis remains to be confirmed, it has been shown that the presence or activity of SLE in pregnancy appears to make little difference to the prognosis for those patients who have APAs. It seems likely that low-dose aspirin, anticoagulants, and steroids may improve the prognosis but the precise criteria on which to advise such therapy remain to be elucidated.

NEONATAL LUPUS SYNDROME

Neonatal lupus is a syndrome characterized by the presence of cutaneous lupus or congenital heart block (or both) in an infant whose mother has a connective-tissue disease and/or the autoantibodies anti-Ro, anti-La, or anti-U1 RNP. Transient hepatic, hematologic, and, rarely, pulmonary and neurologic abnormalities have also been reported, but are not essential components of the syndrome. The syndrome has been reviewed recently by Petri et al.[122].

Serologic and immunogenetic features

Anti-Ro antibody is strongly associated with the neonatal lupus syndrome. It is found in the majority of mothers (92% of 155 cases reviewed by Petri) and infants with neonatal lupus syndrome if measured before 3 months of age (82% of 83)[122]. Anti-Ro is often associated with anti-La in the same patient, and a small minority have anti-La only[122,126]. Provost has reported two infants with cutaneous neonatal lupus in whom only anti-U1 RNP antibody was present[127]. The reported frequency of these antibodies in pregnant normal and lupus women, and their persistence over time, varies widely, influenced particularly by such factors as patient selection and laboratory method[122]. Studies that employ immunodiffusion or counterimmunoelectrophoresis have found frequencies of anti-Ro of 0.4–1.0% in normal pregnant women and 14–33% in lupus[122].

The risk of mothers with anti-Ro antibodies having babies with neonatal lupus is not precisely known. The mere presence of anti-Ro in the mother is not a good predictor. Lockshin, in a prospective study of 91 infants born to women with SLE or SLE-like disease calculated that a pregnant woman who is identified in advance as having lupus or lupus-like syndrome will have a minimum risk of 3% of bearing a child with definite neonatal lupus, and a maximum risk for possible or definite neonatal lupus of 32% if anti-Ro antibodies are present[124]. None of Lockshin's prospectively reported cases had congenital heart block, but from retrospective data he estimated the risk to be less than 3%, consistent with the data of Ramsey-Goldman et al., who found the overall risk of giving birth to an infant with congenital heart block among women with probable or definite SLE to be 1.7%, and 5% when anti-Ro was present[128]. The incidence in the general population is 1 : 20 000[129].

McCune et al. suggested an even greater risk for subsequent pregnancies when the mother had already borne an infant with neonatal lupus, but their small numbers (3 of 12) made this difficult to substantiate[130]. Esscher and Scott, in their review of 67 probands, found that 22 had affected siblings and suggested that an influence transmitted from the mother was relatively important[131]. However, twin pregnancies in Lockshin's study and in others were often discordant, suggesting that the passive transfer of maternal autoantibody alone is not sufficient to explain neonatal lupus[124,132,133]. The frequency of anti-Ro and anti-La antibodies in mothers of congenital heart block infants is at least 83%[126,133,134].

Maternal HLA-DR3 is strongly associated with neonatal lupus, and to date all reported mothers of neonatal lupus infants with congenital heart block have had HLA-DR3[122]. McNicholl et al. reported a relative risk of 24.1 for the haplotype HLA-B8, DR3, DQ2, and DRw52[135].

There is no particular HLA association in the infants, and studies of HLA phenotypes show that the infants inherit maternal HLA antigens randomly. HLA-DR3 in the infant can be found with both cutaneous and congenital heart block manifestations, so that, in the infant, HLA-DR3 does not account for target organ specificity[122].

Maternal outcome

In her review of 245 published cases, Petri found that at the time of delivery of an infant with neonatal lupus syndrome, 40% of mothers were asymptomatic, 35% had lupus in any of its forms (systemic, discoid, subacute cutaneous), 14% had Sjögren's syndrome (which was often mild), and 11% had other connective-tissue disorders (usually undifferentiated)[122]. Studies that include follow-up periods have reported that most of the asymptomatic mothers eventually developed connective-tissue disease symptoms, although this may, in part, have reflected greater maternal and physician awareness of such symptoms which were often mild[130,131,136]. McCune et al., for example, found 8 of 12 initially asymptomatic mothers developed connective-tissue disease symptoms after an average of 4.5 years[130]. It is not known whether the outcome of females with anti-Ro is influenced by pregnancy.

Fetal outcome

Many of the mothers of neonatal lupus infants have a past history of fetal death. However, because many of these mothers have connective-tissue disease, where the fetal death rate is known to be increased, in order to determine the effects of anti-Ro, anti-Ro negative connective-tissue disease mothers are required as controls. In 155 women with systemic lupus erythematosus there was no difference in the rates of fertility or fetal death between the 47 patients with anti-Ro and the 108 without[128]. Similarly, Lockshin found that anti-Ro did not predict fetal death in lupus[137].

The two dominant manifestations of neonatal lupus are transient cutaneous lupus and congenital heart block. It is unusual for them to occur together. There are more published reports on the latter than the former, although it is likely that neonatal cutaneous lesions may be underestimated and underreported[122].

The onset of cutaneous lupus can be at birth or as late as 5 months with a mean onset at 7 weeks[130]. There is some suggestion that it may be precipitated by sun-exposure[130,138]. By 6 months, most infants have cleared the placentally-transferred maternal anti-Ro antibodies and in most infants inflammatory skin lesions (and the systemic features) have completely subsided, but persisting mild hypopigmentation, atrophy, and telangiectasia have been described[130].

Heart block is usually complete and appears abruptly during the last few weeks of pregnancy, although it has developed as early as 22 weeks[139]. Rarely, other conduction disturbances, myocarditis, and structural defects, particularly patent ductus arteriosus, can occur, although these are not necessarily related to maternal autoantibodies[123,125,130]. Unlike the cutaneous lesions, congenital heart block is a permanent defect, with a significant mortality. In a review of 35 patients with congenital heart block (not confined to neonatal lupus cases) Reid found that all but two required a pacemaker before the age of 50, although most pacemakers were inserted during the second to fourth decades, not in the neonatal period[140]. McCune et al. found that 3 of 14 infants with congenital heart block died in the perinatal period, while 5 of the remaining 11 patients required pacemakers[130].

There are at least seven reports of the late development of connective-tissue disease, particularly SLE, in the neonatal lupus syndrome child[141-146]. Although a formal controlled study has not been reported, it is generally felt that this represents genetic predisposition rather than continuation of a primary disease process. However, more prospective long-term studies are required, because most patients documented to have neonatal lupus syndrome are still children.

OTHER CONNECTIVE-TISSUE DISEASES

Mixed connective-tissue disease

Data concerning pregnancy in MCTD are scanty compared with those for SLE[147-149]. Kaufman and Kitridou reported normal fertility and high fetal mortality both before (14%) and after (76%) the onset of clinical disease in 31 patients compared with 9% in normal controls. Uncontrolled retrospective data suggest that the onset of clinical disease and disease exacerbation are not uncommon during gestation[147]. MCTD appears to carry similar pregnancy risks to SLE in terms of both fetal and maternal outcomes[149].

There is one report of the neonatal lupus syndrome in the offspring of mothers with MCTD who have anti-U1 RNP, but no anti-Ro in their blood[150].

Systemic sclerosis

Systemic sclerosis is comparatively rare, often begins after the childbearing years, and may lead to reduced fertility. Although there is a comparatively large literature, much of this comprises single case reports that are presumably selected for their interest, severity, and complications rather than being representative of the general scleroderma population. There are, however, a number of retrospective studies, three of which are case-controlled[151-153] but prospective controlled data are still awaited.

Effect of scleroderma on pregnancy

Several reports suggest that fertility may be reduced in at least some patients with scleroderma[152-154]. However, Giordino et al. from Naples reported 299 pregnancies in 80 women in a clinic population of 86 with scleroderma, compared with 332 pregnancies in 82 of 86 controls[151].

Fifty of the 299 pregnancies (16.7%) reported by Giordino ended in spontaneous abortion compared with 32 of 33 controls (9.6%)[151]. Silman and Black, in a retrospective postal questionnaire study of 115 case-control pairs, found that women with scleroderma had twice the rate of spontaneous abortion and multiple abortions were more frequently reported in the women with scleroderma[152]. These results appeared to be confirmed in an extension of this postal study to 493 pregnancies in 186 women[155]. This increased abortion rate was present prior to the clinical onset of scleroderma, as also has been described in a retrospective study of SLE[82]. The problems inherent in interpreting such data are as described in the section on SLE. In a more detailed study of fetal outcome, Steen found significantly more "small for dates" babies and slightly more premature deliveries but no increase in spontaneous miscarriage or perinatal death compared with rheumatoid arthritis patients and normal controls. As in Silman's study, the adverse outcomes occurred both before and after the onset of clinical disease and were found exclusively in women with limited cutaneous involvement[153].

Scleroderma involvement of the uterine cervix or perineal skin sufficient to cause difficulty with delivery has been described but is uncommon[156,157].

Effect of pregnancy on scleroderma

Steen found that the less-severe manifestations of scleroderma, including Raynaud's phenomenon, digital ulcers, and joint symptoms, were not influenced by pregnancy, although there are reports of skin softening in some patients[153,154,158]. The most significant influence on maternal prognosis is renal involvement. In a series of 21 case reports reviewed by Black and Stevens, all were normotensive at the onset of pregnancy but 10 patients developed renal disease during pregnancy and one in the postpartum period. Seven of the 9 patients with toxemia had biopsy-proven renal scleroderma. Five or possibly 7 of the 9 deaths in the series were due to renal disease[159]. On the other hand, in Steen's own clinic series, renal crisis developed in 4 of 23 women (17%) with diffuse cutaneous scleroderma who had one or more pregnancies during their disease course, compared with 25 of 116 patients (22%) who were not pregnant during the disease course. This difference was not statistically significant[153]. In two instances, renal crisis developed during pregnancy itself and ultimately proved fatal. The frequency of renal crisis occurring during the pregnant versus the nonpregnant state was not significantly different even when the duration of time at risk was taken into account. Furthermore, there was no increase in preeclampsia or hypertension during pregnancy. These observations suggest that even with diffuse cutaneous involvement, pregnancy itself does not increase the already present risk of developing renal crisis. In an earlier study, Steen et al. found rapidly progressive diffuse skin involvement to be a risk factor for developing renal crisis and suggested that pregnancy is unwise in this situation[153]. There are a few reports that captopril may alter the course of renal crisis in pregnancy[153].

The effect of pregnancy on long-term maternal prognosis is unknown. Steen found no differences in survival rates for women with a similar disease subtype (diffuse or limited scleroderma) and of a similar age, with versus without concomitant pregnancy. Although it seems possible that those patients who chose to become pregnant and were able to do so had milder illness, this was not apparent in their series[153].

Relapsing polychondritis (RP)

There is a distinct paucity of information regarding RP in pregnancy. We have recently encountered a 26-year-old patient with RP who had four pregnancies, each of which resulted in the birth of a normal healthy infant[160]. The first and fourth pregnancies were unremarkable. The first sign of eye disease (iritis) occurred between the first two pregnancies. In, as well as, between the second and third she experienced ocular inflammation (scleritis, iritis). Just prior to, and again during, her third pregnancy, she developed episodes of inflammatory chondritis affecting the cartilaginous portion of the ear but sparing the lobule. While it is not possible to generalize from a single case, in this instance the presence of symptoms of RP during one pregnancy did not predict their recurrence in the next pregnancy. Furthermore, in spite of active hydrocortisone-dependent disease during the period of fetal organogenesis, and a rather low initial APGAR score at delivery requiring a period of resuscitation, the final outcome of the third pregnancy was also a normal healthy infant.

MISCELLANEOUS RHEUMATIC DISORDERS

Carpal tunnel syndrome

Two retrospective self-report questionnaire reviews of over 1000 pregnancies each found hand symptoms during pregnancy in around

35%[161,162]. McLennan et al.[162] found similar though less severe symptoms in 30% of nonpregnant premenopausal controls. In 69%, hand symptoms were generalized and in 20% they corresponded to a classical median nerve symptom distribution (carpal tunnel syndrome), while in 12% the symptoms were in the distribution of the ulnar nerve[162]. Voitk et al. found that in 20% the distribution was indefinite, 74% corresponded to the median nerve, and 6% to the ulnar nerve territory[161]. In both of the series, symptoms were bilateral in most cases, commenced in the third trimester, correlated with manifestations of preeclampsia, and tended to recur in subsequent pregnancies. The treatment utilized in both series was quite conservative, although a small number of patients in each reported quite significant pain and disability. While outcome following pregnancy was not specifically addressed, both authors claimed that carpal tunnel syndrome spontaneously resolved with delivery[161,162]. Melvin followed up 15 patients after delivery with clinical and electrophysiologic criteria of carpal tunnel syndrome. Five still had carpal tunnel syndrome at 5 months, two at 10 months, and one had distal median nerve sensory latency persisting at 20 months. Two patients in this series were treated surgically[163]. The proportion receiving surgery seems to vary according to the specialty concerned[164].

Low back pain

There are no precise criteria for pregnancy backache. It is generally accepted as coming on after the fifth month, due to a number of possible causes including strains of the gravid uterus on sacroiliac joint ligaments softened by hormonal changes, hyperextension of the lumbar spine with hypotonicity of the muscles of the back and abdominal wall, and lumbar disc protrusions[25,165].

In a study of 180 women, pregnancy backache occurred in almost 50% and was severe in one-third of these especially at night. The prevalence of backache increased with maternal age and parity, but there was no association with the patient's weight or the baby's birth weight. Many of the women reported experiencing similar backache during labor[166].

The relationship of pregnancy backache to future maternal low back pain remains unknown.

Gonococcal arthritis

Pregnancy is a predisposing factor for disseminated gonococcal infection, possibly due to local mucosal factors[167]. The peak incidence is in the third trimester[168]. Tenosynovitis and skin lesions are common, but a minority of patients develop suppurative arthritis[169]. Both subsets respond well to prompt institution of standard antibiotic regimens with no evidence of an unfavorable effect on the pregnancy[167]. Follow-up does not usually reveal residual maternal joint disease or deformity[168]. Gonococcal infection left untreated, however, will cause cartilage destruction and significant secondary degenerative arthritis[169].

ANTIRHEUMATIC DRUGS IN PREGNANCY AND LACTATION

The effects of antirheumatic drugs on fertility are variable. There is no evidence, for example, that aspirin, the newer NSAIDs, systemic corticosteroids, or antimalarials adversely affect fertility[170]. In contrast, methotrexate[171], and to a greater extent cyclophosphamide, may reduce fertility and the latter may result in sterility[172-175]. The risk to fertility from azathioprine therapy is less certain but may be negligible. It is preferable to discontinue any disease-modifying antirheumatic drugs (DMARDs) at least 3 months prior to conception. This is partly due to concern regarding the potential effects of these drugs on the conceptus and partly because any adverse effects on fertility tend to diminish as a function of time after discontinuation of drug treatment.

The exposure of a pregnant woman to an antirheumatic drug poses a potential risk to fetal health. Since many antirheumatic drugs find application in nonmusculoskeletal conditions, the relevant literature is read across many disciplines and is found in the basic science, general medical, obstetric, and rheumatologic journals. All recent reviews express concern about the exposure of pregnant and lactating women to antirheumatic drugs[170,176,177], only some providing estimates of risk relevant to those patients with active disease in whom drug therapy may be unavoidable. A recent review of the topic by Roubenoff et al.[170] stands apart from other reviews in that a defined protocol was followed in selecting and appraising those articles on which subsequent prevalence estimates were based. In particular, the authors made attempts to rate the strength of the evidence, to check their interrater reliability ($\kappa = 0.75$), and to compare the prevalence rates of congenital malformation to those in the general population and provide 95% confidence intervals. No significant therapeutic developments have occurred since that review, which includes not only human but also animal studies. In general, one has to be cautious in extrapolating findings from animal studies to humans, and from one human disorder to another. The interpretation of the Roubenoff data is complex and a number of factors need to be taken into consideration. These include comorbidity (i.e., some patients had nonmusculoskeletal disease) and concomitant medication (i.e., some patients were receiving more than one medication or were on more than one antirheumatic drug). These other diseases and other drugs, or drug combinations, may themselves have determined the observed prevalence rates rather than the index drugs themselves. Furthermore, the maximum dose, dosing schedule, and time of administration with respect to pregnancy (i.e., before versus during) often differ and this may distort any dose-dependent or time-dependent effects. Many of the estimates were derived by pooling data from diverse sources.

The hazards of meta-analysis are well known[178]. Indeed, apart from the large population surveys, some of the published reports may reflect a positive reporting bias[179]. The referral filters through which patients passed in order to reach the care of subspecialists may also have served to increase event rates in studies based at tertiary referral centers[179]. Furthermore, the Roubenoff study was based on live births and excluded stillbirths. It also used an index for congenital abnormality rates in the general population that was derived from a data source being neither population-based nor a random sample[170]. Such estimates for congenital malformation may show as much as a threefold country-to-country variation[170]. A further limitation of the Roubenoff data is the inclusion of case reports[170]. These cases contribute disproportionately more heavily to the numerator of the prevalence calculation than to the denominator. As a result, the prevalence rates are conservatively high. Indeed, an inspection of the data indicates that all the calculated prevalence rates, with the exception of methotrexate, are increased above the 2.0–3.5 rate for congenital malformation per hundred live births in the general population (Table 3). However, the 95% confidence intervals are large for some drugs. Nevertheless, they do not all overlap the specified "normal range." In particular, aspirin-, indomethacin-, chlorambucil-, and cyclophosphamide-related toxicities are elevated. The authors themselves were cognizant of the potential problems of their method of analysis and are to be complimented for discussing them exhaustively and cautioning readers appropriately. In particular, the data on aspirin and indomethacin are surprising, until one utilizes the authors' rating scores, which reflect the relative scientific strength of each piece of evidence. In other instances, the results of the larger and methodologically more robust studies suggest the absence of any causal association between these drugs and teratogenicity[180-182]. The elevated prevalence rates, observed with these and other drugs, likely represent the absolute upper limit, the true value falling somewhere between these values and those in the general population (once various sources of bias are accounted for). In essence, therefore, it is prudent to be cautious in prescribing these drugs in pregnancy since there is no irrefutable evidence that the antirheumatic drugs are safe (i.e., free of teratogenic potential).

These and other data sources provide some indication of the prognostic issues relating to adverse drug outcomes, even though accurate rates of occurrence elude exact definition. Clearly, the data on aspirin and indomethacin are more extensive than those on the other, newer NSAIDs[183,185]. Thus, in spite of the fact that in large dosages salicylates have been associated with an increased incidence of prolongation of gestation, prematurity, prolonged labor, and greater blood loss during pregnancy and delivery (Table 4), they remain the drugs of choice for treating arthritis in pregnancy[176]. The newer NSAIDs may also prolong gestation and labor and, like salicylates, have infrequently been

Table 3. Estimated prevalence rates of congenital malformation in women receiving antiinflammatory and immunosuppressive drugs, based on published reports

Drug	No. of live births	No. malformed	Rate[a]	95% CI+[b]
Aspirin[c]	5128	349	6.8	6.1-7.6
Indomethacin	230	26	7.0	4.0-11.3
Prednisone	562	25	4.4	2.9-6.6
Chlorambucil	6	2	33.3	6.8-96.4
Cyclophosphamide	9	2	22.2	10.2-44.0
Azathioprine	487	21	3.7	1.5-7.6
Antimalarials	188	7	4.5	1.9-8.7
D-Penicillamine	93	4	4.3	1.2-10.9
Gold	11	1	9.1	2.3-50.7
Methotrexate	290	10	3.4	1.7-6.3

No conclusions should be drawn from this table without consulting the appropriate sections in the text.

[a] Rate per 100 live births. For comparison, the rate of all congenital malformations in the general population is 2.0 to 3.5 per 100 live births. Neonatal hemorrhage, respiratory distress syndrome, and neonatal jaundice are not considered malformations.

[b] 95% confidence intervals calculated using the Poisson distribution.

[c] Based solely on reference 22. Control group (no aspirin exposure) had a congenital malformation rate of 6.9.

From ref. 170 with permission of the authors and the publisher (*Seminars in Arthritis and Rheumatism*).

associated with neonatal bleeding[183]. If possible these drugs should be discontinued a few weeks prior to delivery. This, however, is not always possible. In spite of early concerns regarding an association between systemic corticosteroids and cleft lip and cleft palate[186,187], more recent human data on systemic corticosteroids (i.e., prednisone, prednisolone) have failed to show any teratogenic effects[188-193] or increase in fetal mortality or infection[189,192-194]. It is possible that they may reduce birth weight to a small extent, but this finding remains unconfirmed at the present time[195]. Systemic corticosteroid drugs are regarded as being relatively safe in pregnancy in small doses up to 10 mg prednisone per day. In higher doses there is an increased risk of adrenal suppression[85,196,197]. Systemic corticosteroid drugs should only be used in pregnancy when absolutely necessary. Gold and D-penicillamine find their greatest application in the treatment of rheumatoid disease. The experience with intramuscular gold far exceeds that with oral gold at the present time. Owing to the ameliorating effects of pregnancy on RA, it is often possible to discontinue these drugs during pregnancy or prior to a planned pregnancy. It has been suggested by Ostensen and Husby that intramuscular gold may be given with caution during pregnancy, but D-penicillamine should be avoided (Table 4). D-Penicillamine has been taken in pregnancy not only by arthritis patients but also by those with Wilson's disease and cystinuria. In general, it has proven safe[170], but there are case reports of cutis laxa occurring in children when mothers were treated for their condition with D-penicillamine[198-202]. As a result the debate is ongoing[170,176,177,203]. Antimalarial drug therapy during pregnancy is particularly concerning since it is recognized that this class of drugs can produce chromosomal damage[204] and is concentrated in the fetal uveal tract[205]. However, reports are conflicting, some not showing any evidence of teratogenicity or retinopathy[206-210]. Since the effect on chromosomes is not one of addition or deletion, it is not possible to detect it with routine testing. These effects, together with past experience with antimalarial drugs in the adult population, have led to their almost uniform avoidance during pregnancy. Sulfasalazine has been more extensively studied in pregnant and lactating women with inflammatory bowel disease than with arthritis. In a recent review, Brooks and Needs concluded that there was overwhelming evidence that sulfasalazine treatment was not associated with any increased incidence of fetal malformation[177]. The experience with immunosuppressive and cytotoxic medications is comparatively sparse, although experience, particularly with azathioprine and lately with methotrexate, is growing. It is likely that the teratogenic potential of chlorambucil and cyclophosphamide may exceed that of either azathioprine or methotrexate. However, none of these drugs is regarded as entirely safe in pregnancy at the present time. Ostensen and Husby consider that methotrexate and cyclophosphamide should be avoided while azathioprine might be given with caution (Table 4)[176].

The data of Roubenoff et al. suggest that fetal death is a rare event during antirheumatic drug therapy, there being relatively few reports of fetal wastage[170]. However, their analysis excluded stillbirths, and, since fetal abnormality may result in stillbirth, the true rates of fetal abnormality and fetal wastage remain poorly defined. The fact of the matter is that we really do not know what the exact risks of drug therapy in pregnancy are at the present time. They are probably least for NSAIDs and systemic corticosteroids and greatest for cytotoxic DMARDs. Progression in this area of therapeutics is only likely to occur as a result of a concerted multidisciplinary approach based on either a drugs-in-pregnancy register or large population databases. At present there are four therapeutic principles to be followed: (1) Owing to the often spontaneous nature of conception, it is wise to fully inform every potentially fertile patient of the relevant information relating to these drugs in pregnancy. (2) An attempt should be made to discontinue DMARD therapy at least 3 months prior to conception. (3) If drug therapy is required during pregnancy, then the dosage prescribed should be as low as possible (i.e., that which permits adequate control of the disease). (4) It should be recognized that an active systemic rheumatic disease with major organ involvement may pose a greater threat to the mother, and indirectly to her fetus, than the drug therapy she requires to control her disorder.

The use of antirheumatic drugs during lactation is an additional problem, particularly for RA patients who wish to continue breast-feeding, and in whom the disease so often relapses within a few short

Table 4 Antirheumatic drug treatment during pregnancy

Drug	Reported side-effects	Comments
Salicylates	Prolonged gestation and labor Maternal bleeding Neonatal bleeding Respiratory distress in neonate	Can be given in low dose $\leqslant$ 3g/d, stop treatment 4 weeks prior to delivery
Nonsteroidal anti-inflammatory drugs	Prolonged gestation and labor Premature closure of d. arteriosus Pulmonary hypertension and gastrointestinal bleeding in neonate Renal dysfunction in neonate	May be given in the lowest possible dose, stop treatment 4–2 weeks prior to delivery
Chloroquine	Hearing loss in neonate (single case report)	Not recommended
Gold	None reported in humans	May be given with caution
Penicillamine	Cutis laxa in neonate	Not recommended
Azathioprine	Intrauterine growth retardation and intrauterine virus infection	May be given with caution
Methotrexate and cyclophosphamide	Congenital malformations	Not recommended
Glucocorticosteroids	Cleft palate, adrenal insufficiency (?)	May be given in small doses

Adapted from ref. 176 with permission of the author of the *Scandinavian Journal of Rheumatology*.

weeks of delivery. Salicylates, many of the new NSAIDs and some DMARDs have been detected in variable amounts in breast milk[176]. The clinical decision, therefore, is whether to suppress lactation and transfer the infant to bottle feeding, in order to increase the therapeutic options of the treating physician, or to permit continued breast feeding and give concomitant systemic antirheumatic drugs. Ostensen and Husby have rated low-dose salicylates ($<$ 3 g daily), ibuprofen, ketoprofen, naproxen, diclofenac, mefenamic acid, flufenamic acid, and phenylbutazone as being devoid of risk during lactation[176]. They are less certain about piroxicam[211], and have noted convulsions occurring in a breast-fed infant whose mother received indomethacin (Table 5)[212]. In spite of this, it is recommended that NSAIDs should be given only if necessary and then in the lowest possible dose and where applicable on an intermittent schedule. Systemic corticosteroid drugs also enter breast milk in small quantities. Although the effects are uncertain, Brooks and Needs have noted that with standard doses of prednisolone used in the rheumatic diseases, there is little chance of an infant receiving significant amounts[177]. Large quantities of cyclophosphamide have been found in breast milk[213], and this drug is certainly contraindicated during lactation. In contrast, only small quantities of gold, antimalarials, azathioprine, and methotrexate appear in breast milk[176,177,214-217]. Up to 30% of a single dose of sulfasalazine appears in

Table 5 Nonsteroidal anti-inflammatory drugs in breast milk

Drug	Concentration in breast milk	Effect on nursing infant
Salicylates	4–50% of maternal serum level	No risk of < 3 g/d
Diflunisal	2–7% of maternal serum level	Effect not known
Diclofenac	Small amounts	No risk
Ketoprofen	Small amounts	No risk
Ibuprofen	1% of maternal serum level	No risk
Naproxen	1% of maternal serum level	No risk
Mefenamic acid	Trace amounts	No risk
Flufenamic acid	Trace amounts	No risk
Indomethacin	Exceeds maternal serum level	Contraindicated
Sulindac	Not studied	Effect not known
Phenylbutazone	Small amounts	No risk
Piroxicam	1% of maternal serum level	Probably no risk

Adapted from ref. 176 with permission of the author and the *Scandinavian Journal of Rheumatology*.

breast milk[177]. However, a 7-day study has failed to show any significant displacement of bilirubin from protein binding sites[218]. The decision to use these agents very much depends on the severity of disease, the availability or nonavailability of therapeutic alternatives, and the dose of DMARD therapy being contemplated. In general we prefer to avoid all of these agents during lactation, including D-penicillamine (about which there is little or no information). While collecting data on the ingress of drugs into breast milk is relatively easy, accumulating data on adverse effects on breast-fed infants is much more difficult. This has resulted in our knowledge being limited, and excessively influenced by single case reports of adverse events. This has a biasing effect, tending to augment apparent risks. Data will be difficult to obtain in this area as physicians may prefer to suppress lactation, bottle feed the infant, and thereby increase their therapeutic options. Increased knowledge of DMARD therapy in lactations is likely to come slowly from cases with severe disease requiring treatment and in whom the mother insists on breast feeding. In order to avoid numerator/denominator discrepancies, accurate data will most likely come from prospective studies using registers or other population databases.

We have not attempted to present every case report found in the literature in this overview, since such reports do not constitute proof of a causal relationship between exposure and outcome. Readers interested in pursuing specific drugs or specific outcomes are referred to several recent overviews for more detailed information[170,176,177]. Nevertheless, case reports indicate a need for caution in prescribing and provide justification for further studies in this area of therapeutics.

References

1. Fries, J. F. (1983). Toward an understanding of patient outcome measurement. *Arthritis Rheum.*, **26**, 297-704
2. Hench, P. S. (1938). A meliorating effect of pregnancy on chronic atrophic (infectious) rheumatoid arthritis, fibrositis and intermittent hydrarthrosis. *Proc. Mayo Clin.*, **13**, 161-167
3. Bellamy, N. (1982). In vitro studies on immunoregulation with special reference to rheumatoid arthritis. MD Thesis, Glasgow University, pp. 9-14
4. A committee of the American Rheumatism Association. (1959). Revision of diagnostic criteria for rheumatoid arthritis. *Arthritis Rheum.*, **2**, 16-20
5. Mitchell, D. M., Spitz, P. W., Young, D. Y., Bloch, D. A., McShane, D. J. and Fries, J. F. (1986). Survival prognosis and causes of death in rheumatoid arthritis. *Arthritis Rheum.*, **29**(6), 706-714
6. Ehrlich, G. E. (1978). Restoring arthritics first loss. *Sexual Medicine Today*, **2**, 6-8
7. Yoshino, S. and Uchida, S. (1981). Sexual problems of women with rheumatoid arthritis. *Arch. Phys. Med. Rehabil.*, **62**, 122-123
8. Kay, A. and Bach, F. (1965). Subfertility before and after the development of rheumatoid arthritis in women. *Ann. Rheum. Dis.*, **24**, 169-173
9. Hargreaves, E. R. (1958). A survey of rheumatoid arthritis in west Cornwall. A report to the Empire Rheumatism Council. *Ann. Rheum. Dis.*, **17**, 61-75
10. Klipple, G. L. and Cecere, F. A. (1989). Rheumatoid arthritis and pregnancy. *Rheum. Dis. Clin. North Am.*, **15**(2), 213-239
11. Silman, A. J. (1986). Is pregnancy a risk factor in the causation of rheumatoid arthritis. *Ann. Rheum. Dis.*, **45**, 1031-1034
12. Oka, M. (1953). Effect of pregnancy on the onset on course of rheumatoid arthritis. *Ann. Rheum. Dis.*, **73**, 227-229
13. Oka, M. and Vainio, U. (1966). Effect of pregnancy on the prognosis and serology of rheumatoid arthritis. *Acta Rheum. Scand.*, **12**, 47-52
14. Felbo, M. and Snorrason, E. (1961). Pregnancy and the place of therapeutic abortion in rheumatoid arthritis. *Acta Obstet. Gynecol. Scand.*, **40**, 116-126
15. Betson, J. R. and Dorn, R. V. (1964). Forty cases of arthritis and pregnancy. *J. Int. Coll. Surg.*, **42**(5), 521-526
16. Kaplan, D. and Diamond, H. (1965). Rheumatoid arthritis and pregnancy. *Clin. Obstet. Gynecol.*, **8**(2), 286-303
17. Morris, W. I. C. (1969). Pregnancy in rheumatoid arthritis and systemic lupus erythematosus. *Aust. N. Z. J. Obstet. Gynaecol.*, **9**, 136-144
18. Persellin, R. H. (1977). The effect of pregnancy on rheumatoid arthritis. *Bull. Rheum. Dis.*, **27**(9), 922-927
19. Neely, N. T. and Persellin, R. H. (1977). Activity of rheumatoid arthritis during pregnancy. *Texas Med.*, **73**, 59-63
20. Cecere, F. A. and Persellin, R. H. (1981). The interaction of pregnancy and the rheumatic diseases. *Clin. Rheum. Dis.*, **7**(3), 747-768
21. Unger, A., Kay, A., Griffin, A. J. and Panayi, G. S. (1983). Disease activity and pregnancy associated alpha-2-glycoprotein in rheumatoid arthritis during pregnancy. *Br. Med. J.*, **286**, 750-752
22. Ostensen, M., Aune, B. and Husby, G. Effect of pregnancy and hormonal changes on the activity of rheumatoid arthritis. *Scand. J. Rheumatol.*, **12**, 69-72
23 Ostensen, M. and Husby, G. (1983). A prospective clinical study of the effect of pregnancy on rheumatoid arthritis and ankylosing spondylitis. *Arthritis Rheum.*, **26**(9), 1155-1159
24. Harris, C. J. (1985). Rheumatoid arthritis and the pregnant woman. *Am. J. Nursing*, **85**, 414-417

25. Urowitz, M. B. and Gladman, D. D. (1982). Rheumatic diseases. In Burrow G. N. and Farris, T. F. (eds.) *Medical Complications During Pregnancy*, pp. 474-497 (Philadelphia: W. B. Saunders)
26. Sibley, J. T. (1986). Pregnancy and benign rheumatoid nodules. *Am. J. Med.*, **81**, 1124
27. Mor-Yosef, S., Navot, D., Rabinovwitz, R. and Schenker, J. G. (1984). Collagen diseases in pregnancy. *Obstet Gynecol. Surv.*, **39**(2), 67-84
28. Kaplan, D. (1986). Fetal wastage in patients with rheumatoid arthritis. *J. Rheumatol.*, **13**, 875-877
29. Silman, A. J., Roman, E., Beral, V. and Brown, A. (1988). Adverse reproductive outcomes in women who subsequently develop rheumatoid arthritis. *Ann. Rheum. Dis.*, **47**, 979-981
30. Siamopoulou-Mavridou, A., Manoussakis, M. N., Maviridis, A. K. and Moutsopoulos, H. M. (1988). Outcome of pregnancy in patients with autoimmune rheumatic disease before the disease onset. *Ann. Rheum. Dis.*, **47**, 982-987
31. McHugh, N. J., Reilly, P. A. and McHugh, L. A. (1989). Pregnancy outcome and autoantibodies in connective tissue disease. *J. Rheumatol.*, **16**, 42-46
32. Duhring, J. L. (1970). Pregnancy, rheumatoid arthritis and intra uterine growth retardation. *Am. J. Obstet. Gynecol.*, **108**(2), 325-326
33. Bulmash, J. M. (1979). Rheumatoid arthritis and pregnancy. *Obstet. Gynaecol. Annu.*, **8**, 223-276
34. Thurnau, G. R. (1983). Rheumatoid arthritis. *Clin. Obstet. Gynaecol.*, **26**(3), 558-578
35. Nicholas, N. S. (1988) Rheumatic diseases in pregnancy. *Br. J. Hosp. Med.*, **39**, 50-53
36. Persellin, R. H., Wiginton, D. A. F., Rutstein, J. E. *et al.* (1982). Pregnancy alpha-glycoprotein (PAG) and rheumatoid arthritis (RA) activity: a prospective analysis during gestation. *Arthritis Rheum.*, **25** (Suppl. April), 56
37. Unger, A., Kay, A., Griffin, A. J. *et al.* (1983). Disease activity and pregnancy associated alpha-2-glycoprotein in rheumatoid arthritis during pregnancy. *Br. Med. J. (Clin. Res.)*, **5**, 750-752
38. Ostensen, M., von Schoultz, B. and Husby, G. (1983). Comparison between serum alpha-2-pregnancy-associated globulin and activity in rheumatoid arthritis and ankylosing spondylitis during pregnancy. *Scand. J. Rheumatol.*, **12**, 315-318
39. Wallace, D. J., Goldfinger, D. and Klinenberg, J. R. (1987). Use of autologous pregnancy plasma to treat a flare of juvenile rheumatoid arthritis: a case report and literature review. *J. Clin. Apheresis*, **3**(4), 216-218
40. Bango, M. Y., Garcia Paez, J. M., Solovera, J. J. *et al.* (1985). Adult onset Still's disease: a case with onset during pregnancy. *Arthritis Rheum.*, **28**(8), 957
41. Katz, W. E., Starz, T. W. and Winkelstein, A. (1990). Recurrence of adult Still's disease after pregnancy. *J. Rheumatol.*, **17**, 373-374
42. Stein, G. H., Cantor, B. and Panush, R. S. (1980). Adult Still's disease associated with pregnancy. *Arthritis Rheum.*, **23**(2), 248-250
43. Masi, A. T. and Medsger, T. A. (1979). A new look at the epidemiology of ankylosing spondylitis and related syndromes. *Clin. Orthop.*, **143**, 15
44. Hart, F. D. (1980). Clinical features and complications. In Moll, J. M. H. (ed.) *Ankylosing Spondylitis*, p. 52. (Edinburgh: Churchill Livingstone)
45. Hart, F. D. (1980). Bechterew's syndrome in women: is it different from that in men? *Scand. J. Rheumatol.*, **Suppl. 32**, 38-40
46. Marks, S. H., Barnett, M. and Calin, A. (1983). Ankylosing spondylitis in women and men: A case-control study. *J. Rheumatol.*, **10**, 624-628
47. Ostensen, M. and Husby, G. (1989). Ankylosing spondylitis and pregnancy. *Rheum. Dis. Clin. North Am.*, **15**, 241-254
48. Ostensen, M., Romberg, O. and Husby, G. (1982). Ankylosing spondylitis and motherhood. *Arthritis Rheum.*, **25**, 140-143
49. Husby, G., Ostensen, M. and Gran, J. T. (1988). Ankylosing spondylitis and pregnancy. *Clin. Exp. Rheumatol.*, **6**, 165-167
50. Ostensen, M. (1988). Pregnancy in psoriatic arthritis. *Scand. J. Rheumatol.*, **17**, 67-70
51. Van der Linden, S. M., Valkenburg, H. A., de Jongh, B. M. and Cats, A. (1984). The risk of developing ankylosing spondylitis in HLA-B27 positive individuals: a comparison of relatives of spondylitis patients with the general population. *Arthritis Rheum.*, **27**, 241-249

52. Van der Linden, S. M. and Khan, M. A. (1984). The risk of ankylosing spondylitis in a HLA-B27 positive individual: A reappraisal. *J. Rheumatol.*, **11**, 727-728
53. Calin, A., Marder, A., Beckss, E. and Burns, T. (1983). Genetic differences between B27 positive patients with ankylosing spondylitis and B27 positive healthy controls. *Arthritis Rheum.*, **26**, 1460-1464
54. Calin, A. (1984). Comment on Van der Linden article. *Arthritis Rheum.*, **27**, 1438
55. McHugh, N. and Laurent, M. R. (1986). Psoriatic arthritis and pregnancy. *Br. J. Rheumatol*, **25** (suppl.), 47 (Abstract)
56. Liang, M. H., Socher, S. A., Roberts, W. N. and Esdaile, J. M. (1988). Measurement of systemic lupus erythematosus activity in clinical research. *Arthritis Rheum.*, **31**, 817-825
57. Liang, M. H., Socher, S. A., Larson, M. G. and Schur, P. H. (1989). Reliability and validity of six systems for the clinical assessment of disease activity in systemic lupus erythematosus. *Arthritis Rheum.*, **32**, 1107-1118
58. Lockshin, M. D., Reinitz, E., Druzin, M. L., Murrman, M. and Estes, D. (1984). Lupus pregnancy: case control study demonstrating absence of lupus exacerbation during or after pregnancy. *Am. J. Med.*, **77**, 893-898
59. Lockshin, M. D. (1989). Pregnancy does not cause systemic lupus erythematosus to worsen. *Arthritis Rheum.*, **32**, 665-670
60. Lockshin, M. D. and Levy, R. A. (1989). Effect of pregnancy on rheumatic diseases. In *Proceedings XVII ILAR Congress of Rheumatology*, Rio de Janeiro, Brazil, p. 174
61. Gatenby, P. A. (1989). Systemic lupus erythematosus and pregnancy. *Aust. N. Z. J. Med.*, **19**, 261-278
62. Urowitz, M. B. (1989). Lupus and pregnancy studies. In *Proceedings: Second International Conference on Systemic Lupus Erythematosus*, Singapore.
63. Ramsey-Goldman, R. (1988). Pregnancy in systemic lupus erythematosus. *Rheum. Dis. Clin. North Am.*, **14**, 169-185
64. Mintz, G., Niz, J., Gutierrez, G. et al. (1986). Prospective study of pregnancy in systemic lupus erythematosus. *J. Rheumatol.*, **13**, 732-739
65. Meehan, R. T. and Dorsey, J. K. (1987). Pregnancy among patients with systemic lupus erythematosus receiving immunosuppressive therapy. *J. Rheumatol.*, **14**, 252-258
66. Burkett, G. (1989). Lupus nephropathy and pregnancy. *Clin. Obstet. Gynecol.*, **28**, 310-323
67. Siegall, M., Gwon, N., Lee, S. L., and Wong, W. (1969). Survivorship in systemic lupus erythematosus: relationship to race and pregnancy. *Arthritis Rheum.*, **12**, 117-125
68. Friedman, E. A. and Rutherford, J. W. (1956). Pregnancy and lupus erythematosus. *Obstet. Gynecol.*, **8**, 601-609
69. Fraga, A., Mintz, G., Orozco, J. and Orozco, J. H. (1974). Sterility and fertility rates, fetal wastage and maternal morbidity in systemic lupus erythematosus. *J. Rheumatol.*, **1**, 293-298
70. Tozman, E. C. S., Urowitz, M. D. and Gladman, D. D. (1980). Systemic lupus erythematosus and pregnancy. *J. Rheumatol.*, **7**, 624-632
71. Estes, D. and Larson, D. L. (1965). Systemic lupus erythematosus and pregnancy. *Clin. Obstet. Gynecol.*, **8**, 307-321
72. Dubois, E. L. (1974). The clinical picture of systemic lupus erythematosus. In Dubois, E. L. (ed.) *Lupus Erythematosus*, pp. 324-330, 371-379, 612. (Los Angeles: University of Southern California Press)
73. Martinez-Cordero, E., Reyes, P. A., Porias, H., Hernandez, A., Romo, J. and Katona, G. (1982). Systemic lupus erythematosus and amenorrhea. Hormonal profile and pathogenic significance. *Arthritis Rheum.*, **25**, 581
74. Zurier, R. B. (1987). Systemic lupus erythematosus and pregnancy. In Lahita, R. G. (ed.) *Systemic Lupus Erythematosus*, p. 545 (New York: Wiley)
75. Lockshin, M. D., Harpel, P. C., Druzin, M. L., Becker, C. G., Klein, R. F., Watson, R. M., Elkon, K. B. and Reinitz, E. (1985). Lupus pregnancy. II. Unusual pattern of hypocomplementemia and thrombocytopenia in the pregnant patient. *Arthritis Rheum.*, **28**, 58-66

76. Buyon, J. P., Cronstein, B. N., Morris, M., Tanner, M. and Weissman, G. (1986). Serum complement values (C3 and C4) to differentiate between systemic lupus activity and pre-eclampsia. *Am. J. Med.*, **81**, 194-200
77. Lockshin, M. D., Qamar, T. and Druzin, M. L. (1987). Hazards of lupus pregnancy. *J. Rheumatol.*, **14** (suppl. 13), 214-217
78. Hayslett, J. P. and Lynn, R. I. (1980). Effect of pregnancy in patients with lupus nephropathy. *Kidney Int.*, **18**, 207-220
79. Houser, M. T., Fish, A. J., Williams, P. P. and Michael, A. F. (1980). Pregnancy and systemic lupus erythematosus. *Am. J. Obstet. Gynecol.*, **138**, 409-413
80. Jungers, P., Dougados, M., Pelissier, C., Kuttenn, F., Tron, F. and Lesaure, P. (1982). Lupus nephropathy and pregnancy. *Arch. Intern. Med.*, **142**, 771-776
81. Mund, A., Simson, J. and Rothfield, N. (1963). Effect of pregnancy on course of systemic lupus erythematosus. *J. Am. Med. Assoc.*, **183**, 917-920
82. Grigor, R. R., Shervington, P. C., Hughes, G. R. V. and Hawkins, D. F. (1977). Outcome of pregnancy in system lupus erythematosus. *Proc. R. Soc. Med.*, **70**, 99-100
83. Chesley, L. C. (1978). *Hypertensive Disorders in Pregnancy*, pp. 504-508. (New York, Appleton-Century-Crofts)
84. Mintz, G. and Rodriguez-Alvarez, E. (1989). Systemic lupus erythematosus. *Rheum. Dis. Clin. North Am.*, **15**, 255-274
85. Fine, L. G., Barnett, E. V., Danovitch, G. M., Nissenson, A. R., Conolly, M. E., Lieb, S. M. and Barrett, C. J. (1981). Systemic lupus erythematosus in pregnancy. *Am. Intern. Med.*, **94**, 667-677
86. Kistner, R. W. (1971). In Kistner, R. W. (ed.) *Gynecology Principles and Practice*, 2nd Edn., p. 500. (Chicago: Year Book Medical Publishers)
87. Abramowsky, C. R., Vegas, M. E., Swinehart, G. and Gyues, M. T. (1980). Decidual vasculopathy of the placenta in lupus erythematosus. *N. Engl. J. Med.*, **303**, 668-672
88. Dkombroski, R. A. (1989). Autoimmune disease in pregnancy. *Med. Clin. North Am.*, **73**, 605-621
89. Gimovsky, M. L., Benner, P., Mosntoro, M. *et al.* (1983). Successful pregnancy in a patient with systemic lupus erythematosus, renal transplantation and chronic renal failure. *J. Reprod. Med.*, **28**, 677-680
90. Asherson, R. A., Derksen, R. H. W. M., Harris, E. N., Bouma, B. N., Gharavi, A. E., Kater, L. and Hughes, G. R. V. (1987). Chorea in systemic lupus erythematosus and "lupus-like" disease: Association with antiphospholipa antibodies. *Semin. Arthritis Rheum.*, **16**, 253-259
91. Boey, M. L., Colaco, C. B., Gharavi, A. E., Elkon, K. B., Loizou, S. and Hughes, G. R. V. (1983). Thrombosis in systemic lupus erythematosus: striking association with the presence of circulating lupus anticoagulant. *Br. Med. J.*, **287**, 1021-1023
92. Gastineau, D. A., Kazmier, F. J., Nichols, W. L. and Bowie, E. J. (1985). Lupus anticoagulant: An analysis of the clinical and laboratory features of 219 cases. *Am. J. Hematol.*, **19**, 265-275
93. Much, J. R., Herbst, K. D. and Rappaport, S. I. (1980). Thrombosis in patients with the lupus anticoagulant. *Ann. Intern. Med.*, **92**, 156-159
94. Hughes, G. R. V. (1983). Thrombosis, abortion, cerebral disease and lupus anticoagulant. *Br. Med. J.*, **287**, 1088-1089
95. Eswaran, K. and Rosen, S. W. (1985). Recurrent abortions, thromboses, and a circulating anticoagulant. *Am. J. Obstet. Gynecol.*, **151**, 751-752
96. Branch, W. D., Scott, J. R., Kochenour, N. K. *et al.* (1985). Obstetric complications associated with the lupus anticoagulant. *N. Engl. J. Med.*, **313**, 1322-1326
97. Weinstein, C., Miller, M. H., Axtens, R., Buchanan, R. and Littlejohn, G. O. (1987). Livedo reticularis associated with increased titres of anticardiolipin antibodies in systemic lupus erythematosus. *Arch. Dermatol.*, **123**, 596-600
98. Kalunian, K. C., Peter, J. B., Middlekauf, H. R., Sayre, J., Ando, D. G., Mangotich, M. and Hahn, B. H. (1988). Clinical significance of a single test for anticardiolipin antibodies in patients with systemic lupus erythematosus. *Am. J. Med.*, **85**, 602-608
99. Chartash, E. K., Paget, S. A. and Lockshin, M. D. (1986). Lupus anticoagulant

associated with aortic and mitral valve insufficiency. *Arthritis Rheum.*, **29**, 595 (Abstract)
100. Khamashta, M. A., Oliver, J. M., Gil, A., Fernando, Z., de Soria, R., Dominquez, F. J. and Vasquez, J. J. (1988). High frequency of subclinical mitral valve dysfunction in patients with SLE: a prospective doppler and echocardiographic study. *Br. J. Rheumatol*, **27** (suppl. 2), 73
101. Mackworth-Young, C. G., Loizou, S. and Walport, M. J. (1989). Primary antiphospholipid syndrome: features of patients with raised anticardiolipin antibodies and no other disorder. *Ann. Rheum. Dis.*, **48**, 362–367
102. Alarcon-Segovia, D. (1988). Pathogenetic potential of antiphospholipid antibodies. *J. Rheumatol.*, **15**, 890–893
103. Lockshin, M. D., Qamar, T., Druzin, M. L. and Goei, S. (1987). Antibody to cardiolipin, lupus anticoagulant and fetal death. *J. Rheumatol.*, **14**, 259–262
104. Pattison, N. S., McKay, E. J., Liggins, G. C. and Lubbe, W. F. (1987). Anticardiolipin antibodies: their presence as a marker of lupus anticoagulant in pregnancy. *N. Z. Med. J.*, **100**, 61–63
105. Lockshin, M. D., Druzin, M. L., Goei, S., Qamar, T., Magid, M. S., Jovanovic, L. and Ferene, M. (1985). Antibody to cardiolipin as a predictor of fetal distress or death in pregnant patients with systemic lupus erythematosus. *N. Engl. J. Med.*, **313**, 152–156
106. Cronin, M. E., Biswas, R. M., Van der Stracton, C., Fleisher, T. A. and Klippel, J. M. (1988). IgG and IgM anticardiolipin antibodies in patients with lupus with anticardiolipin antibody associated clinical syndromes. *J. Rheumatol.*, **15**, 795–798
107. Hughes, G. R. V., Harris, E. N. and Gharavi, A. E. (1986). The anticardiolipin syndrome. *J. Rheumatol.*, **13**, 486–489
108. Harris, E. N., Gharavi, A. E., Patel, S. P. and Hughes, G. R. V. (1987). Evaluation of the anticardiolipin antibody test: report of an international workshop held 4 April 1986. *Clin. Exp. Immunol.*, **68**, 215–222
109. Petri, M., Rheinschmidt, M., Whiting-O'Keefe, Q., Hellman, D. and Corash, L. (1987). The frequency of lupus anticoagulant in systemic lupus erythematosus: a study of 60 consecutive patients by activated partial thromboplastin time, Russell viper venom time, and anticardiolipin antibody level. *Ann. Intern. Med.*, **106**, 524–530
110. Lechner, K. (1987). Lupus anticoagulants and thrombosis. In Verstraete, M., Vermylen, J., Lijneu, R. and Arnaut, J. (eds.) *Thrombosis and Hemostasis*, pp. 525–547 (Leuven: International Society on Thrombosis and Hemostasis and Leuven, University Press)
111. Lockshin, M. D. (1989). Anticardiolipin antibodies and pregnancy. *Proceedings XVII ILAR Congress of Rheumatology*, Rio de Janeiro, Brazil, pp. 43–45
112. Petri, M., Golbus, M., Anderson, R., Whiting-O'Keefe, Q. Corash, L. and Hellman, D. (1987). Antinuclear antibody, lupus anticoagulant, and anticardiolipin antibody in women with idiopathic habitual abortions. *Arthritis Rheum.* **30**, 601–606
113. Cowchock, S., Fort, J., Munoz, S., Norberg, R. and Maddrey, W. (1988). False positive ELISA tests for anticardiolipin antibodies in sera from patients with repeated abortion, rheumatologic disorders and primary biliary cirrhosis: correlation with elevated polyclonal IgM and implications for patients with repeated abortion. *Clin. Exp. Immunol.*, **73**, 289–294
114. Hughes, G. R. V., Asherson, R. A. and Khamashta, M. A. (1989). Antiphospholipid syndrome: linking many specialties. *Ann. Rheum. Dis.*, **48**, 355–356
115. Lubbe, W. F. and Liggins, G. C. (1985). Lupus anticoagulant and pregnancy. *Am. J. Obstet. Gynecol.*, **153**, 322–327
116. Branch, D., Scott, J., Kochenaur, N. and Hershgold, E. (1985). Obstetric complications associated with the lupus anticoagulant. *N. Engl. J. Med.*, **313**, 1322–1326
117. Hanly, J. G., Gladman, D. D., Rose, T. H., Laskin, C. A. and Urowitz, M. B. (1988). Lupus pregnancy. A prospective study of placental changes. *Arthritis Rheum.*, **31**, 358–366
118. Stafford-Brady, F. J., Gladman, D. D. and Urowitz, M. B. (1988). Successful pregnancy in systemic lupus erythematosus with an untreated lupus anticoagulant. *Arch. Intern. Med.*, **148**, 1647–1648
119. Trudinger, B. J., Stewart, G. J., Cook, C. M., Connelly, A. and Exner, T. (1988).

Monitoring lupus anticoagulant-positive pregnancies with umbilical artery flow velocity waveforms. *Obstet. Gynecol.*, **72**, 215-218

120. Harris, E. N. (1988).Third International Antiphospolipid Conference: barbecues, rum punches, and kaps. *Ann. Rheum. Dis.*, **47**, 612-614
121. Walport, M. J. (1989). Pregnancy and antibodies to phospholipids. *Ann. Rheum. Dis.*, **48**, 795-797
122. Petri, M., Watson, R. and Hochberg, M. L. (1989). Anti-Ro antibodies and neonatal lupus. *Rheum. Dis. Clin. North Am.*, **15**, 335-360
123. Provost, T. T., Watson, R., Garther, K. K. and Harley, J. B. (1987). The neonatal lupus erythematosus syndrome. *J. Rheumatol.*, **14**, 199-207
124. Lockshin, M. D., Bonfa, E., Elkon, K. and Druzin, M. L. (1988). Neonatal risk to newborns of mothers with systemic lupus erythematosus. *Arthritis Rheum.*, **31**, 697-701
125. Buyon, J. P., Sweisky, S. H., Fox, H. E., Bierman, F. Z. and Winchester, R. J. (1987). Intrauterine therapy for presumptive fetal myocarditis with acquired heart block due to systemic lupus erythematosus. *Arthritis Rheum.*, **30**, 44-49
126. Taylor, P. V., Taylor, K. F., Norman, A., Griffiths, S. and Scott, J. S. (1988). Prevalence of maternal Ro (SS-A) and La (SS-B) autoantibodies in relation to congenital heart block. *Br. J. Rheumatol.*, **27**, 128-132
127. Provost, T. T., Watson, R. M., Gammon, W. R., Radowsky, M., Harley, J. B. and Reichlin, M. (1987). The neonatal lupus syndrome associated with U1 RNP (nRNP) antibodies. *N. Engl. J. Med.*, **316**, 1135-1138
128. Ramsey-Goldman, R., Hom, D., Deng, J. S., Ziegler, G. C., Kahl, L. E., Steen, V. D., La Porte, R. E. and Medsger, J. A. (1986). Anti-SS-A antibodies and fetal outcome in maternal systemic lupus erythematosus. *Arthritis Rheum.*, **29**, 1269-1273
129. Michaelsson, M. and Engle, M. A. (1972). Congenital complete heart block: An international study of the natural history. *Cardiovasc. Clin.*, **4**, 85-101
130. McCune, A. B., Weston, W. L. and Lee, L. A. (1987). Maternal and fetal outcome in neonatal lupus erythematosus. *Ann. Intern. Med.*, **106**, 518-523
131. Esscher, E. and Scott, J. S. (1979). Congenital heart block and maternal systemic lupus erythematosus. *Br. Med. J.*, **1**, 1235-1238
132. Harley, J. B., Kaine, J. L., Fox, O. F., Reichlin, M. and Gruber, B. (1985). Ro (SS-A) antibody and antigen in a patient with congenital complete heart block. *Arthritis Rheum.*, **28**, 1321-1325
133. Callen, J. P., Fowler, J. F., Kulick, K. B., Stelzer, G. and Smith, S. Z. (1985). Neonatal lupus erythematosus occurring in one fraternal twin: serologic and immunogenetic studies. *Arthritis Rheum.*, **28**, 271-275
134. Scott, J. S., Maddison, P. J., Taylor, P. V., Esscher, E., Scott, O. and Skinner, R. P. (1983). Connective tissue disease, antibodies to ribonucleoprotein and congenital heart block. *N. Engl. J. Med.*, **309**, 209-212
135. McNicholl, J. M., Provost, T. T., Bias, W.-B., Harley, J. B., Reichlin, M. and Alexander, E. L. (1988). Immunogenic relationship between anti-Ro (SS-A) positive Sjogrens syndrome/lupus erythematosus patients and mothers of infants with neonatal lupus erythematosus. *Arthritis Rheum.*, **31**, 594
136. Kasinath, B. S. and Katz, A. I. (1982). Delayed maternal lupus after delivery of offspring with congenital heart block. *Arch. Intern. Med.*, **142**, 2317
137. Lockshin, M. D., Harpel, P. C., Druzin, M. C., Becker, C. G., Klein, R. F., Watson, R. M., Elkon, K. B. and Reinitz, E. (1985). Lupus pregnancy. II. Unusual pattern of hypocomplementemia and thrombocytopenia in the pregnant patient. *Arthritis Rheum.*, **28**, 58-66
138. Watson, R. M., Lane, A. T., Barnett, N. K., Bias, W. B., Arnett, F. C. and Provost, T. T. (1984). Neonatal lupus erythematosus. A clinical, serological and immunogenetic study with review of the literature. *Medicine (Baltimore)*, **63**, 362-378
139. Maddison, P. J. (1988). The neonatal lupus syndrome. *Clin. Exp. Rheumatol.*, **6**, 173-178
140. Reid, J. M., Coleman, E. N. and Doig, W. (1982). Complete congenital heart block. Report of 35 cases. *Br. Heart J.*, **48**, 236-240
141. McCune, C. M., Mantakas, M. E., Tingelstad, J. B. and Ruddy, S. (1977). Congenital heart block in newborn of mothers with connective tissue disease. *Circulation*, **56**, 82-90

142. Lanham, J. G., Walport, M. J. and Hughes, G. R. V. (1983). Congenital heart block and familial connective tissue disease. *J. Rheumatol.*, **10**, 823-825
143. Waterworth, R. F. (1980). Systemic lupus erythematosus occurring with congenital complete heart block. *N. Z. Med. J.*, **92**, 311-312
144. Brustein, D., Rodriquez, J. M. and Minkin, F. (1977). Familial lupus erythematosus. *J. Am. Med. Assoc.*, **238**, 2294
145. Jackson, R. and Gulliver, M. (1979). Neonatal lupus erythematosus progressing into systemic lupus erythematosus: a 15 year follow-up. *Br. J. Dermatol.*, **101**, 81-86
146. Fox, J. R., McCuistion, C. H. and Schooch, E. P. (1979). Systemic lupus erythematosus: association with previous neonatal lupus erythematosus. *Arch. Dermatol.*, **115**, 340
147. Kaufman, R. L. and Kitridou, R. C. (1982). Pregnancy in mixed connective tissue disease: comparison with systemic lupus erythematosus. *J. Rheumatol.*, **9**, 549-555
148. Bennett, R. M. and O'Connell, D. (1980). Mixed connective tissue disease: a clinicopathologic study of 20 cases. *Semin. Arthritis Rheum.*, **10**, 25-31
149. Kitridou, R. C. (1988). Pregnancy in mixed connective tissue disease, polydermatomyositis and scleroderma. *Clin. Exp. Rheumatol.*, **6**, 173-178
150. Provost, T. T., Watson, R., Gammon, W. R., Radowsky, M., Harley, J. B. and Reichkin, M. (1987). The neonatal lupus syndrome associated with U. RNP (nRNP) antibodies. *N. Engl. J. Med.*, **316**, 1135-1138
151. Giordino, M., Valentini, G., Lupolis, S. and Giordano, A. (1985). Pregnancy and systemic sclerosis. *Arthritis Rheum.*, **28**, 237-238
152. Silman, A. J. and Black, C. (1988). Increased incidence of spontaneous abortion and infertility in women with scleroderma before disease onset: a controlled study. *Ann. Rheum. Dis.*, **47**, 441-444
153. Steen, V. D., Conte, C., Day, N., Ramsey-Goldman, R. and Medsger, T. A. (1989). Pregnancy in women with systemic sclerosis. *Arthritis Rheum.*, **32**, 151-157
154. Ballou, S. P., Morley, J. J. and Kashnor, I. (1984). Pregnancy and systemic sclerosis. *Arthritis Rheum.*, **27**, 295-298
155. Englert, H., Black, C. M. and Silman, A. (1988). Pregnancy outcome in patients with scleroderma. *Br. J. Rheumatol.*, **27** (abs. suppl. 2), 75
156. Stevener, M. A. and Ng, A. B. P. (1970). Scleroderma of the uterine cervix. *Am. J. Obstet. Gynecol.*, **107**, 965-966
157. Johnson, T. R., Banner, E. A. and Winkelmann, R. K. (1964). Scleroderma and pregnancy. *Obstet. Gynecol.*, **23**, 467-469
158. Scarpinato, L. and MacKenzie, A. H. (1985). Pregnancy and systemic sclerosis: case report and review of the literature. *Cleve. Clin. Q.*, **52**, 207-211
159. Black, C. M. and Stevens, W. M. (1989). Scleroderma. *Rheum. Dis. Clin. North Am.*, **15**, 193-212
160. Bellamy, N. and Dewar, C. L. (1990). Relapsing polychondritis in pregnancy. *J. Rheumatol.* (in press)
161. Voitk, A. J., Mueller, J. C., Farlinger, D. E. and Johnston, R. V. (1987). Carpal tunnel syndrome in pregnancy. *Can. Med. Assoc. J.*, **128**, 277-281
162. McLennan, G., Oats, J. N. and Walstab, J. E. (1987). Survey of hand symptoms in pregnancy. *Med. J. Aust.*, **147**, 542-544
163. Melvin, J. L., Burnett, C. N. and Johnson, E. W. (1969). Median nerve conduction in pregnancy. *Arch. Phys, Med. L.*, **50**, 75-80
164. Tobin, S. M. (1967). Carpal tunnel syndrome in pregnancy. *Am. J. Obstet. Gynecol.*, **97**, 493-498
165. Golding, D. N. (1982). Some problems of backache in women. In Hill A. G. S. (ed.) *Topical Reviews in Rheumatic Disorders*, pp. 203-213. (Bristol: John Wright and Sons)
166. Mantle, M. J., Greenwood, R. M. and Currey, H. L. F. (1977). Backache in pregnancy. *Rheumatol Rehabil.*, **16**(2), 95-101
167. O'Brien, J. P., Goldenberg, D. L. and Rice, P. A. (1983). Disseminated gonococcal infection: a prospective analysis of 49 patients and a review of pathophysiology and immune mechanisms. *Medicine*, **62**, 395-406
168. Taylor, H. A., Bradford, S. A. and Patterson, S. P. (1966). Gonococcal arthritis in pregnancy. *Obstet. Gynecol.*, **27**, 776-782

169. Eisenstein, B. I. and Masi, A. T. (1981). Disseminated gonococcal infection (DGI) and gonococcal arthritis (GCA): I. Bacteriology, epidemiology, host factors, pathogen factors, and pathology. *Semin. Arthritis Rheum.*, **10**(3), 155-172
170. Roubenoff, R., Hoyt, J., Petri, M. *et al.* (1988). Effects of anti-inflammatory and immunospressive drugs on pregnancy and fatality. *Semin. Arthritis Rheum.*, **18**(2), 88-110
171. Rustin, G. J., Both, M., Dent, J. *et al.* (1984). Pregnancy after cytotoxic chemotherapy for gestational trophoblastic tumours. *Br. Med. J.*, **288**, 103-105
172. Warne, G. L., Farley, K. F., Hobbs, J. B. *et al.* (1973). Cyclophosphamide-induced ovarian failure. *N. Engl. J. Med.*, **289**, 1159-1162
173. Uldall, P. R., Kerr, D. N. S. and Tacchi, D. (1972). Sterility and cyclophosphamide. *Lancet*, **1**, 693-694
174. Kumar, R., McEvoy, J., Biggart, J. D. *et al.* (1972). Cyclophosphamide and reproductive function. *Lancet*, **1**, 1212-1214
175. Kayama, H., Wada, T., Nishizawa, Y. *et al.* (1977). Cyclophosphamide-induced ovarian failure and its therapeutic significance with patients with breast cancer. *Cancer*, **39**, 1403-1409
176. Ostensen, M. and Husby, G. (1985). Anti-rheumatic drug treatment during pregnancy and lactation. *Scand. J. Rheumatol.* **14**, 1-7
177. Brooks, P. M. and Needs, C. J. (1989). The use of antirheumatic medication during pregnancy and in the puerperium. *Rheum. Dis. Clin. North Am.*, **15**(4), 789-806
178. Boissel, J. P., Blanchard, J., Panak, E. *et al.* (1989). Considerations for the meta-analysis of randomized clinical trials. *Controlled Clinical Trials*, **10**, 254-281
179. Sackett, D. L. (1979). Bias in analytic research. *J. Chronic Dis.*, **32**, 51-63
180. Slone, D., Heinonen, O. P., Kaufman, D. W. *et al.* (1976). Aspirin and congenital malformations. *Lancet*, **1**, 1373-1375
181. Dudley, D. K. L. and Hardie, M. J. (1985). Fetal and neonatal affects of indomethacin as a tocolytic agent. *Am. J. Obstet. Gynecol.*, **151**, 181-184
182. Niebyl, J. R. and Witter, F. R. (1986). Neonatal outcome after indomethacin treatment for preterm labour. *Am. J. Obstet. Gynecol.*, **155**, 747-749
183. Wilkinson, A. R., Aynsley-Green, A. and Mitchell, M. D. (1971). Persistent pulmonary hypertension and abnormal prostaglandin E levels in preterm infants after maternal treatment with naproxen. *Arch. Dis. Child.*, **54**, 942-945
184. Wilkinson, A. R. (1980). Naproxen levels in preterm infants after maternal treatment. *Lancet*, **2**, 591-592
185. Alun-Jones, E., Williams, J. and Clwyd, G. (1986). Hyponatremia and fluid retention in a neonatal associated with maternal naproxen overdosage. *Clin. Toxicol.*, **24**, 257-260
186. Bongiovanni, A. M. and McPadden, A. J. (1960). Steroids during pregnancy and possible fetal consequences. *Fertil. Steril.*, **11**(2), 181-186
187. Serment, M. M. H., Charpin, J., Tessier, G. *et al.* (1968). Corticotherapie et grossesse. *Bull. Fed. Soc. Gynecol. Langue Francaise*, **20**, 159-161
188. Jefferies, W. M. and Levy, R. P. (1959). Treatment of ovarian dysfunction with small doses of cortisone or hydrocortisone. *J. Clin. Endocrinol. Metab.*, **19**, 1069-1080
189. Walsh, S. D. and Clark, F. R. (1967). Pregnancy in patient on long term corticosteroids therapy. *Scott. Med. J.*, **12**, 302-306
190. Oakey, R. E. (1970). The interpretation of urinary estrogen and pregnanediol excretion in pregnant women receiving corticosteroids. *J. Obstet. Gynecol.*, **77**, 922-927
191. Schatz, M., Patterson, R., Zeitz, S. *et al.* (1975). Corticosteroid therapy for the pregnant asthmatic patient. *J. Am. Med. Assoc.*, **233**, 804-807
192. Taeusch, H. W., Frigoletto, F., Kitzmiller, J. J. *et al.* (1979). Risk of respiratory distress syndrome after prenatal dexamethasone treatment. *Paediatrics*, **63**, 64-72
193. Collaborative Group on Antenatal Steroid Therapy (1981). Effect of antenatal dexamethasone administration on the prevention of respiratory distress syndrome. *Am. J. Obstet. Gynecol.*, **141**, 276-286
194. Yackel, D. B., Kempers, R. D. and McConahey, W. M. (1966). Adrenocorticosteroid therapy in pregnancy. *Am. J. Obstet. Gynecol.*, **96**, 985-989

195. Reinsch, J. M. and Simon, M. J. (1978). Prenatal exposure to prednisone in humans and animals retards intrauterine growth. *Science*, **202**, 436-438
196. Oppenheimer, E. H. (1964). Lesions in the adrenals of an infant following maternal corticosteroid therapy. *Bull. Johns Hopkins Hosp.*, **114**, 146-151
197. Taeusch, H. W., Kamali, H., Hehre, A. *et al.* (1977). Dexamethasone and its effect on adrenal function in prematures. *Pediatr. Res.*, **11**, 432
198. Lyle, W. H. (1978). Penicillamine in pregnancy. *Lancet*, **1**, 606-607
199. Mjolnerod, O.-K., Rasmussen, K., Dommerud, S. A. *et al.* (1971). Congenital connective-tissue defect probably due to D-penicillamine treatment in pregnancy. *Lancet*, **1**, 673-674
200. Solomon, L., Abrams, G. Dinneser, M. *et al.* (1977). Neonatal abnormalities associated with D-penicillamine treatment during pregnancy. *N. Engl. J. Med.*, **296**, 54-55
201. Lenares, A., Zarrazz, J. J., Rodriquez-Alarcon, J. *et al.* (1977). Reversible cutis laxa due to maternal D-penicillamine treatment. *Lancet*, **2**, 43
202. Harpey, J. P., Jaudon, M. C., Clavel, J. P. *et al.* (1983). Cutis laxa and low serum zinc after antenatal exposure to penicillamine. *Lancet*, **2**, 144-145
203. Endres, W. (1981). D-Penicillamine in pregnancy — to ban or not to ban. *Med. Klin.Wochenschr.*, **59**, 535-537
204. Neel, W. A., Panaye, G. S., Duthie, J. J. R. *et al.* (1973). Action of chloroquine phosphate in rheumatoid arthritis. II. Chromosone damaging effect. *Ann. Rheum. Dis.*, **32**, 547-550
205. Ullberg, S., Lindquist, N. J. and Sjostrand, S. E. (1970). Accumulation of chororetinotoxic drugs in the fetal eye. *Nature*, **227**, 1257-1258
206. Merwin, C. F. and Winkelmann, R. K. (1962). Anti-malarial drugs in the therapy of lupus erythematosus. *Mayo Clin. Proc.*, **37**, 253-268
207. Dziubinski, E. H., Winkelmann, R. K. and Wilson, R. B. (1962). Systemic lupus erythematosus and pregnancy. *Am. J. Obstet. Gynecol.*, **84**, 1873-1877
208. Stone, C. T. (1962). Antimalarial drugs in the treatment of rheumatoid arthritis. *Tex. J. Med.*, **58**, 809
209. Fraga, A., Mintz, G., Orozco, J. and Orozco, J. H. (1974). Sterility and fertility rates, fetal wastage and maternal morbidity in systemic lupus erythematosus. *J. Rheumatol.*, **1**, 293-298
210. Park, A. L. (1988). Antimalarial drugs, systemic lupus erythematosus and pregnancy. *J. Rheumatol.*, **15**, 607-610
211. Ostensen, M. (1983). Piroxicam in human breast milk. *Eur. J. Clin. Pharmacol.*, **25**, 829
212. Eeg-Olofsson, O., Malmros, I., Elwin, C. E. *et al.* (1978). Convulsions in a breast-fed infant after maternal indomethacin. *Lancet*, **2**, 215
213. Wiernik, P. H. and Duncan, J. H. (1971). Cyclophosphamide in human milk. *Lancet*, **1**, 912
214. Blau, S. P. (1973). Metabolism of gold during lactation. *Arthritis Rheum.*, **16**, 777-778
215. Merland, R. and Creste, M. (1951). Study of the elimination and estimation of nivaquine in human milk. *Med. Trop.*, **11**, 793-795
216. Anderson, P. O. (1977). Drugs and breast feeding — a review. *Drug Int. Clin. Pharm.*, **11**, 208-223
217. Johns, D. G., Rutherford, L. D., Leighton, P. C. *et al.* (1972). Secretion of methotrexate into human milk. *Am. J. Obstet. Gynecol.*, **112**, 978-980
218. Esbjorner, E., Jarnerot, G. and Wranne, L. (1986). Sulphasalazine and sulphapyridine levels in children of mothers treated with sulphasalazine during pregnancy and lactation. *Acta Paediatr. Scand.*, **76**, 137-142

15
Fibromyalgia

F. WOLFE

Musculoskeletal aching and concomitant soft-tissue rheumatism are the most common rheumatic disorders. They are rarely identified as "diseases" or "disorders" in population surveys because of the difficulty in reliable diagnosis[1,2]. Clinicians have similar troubles. Pain in the arm, leg, buttock, or chest, for example, is often difficult to understand and explain, and can be attributed to disk disorders, neuritis, bursitis, tendonitis, myositis, arthritis, myofascial pain, and psychologic disturbance. Few validation studies relating to diagnostic accuracy have been performed in these conditions and, although they remain common in the clinic, their vagueness and lack of adequate definition and validated criteria has generally excluded them as subjects for valued research.

Fibromyalgia, a disorder of generalized musculoskeletal pain, has been plagued by similar problems. From the point of view of face credibility, fibromyalgia (fibrositis) has been suspect. It does not fit within the general biomedical model of disease. It has no clearly understood pathophysiology; it has been linked to psychological abnormality[3-7], and the diagnostic term has been applied to so many disparate local and generalized muscular and nonmuscular conditions that it lacked specificity and useful meaning.[8] Even the widely used (and actually quite good[9]) criteria of Yunus *et al.* with their emphasis on anxiety, headache, modulation of symptoms with weather, vacation, noise, etc., seemingly added to the face *in*credibility of the syndrome. What has driven research into the syndrome, however, is the sheer number of rheumatic disease patients with generalized pain[10,11]. What has made research possible is a change in the research model from individual case reports and small uncontrolled studies to scientifically and epidemiologically sound descriptive reports[6,9,12-23], case control studies[24-27], and randomized clinical trials[28-33].

The modern era of fibromyalgia research began less than 15 years ago when Smythe and Moldofsky proposed diagnostic criteria for the syndrome and identified its chief characteristics[34]. Although subsequent reports further described characteristics of fibromyalgia patients they did not substantially alter the Smythe–Moldofsky definition. A recent 16-center study of 558 patients and controls reemphasized the definition of fibromyalgia: A disorder of widespread pain, multiple tender points (at least 11 of 18), frequently associated with non-refreshed sleep, fatigue, and morning stiffness[35]. This definition growing out of the Smythe–Moldofsky paper represents *the* definition of fibromyalgia[35].

The multicenter study, while establishing new, sensitive, and specific criteria for the syndrome[35], also tested the sensitivity and specificity of the previous criteria sets of Yunus[9], Bennett, Clark, and Campbell[25,26,36], Goldenberg[33], Smythe and Moldofsky[34], and Wolfe *et al.*[17] Although these criteria differed from each other in various ways, all had adequate sensitivity and specificity for the purposes for which they were used. Thus, research based on these criteria appears valid. An important corollary is that non-criteria-based fibromylagia research as well as those studies that do not exclude the older definitions of fibromyalgia (fibrositis) as a local disorder should not be considered to deal with fibromyalgia. Such reports will not be considered here. Other scientific problems within fibromyalgia research have been considered previously[8].

The consequence of specific criteria and definition is that the first studies of the syndrome did not appear in the literature until 1981, and that what we know about the syndrome and its prognosis has accumulated in less than 10 years. Our knowledge of the epidemiology and natural history of the disorder is clearly limited.

THE NATURAL HISTORY OF FIBROMYALGIA

Onset

Most studies of fibromyalgia have identified patients who have had the syndrome for many years, and little is known about early fibromyalgia except when the syndrome follows trauma. It appears, however, that five groups of fibromyalgia patients can be identified: (1) those who are identified as having fibromyalgia in childhood[37,38]; (2) those who have a long history of various musculoskeletal complaints but who develop frank fibromyalgia in adult life; (3) those whose musculoskeletal symptoms develop insidiously during adult life; (4) those who develop the syndrome suddenly, apparently after some inciting event such as infection or surgery; and (5) those who develop the disorder following trauma.

Childhood fibromyalgia has been described in only one report of 33 cases by Yunus *et al.*, where it was found to be similar in all of its features to the adult syndrome[37]. The authors noted that "depression" and "anxiety" were present in 55% and 70% of patients, respectively. They also noted the absence of nocturnal leg cramps, but hypothesized that "muscle spasm" forms a pathologic basis for the syndrome. Family dynamics and psychosocial status were not evaluated in this report, and no data on possible initiating events were presented. The same authors noted that 28% of all their fibromyalgia patients had disease onset between ages 9 and 15[9].

More commonly fibromyalgia appears to develop gradually during adult life, but those with the syndrome frequently note childhood symptoms. Fifty-six percent of adult patients reported "growing pains" and 64% reported "leg aches." Among controls in this series such symptoms were noted in 29% and 29%, respectively ($p < 0.001$)[16]. Fifty-five percent of patients were unable to state any precipitating "cause" for their symptoms[16].

Among factors that initiated symptoms of fibromyalgia, infection was reported in 18% in one series[14], and viral infection in 55% in another[39]. Trauma is an important antecedent of fibromyalgia, and has been reported in about 22% of patients[14,16]. Most often the syndrome follows an "event", which may be a "fall", "back strain", or "whiplash-like auto injury." Pain is noted locally in the neck and shoulder region, but is soon noted in the arm, with subsequent spread to the contralateral side and then generally throughout the body. A similar pattern of dispersion has been noted in the so-called "repetitive strain syndrome". This syndrome and its evolution into fibromyalgia has been described in detail in excellent reports by Littlejohn[40,41].

Except for those cases that follow upon an event (infection or trauma), the exact time of development or mode of development is uncertain since the diagnosis of fibromyalgia, unlike that of RA, for example, requires a physician-observer. Back pain, for example, was reported by 55% of Bengstsson's patients prior to the diagnosis of fibromyalgia, and only 29% noted a sudden onset of symptoms[14]. Whether the onset of the disorder should be declared to be from the time of the first musculoskeletal pain (or when multiple regions become painful) or to the time of diagnosis is not known. Nor is it known whether musculoskeletal symptoms such as back pain "prior to diagnosis" are in fact part of the syndrome or isolated, unrelated events. The inability to accurately ascertain the date of onset of the syndrome limits our knowledge of its natural history.

Clinical course

There are no data concerning fibromyalgia in the community, and community patients may differ from those seen in specialty clinics where the syndrome appears severe and unremitting. Figure 1 illustrates the "fibromyalgia funnel," and suggests that milder, treatment-responsive and remittent disease may exist in the community. As with most chronic pain disorders, patients who find their way to specialty clinics are usually systematically different from community patients in clinical features such as pain levels, physical findings, and psychological behavior, and in coping and support mechanisms[8].

Only a few studies have examined aspects of the natural history of the syndrome, and these studies have all identified patients attending

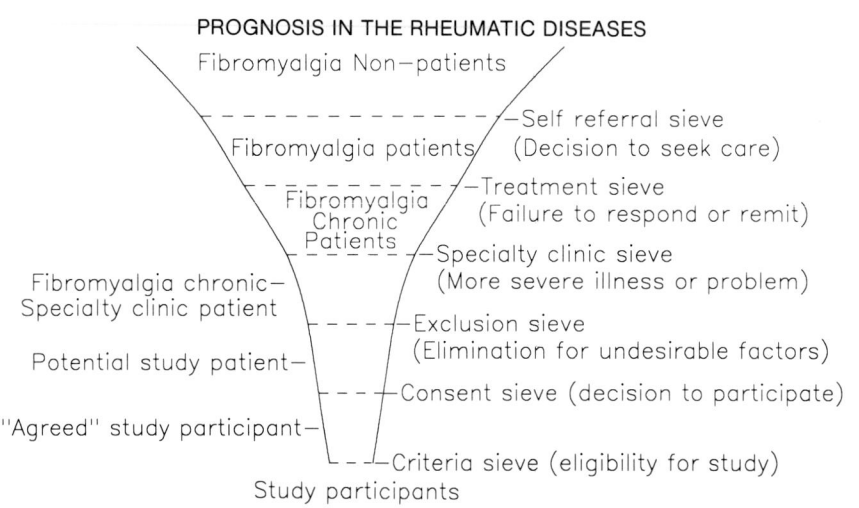

```
                PROGNOSIS IN THE RHEUMATIC DISEASES
              Fibromyalgia Non-patients
            -----------------/-Self referral sieve
              Fibromyalgia patients  (Decision to seek care)
                ----------/-Treatment sieve
                 Fibromyalgia     (Failure to respond or remit)
                   Chronic
                   Patients /-Specialty clinic sieve
   Fibromyalgia chronic-            (More severe illness or problem)
   Specialty clinic patient
                        -----/-Exclusion sieve
     Potential study patient-     (Elimination for undesirable factors)
                         ----/-Consent sieve (decision to participate)
   "Agreed" study participant-
                            ---/-Criteria sieve (eligibility for study)
              Study participants
```

Figure 1 The "fibromyalgia funnel". Hypothetical model of course of fibromyalgia patients in their passage from community nonpatients to study subjects. From Wolfe[8] (with permission)

specialty rheumatic disease clinics[12,13,22,42]. Symptoms appear to be constant over time and remissions uncommon. Hawley and associates followed 75 patients monthly over a 12-month period using self-assessed measures of pain, global severity, functional disability, stiffness, and sleep[13]. As noted in Figures 2 and 3, fibromyalgia patients appear to vary widely in their levels of pain and global severity, but these levels as well as the levels of the other variables assessed did not change significantly over the 12-month period as judged by repeated measures analyses. Felson and Goldenberg interviewed 39 patients at yearly intervals for 2 years beginning in 1983[22]. More than 60% of patients reported moderate to severe symptoms of pain and global symptoms over the three surveys in spite of receiving treatment for the disorder. At the final assessment, approximately 3.1 years after diagnosis, 92% of patients had pain complaints. Our group studied 81 previously diagnosed fibromyalgia patients concerning remission of symptoms. The mean duration of symptoms was greater than 12 years. At interview none of the 81 patients was in remission, although 23% reported remissions in the past. The median duration of remission was 12 months, a duration that represented 21% of the time course of the illness for the subjects achieving remissions. Stated in terms of the 81 patients studied, a remission of at least 12 months occurred in only 10.5% of patients during the 12-year disease course[16]. As noted above, data such as these derived from clinic patients may not accurately reflect the status of those in the community.

Outcome measures

Limited data are available concerning outcome variables in the syndrome. No prospective longitudinal studies have been reported,

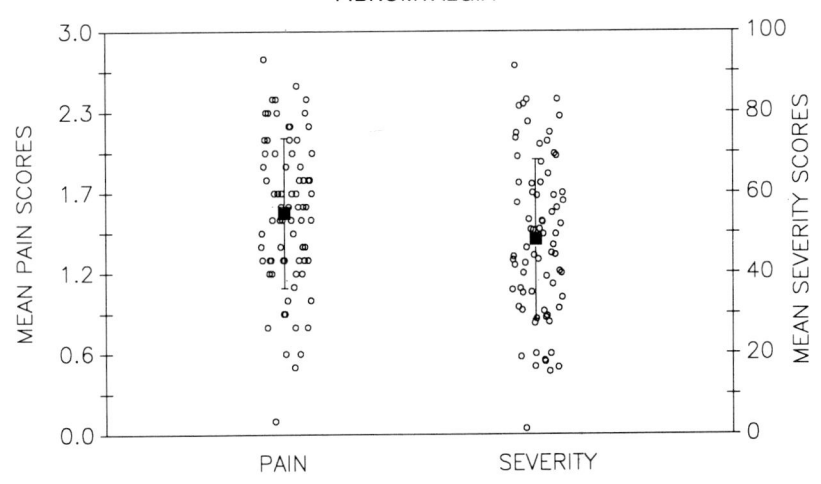

Figure 2 Means of 12-month scores of severity and pain for 75 patients with fibromyalgia. Error bars are standard deviations. From Hawley et al.[13] (with permission)

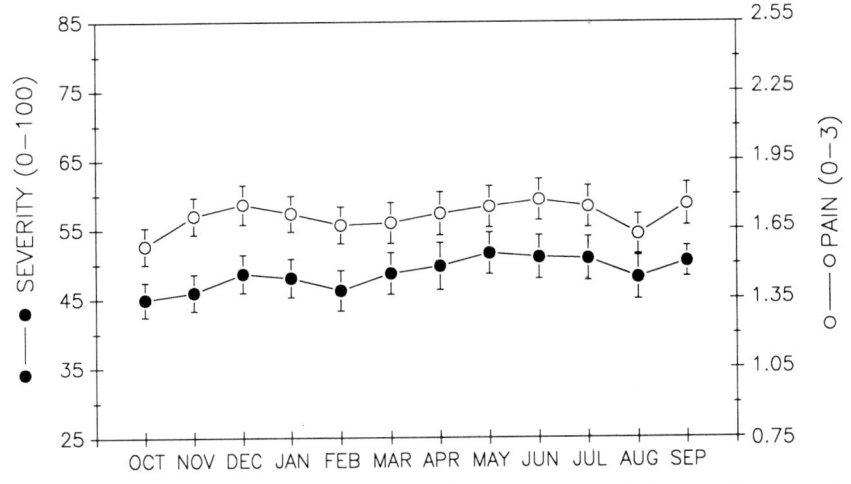

Figure 3 Mean scores for severity and pain for 75 patients with fibromyalgia over 12 months. Error bars are SEM. From Hawley et al.[13] (with permission)

although a multicenter study is in progress through the ARAMIS databank system[43].

Pain and psychological status are the two outcome measures that have been studied most thoroughly. Pain levels are higher in fibromyalgia than in other rheumatic diseases with the exception of low back pain where self-report scores of pain are similar[44]. In addition, the distribution of pain is more widespread compared with other rheumatic conditions[45]. Pain scores using a variety of instruments were found to be greater in fibromyalgia than in rheumatoid arthritis in all studies but one where scores were equal to RA[45]. Within a group of RA patients those with fibromyalgia had higher levels of pain than rheumatoid arthritis patients without fibromyalgia[19]. In general, fibromyalgia scores are similar among centers. In our series the mean pain score using a visual analog pain scale (0–3) was 1.7 (0.55 SD)[13].

Psychological status has been the subject of numerous cross-sectional investigations. Test scores using a variety of instruments are more abnormal in fibromyalgia patients than in normals or in rheumatic disease controls[3-7]. The meaning of these observations has been the subject of debate. Most of the psychological instruments used to assess status suffer from "criterion contamination" in that they rate as psychological abnormality symptoms such as fatigue, difficulty with function, headache, sleep abnormality, and poor health compared to others[46,47]. Even so, fibromyalgia patients have more abnormal scores on instruments with minimal contamination[4,6], and nonfibromyalgia-related questions in the Minnesota Multiphasic Personality Index[48]. The psychological status of fibromyalgia patients in the community is not known, but may be considerably different from those patients seen in the clinic. Evidence for this comes from recent studies in the irritable bowel syndrome where similar clinic "psychological abnormality" is well known. Community "nonpatients" who satisfied IBS criteria were psychologically normal in comparison with community healthy controls[49,50]. Clark[26] found persons with fibromyalgia to be without psychological abnormality compared with controls when selected at random on the basis of fibromyalgia symptoms from patients attending a general medical clinic for other conditions.

The weight of evidence suggests that patients with a chronic pain problem will have greater levels of anxiety and depression than those without pain, and that patients who self-select to seek chronic medical care represent a still more psychologically distressed subset of all patients.

Functional ability in fibromyalgia has been the subject of several recent investigations using the Stanford Health Assessment functional disability index[13,44,51]. Functional scores were abnormal in 28 fibromyalgia patients participating in a study of physical ability using a computerized work testing instrument (BTE-Baltimore Therapeutic Instrument Co, Baltimore, MD). The HAQ scores were 0.9 (0.61 SE) vs. 14 (0.12 SE) for RA patients and 0.0 (0.13 SE) for normal controls[51]. In a series of 75 fibromyalgia patients the mean HAQ FDI was 1.1 (0.70 SD)[13]. The mean FDI for 572 fibromyalgia patients attending an outpatient clinic was 0.9 (0.65 SD) compared with scores for 1285 RA patients of 1.1 (0.68 SD), 1068 low back pain patients of 0.6 (0.57 SD), 744 knee osteoarthritis of 0.7 (0.57), and 493 hand osteoarthritis patients of 0.5 (0.54 SD)[44].

Fibromyalgia patients "look well" when seen in the clinic. Given the abnormality in psychological scores discussed above, concern has been raised as to whether the stated disability arises on the basis of physical or psychological abnormality or both. Jacobsen found evidence of abnormal muscle strength in fibromyalgia patients using a CYBEX machine[15]. Recent reports from the University of Oregon[52] indicate that fibromyalgia patients are poorly physically conditioned and have reduced muscle blood flow as measured by xenon-133 clearance. Observation of fibromyalgia patients during work testing indicated the dysfunction appeared to be on the basis of pain experienced during the work testing tasks[51]. In addition, HAQ FDI prework test scores were correlated with work ability ($r=0.61$) in this study. Regardless of the mechanism of dysfunction the available data suggest clinically important levels of dysfunction in many fibromyalgia patients.

Work disability has also been investigated[12,14,42,51]. Cathey reported on 81 patients from Wichita[53]. The sample was 90% female. Among the 37% who were employed the mean work loss per year was 9.8 days, compared with 8.0, 7.4, and 5.2 from US statistics for low back pain, rheumatoid arthritis, and osteoarthritis, respectively[54]. In contradistinction to days lost from work, only 6% of fibromyalgia patients received disability payments compared to 6%, 24%, and 29% with low back pain, RA, and OA, respectively, in the national sample. A subsequent study from the Wichita group using a larger sample ($n=176$) found 5 (16.55 SD) days lost from work during a 6-month period. Nine (9.3%) of patients considered themselves disabled, but only 5.7% received disability payments from any source. Seventeen percent of patients reported that they stopped working because of fibromyalgia, while 30.4% stated that they changed jobs because of the syndrome.

A recent study from the Boston group[42] compared 73 fibromyalgia patients and 186 rheumatoid arthritis patients. Thirty-three percent of fibromyalgia patients and 26% of those with RA reported changing jobs because of their illness, and 22% reported themselves as being disabled. Bengstsson, studying Swedish patients, reported on 55 with fibromyalgia[14]. Fifty-five percent reported being unable to manage household work alone, and 24% were receiving pensions.

As with other outcome measures in fibromyalgia, the available data derive from patients with more severe disease attending outpatient specialty clinics, and are almost certainly different from those with the syndrome in the community. Even so, the public health impact of such data is striking. As many as 20% of new patients seen in rheumatology clinics have the syndrome[9], as do 2.1% of patients in family practice clinics[55].

Iatrogenic factors have not been studied in fibromyalgia. Anecdotal reports and clinical studies[9] have stressed the inappropriate interventions and investigations that have been undertaken to establish diagnosis or to treat the wrong syndrome when the diagnosis was not established correctly. We have noted patients treated with second-line drugs and corticosteroids for inappropriately diagnosed rheumatoid arthritis or systemic lupus erythematosus. The extent of such problems has not been studied quantitatively, but Cathey[12] noted that 11 of 81 fibromyalgia patients had undergone low back surgery and 2 of 81 surgery on the cervical spine. It is interesting that the usual treatments for fibromyalgia, which include tricyclic compounds, exercise, and analgesics, probably will not result in many clinically important adverse reactions. Short-term studies of NSAIDs have failed to show benefit[31,35].

Utilization of medical services and *direct and indirect costs* related to diagnosis and treatment of the fibromyalgia syndrome have only been reported once[12]. Cathey noted very high lifetime rates of hospitalization. She also noted that physician, chiropractic, and physical and occupational therapy visits were common. Patients averaged 3.5 (0.74 SE) visits to MDs for treatment of fibromyalgia during a 1-year period. More than 90% had used NSAIDs or analgesics during the study period, and the mean number of drugs (for any condition) being used at the end of the study years was 3.8 (2.0 SD).

There are no data relating to mortality in the syndrome, but anecdotally there has been no suggestion of increased mortality rates.

Fibromyalgia and concomitant disease. Fibromyalgia probably occurs most frequently within the setting of another musculoskeletal disorder[16]. Fibromyalgia has been designated as "primary" when the symptoms and physical findings of the patient derive almost entirely from fibromyalgia, and "secondary" or "concomitant" when a second illness "causes" or is associated with fibromyalgia. Difficulties with such terminology and the finding that primary and secondary or concomitant patients cannot be distinguished from each other as the level of diagnostic criteria have led the fibromyalgia criteria committee in their American College of Rheumatology 1990 criteria for the classification of fibromyalgia to recommend that at the diagnostic level the distinction between primary and secondary or concomitant fibromyalgia be abolished[35]. To date no studies have investigated the effect of treatment of the underlying disorder on the symptoms and physical findings of fibromyalgia, but it seems likely that such treatment could lead to a reduction of fibromyalgia symptomatology.

The choice of outcome measures (Table 1)

The lack of longitudinal data in fibromyalgia means that we have no evidence how any of the clinical or putative outcome measures may perform over time. *Pain* is the most important factor in most rheumatic conditions and certainly is a cardinal factor in fibromyalgia. *Functional disability* has been shown to strongly correlate to overall severity, after controlling for the effect of pain[13]. But unlike conditions like rheumatoid arthritis, where the combination of ongoing inflammation *and* structural loss leads to loss of function, structural abnormality is not generally present in fibromyalgia. Therefore, it is possible that disability will not progress over time. Until longitudinal data are available the long-term meaning and the value of functional measures will remain uncertain. But given the strong correlation between functional assessment and work performance, functional ability measurements are strong candidates for appropriate outcome determination. *Psychological function* seems another appropriate health status measure in

Table 1 Important study variables in the fibromyalgia syndrome

Outcome measures

1. Pain: Visual analog scales (VAS) and pain drawings
2. Functional disability (HAQ and similar instruments)
3. Psychological measurements
4. Utilization of medical services
5. Employment status
6. Sleep disturbance (may be primarily a process measure)

Process measures

1. Sleep disturbance
2. Stiffness
3. Fatigue

this syndrome, and remains correlated with global severity after adjustment for pain and dysfunction[13]. *Utilization of medical services* measures the cost of an illness and serves as a surrogate for its severity. Appropriate management or control of the syndrome should reduce expenditures. Service utilization appears to be an excellent measure of direct severity of illness. Similarly, *employment-related variables* should provide markers for the overall effect of fibromyalgia on the individual. Sleep disturbance, along with fatigue and morning stiffness, are core features of the fibromyalgia syndrome, but probably represent process rather than outcome measures.

Prognosis and future perspectives

Relatively nothing is known about long-term prognosis in this syndrome, primarily owing to the lack of longitudinal reports. Therapy may influence signs and symptoms in short-term reports[28,30,32,56,57], but treatment effects are minimal. Moreover, there are no long-term data on fibromyalgia treatment. The few studies that have examined the syndrome over periods of 1 to 2 years have found persistence of symptoms[13,22].

There is no doubt that there are identifiable factors that influence prognosis in fibromyalgia (Table 2). Candidate factors include psychosocial variables such as education, social class, psychological status, social and family support; antecedent "triggering" events, areas of pain involvement, physical stamina and status, coexistent osteoarthritis, age at onset, response to treatment, and probably many more. The value of such factors and others awaits longitudinal studies.

Current goals in fibromyalgia treatment include reduction in pain, decreased medical visits, the development of self-sufficiency, and reduction in anxiety and depression. In the short and medium term the outcome measures noted above appear appropriate in the assessment of outcome in this disorder.

Table 2 Factors that might influence prognosis in the fibromyalgia syndrome

1. Education level	7. Physical stamina
2. Social class	8. Physical training and status
3. Psychological status	9. Coexistent osteoarthritis
4. Social and family support	10. Age at onset
5. "Triggering" event	11. Sympathetic (hyper)activity
6. Areas of pain involvement	12. Response to therapy

References

1. Cobb, S. (1971). *The Frequency of Rheumatic Diseases*. (Cambridge, Mass.: Harvard University Press)
2. Lawrence, R. C., Hochberg, M. C., Kelsey, J. L. et al. (1989). Estimates of the prevelance of selected arthritic and musculoskeletal diseases in the United States. *J. Rheumatol.*, **16**, 427–441
3. Goldenberg, D. L. (1986). Psychologic studies in fibrositis. *Am. J. Med.*, **81**, 67–70
4. Hawley, D. J. and Wolfe, F. (1988). Anxiety and depression in patients with RA: A prospective study of 400 patients. *J. Rheumatol.*, **15**, 932–941
5. Payne, T. C., Leavitt, D. C., Garron, D. C. et al. (1982). Fibrositis and psychologic disturbance. *Arthritis Rheum.*, **25**, 213–217
6. Scudds, R. A., Rollman, G. B., Harth, M. and McCain, G. A. (1987). Pain perception and personality measures as discriminators in the classification of fibrositis. *J. Rheumatol.*, **14**, 563–569
7. Wolfe, F., Cathey, M. A., Kleinheksel, S. M. et al. (1984). Psychological status in primary fibrositis and fibrositis associated with rheumatoid arthritis. *J. Rheumatol.*, **11**, 500–506
8. Wolfe, F. (1990). Methodologic and statistical problems in the epidemiology of fibromyalgia. In Ewad, E. and Fricton, J. R. (eds.) *Myofascial Pain and Fibromyalgia*, Chap. 8, pp. 147–163. (New York: Raven Press)
9. Yunus, M. B., Masi, A. T., Calabro, J. J., Miller, K. A. and Feigenbaum, S. L. (1981). Primary fibromyalgia (fibrositis): clinical study of 50 patients with matched normal controls. *Semin. Arthritis Rheum.*, **11**, 151–171
10. Bennett, R. M. (1987). Fibromyalgia (editorial). *J. Am. Med. Assoc.*, **257**, 2802–2803
11. Goldenberg, D. L. (1987). Fibromyalgia syndrome. An emerging but controversial condition. *J. Am. Med. Assoc.*, **257**, 2782–2787
12. Cathey, M. A., Wolfe, F., Kleinheksel, S. M. and Hawley, D. J. (1986). Socioeconomic impact of fibrositis. A study of 81 patients with primary fibrositis. *Am. J. Med.*, **81**, 78–84
13. Hawley, D. J., Wolfe, F. and Cathey, M. A. (1988). Pain, functional disability, and psychological status: a 12 month study of severity in fibromyalgia. *J. Rheumatol.*, **15**, 1551–1556
14. Bengtsson, A., Henriksson, K. G., Jorfeldt, L., Kagedal, B., Lennmarken, C. and Lindstrom, F. (1986). Primary fibromyalgia. A clinical and laboratory study of 55 patients. *Scand. J. Rheumatol.*, **15**, 340–347
15. Jacobsen, S. and Danneskiold Samse, B. (1987). Isometric and isokinetic muscle strength in patients with fibrositis syndrome. New characteristics for a difficult definable category of patients. *Scand. J. Rheumatol.*, **16**, 61–65
16. Wolfe, F. (1986). The clinical syndrome of fibrositis. *Am. J. Med.*, **81**, 7–14
17. Wolfe, F., Hawley, D. J., Cathey, M. A., Caro, X. and Russel, I. J. (1985). Fibrositis: symptom frequency and criteria for diagnosis. An evaluation of 291 rheumatic disease patients and 58 normal individuals. *J. Rheumatol.*, **12**, 1159–1163
18. Wolfe, F. and Cathey, M. A. (1985). The epidemiology of tender points: A prospective study of 1520 patients. *J. Rheumatol.*, **12**, 1164–1168

19. Wolfe, F., Cathey, M. A. and Kleinheksel, S. M. (1984). Fibrositis (fibromyalgia) in rheumatoid arthritis. *J. Rheumatol.*, **11**, 814-818
20. Wolfe, F. and Cathey, M. A. (1983). Prevalence of primary and secondary fibrositis. *J. Rheumatol.*, **10**, 965-968
21. Dinerman, H., Goldenberg, D. L. and Felson, D. T. (1986). A prospective evaluation of 118 patients with the fibromyalgia syndrome: prevalence of Raynaud's phenomenon, sicca symptoms, ANA, low complement, and Ig deposition at the dermal-epidermal junction. *J. Rheumatol.*, **13**, 368-373
22. Felson, D. T. and Goldenberg, D. L. (1986). The natural history of fibromyalgia. *Arthritis Rheum.*, **29**, 1522-1526
23. Simms, R. W., Goldenberg, D. L., Felson, D. T. and Mason, J. H. (1988). Tenderness in 75 anatomic sites. Distinguishing fibromyalgia patients from controls. *Arthritis Rheum.*, **31**, 182-187
24. Ahles, T. A., Yunus, M. B., Riley, S. D., Bradley, J. M. and Masi, A. T. (1984). Psychological factors associated with primary fibromyalgia syndrome. *Arthritis Rheum.*, **27**, 1101-1106
25. Campbell, S. M., Clark, S., Tindall, E. A., Forehand, M. E. and Bennett, R. M. (1983). Clinical characteristics of fibrositis. I. A "blinded," controlled study of symptoms and tender points. *Arthritis Rheum.*, **26**, 817-824
26. Clark, S., Campbell, S. M., Forehand, M. E., Tindall, E. A. and Bennett, R. M. Clinical characteristics of fibrositis. II. A "blinded," controlled study using standard psychological tests. *Arthritis Rheum.*, **28**, 132-137
27. Littlejohn, G. O., Weinstein, C. and Helme, R. D. (1987). Increased neurogenic inflammation in fibrositis syndrome. *J. Rheumatol.*, **14**, 1022-1025
28. Bennett, R. M., Gatter, R. A., Campbell, S. M., Andrews, R.-P., Clark, S. R. and Scarola, J. A. (1988). A comparison of cyclobenzaprine and placebo in the management of fibrositis: A double-blind controlled study. *Arthritis Rheum.*, **31**, 1535-1542
29. Clark, S., Tindall, E. and Bennett, R. M. (1985). A double blind crossover trial of prednisone versus placebo in the treatment of fibrositis. *J. Rheumatol.*, **12**, 980-983
30. McCain, G. A., Bell, D. A., Mai, F. M. and Halliday, P. D. (1988). A controlled study of the effects of a supervised cardiovascular fitness training program on the manifestations of fibromyalgia. *Arthritis Rheum.*, **31**, 1135-1141
31. Yunus, M. B., Masi, A. T. and Aldag, J. C. (1989). Short term effects of ibuprofen in primary fibromyalgia syndrome: A double blind, placebo controlled trial. *J. Rheumatol.*, **16**, 527-532
32. Carette, S., McCain, G. A., Bell, D. A. and Fam, A. G. (1986). Evaluation of amitriptyline in primary fibrositis. A double- blind, placebo-controlled study. *Arthritis Rheum.*, **29**, 655-659
33. Goldenberg, D. L., Felson, D. T. and Dinerman, H. (1986). A randomized, controlled trial of amitriptyline and naproxen in the treatment of patients with fibromyalgia. *Arthritis Rheum.*, **29**, 1371-1377
34. Smythe, H. A. and Moldofsky, H. (1977). Two contributions to understanding of the "fibrositis" syndrome. *Bull. Rheum. Dis.*, **28**, 928-931
35. Wolfe, F., Smythe, H. A., Yunus, M. B. *et al.* (1990). The American College of Rheumatology 1990 criteria for the classification of fibromyalgia. *Arthritis Rheum.*, **33**, 160-172
36. Bennett, R. M. (1981). Fibrositis: misnomer for a common rheumatic disorder. *West. J. Med.*, **134**, 405-413
37. Yunus, M. B. and Masi, A. T. (1985). Juvenile primary fibromyalgia syndrome. A clinical study of thirty-three patients and matched normal controls. *Arthritis Rheum.*, **28**, 138-145
38. Calabro, J. J. and Perry, R. F. (1986). Juvenile primary fibromyalgia syndrome [letter]. *Arthritis Rheum.*, **29**, 452-453
39. Buchwald, D., Goldenberg, D. L., Sullivan, J. L. and Komaroff, A. L. (1987). The "chronic, active Epstein-Barr virus infection" syndrome and primary fibromyalgia. *Arthritis Rheum.*, **30**, 1132-1136
40. Littlejohn, G. E. (1986). Repetitive strain syndrome: an Australian experience (editorial). *J. Rheumatol.*, **13**, 1004-1006

41. Littlejohn, G. O. (1989). Fibrositis/fibromyalgia in the workplace. *Rheum. Dis. Clin. N. Am.*, **15**, 45-60
42. Mason, J. H., Simms, R. W., Goldenberg, D. L. and Meenan, R. F. (1989). The impact of fibromyalgia on work: a comparison with RA. *Arthritis Rheum.*, **32**, S197-S197 (Abstract)
43. Fries, J. F. (1984). The chronic disease data bank: first principles to future directions. *J. Med. Philos.*, **9**, 161-180
44. Wolfe, F. (1989). A brief health status instrument: CLINHAQ. *Arthritis Rheum.*, **32**, S99 (Abstract)
45. Leavitt, F., Katz, R. S., Golden, H. E., Glickman, P. B. and Layfer, L. F. (1986). Comparison of pain properties in fibromyalgia patients and rheumatoid arthritis patients. *Arthritis Rheum.*, **29**, 775-781
46. Smythe, H. A. (1984). Problems with the MMPI [editorial]. *J. Rheumatol.*, **11**, 417-418
47. Pincus, T., Callahan, L. F., Bradley, L. A. and Wolfe, F. (1986). Elevated MMPI scores for hypochondriasis, depression and hysteria in patients with rheumatoid arthritis reflect disease rather than psychological status. *Arthritis Rheum.*, **29**, 1456-1466
48. Leavitt, F. and Katz, R. S. (1989). Is the MMPI invalid for assessing psychological disturbance in pain related organic conditions. *J. Rheumatol.*, **16**, 521-526
49. Drossman, D. A., McKee, D. C., Sandler, R. S., Mitchell, C. M., Lowman, B. C. and Burger, A. L. (1988). Psychosocial factors in the irritable bowel syndrome. *Gastroenterology*, **95**, 701-708
50. Whitehead, W. E., Bosmajian, L., Zonderman, A. B., Costa, Jr., P. G. and Schuster, M. M. (1988). Symptoms of psychologic distress associated with irritable bowel syndrome. *Gastroenterology*, **95**, 709-714
51. Cathey, M. A., Wolfe, F., Kleinheksel, S. M., Miller, S. and Pitetti, K. H. (1988). Functional ability and work status in patients with fibromyalgia. *Arthritis Care Res.*, **1**, 85-98
52. Bennett, R. M., Clark, S. R., Goldberg, L. et al. (1989). Aerobic fitness in patients with fibrositis: A controlled study of respiratory gas exchange and ^{133}xenon clearance from exercising muscle. *Arthritis Rheum.*, **32**, 454-460
53. Caro, X. J. (1986). Immunofluorescent studies of skin in primary fibrositis syndrome. *Am. J. Med.*, **81**, 43-49
54. Kramer, J. S., Yelin, E. H. and Epstein, W. V. (1983). Social and economic impacts of four musculoskeletal conditions. *Arthritis Rheum.*, **26**, 901-907
55. Hartz, A. and Kirchdoerfer, E. (1987). Undetected fibrositis in primary care practice. *J. Fam. Pract.*, **25**, 365-369
56. Goldenberg, D. L. (1989). Treatment of fibromyalgia syndrome. *Rheum. Dis. Clin. N. Am.*, **15**, 61-71
57. Wolfe, F. (1988). Fibromyalgia: whither treatment? *J. Rheumatol.*, **15**, 1047-1049

16
Low back pain

I. K. Y. TSANG

Low back pain is a problem of great medical, social, and economic concern. Each year, 2–5% of the population develop low back pain[1,2]. This means that about 80% of all people will experience low back pain at some stage during their adult life[3,4]. Svensson showed that almost 70% of 40- to 47-year-old men in Göteborg, Sweden had experienced low back pain. Fifty percent of these men, as a result, had missed work at least once[1]. In Great Britain between 1960 and 1970, low back pain caused 3.6% of all sickness absence days and the number of sickness absence periods per 1000 persons was 11 days for women and 22.6 days for men[5].

Despite the prevalence of this problem, in most cases of low back pain the precise causes cannot yet be identified. Many patients are, therefore, grouped together in a single poorly defined category casually termed lumbago, back strain, or low back pain. A study was made of first attacks of acute low back pain seen by general practitioners in England[6]. In their report, Dillane et al. stated that the specific cause of the attacks was unknown in 79% in men and in 89% in women. The diagnosis of "strain" was made in 11% of the attacks in men and 4% in women. This term is nonspecific and cannot actually be regarded as a diagnosis. In only 8% of men and 6% of women was there a proven diagnosis of disk prolapse. The remaining 2% of cases in men and 1% in women were attributed to other less common and sometimes more serious lesions, such as neoplasms or inflammatory joint disease. The numbers produced in this study indicated that about 90% of first-attack low back pain patients were undiagnosed by their general practitioners. Clinicians, however, must keep in mind the 10% for whom a diagnosis could be made. Such a diagnosis may uncover a serious condition.

As with diagnosis, difficulty is encountered identifying the prognosis of low back pain. This can be explained by the following: (1) Since the cause of most cases of low back pain is nonspecific, it is unlikely that any particular treatment will show a major effect when applied indiscriminately to all patients with low back pain. (2) The assessment of the effect of a treatment lies in the measurement of the outcome of the patient's low back pain. This measurement can be in the form of pain medication requirement, return to work, or improvement of functional level. If measurements are used inappropriately, the true effect of a treatment may not be detected. (3) Despite the volume of literature on the study of low back pain, only a few studies are well designed and controlled. The Quebec Task Force on Spinal Disorders illustrates this point clearly[7].

Prognosis is better defined for those disorders that can be distinctly diagnosed, such as spondylolysis, spondylolisthesis, spinal stenosis, and herniated lumbar discs.

SPONDYLOLYSIS AND SPONDYLOLISTHESIS

Four to five percent of the population in most western countries have spondylolysis, but only half of these have spondylolisthesis. In the instance of spondylolisthesis, the slip generally does not exceed 25-30%. There is a strong tendency for familial aggregation. Five etiologic categories of spondylolisthesis are currently identified: dysplastic, isthmic, degenerative, traumatic, and pathologic[8]. It is uncommon for spondylolysis to be symptomatic in children and adolescents. Physicians should resist the temptation to credit it exclusively as the cause of symptoms. Rather, one should vigorously explore other causes of low back pain. The differential diagnosis includes discitis, osteoid osteoma, spinal cord tumor, herniated disk, and muscle and neurologic disorders. As uncommon as these conditions are in childhood and adolescence, they are equally as common as symptomatic spondylolysis in childhood and adolescence. On the rare occasion that spondylolysis is symptomatic, restriction of vigorous activities, and back and abdominal strengthening exercises are usually successful in controlling symptoms[9,10].

Spondylolisthesis is a problem for 5% of the general population. Although the lesion occurs in the growth years, very few individuals develop symptoms during childhood and adolescence. If symptoms do occur, their onset usually coincides with the adolescent growth spurt.

In adult patients with symptomatic spondylolisthesis, degenerative changes and nerve root irritation are the prime sources of the symptoms. These patients usually respond to conservative treatments. It should be noted that flexion exercise is considered superior to extension exercise[11].

SPINAL STENOSIS

Nonoperative treatments, nonsteroidal anti-inflammatory drugs, and exercise programs to strengthen abdominal muscles and reduce lumbar lordosis, are usually effective in patients with no neurologic abnormalities. For lateral recess stenosis, some studies have shown conservative treatments are also effective, at least initially. Rest, analgesics, muscle relaxants, local heat, and other physical modalities of pain control are used in the acute stage. Postural exercises, lumbosacral corset, and transcutaneous nerve stimulation can be used between acute attacks. Although no controlled studies have demonstrated its efficacy, spinal bracing seems warranted in patients whose osteoporotic compression fractures or spondylolisthesis have caused spinal stenosis.

In patients with progressive neurologic involvement, surgery may be indicated. Most studies report "good" or "excellent" surgical results in about 80-85% of lumbar spinal stenosis cases. It must be realized, however, that degenerative disease is the most common cause of spinal stenosis, and surgical treatment only alleviates compression on neural contents and does not alter the underlying osteoarthrosis. Postoperatively, many patients are not able to return to work that requires lifting, walking long distances, standing, sitting for long periods, or riding in an automobile for long distances. Of the various symptoms, back pain is the least improved after surgery. One retrospective study of 81 patients undergoing laminectomy for lumbar stenosis reported good results in 95% of patients and a reoperation rate of 7%. The most common cause of an unsatisfactory result was inadequate decompression of spinal contents. Although there was only a 15-20% short-term failure rate after decompressive procedures, there was about a 50% failure rate within 10 years of surgery. The longer the duration of the disease and the more severe the preoperative symptoms, the worse the postoperative results. Preoperative sphincter disturbance, psychosomatic disorders, insurance or medical-legal issues, and poor patient selection have all been associated with poor surgical results. Old age, per se, is not necessarily a factor in negative spinal surgery outcome[12].

HERNIATED LUMBAR DISK

Nonsurgical treatment is successful for 80-90% of patients with herniated lumbar disk[13]. Many surgical techniques have been devised for patients who suffer from lumbar disk herniations, but few have been examined in carefully controlled studies[14-16]. Progressive neurologic involvement is a definite indication for surgical intervention. A less certain indication is pain that interferes with the patient's desired lifestyle. Selection of patients for lumbar disk surgery represents the most important step in surgical management[17,18]. This selection process is not difficult when consistent clinical symptoms, signs, and confirmatory imaging studies are present. Unfortunately, much of the patient selection for surgical treatment is based on overdiagnosis and subsequent overtreatment of disk herniation. Such unwarranted treatment results in added health care costs and has a significant adverse impact on outcome[14,15]. Less invasive treatment approaches such as chymopapain have proven to be ineffective. Equally important to signs and symptoms are preoperative psychological evaluations. These have been demonstrated to have direct correlation to surgical outcome[2,19-21].

THE ROLE OF SURGERY FOR HERNIATED LUMBAR DISK

In a prospective, randomized, 10-year follow-up study, Weber compared the outcome of surgically and nonsurgically treated patients with lumbar disk herniation[22]. He demonstrated that both surgical and non-surgical treatment could result in satisfactory recovery from this condition. It can be concluded that most patients with lumbar disk herniation can expect a spontaneous improvement, if they can wait long enough.

Green showed that only 7-12% of patients required surgery for sciatica, and a very high proportion of the surgeries were successful[23]. Shannon and Paul showed that only 2% of males and 6% of females suffered severe intractable pain following laminectomy[24]. Although the results of first-time surgery are encouraging, repeated surgery has a very bad record[18]. Nachemson pointed out that with a third procedure there is only a 5% chance of success. Selecki et al.[25] found that only 8% of patients with multiple operation had satisfactory results. Waddell et al.[26] indicated that by all standards the results of repeat back surgery for degenerative lumbar disk disease in compensation patients were poor. With successive low back operations the results rapidly deteriorated. A second surgery made 40-50% of patients better but made 20% worse. A third surgery made 20-30% of patients better but 25% worse. A fourth made only 10-20% of patients better but 45% worse. Unless there is clear evidence of new disk prolapse, repeat back surgery is unlikely to improve the patient's condition.

The timing of any surgical intervention is particularly important for patients with nerve root compression. The prognosis for return of normal nerve function deteriorates after 3 months of nerve root compression[27]. Wall et al.[28] demonstrated the multiple changes that occur after nerve damage. Some believe that these changes are the reason for persistent severe symptoms after a correct operation by an experienced surgeon to decompress nerve roots entrapped in the bony canal. Further study is needed to define more clearly the optimum time for nerve root decompression and functional recovery.

Of the 80% of the population who develop low back pain, only a small proportion can attribute their pain to the specific causes mentioned above. For the others, it is not possible to provide a firm diagnosis. It is likely that a number of different pathologic processes are responsible for the production of their low back pain. The natural history of the symptom is extremely variable; some patients are better within days, while others complain of back pain for years. For most patients with acute low back pain, the prognosis is well established. Eighty to ninety percent of patients with acute attacks recover in about 6 weeks, irrespective of the administration or type of treatment[3,5,29]. In a 3-year follow-up study of 31 chronic idiopathic low back pain patients, Lankhorst et al.[30] found significant spontaneous improvements in pain and disability scores. Unfortunately, recurrences were frequent and were reported in 30–70% of affected persons[1,3,31,32].

The group of patients with low back pain who (1) fail to respond to treatment, (2) do not return to their normal activities quickly, and (3) cannot be diagnosed accurately, have chronic complaints but no objective findings. These patients usually make a lasting impression on the physician, creating the illusion that they constitute the majority of his low back pain patients. In fact, they only represent a small percentage of the total low back pain population. The prognosis for this group has not been well established. Wiesel, Feffer, and Borenstein found that of the 5362 patients with a primary complaint of lumbosacral pain presented to The George Washington University Low Back Clinic, 98% had a definite diagnosis and/or got better without a specific diagnosis[33]. There were only 109 (2%) who failed to improve with treatment and/or for whom no specific diagnosis could be reached to explain their complaints. Of this group, 10% were eventually found to have an underlying medical problem. It was recommended that patients with unexplained chronic low back pain should undergo a thorough general medical examination initially and be reassessed on a periodic basis[33]. Pary et al.[34] also advocate that it is imperative, when seeing a patient with intractable low back pain, to make sure that a lesion in the bony canal has not been missed.

Episodes of acute low back pain are chronic and incapacitating in a minority of cases. This group has proven particularly refractory to traditional medical and surgical interventions. Alternative treatment modalities are needed; for example, multidisciplinary treatment programs. These programs are based on principles of operant conditioning. An integral component is a gradually progressive, structured exercise program. A wide variety of cognitive behavioral pain management strategies are generally taught. The literature reviewed suggests that such treatment achieves favorable outcomes in both the short and long terms in a majority of cases. Unfortunately, comparison of studies is difficult owing to the lack of common measures. Many of the studies were based on samples of a few dozen cases and thus were limited in their general application. Cairns, Mooney, and Crane[35] report that of 100 patients with chronic low back pain in their multidisciplinary treatment program, about 75% of their inpatients and 50% of their outpatients showed initial decreases in pain and increases in activity at the time of discharge. These improvements eroded over time. By 1 year after discharge, only about 50% of their inpatients remained improved. The outpatient program appeared to have a more durable effect regarding pain (92%) and activity (95% increase maintained), even though fewer outpatients reported they were improved at discharge. On follow-up, 15% of the inpatients stated they were working, whereas 52% of the outpatients returned to work.

Using a variety of psychologic and functional performance instruments, McArthur et al.[36], studied 702 consecutive admissions to their Multidisciplinary Chronic Low Back Pain Program at admission, discharge, and 1-month follow-up. Sixty-seven percent completed four or more weeks of the program and were considered to have graduated. McArthur et al. found that the psychological profiles demonstrated a substantial degree of disability at admission, this being significantly reduced at follow-up. Both behavioral and cognitive aspects of performance improved as a direct function of the length of stay in the treatment program. This was evidenced by objective assessments of patients' physical abilities and verbalizations. The improvements continued modestly through to follow-up. Composite indices of improvement demonstrated favorable outcomes for no less than 4 and as high as 9 in every 10 participants. In a separate article[37], the same authors reported the results of a long-term follow-up in the same group of patients. Evidence gathered at 12 months following treatment of a sample of 42 men and 36 women graduates from their program showed that 45% had returned to work. A relationship was demonstrated between return to work and pain ratings, medication use, and utilization of physician services for pain during the intervening year. Longer-term follow-ups were conducted by telephone interviews. Six aspects concerning the individual's status at follow-up were selected for analysis. These were: (1) return to work, (2) litigation, (3) pain rating, (4) activity restricted by pain, (5) drug use for pain, and (6) hospitalization for pain. In general, the results found for each variable examined over 5 years of follow-up pointed to progressive improvement. Favorable outcomes on all measures were observed, and the proportion of respondents who appeared to be chronically suffering decreased steadily across serial observations. The problem with this study is that the interviews were simplified, and the outcomes were not appraised; for example, the study did not specify the actual nature of employment, the appropriateness of that employment for the respondent, or how satisfied the respondent was with the position.

PREDICTORS OF OUTCOME

Efforts have been made to identify job performance variables as possible predictors of potentially costly back injuries in an uninjured industrial population. Such predictors might be termed primary predictors, in that they identify the percentage of an uninjured population likely to develop a low back pain incident. Secondary predictors identify those with acute low back pain incident likely to develop chronic difficulties, while tertiary predictors look at success or failure in chronic patients.

Since the early 1920s, radiographic examinations have been used as a preemployment screen to identify susceptible employees and thereby protect them from back injuries. Despite these efforts, the magnitude of the industrial back injury problem has not diminished. The relationship of radiographic abnormalities to back problems is now considered questionable[38-41]. Interest has grown in evaluating other individual employee factors for their relationship to subsequent low back injury. These include age, sex, anthropomorphic measurements, psychosocial factors, and physical capacities.

Spinal aging, as expressed in degenerative changes, is noted early in adulthood and continues to increase with age. Back pain also begins to appear in early adulthood, with the peak incidence in the 30–50-year-old population[42,43]. In contrast to anatomic spinal aging, back problems seem to subside in the older population. Bigos et al. conducted a retrospective analysis of injuries occurring among a group of 31 200 employees of the Boeing Company: 4645 injury claims were made by 3958 different employees over a 15-month period. Nine hundred of these claims were back injuries[44]. Claims were categorized according to severity, as judged by the sum of the medical costs together with indemnity costs. High-cost claims were defined as those with a total cost greater than $10 000 and low-cost claims as those with a total cost less than $10 000. They found that employees younger than 25 years of age had a statistically significant increased risk of back injury. These claims tended to be low-cost. While the 31–40-year age group had a lower injury rate, this group was most susceptible to high-cost back injuries. Newer employees tended to have a significantly increased risk of back injury. Women had fewer injuries than men but a statistically significant increased risk of becoming a high-cost injury claim. Bigos et al. also observed a correlation between incidence of back injuries and poor employee appraisal rating evaluated by the employee's supervisor within 6 months before the injury.

In the identification of secondary predictors, Lanier and Stockton[45] found that a history of anxiety or depression was a significant predictor for poor outcome among patients not involved in manual labor. Cigarette smoking was also found to be related to greater long-term disability. Among the manual laborers, the number of hours of manual labor performed daily was a strong predictor of poor outcome. For both groups, the number of days off work prescribed by the physician was significantly related to greater absenteeism from work. The influence of physician behavior on absenteeism from work by patients with low back pain was also emphasized by Deyo et al.[15]. They demonstrated that absenteeism from work could be significantly and safely reduced if physicians prescribed only 2 days of bed rest instead of longer periods for acute low back pain.

Thomas studied a group of 200 patients who were presented in general practice with symptoms but no abnormal physical signs and in whom no definite diagnosis was made[46]. He demonstrated that 2 weeks after consultation, 64% of those who received a positive consultation got better, while 39% of those who received a negative consultation improved. A positive consultation is a consultation in which the patient was given a firm diagnosis and told confidently that he would be better in a few days. A negative consultation was an artificial consultation, devised so that no firm assurance was given.

The number of days absent from work was greater if particular symptoms or signs were present — buttock pain, thigh pain, leg pain, limited flexion, and limited extension. The presence of these symptoms and signs did not, however, affect the return to normal duties at 1 month after the injury[47,48].

A wide range of clinical features of patients at time of presentation were analyzed to see whether they were related to the outcome of the episode of low back pain[48-51]. Features that were not related to poor outcome included age, height, weight, obesity, the primary site of pain, and type of occupation. Pain rating scale was not identified as a significant prognostic feature. Significant independent prognostic risk factors for poor outcome that were identified were: (1) straight-leg raising limited to less than 60 degrees in either leg, (2) gradual onset of pain, (3) duration of pain more than 1 week prior to consultation, and (4) previous history of low back pain. Previous history of low back pain, limited straight-leg raise, and leg pain were also identified as risk indicators for recurrence[51]. Although loss of spinal motion is generally associated with increases in reported pain and decreases in functional capacity, Lankhorst et al., in their 3-year follow-up study[30], found that in the long run (3 years), a decrease in spinal motion accompanies decreasing pain and improving functional capacity. A progressive improvement of active straight-leg raising was also observed.

Specific predictive factors of chronicity and treatment success or failure (tertiary predictors) once the chronic low back pain is established remain inconclusive.

It has been proposed that low back pain is a learned behavior[19,52,53]. Pain behaviors, while elicited by antecedent physical lesions, are subject to subsequent consequences. When the pain behavior is followed by a positive consequence, that behavior is more likely to occur in the future; that is, the behavior will be strengthened or increased in rate of occurrence. The pain behavior is likely to occur less frequently in the future or decrease in strength if the positive consequence is removed or when the pain behavior meets with a negative consequence.

It is interesting to note that decrease in pain is unrelated to all other treatment outcomes. Pain level on admission and discharge may be of concern in terms of "relief of suffering," but decrease in pain does not necessarily result in return to work, increase in activity, decrease in medication, or cessation of requirement for further treatment[35].

It has been observed[50] that pain and functional impairment are poorly correlated with sickness absence. Fordyce et al., in their follow-up of 36 patients with chronic pain, showed that increase in activity occurred despite the fact that there was no decrease in pain[53]. This suggests that other factors are also involved. These may be social or economic in nature.

While there is no evidence in the literature that returning to work is beneficial, there is also no evidence to support the beneficial nature of bed rest for low back pain patients. The longer patients are away from work, the less is their chance of being rehabilitated to active life. The probability of returning to work has been estimated to be about 50% after an absence from work of 26 weeks. This probability drops to about 25% for an absence of 52 weeks[52].

In most treatment programs the expectation for patients returning to work is lower in cases involving litigation and compensation. In the study done by Cairns et al.[35] of those outpatients who had returned to work at 1 year follow-up, 42% were involved in Workers' Compensation litigation. This suggests that litigation may not limit return to work as much as expected; but, in another study, only two of the 20 inpatients receiving Workers' Compensation payments returned to work. Compensation factors have been considered among the strongest factors relating to chronic pain disability[19]. A large majority of patients remaining on some form of compensation or disability payment actually reported their general disability was worse, while very few saw themselves as less disabled. Conversely, almost half the patients who had settled their claims had, in some way, improved. It should be noted that half the patients did not improve after their claim had been settled. Talo et al. studied Workers' Compensation patients as well as patients engaged in litigation, and examined the effects of active and completed litigation on their treatment results[54]. They found no difference between the groups in organic and psychologic pathology. Significant improvement in outcome measures was found for the total group, but the Workers' Compensation claimants with active or completed litigation improved less than the total group. The claimants with completed litigation, however, returned to work more often than those with active litigation. Unfortunately, data for the group with other active litigation were not shown because the sample size was too small. The results of this study suggest that the compensation system, itself, and legal factors can be obstacles to the rehabilitation of patients with chronic low back pain[54].

Judicious use of primary, secondary, and tertiary predictors of outcome can aid in treatment choice. Studies[35] suggest that it is possible to develop a rational method for selecting patients for treatment in inpatient or outpatient programs using these predictors.

FUNCTIONAL IMPAIRMENT AND DISABILITY

Pain and disability must be differentiated. Disability may be judged by its effect on a patient's way of life, but pain is personal, an entirely subjective experience that language can not adequately communicate. It is also important to differentiate physical impairment and disability. Physical impairment is an anatomic or pathologic abnormality leading to loss of normal body ability, while disability is diminished capacity for everyday activities or the limitation of a patient's performance compared with a fit person's of the same age and sex. Physical impairment is an objective structural limitation and disability is a subjectively reported loss of function. The majority of patients with low back pain and even those with physical impairment never seek medical treatment, preferring to cope with the problem on their own. This is because many everyday symptoms are interpreted as a minor and temporary nociceptive stimulus that generates little anxiety. It is usually managed either by ignoring the affected part or modifying activity in expectation of natural resolution. It generally causes little disability. Seeking medical treatment appears to depend on the symptoms, the availability and expectations of treatment, and on learned and cultural patterns of illness behavior. The physician's response to the patient's condition is greatly influenced by the perceived distress and illness behavior exhibited by the patient. It is not so much dependent upon the facts of the actual physical disorder. It has been noted that 43% of occupational low back patients were able to return to alternative duties without any absence from work. The majority (82%) had returned to work in fewer than 5 days. At 5-year follow-up, 93% of patients were in work, but 70% stated that they were still suffering back pain. Fewer than one-third of patients were receiving medical or other treatment at the time of follow-up[47]. Other data also suggest that even those people with chronic back pain are able to return to the work force if they are provided with an appropriate early multidisciplinary rehabilitation program[47,53,55,56]. This further supports the necessity of differentiating between physical impairment and disability in the management of low back pain patients.

CONCLUSION

Low back pain is common. In its acute form it carries a very clear prognosis. Recurrence is not uncommon. Preventive methods have been tried in various industries with limited success. In the small percentage of chronic low back pain sufferers the prognosis is uncertain or poor. In most cases of low back pain, we have neither a biomechanical or pathologic understanding of the disease process nor knowledge of the anatomic source of the pain[4]. Diagnosis is, therefore, nominal at the best, keeping in mind the small percentage of low back pain that may be attributed to specific causes. There is no definite evidence that any treatment for low back pain is superior to a combination of natural history and the placebo effect. Physical treatment, particularly potentially harmful procedures such as surgery, should only be applied to those cases of definite pathology that are likely to benefit. When managing patients with chronic low back pain, we must consider the difference between low back pain and low back disability. We must distinguish pain from disability and the symptoms and signs of illness behavior from those of physical disease. Patients must be made to understand that a magic cure for all low back pain is unlikely. Both the physician and patient should realize that a doctor's role is merely to teach a patient how to get better. It is the patient's responsibility to follow these instructions and make himself better.

Appropriate treatment for low back pain should concentrate on active rehabilitation aiming at early return to normal life. The main theme of management of low back pain, acute or chronic, must change from rest to rehabilitation and restoration of function.

References

1. Biering-Sorensen, F. (1982). A prospective study of low back pain in a general population. 1. Occurrence, recurrence and aetiology. 2. Location, character, aggravating and relieving factors. *Scand. J. Rehabil. Med.*, **15**, 71-88
2. Nachemson, A. (1985). Advances in low back pain. *Clin. Orthop. Related Res.*, **200**, 266-278
3. Horal, J. (1969). The clinical appearance of low back disorders in the city of Gothenberg, Sweden: comparisons of incapacitated probands with matched controls. *Acta Orthop. Scand.* (suppl. 118), 1-74
4. Nachemson, A. (1976). The lumbar spine. An orthopaedic challenge. *Spine*, **1**, 59-71
5. Benn, R. T. and Wood, P. H. N. (1975). Pain in the back: An attempt to estimate the size of the problem. *Rheum. Rehabil.*, **14**, 121-128
6. Dillane, J. B., Fry, J. and Kalton, G. (1966). Acute back syndrome: a study from general practice. *Br. Med. J.*, **2**, 82-84
7. Quebec Task Force on Spinal Disorders. (1987). Scientific approach to the assessment and management of activity-related spinal disorders: A monograph for clinicians. *Spine*, **12** (suppl. 1), S9-S11
8. Wiltse, L. L., Newman, P. H. and MacNab, I. (1976). Classification of spondylolysis and spondylolisthesis. *Clin. Orthop.*, **117**, 23-29
9. Pizzutillo, P. D. and Hummer, C. D. III (1989). Nonoperative treatment for painful adolescent spondylolysis or spondylolisthesis. *J. Pediatr. Orthop.*, **9**, 538-540
10. Hensinger, R. N. and MacEwen, G. D. (1982). Congenital anomalies of the spine. In Rothman, R. H. and Simeone, F. A. (eds.) *The Spine*, pp. 188-315 (Philadelphia; W. B. Saunders)
11. Sinake, M., Lutness, M. P., Ilstrup, D. M., Chu, C. and Gramse, R. R. (1989). Lumbar spondylolisthesis: retrospective comparison and three-year follow-up of two conservative treatment programs. *Arch. Phys. Med. Rehabil.*, **70**, 594-598
12. Moreland, L. W., Lopez-Mendez, A. and Alarcon, G. (1989). Spinal stenosis: a comprehensive review of the literature. *Semin. Arthritis Rheum.*, **19**, 127-149
13. Troup, J. D. G. (1981). Straight-leg-raising (SLR) and the qualifying tests for increased root tension: their predictive value after back and sciatic pain. *Spine*, **6**, 526-527
14. Deyo, R. A. (1983). Conservative therapy for low back pain, distinguishing useful from useless therapy. *J. Am. Med. Assoc.*, **250**, 1057-1062
15. Deyo, R. A., Diehl, A. K. and Rosenthal, M. (1986). How many days of bed rest for acute low back pain? *N. Engl. J. Med.*, **315**, 1064-1070
16. Bergquist-Ullman, M. and Larsson, U. (1977). Acute low back pain in industry: a controlled prospective study with special reference to therapy and confounding factors. *Acta Orthop. Scand.*, **170**, 1-117
17. Spangfort, E. V. (1972). The lumbar disc herniation: a computer-aided analysis of 2504 operations. *Acta Orthop. Scand.*, **142** (suppl.), 1-95
18. Spengler, D. M., Freeman, C. and Westbrook, R. (1980). Low back pain following multiple lumbar spine procedures: failure of initial selection? *Spine*, **5**, 356-360
19. Nachemson, A. (1983). Work for all (for those with low back pain as well). *Clin. Orthop. Related Res.*, **179**, 77-85
20. Beals, R. K. and Hickman, N. W. (1972). Industrial injuries of the back and extremities: comprehensive evaluation — an aid in prognosis and management. A study of one hundred and eighty patients. *J. Bone Joint Surg.*, **54A**, 1593-1611
21. Ransford, A. O., Cairns, D. and Mooney, V. (1976). The pain drawing as an aid to the psychologic evaluation of patients with low back pain. *Spine*, **1**, 127-134

22. Weber, H. (1983). Lumbar disc herniation: a controlled, prospective study with ten years of observation. *Spine*, **8**, 131-140
23. Green, L. N. (1975). Dexamethasone in management of symptoms due to herniated lumbar disc. *J. Neurol. Neurosurg. Psychiatry*, **38**, 1211-1221
24. Shannon, N. and Paul, E. A. (1979). L4/5 and L5/S1 disc protrusion — analysis of 323 cases operated on over 12 years. *J. Neurol. Neurosurg. Psychiatry*, **42**, 804-809
25. Selecki, B. P., Ness, T. D., Limbers, P., Blum, P. W. and Stening, W. A. (1975). The surgical management of low back pain and sciatic syndrome in disc disease or injury: results of a joint neurosurgical and orthopaedic project. *Aust. N. Z. J. Surg.*, **45**, 183-191
26. Waddell, G., Kummel, E. G., Lotto, W. N., Graham, J. D., Hall, H. and McCulloch, J. A. (1979). Failed lumbar disc surgery and repeat surgery following industrial injuries. *J. Bone Joint Surg.*, **61A**, 201-207
27. Hakelius, A. (1970). Prognosis in sciatica: a clinical follow-up of surgical and non-surgical treatment. *Acta Orthop. Scand.*, **129** (suppl.) 5-76
28. Wall, P. D. and Devor, M. (1978). Physiology of sensation after peripheral nerve injury regeneration and neuroma formation. In Waxman, S. G. (ed.) *Physiology and Pathology of Axons*. (New York: Raven Press)
29. Rowe, M. L. (1969). Low back pain in industry. *J. Occup. Med.*, **11**, 161-169
30. Lankhorst, G. J., Van de Stadt, R. J. and Van der Korst, J. K. (1985). The natural history of idiopathic low back pain: a three-year follow-up study of spinal motion, pain and functional capacity. *Scand. J. Rehabil. Med.*, **17**, 1-4
31. Wilson, R. N. (1964). A ten-year follow-up of cases of low back pain. *Practitioner*, **192**, 657-660
32. Hakelius, A. (1970). Prognosis in sciatica: a clinical follow-up of surgical and non-surgical treatment. *Acta Orthop Scand.* (suppl. 129), 1-76
33. Wiesel, S. W., Feffer, H. L. and Borenstein, D. G. (1988). Evaluation and outcome of low-back pain of unknown etiology. *Spine*, **13**, 679-680
34. Wynn Parry, C. B., Girgis, F., Moffat, B. and Bhalla, A. K. (1988). The failed back: a review. *J. R. Soc. Med.*, **81**, 348-351
35. Cairns, D., Mooney, V. and Crane, P. (1984). Spinal pain rehabilitation: inpatient and outpatient treatment results and development of predictors for outcome. *Spine*, **9**, 91-95
36. McArthur, D. L., Cohen, M. J., Gottlieb, H. J., Naliboff, B. D. and Schandler, S.L. (1987). Treating chronic low back pain: I. Admission to follow-up. *Pain*, **29**, 1-22
37. McArthur, D. L., Cohen, M. J., Gottlieb, H. J., Naliboff, B. D. and Schandler, S. L. (1987). Treating chronic low back pain: II. Admission to follow-up. *Pain*, **29**, 23-38
38. LaRoca, H. and MacNab, I. (1969). Value of pre-employment radiographic assessment of the lumbar spine. *Can. Med. Assoc. J.*, **101**, 383-388
39. Fullenlove, T. M. and Williams, A. J. (1957). Comparative roentgen findings in symptomatic and asymptomatic backs. *J. Am. Med. Assoc.*, **168**, 572-574
40. Torgeson, W. R. and Dotler, W. E. (1976). Comparative roentgenographic study of the asymptomatic and symptomatic lumbar spine. *J. Bone Joint Surg.*, **58A**, 850-853
41. Magora, A. and Schwartz, A. (1976). Relation between the low back pain syndrome and x-ray findings. 1. Degenerative osteoarthritis. *Scand. J. Rehabil. Med.*, **8**, 115-125
42. Heliovaara, M., Knekt, P. and Aromaa, A. (1987). Incidence and risk factors of herniated lumbar intervertebral disc or sciatica leading to hospitalization. *J. Chronic Dis.*, **40**, 251-258
43. Lawrence, J. S. (1969). Disc degeneration: its frequence and relationship to symptoms. *Ann. Rheum. Dis.*, **28**, 121-138
44. Bigos, S. J., Spengler, D. M., Martin, N. A., Zeh, J., Fisher, L. and Nachemson, A. (1986). Back injuries in industry: a retrospective study. III. Employee related factors. *Spine*, **11**, 252-256
45. Lanier, D. C. and Stockton, P. (1988). Clinical predictors of outcome of acute episodes of low back pain. *J. Family Pract.*, **27**, 483-489
46. Thomas, K. B. (1987). General practice consultations: is there any point in being positive? *Br. Med. J.*, **294**, 1200-1202

47. Piterman, L. and Dunt, D. (1987). Occupational lower-back injuries in a primary medical care setting: a five-year follow-up study. *Med. J. Aust.*, **147**, 276-279
48. Pedersen, P. A. (1981). Prognostic indicators in low back pain. *J. R. Coll. Gen. Pract.*, **31**, 209-216
49. Hull, F. M. (1982). Diagnosis and prognosis of low back pain in three countries. *J. R. Coll. Gen. Pract.*, **6**, 352-356
50. Roland, M. and Morris, R. (1983). A study of the natural history of low back pain part 2: development of guidelines for trials of treatment inprimary care. *Spine*, **8**, 145-150
51. Biering-Sorensen, F., Thomsen, C. E. and Hilden, J. (1989). Risk indicators for low back trouble. *Scand. J. Rehab. Med.*, **21**, 151-157
52. Waddell, G. (1987). A new clinical model for the treatment of low back pain. *Spine*, **12**, 632-644
53. Fordyce, W. E., Fowler, R. S. Jr, Lehmann, J. F., DeLateur, B. J., Sand, P. L. and Trieschmann, R. B. (1973). Operant conditioning in the treatment of chronic pain. *Arch. Phys. Med. Rehabil.*, **54**, 399-408
54. Talo, S., Hendler, N. and Brodie, J. (1989). Effects of active and completed litigation on treatment results: workers' compensation patients compared with other litigation patients. *J. Occup. Med.*, **31**, 265-269
55. Wiesel, S. W., Feffer, H. L. and Rothman, R. H. (1984). Industrial low back pain: a prospective evaluation of a standardized diagnostic and treatment protocol. *Spine*, **9**, 199-203
56. Fordyce, W. E., Brockway, J. A., Bergman, J. A. and Spengler, D. (1986). Acute back pain, a control group comparison. *J. Behav. Med.*, **9**, 127-140

17
Prediction of the clinical efficacy of and intolerance to antirheumatic drug therapy

P. M. BROOKS and W. W. BUCHANAN

PROGNOSIS FOR CLINICAL EFFICACY

Prognostics do not always prove prophecies — at least the wise prophets make sure of the event first.
Horace Walpole (1717-1797)

The prediction of a positive or negative outcome of antirheumatic drug therapy is made particularly difficult by the large number of medications available. In addition to simple analgesics, such as acetaminophen (paracetamol) and salicylates, some 100 or so nonsteroidal antiinflammatory analgesic agents (NSAIDs) are marketed worldwide or are at an advanced stage of development[1]. Some of these NSAIDs have now been licensed for purchase "over the counter" but no less than 17 have had to be withdrawn due to side-effects[1]. It has been estimated that approximately $1000 million is spent on nonsalicylate antiinflammatory analgesics each year in the United States[2] entailing no fewer than 700 000 prescriptions[3]. Cogent arguments in favor of early use of slow-acting antirheumatic drugs (SAARDs) in the treatment of rheumatoid arthritis[4] have been persuasive not only for single agents but also for combinations of SAARDs[5]. Although most rheumatologists maintain that oral corticosteroids should rarely be used to treat patients with rheumatoid arthritis[6], some 10-25% of such patients attending hospital outpatient clinics will be receiving these drugs[6-9]. It has been suggested that small doses of oral corticosteroids can be used to treat active rheumatoid arthritis without fear of significant side-effects[10,11], even in elderly patients[12,13]. The encouraging results seen initially following the use of 1 g of intravenous methylprednisolone[14,15] have waned somewhat since the demonstration of equivalent short-term clinical effects using 1 g oral prednisolone[16] and the fact that clinical and immunologic response is transient[17-19].

Whether a dose as large as 1 g of prednisolone is required is unclear[14] but side-effects are relatively common[15,16]. Realization that retinopathy is rare with low-dose hydroxychloroquine[20,21] has led to a recent increase in the use of this drug[22]. Sulfasalazine, originally introduced by the late Dr Nanna Svartz in Sweden in the 1940s[23] and initially discredited by Sinclair and Duthie[24], has recently been shown, in several well-conducted studies, to be effective in the treatment of rheumatoid arthritis[25-28]. Methotrexate, likewise originally shown to be effective in psoriatic arthritis[29], has recently been found useful in rheumatoid arthritis[30,31], and other connective-tissue diseases such as dermatomyositis[32]. Other cytotoxic drugs such as azathioprine and cyclophosphamide have been shown to be not only effective in rheumatoid arthritis[33-36] and systemic lupus erythematosus[37-40], but in the case of cyclophosphamide also life-saving in several previously incurable diseases such as systemic vasculitis and Wegener's granulomatosis[41-47]. These drugs do, however, have a spectrum of serious side-effects[41,48]. Cyclosporin A has also recently been shown to be effective in refractory rheumatoid arthritis[49-51]. Several other drugs have been tested in rheumatoid arthritis but have been abandoned because of insufficient efficacy or potential toxicity, including captopril[52], dapsone[53,54], phenytoin[55,56], levamisole[57-59], and thalidomide[60]. Levamisole has also been found ineffective in systemic lupus erythematosus[61]. Etretinate has been shown to be effective in the treatment of psoriatic arthritis but side-effects, especially with high doses, may preclude its use[62].

Other than simple analgesics and NSAIDs, the only drug to be specifically developed for the treatment of rheumatoid arthritis and other inflammatory arthropathies in the past quarter of a century has been the oral gold compound auranofin, which has been shown to be effective but perhaps less so than injectable gold[63-67]. Nevertheless, a variety of nondrug therapies have been researched in patients with rheumatoid arthritis, with varying degrees of success, including dietary supplementation with fish oils[68-70], high-dose gamma globulins[71], interferon gamma[72], thymopoietin[73,74], apheresis[75], thoracic duct drainage[71,76], and total lymphoid irradiation[77,78]. Of these various therapeutic modalities, apheresis perhaps holds the most promise, especially in patients with rheumatoid arthritis with vasculitis[75], although it is disappointing that a randomized trial of this modality in SLE failed to demonstrate clinical benefit, despite reduction in serum levels of immunoglobulins, circulating immune complexes and anti-DNA antibody titers[79]. Future therapies might evolve from biologicals such as lymphokines and monoclonal antibodies[80] and rDNA products[81].

Perhaps the greatest advance in the drug treatment of rheumatic disorders, other than septic arthritis, has been in the control of acute and chronic tophaceous gouty arthritis, especially the latter, with the advent of uricosuric drugs and allopurinol[82,83]. The paradox in this condition is that patients are remarkably noncompliant in taking their medications[84]. Moreover, physicians seem equally reluctant to abandon time-honored colchicine for the treatment and prevention of acute gout[85], despite the fact that severe and fatal reactions have been reported[86,87] and NSAIDs have been shown to be equally effective[88].

Prediction of efficacy

Simple analgesics

Despite the fact that some 20-50% of patients with rheumatoid arthritis either self-administer or are prescribed simple analgesics in addition to their other drugs[89-93], controversy still exists as to their efficacy[94,95]. Nuki[96] considered simple analgesics to be of no benefit in inflammatory polyarthritis, whereas others[97-99] have recommended their use. Freemont-Smith and Bayles[100] were the first to show that codeine, propoxyphene, and even meperidine were less effective than salicylates as analgesics in rheumatoid arthritis. Other workers found acetaminophen either alone[101,102] or combined with aspirin[103] and pentazocine[104] to be without effect. On the other hand, Huskisson[97] clearly showed that acetaminophen, codeine, propoxyphene, and pentazocine all had analgesic effects in patients with rheumatoid arthritis, as have others in both this disease and osteoarthritis[105,106]. Of the various analgesics that Huskisson[97] tested, the combination of acetaminophen and propoxyphene (distalgesic) appeared to work best. Perhaps this was why Gibson and Clark[93] found this to be the most frequently prescribed analgesic to patients with rheumatoid arthritis in London, England, where Huskisson works. Recently, Emery and Gibson[108] have shown that mefopam, a simple analgesic, is effective in patients with rheumatoid arthritis.

Why there should be such discrepancies between different workers on the efficacy of simple analgesics in inflammatory joint disease is not clear. Severity of disease and the time over which observations were made (6 hours in the case of the studies of Huskisson[97] and 2 weeks in the studies of Lee and his colleagues[101,102], for example), might be factors. Whatever the reason, there is an urgent need to solve this controversy since simple analgesics such as acetaminophen and propoxyphene are not without their side-effects, especially in elderly patients who are perhaps the most frequent users[109]. There is evidence that morphine and meperidine might be more effective in the elderly[110] which might, however, be due to higher blood concentrations, either as a result of impaired hepatic biotransformation or alteration in protein-binding or volume of distribution[111,112]. Whether the elderly respond better to analgesics than younger people because of an alteration in pain threshold[113] is not clear. A recent study has shown that paracetomol and low-dose indomethacin is as efficacious as high-dose indomethacin in patients with rheumatoid arthritis emphasizing the adjunctive effect of simple analgesics[107].

NSAIDs

Prediction of response to NSAIDs is not determined by the *in vitro* potency of cyclooxygenase inhibition, since the same dose of sodium salicylate, a weak inhibitor, is equipotent in its analgesic effects in patients with rheumatoid arthritis to acetylsalicylic acid, a potent inhibitor[114]. The only variable which Lee *et al.*[115] found to predict outcome of NSAID administration in terms of analgesia in patients with rheumatoid arthritis was the amount of pain the patient had when treatment was commenced, those with severe pain having greater pain relief than those with mild pain. It is of interest that McLagan[116] observed a similar response when he used salicin in patients with acute rheumatic fever over 100 years ago. In the study of Lee *et al.*[115], neither age nor sex, duration of arthritis, nor previous therapy appeared to be important predictors of response to NSAID therapy. However, it is to be noted that in this, the only study of its kind to our knowledge, the extremes of age — the very old and the very young — were not represented. In addition, the study only assessed the immediate response, i.e., over a 2-week period. There is little evidence from other studies that sex is an important variable in determining outcome to NSAIDs.

Variability in response to NSAIDs was first suggested by Huskisson *et al.*[117] and the study of Scott *et al.*[118] certainly showed that differences between patients were greater than differences between drugs. No differences in pharmacokinetic disposition of NSAIDs between so-called "responders" and nonresponders has been found[119-122]. A recent study by our group[123], has, however, failed to confirm evidence for such a phenomenon, which probably is based on a *post hoc ergo procter hoc* fallacy[124]. The distribution in response to different NSAIDs reported by Huskisson *et al.*[117] conforms to a normal Gaussian distribution and shows no evidence of bimodality. None of the papers, other than our own[123], has tested patients on more than one occasion to determine concordance and discordance in clinical effect. If, indeed, responders and nonresponders to NSAIDs exist, it is surprising that the phenomenon should be confined to rheumatoid arthritis and not occur in acute rheumatic fever or acute gouty arthritis. Lack of efficacy on long-term therapy with NSAIDs may likewise be simply due to increase in disease activity, rather than loss of effect of the drug, although further investigation of this phenomenon is required. Some drugs, such as salicylates, induce their own biotransformation[125] with resulting fall in plasma plateau concentrations after 2–3 months[126,127]. The reductions, however, in plasma salicylate concentrations that have been reported[126,127] appear to us to be too small to be meaningful clinically. A range of 1.1–2.2 mmol/l is widely stated to be optimal for the anti-inflammatory effect of salicylate, but plasma concentrations of salicylate do not correlate particularly well with clinical outcome in rheumatoid arthritis[128]. Indeed, prediction of outcome to NSAID therapy cannot be made on plasma concentrations of the drugs, for although therapeutic ranges for salicylate and phenylbutazone[129] have been suggested, no correlation has been found between the plasma concentrations achieved with therapeutic doses of these drugs and clinical outcome[120,121,128,130-132]. Dose–response relationships have been demonstrated with naproxen[133,134], fenclofenac[135], and carprofen[136]. Again, although it is widely accepted that 3 g of aspirin daily is required to achieve anti-inflammatory effect, this is based on the single report of Boardman and Hart[137] using a rather insensitive outcome measure of digital joint circumference. Short-term clinical therapeutic trials of NSAIDs have shown little evidence that any one is superior to any other or, indeed to aspirin[138], but what is needed to allow comparison of the therapeutic value of different NSAIDs are long-term studies, of which there have now been several[139-142]. Although Fries and his colleagues[141] found only minor differences between different NSAIDs, the studies of the Glasgow Group[138,139] showed considerable variation in outcome. Overall it would appear from these two latter studies that only 40% of patients can be expected to continue with the same NSAID therapy over a period of 6 months. Although overall efficacy and toxicity are approximately the same, between 5% and 15% of patients discontinue therapy because of upper gastrointestinal symptoms, and an even greater number (15–60%) because of lack of effect. None of the authors who have conducted long-term studies of NSAID therapy has indicated any predictive clinical or laboratory findings that might help to determine how the patient might respond. Nevertheless, patient acceptance is a reasonable test of the therapeutic usefulness of NSAIDs[138,139]. We need more such studies and fewer short-term double-blind randomized trials.

The nature of the tablets or capsules, and how often they have to be taken, would appear to be potentially important in predicting outcome of NSAID therapy. Thus, a tablet or capsule that is difficult to swallow or has to be taken frequently, would appear likely to result in noncompliance, and there is evidence of this[145], especially for salicylates[144]. Side-effects might also be expected to result in failure of NSAID therapy and indeed do so when severe, as shown in the studies of Capell and her colleagues[138,139]. However, mild side-effects, such as cerebral symptoms from indomethacin, might have the opposite effect since Max *et al.*[147] have shown that toxic symptoms augment analgesic effect. Whether the color of an NSAID tablet or capsule might influence outcome is not known, although Huskisson[97] showed that a red placebo analgesic was more potent than one of yellow, green, or blue color. Others have shown that green was the preferred color for anxiety and yellow for depression[148]. There is little evidence that NSAIDs affect progress of erosive damage to joints, although benoxaprofen and fenclofenac (both now withdrawn because of toxicity) were claimed to do so favorably[149,150]. However, there is still considerable disagreement as to the effect of NSAIDs on cartilage metabolism *in vitro* and *in vivo*[151]. The problem with most of these data is that they are obtained from studies on animal models, although recently Herman *et al.*[152] have shown some NSAIDs to have differential effects on cartilage obtained from patients with osteoarthritis and rheumatoid arthritis.

Pharmacokinetics

Pharmacokinetic disposition of antirheumatic drugs plays a surprisingly small part in prediction of adverse reactions which, to a very large extent, are idiosyncratic in nature[153]. With the possible exception of salicylates, there is little evidence that monitoring serum concentrations of NSAIDs is of any value[154-158] or is cost-effective[159]. Serum concentrations of indomethacin do, however, correlate with headache[160]. Despite the fact that aspirin has been implicated as a causative factor in Reye's syndrome, several authors still recommend the use of this drug in juvenile rheumatoid arthritis[161-163] with monitoring of serum salicylate concentrations[164-166]. Considerable variability in steady-state plasma salicylate concentrations has been observed both in children and in adult patients with rheumatoid arthritis when prescribed the same dose on a weight basis[167,168]. As a result, many authors[169,170] do not recommend routine monitoring of serum salicylate concentrations. The onset of tinnitus has been used as a clinical indicator of toxicity but this is extremely unreliable in patients with impaired hearing, such as the elderly[171-173]. Only small differences have been observed in pharmacokinetic disposition of salicylates in the elderly; however, it should be noted that toxic effects occur at lower salicylate doses in these patients[174-177]. Phenylbutazone-induced aplastic anemia is probably idiosyncratic[178] but has been noted to occur more frequently in females over 50 years of age[179]. O'Malley et al.[180] reported that elderly people had a slower elimination rate of phenylbutazone and it is possible that the aplastic anemia in the elderly is related to higher drug concentration. In patients who develop phenylbutazone-induced aplastic anemia, Cunningham et al.[181] made the fascinating observation that acetanilide, which is oxidized by the same enzyme system as phenylbutazone, had a slower elimination. Measurement of serum phenylbutazone concentrations might, therefore, have had potential value is predicting aplastic anemia in patients receiving this drug. Side-effects of corticosteroids are dose-dependent, but measurement of plasma concentrations has not been used to predict side-effects[182].

The mean steady-state plasma gold concentration does not correlate with oral doses of auranofin[183] and blood gold concentrations are not related to toxicity of this drug or injectable gold[184]. Plasma concentrations of methotrexate remain of pharmacologic significance for only a brief period of time when the drug is prescribed in weekly doses[185]. However, Edelman et al.[186] have suggested that those patients who have a plasma concentration of methotrexate exceeding 0.01 µM at 24 h after 10 mg intramuscularly are more likely to be at risk of side-effects. Hepatic tissue concentrations of methotrexate polyglutamates have been shown to correlate with tissue folate levels, which can be restored with folinic acid[185]. It is possible, therefore, that measurement of methotrexate polyglutamates in the liver might help to predict subsequent fibrosis.

Monitoring of free drug concentrations has not been widely pursued, despite its obvious rationale[187-189]. Serum concentrations of free drug may be increased in the elderly as a result of hypoalbuminemia[190], and the presence of uremia has been shown to increase free salicylate concentrations by a factor of 2[191]. The protein binding of salicylate follows Michaelis–Menten kinetics so that a greater proportion of free salicylate is present in higher concentrations[174]. However, in practice Gurwich et al.[192] found that the free concentration correlated with the total concentration of salicylate, thus making little point of measuring unbound fraction. Gold is highly bound to albumin, although Rudge et al.[193] found no correlation between free plasma and urinary gold concentration and toxic effects, but Heath[194] recently reported a strong association between free plasma gold concentration and toxicity.

Many drugs are prescribed as racemates, including many of the NSAIDs and second-line agents[195]. Although both hepatic biotransformation and renal clearance are stereoselective, differences in R and S enantiomers of NSAIDs are too small to be of any clinical significance[196]. However, it is of interest that the coenzyme, a thioester of carboxylic acids, can replace the natural fatty acid in triglycerols to form "hybrid" triglycerides[197,198]. Williams et al.[199] have shown that the R, but not the S, isomer of ibuprofen is taken up by adipose tissue. Conceivably the accumulation of R isomers of carboxylic acids could perturb membrane function. It is tempting to speculate that such stereoselective accumulation in brain might explain the meningitis syndrome associated with ibuprofen[200]. However, this cannot be the sole explanation since the syndrome has also been described with sulindac[201], tolmetin[202], and cotrimoxazole[203].

The implications of acetylator status on drug biotransformation have already been discussed. Genetic variation has also been demonstrated with the cytochrome P450-dependent mixed-function oxidase system[204] and there is evidence that some of these enzymes might be diminished in the elderly[205]. However, much of the data are conflicting; some workers, for instance, find the plasma half-life of phenylbutazone to be increased[180], whereas others[206] find it decreased. The clearance of some NSAIDs such as ibuprofen[207] and ketoprofen[208] is decreased in elderly subjects although, because these drugs have a short plasma half-life, clinical relevance is unclear. However, for those NSAIDs with long plasma half-lives, changes in elderly people might be of importance. For example, piroxicam, which has an average plasma half-life of 50 hours, has been shown by some workers to have an increased half-life in elderly people, possibly resulting in increased plasma concentrations[209-212]. This, however, has not been confirmed by other groups[213-215]. Old age only accounts for a small amount of the variation in plasma half-life[211,216] and many other factors affect drug disposition[217]. At present there seems no indication for measuring the ability of the P450 enzyme system to biotransform drugs, since the half-life of marker drugs such as antipyrine might not predict an increase in a drug which is biotransformed, even by the same enzymes[218,219].

Conjugative processes of drug biotransformation are not, however, affected by aging. However, 2-arylpropionic acids which form acyl glucuronides might have their plasma half-life prolonged especially in the presence of renal failure[220]. Such drugs include benoxaprofen, diflunisal, ketoprofen, and naproxen. The acyl glucuronide can be hydrolyzed back to the parent drug. The "futile" cycle, as it has aptly been named[221,222], might well have been the cause of the hepatic and renal complications in elderly patients prescribed benoxaprofen[223].

All of the NSAIDs, with the exception of azapropazone which is 70% excreted unchanged in the urine, undergo extensive hepatic biotransformation with less than 10% being excreted unchanged. With the exception of azapropazone and those NSAIDs which form acyl glucuronides, renal failure has little effect on their disposition.

The one drug which might result in serious and fatal side-effects with renal failure is allopurinol[244]. This drug has a short plasma half-life of between 60 and 90 minutes but is metabolized to oxypurinol, which is also an inhibitor of xanthine oxidase and has a prolonged plasma half-life of 15 hours. Allopurinol is excreted in the urine by glomerular filtration and oxypurinol is secreted and reabsorbed by the tubules in the same way as urates. In renal failure, the half-life of oxypurinol is significantly prolonged and it is this which causes the adverse reaction. Diuretics also potentiate the effects of renal insufficiency[225-227]. The reaction consists of fever, maculopapular rash, jaundice, leukocytosis, and eosinophilia and deterioration in renal function and a high mortality. The reaction can be predicted from assessment of the degree of renal dysfunction and can be avoided by reducing the dose of allopurinol.

Slow-acting anti-rheumatic drugs (SAARDs)

Despite the fact that numerous clinical trials have shown different SAARDs to be more effective than placebo in rheumatoid arthritis and other inflammatory arthropathies such as psoriatic arthritis[228], there remains considerable doubt as to their long-term overall efficacy[229,230], especially in preventing radiologic progression[231-237]. Patients who demonstrate a fall in erythrocyte sedimentation rate and acute-phase reactants have been considered in short-term trials of SAARDs to show less radiologic progression[238-240], but Scott et al.[232-234] could find no simple relationship between clinical and laboratory assessments and joint damage over a longer period of follow-up. In a review of the literature, Scott and Bacon[234] found only three of nine placebo-controlled trials which reported less joint erosion with SAARDs — two on gold[241,242] and one on cyclophosphamide[234]. Scott and Bacon observed that many studies had reported radiologic changes in patients treated with SAARDs, but none had included a control group. Perhaps the most impressive of these studies is that of Luukkainen[244,245], who followed 100 patients treated with gold for 5-6 years. Those patients who had to stop treatment because of side-effects fared worse in terms of joint damage. Those patients who started on gold therapy early in the course of their disease did better. In contrast, the study by Scott and his colleagues[232] of 88 patients with rheumatoid arthritis treated with prolonged intensive SAARD therapy and followed up for 10 years was more pessimistic, with two-thirds of the patients showing radiologic progression.

Many of the studies reporting radiologic changes in rheumatoid arthritis treated with chrysotherapy or other SAARDs suffer from small numbers, e.g., Sigler et al.[242] and a variety of methods of assessing radiologic joint damage, although many of these methods have been demonstrated to have acceptable reproducibility[246-248]. It should, however, be noted that some workers have been unable to obtain acceptable reproducibility in erosion counts[249] and Fries et al.[250] have made the important point that if observer error is to be reduced then it is important that films be read by pairs of observers. Fries et al.[250] have also pointed out the importance of measuring joint space narrowing, as well as joint erosions, something which is missing from most studies. Perhaps in future it may be useful to use more refined methods of assessing radiologic joint damage, such as image analysis techniques[251], and microfocal radiology[252].

An important point frequently not addressed in long-term assessments of SAARD therapy is patient noncompliance with medication. Pullar et al.[253] found, for instance, using a pharmacologic indicator, that some 42% of patients with rheumatoid arthritis were noncompliant with penicillamine therapy and if this were to apply to other SAARDs it would make a significant difference to efficacy.

It should be noted that it has not been possible to predict the rate of development of new erosions in early rheumatoid arthritis, either using seropositivity or HLA tissue types[254]. Unfortunately, studies on prognostic features that might influence the final outcome of rheumatoid arthritis often do not include drug therapy as a variable[255]. It has been suggested that patients with seronegative rheumatoid arthritis show a better response to low-dose methotrexate therapy but this may be merely the result of seronegative patients having less-severe disease[256]. Weinblatt et al.[257] suggested that patients with rheumatoid arthritis who were DR2 positive were more likely to have a favorable outcome with methotrexate but this has not been confirmed in more extensive studies[258]. Similar responses to gold therapy in HLA-identical siblings with rheumatoid arthritis in terms of efficacy strongly suggest that genetic factors may play an important role in determining outcome to SAARD therapy[259]. This is supported by the observations of O'Duffy et al.[260] that HLA positivity and HLA-DR4 negativity were the best predictors of a favorable response to chrysotherapy in rheumatoid arthritis. However, Carette et al.[261], could not confirm this interesting finding. No clinical or laboratory predictors have been identified in either juvenile or adult rheumatoid arthritis to determine outcome with auranofin therapy[262,263]. No HLA studies have been reported in the outcome of sulfasalazine therapy in rheumatoid arthritis[264] and no

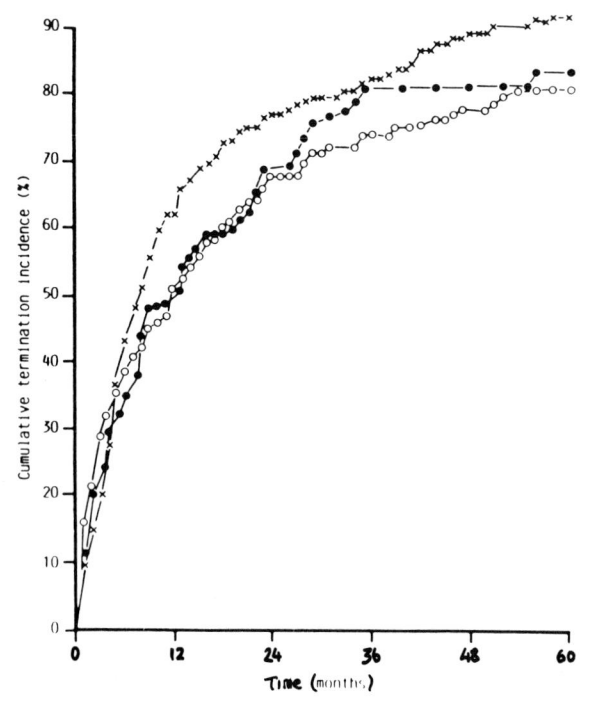

Figure 1 Total treatment termination for three drugs (gold, penicillamine and sulfasalazine) over five years (× gold ● penicillamine, ○ sulfasalazine) (from Situnayake et al.[269] with kind permission of the authors and the Editor of the *Annals of the Rheumatic Diseases*)

relationship to acetylator status has been found[265-267].

Life-table analysis as a method of displaying data is probably the most appropriate means of illustrating the overall outcome and reasons for discontinuation of therapy[268]. This has been admirably done for SAARDs by Situnayake et al.[269], where treatment termination of 317 patients with rheumatoid arthritis followed for 5 years was approximately the same for gold (92%), D-penicillamine (83%), and sulfasalazine (81%) (Figure 1). Ineffectiveness was the reason for termination in more patients receiving sulfasalazine (41%) than the penicillamine (38.1%) or gold (29.5%). In contrast, adverse reactions led to withdrawal especially with gold (57%), rather than with D-penicillamine (41.2%) or sulfasalazine (37%). These results are comparable with other studies, which show that approximately 50% of patients will have been withdrawn from treatment with a particular SAARD by 12 months, mostly owing to side-effects[270-271]. Thompson et al.[271] also showed that about 60% of patients commenced on a SAARD would respond usually by 6 months. However, those patients failing to respond to a second SAARD would only show a 40% response rate to a third SAARD (Figure 2).

A lack of correlation between whole blood gold concentrations and

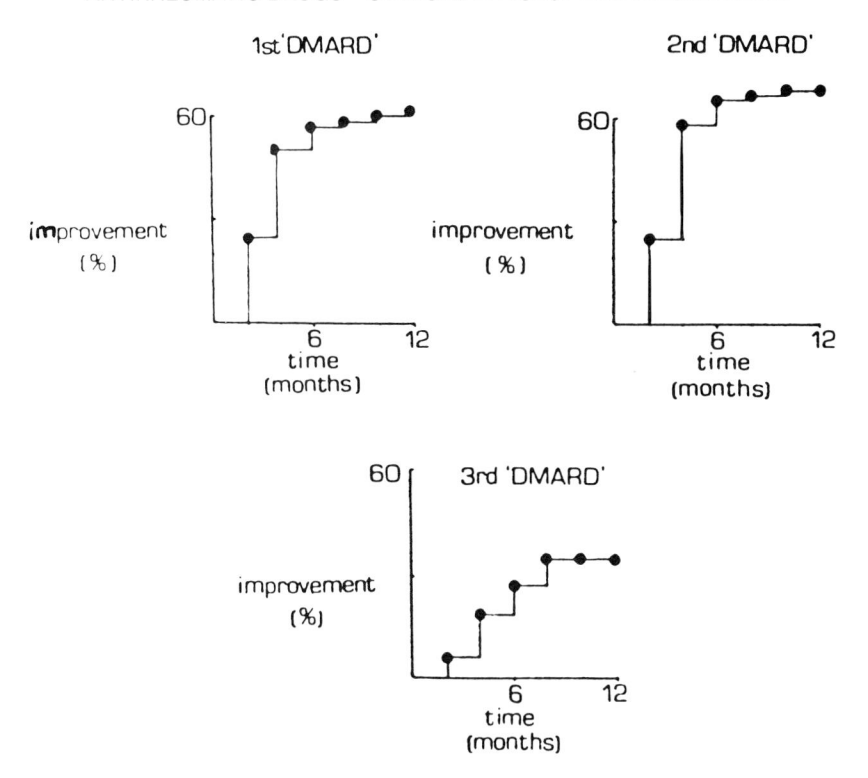

Figure 2 Life tables comparing the probabilities of an improvement occuring after starting treatment with a first, second or third SAARD. The numbers of drug/patient exposures available for analysis, treatment initiation at the two monthly intervals are:
First SAARD: 154, 133, 108, 94, 74, 71 and 64
Second SAARD: 68, 55, 45, 29, 26, 22 and 19
Third SAARD: 22, 17, 13, 10, 7, 7 and 6.
(From Thompson et al.[271] with kind permission of the authors and the Editor of the *British Journal of Rheumatology*)

clinical response has been reported in patients with rheumatoid arthritis. Ahern et al.[272] found no single clinical or laboratory marker which would predict the outcome of discontinuing D-penicillamine treatment in a group of adults with rheumatoid arthritis; however, Rae[273] found that a change in superoxide dismutase activity and plasma and lysate thiol concentrations preceded clinical improvement induced by chrysotherapy.

Whether oral corticosteroids diminish radiologic erosions in rheumatoid arthritis remains controversial[274-277], and clearly requires a properly controlled trial[278].

Steinberg[279] has recently outlined the history of systemic lupus erythematosus, pointing out that in the precorticosteroid era patients usually died of acute lupus. With the advent of low doses (10 - 30 mg/d) of corticosteroids in the late 1940s, many patients had the toxic manifestations of SLE brought under control but often died of renal failure. With the use of high doses of corticosteroids (40–60 mg/d prednisolone) and better medical management, the median survival of patients with renal disease was increased from between 1 and 2½ years[280,281] in the late 1950s, to 5 years in the early 1970s[282-284]. The experience of Steinberg and his colleagues[279] at the National Institutes of Health during the 1970s to the present time has shown an increase in median survival of 10 years for those treated with azathioprine and corticosteroids, and 15 years or greater for those treated with cyclophosphamide. The work of Pollack et al.[280] and Baldwin et al.[281] in the 1960s on defining histologic categories of renal disease did much to help in the assessment of different therapies. In essence, three histologic patterns were described:

1. Focal proliferative lupus nephritis, or glomerulonephritis
2. Diffuse proliferative lupus nephritis or lupus glomerulonephritis
3. Membranous disease

The first pattern was regarded as mild disease capable of responding to low doses of corticosteroids, whereas patients with the second pattern frequently died from renal failure, despite high doses of corticosteroids. Some 20% of patients with membranous disease developed renal failure within 5 years. Thus, the histologic findings on renal morphology dictated therapy, although it soon became apparent that a patient with a mild disease pattern could progress to severe damage. It thus came to be appreciated that a renal biopsy did not represent a final diagnosis, but rather should be reviewed as representing one point in a dynamic process, since in 50% of patients a repeat biopsy will show changes that demand reclassification[285]. Urinalysis is an imperfect but important and useful prognosticator for the type of renal disease. Patients with nephrotic syndrome and massive proteinuria usually have membranous disease. Proteinuria, microscopic hematuria, and casts usually indicate diffuse proliferative or membranoproliferative disease. Red cells and white cells in the absence of infection with a small amount of protein usually predict a focal, segmental, or diffuse glomerular disease. Of greater importance was the realization that the prognosis of the disease, especially the severity of renal involvement, paralleled in general the qualitative properties of anti-DNA antibodies, such as affinity, ability to form precipitates, and ability to fix complement, irrespective of the total amount of anti-DNA and hypocomplementemia[286].

Thus, cyclophosphamide has been found to be the most useful drug in the treatment of severe lupus disease and there is little evidence that high doses of oral corticosteroids are of any real value. The rationale for using high-dose oral corticosteroids is based on a single study done in the 1960s[287]. Patients who received high doses were compared with a group who had received low doses some years previously and who had more severe renal disease. There are no long-term data to determine the usefulness of various drugs and Steinberg points out that short-term changes such as alteration in renal histology and reduction in autoantibodies are insufficient to determine the real value of a drug.

No controlled trial of oral corticosteroid therapy in dermatomyositis or polymyositis has been carried out, but some 90% of patients so treated will improve[288]. The effects of oral corticosteroids may be slow, many patients taking up to 6 months to improve. Patients who receive high doses of corticosteroids, e.g., greater than 50 mg prednisolone per day, tend to do better than those on small doses[289,290]. No single clinical or laboratory prognosticator has been identified in determining outcome of oral corticosteroid therapy in these diseases[291]. Prognosis, however, appears to be worse in those patients in whom treatment is delayed[292]. Retrospective analysis has shown no evidence of increased survival rate of patients treated with oral corticosteroids compared to those not so treated[293,294]. Of the other therapies, including azathioprine, methotrexate, cyclophosphamide, chlorambucil, and mercaptopurine, only the first has been subject to a controlled clinical trial. After 3 months no difference was noted in eight patients who received azathioprine and prednisolone compared to eight patients on prednisolone alone. However, after 3 years the former had greater function and were taking less prednisolone, which five had discontinued. Hydroxychloroquine can be expected to be effective with skin disease, even when associated with malignancy, but not the myositis[295].

One important new observation in polymyositis is the identification of a subset with cytoplasmic and nuclear inclusion[296]. These patients are usually older men who present with a gradual onset and have a much slower progression of their disease. Distal muscles are frequently involved. Such patients respond less well and less rapidly to corticosteroid therapy. As can be seen from the above data, there is a need for carefully planned multicenter studies in these rare connective-tissue diseases to try to identify prognostic factors both clinically and therapeutically.

Prognosis of side-effects

General aspects

Although rheumatologists were well aware that their drugs caused side-effects, the magnitude of the problem only was appreciated following the report by Girdwood in 1974[297] that 50% of deaths from medicaments reported to the Committee of Safety of Medicines in the United Kingdom were due to antirheumatic drugs. Indeed, if the number of prescriptions was taken as the denominator, injectable gold was the most toxic compound in the British Pharmacopoeia. Previous studies had shown that approximately 5% of admissions to a rheumatic disease unit in Glasgow, Scotland, were due to adverse drug side-effects, mostly due to oral corticosteroids[298]. Of 82 patients with rheumatoid arthritis who had died and had autopsies performed, no fewer than 13 (15.9%) of the deaths were considered to be drug-related[299]: the commonest drug to be implicated was again oral corticosteroids, in seven patients (8.5%). In 1966, Reed and Wright[300] reported the combined experience in the United States and United Kingdom of corticosteroid therapy in psoriatic arthritis, and considered that this form of therapy accounted for no less than 50% of deaths. This was at a time, however, when higher doses of corticosteroids were being prescribed. Other studies on the causes of death among patients with rheumatoid arthritis have either confirmed that a significant proportion are drug-related[301-305] or that none was due to drugs[306]. Mortality statistics based on death certificates are notoriously unreliable[307-309]. Deaths of elderly patients on benoxaprofen[310], which led to the removal of the drug[311], have further highlighted the need for accurate data on adverse drug reactions and on whether there may be clinical and laboratory indicators which may predispose a patient to such reactions.

Adverse drug reactions

It is first necessary to consider what we mean by an adverse drug reaction. The World Health Organization[312] has defined it as "one that is noxious, unintended and occurs at doses used in man for prophylaxis, diagnosis or therapy." The problem is that although the definition may be acceptable, the elucidation is more difficult, since the incidence of side-effects will vary greatly according to whether a general or direct question is asked[313]. This may explain, for instance, the marked variation in incidence of dyspepsia with NSAIDs, from 8% to 61%[314]. There is also the problem of "background" dyspepsia occurring spontaneously[315,316] and there are considerable differences among physicians in determining whether a patient has an adverse drug reaction. Algorithms have proved helpful in improving consensus among physicians[317], but have been criticized on the grounds that they merely substitute the opinion of the authors of the algorithm for that of the clinical assessors[318]. The best "hard" data are obtained when discontinuation of therapy is included in the definition, such as has been done in the long-term studies of NSAIDs by Capell and her colleagues[319] and SAARDs by Situnayake and his colleagues[320].

Estimation of risk

Adverse drug reactions are the price we pay for the benefits of modern drugs[312]. This may be so, but it is useful to have an accurate estimate of this price[322]. Spontaneous reporting systems as are currently used in the United States and the United Kingdom serve as early warning systems and do not give an accurate assessment of risk[323]. These must be interpreted cautiously since only some 15–20% of adverse reactions are reported[324,325] and there is a tendency for physicians to report side-effects with new drugs[326]. In addition, other factors influence reporting in these systems, such as reports of a specific side-effect especially with a new drug, particularly if they appear in the lay press[325]. Indeed, several drugs have been removed from the market as a result of sensational news of a rare side-effect, e.g., zomepirac sodium[327], the drug being withdrawn, as Inman[328] has pointed out, because of numbers, not incidence.

Premarketing studies can only be expected to identify commonly occurring adverse reactions, for example, at the 1% level[327], since clinical therapeutic trials of new drugs are performed on "squeaky clean" patients[314,329,330]. Postmarketing surveillance has been advocated to solve the problem[331,332], but the difficulty is, as Fries et al.[333] have pointed out, that if the reaction is rare, say 1 in 100 000, then some 300 000 patients would be required to be seen to be 95% certain of finding a single case — the so-called "rule of three."[334] Enthusiasts of the new discipline of pharmacoepidemiology[330,335,336] should pause to think before entering "where angels fear to tread"! The future of pharmacoepidemiology is at present not clear[337]. Automated databases will not necessarily solve the problem, since they are dependent on data quality and validity[338].

The ideal system would be a follow-up cohort study[339] but this only works if the side-effect is relatively common. The databases collected at Puget Sound, Seattle, Washington, USA[340]; in Saskatchewan, Canada[341], and in Southampton, England[342] are ample testimony to the problem. Fox and Jick[340] found not one renal complication from NSAIDs among 50 000 patients treated with these drugs. Not one blood disorder was identified by Danielson et al.[341] among 41 178 patients receiving phenylbutazone. Inman and Rawson[342] observed a low incidence of serious side-effects among 12 709 patients treated with benoxaprofen, 5058 with fenbufen, 9880 with piroxicam, 8560 with zomepirac, and 10 758 with Osmosin®, a special slow-release form of indomethacin now removed from the market as a result of serious intestinal complications. Indeed, an additional two of these five drugs, benoxaprofen and zomepirac, have also been removed from sale. It is of interest, however, that an increased incidence of acute myocardial infarction was observed following withdrawal of zomepirac[342,343]. If these databases are too small to give meaningful results, then others like the reported 172 patients treated with benoxaprofen without serious side-effects border on the ridiculous[344].

Somewhat surprisingly in this era of computers, biostatistics, and epidemiology, the best alert system of serious side-effects from a new medicament is the published case report. Nineteen of 20 adverse reactions since the thalidomide disaster were identified by an alert physician who published them as case reports[345-347]. However effective this method might be, it does not allow for a proper estimate of incidence[322] and it may result in delay if the side-effect is unusual, as occurred with practolol.

The elderly

Much has recently been written on the problems of adverse reactions to drug therapy in the elderly. Certainly, the magnitude of the problem is now a cause for concern, since just over 1 in 10 of the populations in developed countries is 65 years or older, and one in three of all prescriptions are for this group[348]. A high incidence of adverse drug reactions in elderly patients has been reported by several workers[349] and it is often due to polypharmacy, altered drug pharmacokinetics and pharmacodynamics, multiple pathology, and severity of disease. Multiple drug therapy leads to an increase in adverse drug reactions, not linearly but exponentially, as Nolan and O'Malley[349] have pointed out. The severity of disease is probably just as important as, indeed if not more important than, multiple pathology, and Steel et al.[315] have shown that, when this is taken into account, elderly patients do not necessarily have an increased incidence of adverse drug reactions. Certain illnesses, such as bleeding peptic ulcer, which may result from drug therapy, are more common in elderly persons anyway, the mortality rising sharply after 50 years of age[350]. The Royal College of Physicians of London[351] emphasized in their report on the problems of drug therapy in the elderly that adverse effects were often a result of errors in prescribing. Doctors, in general, are careful in prescribing new drugs, but less so with old ones. In 573 elderly patients admitted to hospital, Gosney and Tallis[352] noted that of 6160 prescriptions, 200 (3.2%) were either contraindicated or had adverse interactions. One hundred and thirty-six patients (3.7%) were affected by these mistakes. Errors in prescribing increase, of course, with increasing number of prescriptions[353]. These problems are particularly evident in long-care institutions were p.r.n. orders are common and where there is often less than ideal supervision of repeat prescriptions[354,355]. Undoubtedly much could be done to improve this situation by involvement of clinical pharmacists in day-to-day prescribing in hospital[356] and in evaluation of drug therapy in general[357]. More could certainly be done by educating elderly patients on the proper use of their medication. Strategies must, however, provide small amounts of specific information, rather than overwhelming the patient with a large number of facts[358]. Elderly patients tend to be highly motivated in taking medicines correctly: it is the young who are less concerned[358]. In the community, more could be done in getting the elderly to use a single pharmacy, and to talk to their pharmacist about their drugs[359].

Until such measures are taken regarding prescribing drug therapy for elderly persons, one can continue to predict an increased incidence of adverse drug reactions in this group. Recently, in lay periodicals, it has been alleged that doctors are not properly educated in pharmacology and geriatric medicine; although one can criticize the journalistic and sensational style in these publications, nevertheless one has to admit in all honesty that they contain more than a grain of truth.

The elderly cannot be defined simply on a chronological basis[360,361]. Many elderly people, especially those under 75 years of age[362], are perfectly fit and healthy, and in terms of adverse drug reactions probably do not differ from younger persons. It is the frail elderly, especially those older than 75 years and with multiple organ failure, who are at particular risk from drug therapy, particularly if they are institutionalized[349].

That the elderly are not homogeneous is seen from the studies of Sheldrake and her colleagues[363] on side-effects of flurbiprofen in patients with rheumatoid arthritis. Those patients over the age of 50 years actually had fewer adverse reactions than those who were younger. However, all of the older patients were otherwise in reasonable health.

Tablet formulations and route of administration

Tablet formulation may influence whether or not side-effects occur. Thus, Osmosin®, a slow-release form of indomethacin, resulted in a high incidence of intestinal perforation and hemorrhage, due to a high concentration of the drug being delivered to the intestinal mucosa[364].

Hort[365] noted that tablets of alclofenac, an NSAID now removed from the market, were associated with a 10.3% incidence of adverse effects, compared to 2.1% with capsules. Similarly, the original formulation of indomethacin as a tablet gave rise to a high incidence of dyspepsia compared to the capsule formulation[366]. The chemistry of drugs may be expected to play a role in causing adverse reactions, and certainly this is true with certain drugs that are chiral[367,368]. However, the 17 NSAIDs withdrawn from the market were not associated with any one structural class.

Genetic predisposition

In 1978, Stastny[369] first reported an association between the HLA-DR4 antigen and rheumatoid arthritis. In the same year, Panayi et al.[370] suggested a genetic predisposition to toxic reactions to chrysotherapy and D-penicillamine. That this is, indeed, the case has been supported by a large corpus of evidence, which has been ably reviewed by Ford[371].

Several workers have reported an association between HLA-DR3 and B8, and to a lesser extent A1 and CW7, and proteinuria induced by gold therapy[372-380] and D-penicillamine[372,374,376,378,381-383]: on the other hand, no such association was found with any HLA phenotype with either gold[384-387] or D-penicillamine. Indeed, the presence of the phenotypes DR2 and DR7 has been considered to be protective for both gold[375,388,389] and D-penicillamine[383,389]. It should be noted, however, that Panayi et al.[370] found a positive association with D-penicillamine-induced proteinuria. Proteinuria with prior gold therapy has been found predictive for the development of this side-effect with D-penicillamine[382,383,390,391] and tends to further support a genetic basis. Proteinuria in rheumatoid arthritis may of course have a number of causes. Gold and D-penicillamine-induced proteinuria, however, has been shown to be due to a membranous nephropathy[392]. Electron microscopy has shown subepithelial electron-dense deposits and fusion of epithelial foot processes, and immunofluorescence has frequently demonstrated granular capillary wall deposits of IgG and C_3[392,393]. Rheumatoid vasculitis, immune membranous nephropathy and systemic lupus erythematosus have all been associated with HLA-B8 and DR3[394-396]. Macrophages, granulocytes and many lymphocytes express surface receptors for the Fc domain of immunoglobulin[387]. Patients who are HLA-B8 and DR3 positive have been shown to have an Fc receptor defect on macrophages, an impaired clearance of immune complexes[398], and slow degradation of antigen by macrophages[399].

Thrombocytopenia occurring with chrysotherapy appears to be of two types: one that occurs soon after commencing therapy and is not dose related, nor associated with platelet antibodies or increased peripheral platelet destruction and responds to corticosteroids; and a second type that is dose-related, occurs usually after a prolonged course, and appears to consist of a toxic effect on the marrow[398-400]. The former, especially, appears to be associated with the DR3 phenotype but also to a lesser extent with A1, B8 and DR4[400-403]. D-Penicillamine-induced thrombocytopenia, however, appears to be associated with A1, B8 and DR4[404], which may be consistent with the view that thrombocytopenia caused by this drug is due to a toxic effect on the marrow[405]. Wooley et al.[373] found no association of thrombocytopenia induced by gold or D-penicillamine with DR3.

Mucocutaneous reactions have been reported to be increased with both gold[377,388] and D-penicillamine[388]. Some workers have also recorded an association between mucocutaneous reactions due to gold and Bw35 phenotype[406,407], whereas others[408,409] have not. Perrier et al.[388] have suggested that DR7 may have a protective role since the prevalence of this antigen was decreased in those patients who developed skin eruptions on gold and D-penicillamine. Neutropenia on gold therapy has been associated with DR4, not DR3[410] which is similar to Felty's syndrome[411,412]. Garlepp et al.[413] have reported an association of Bw35 and DR1 with D-penicillamine-induced myasthenia gravis.

Little has been reported on the association of HLA haplotypes and side-effects with sulfasalazine[414]. However, Tishler et al.[415] observed an association of DR1 and DR7 with increased serum transaminases on inpatients with rheumatoid arthritis treated with methotrexate. This study was performed in Israel, where DR1, and not DR4, is associated with rheumatoid arthritis[417].

The lack of uniform agreement among different workers is due to the fact that many of the studies differ in terms of patient selection and duration of follow-up; in addition, many have too small numbers so that differences do not reach statistical significance.

At the present time, all that can be concluded is that the association of different HLA phenotypes with adverse reactions to gold and D-penicillamine is largely of academic interest. The fact that some studies have shown no association at all between different HLA types and adverse effects of these drugs[418] and that many of those which purport to do so fail to reach statistical significance means that prediction cannot be made with any certainty at a clinical level when a decision is made to treat a patient with these drugs.

Genetic control of metabolism

The control of polymorphic acetylation is determined by a single form of acetyl transferase which affects the biotransformation of many drugs, including isonicotinic acid hydrazide, sulfadimidine, dapsone, hydralazine and procainamide[419,420]. Recently, Grant et al.[421] have shown that the acetylation of caffeine can be used to determine acetylation status, i.e., either a slow or fast acetylation. Patients who are slow acetylators have been shown to be more prone to develop systemic lupus erythematosus when treated with hydralazine[422,423]. However, fast acetylators are not immune[424,425] and Mansilla-Tinoco et al.[426] have recorded the same incidence of serum antinuclear factors in patients who are on continuous hydralazine therapy for 3 years, irrespective of acetylator status. Batchelor et al.[427] have also suggested that hydralazine-induced lupus is associated with HLA-DR genes.

Procainamide is acetylated to N-acetylprocainamide and slow acetylators are more likely to develop a lupus syndrome[428]. The reaction appears to depend on a primary amino group of the procainamide and not on the metabolite[139]. The phenomenon is largely related to dose, since if an adjustment is made so that slow acetylators have the same blood levels as fast acetylators, there is no difference in incidence of the lupus syndrome[430].

The adverse effects of sulfasalazine can be divided into two main categories: first, those which are dose-related, including nausea and vomiting, headache, etc., and rarely hemolytic anemia, and methemoglobinemia; second, the idiosyncratic and hypersensitivity reactions, including rashes, pneumonitis, hepatitis, and bone marrow depression[415,431]. The former appears to be related to acetylator status and is dose-related[432,433]. It is the sulfapyridine moeity which is acetylated[434]. Although adverse drug reactions are much more common in slow acetylators treated with the drug for ulcerative colitis, the relatively small doses used in rheumatoid arthritis make the association weak. It therefore becomes of little clinical importance[433,435].

X-chromosome-linked glucose-6-phosphate dehydrogenase deficiency is the most common enzymopathy associated with hemolytic anemia in man. Some 150 mutant gene products have been identified so far[435]. Some 10% of American Negroes have one of the variants, but this is associated with relatively mild manifestations. People of Mediterranean origin also are commonly affected. A small proportion of persons who have glucose-6-phosphatase deficiency have chronic hemolytic anemia and splenomegaly. A number of drugs may precipitate an acute hemolytic anemia with Heinz bodies. Sulfonamides are one of these drugs so that one might expect sulfasalazine to be implicated. The drug may cause a hemolytic anemia, but so far has not been reported to do so in rheumatoid arthritis as a result of the patient having glucose-6-phosphate dehydrogenase deficiency[414]. Salicylates, acetaminophen, or phenylbutazone have also been implicated to cause clinically significant hemolytic anemia in glucose-6-phosphate dehydrogenase deficiency[436], but most people with enzymopathy have been shown to be able to safely take these drugs[437,438]. However — because of the heterogeneity of G6PD — take care[439].

Poor sulfoxidation in patients with rheumatoid arthritis has been reported to be associated with a ninefold increase in gold toxicity[440].

A number of metabolite disorders have recently been described as causing Reye-like syndrome[441]. In view of the somewhat debatable evidence to incriminate aspirin as a cause of Reye's syndrome, it is intriguing to speculate that the syndrome is due to a genetic enzyme defect, and may be precipitated by aspirin or other drugs.

Interactions

It has been estimated that some 5-10% of adverse reactions to medicaments are due to drug interactions and that these constitute some 2-3% of admissions to hospital[442]. However, the majority of these interactions are fortunately of minor clinical importance[443]. The major relevant clinical interactions are shown in Table 1. The clinically important interactions with antirheumatic drugs are well documented[444-447]. However, the problem is not only in predicting whether in interaction will be of clinical importance[448] but what the likelihood is of a patient having a reaction. To date there is little information on the latter point and certainly few clinical and few laboratory findings to help the physician making a prediction of such an outcome.

Aspirin and NSAIDs

Approximately 40% of patients with rheumatoid arthritis are prescribed two NSAIDs[449-451]. Aspirin has been shown to reduce the plasma concentrations of a number of NSAIDs including diclofenac[452], diflunisal[453], fenbufen[454], fenoprofen[455], flurbiprofen[456], ibuprofen[457], isox-

Table 1 Interactions with NSAIDs

Drug affected	NSAIDs implicated	Effect	Approach to management
A. PHARMACOKINETIC			
Oral anticoagulants	Phenylbutazone Oxyphenbutazone Azapropazone	Inhibition of metabolism of S-warfarin, increasing anticoagulant effect	Avoid NSAIDs if possible. Careful monitoring where unavoidable
Lithium	Probably all NSAIDs	Inhibition of renal excretion of lithium, increasing risk of toxicity	Use sulindac, aspirin if NSAID unavoidable. Careful monitoring of lithium concentration and appropriate dose reduction
Oral hypoglycemic agents	Phenylbutazone Oxyphenbutazone Azapropazone	Inhibition of metabolism of sulfonylurea drugs, prolonging half-life and increasing risk of hypoglycemia	Avoid this group of NSAIDs if possible; if not, monitor blood sugar closely
Phenytoin	Phenylbutazone Oxyphenbutazone	Inhibition of metabolism of phenytoin, increasing plasma concentration and risk of toxicity	Avoid this group of NSAIDs if possible; if not intensify therapeutic drug monitoring
	Other NSAIDs	Displacement of phenytoin from plasma protein, reducing total concentration for the same unbound (active) concentration	Careful interpretation of phenytoin total concentration
Methotrexate (high dose)	Probably all NSAIDs	Reduced clearance of methotrexate (mechanism unclear) increasing plasma concentration and risk of severe toxicity	Simultaneous dosing is contrindicated. Use of NSAIDs between cycles of *chemotherapy* is probably safe

Table 1 Interactions with NSAIDS *continued*

Drug affected	NSAIDs implicated	Effect	Approach to management
Sodium valproate	Aspirin	Inhibition of valproate metabolism increasing plasma concentration	Avoid aspirin; dose monitoring of plasma concentration if other NSAID used
Digoxin	All NSAIDs	Potential reduction in renal function (particularly in very young and very old) reducing digoxin clearance and increasing plasma concentration and risk of toxicity. (No interation if renal function normal)	Avoid NSAIDs if possible; if not, frequent checks of digoxin plasma concentration and plasma creatine
Aminoglycosides	All NSAIDs	Reduction in renal function in susceptible individuals, reducing aminoglycoside clearance and increasing plasma concentration	Close plasma concentration monitoring and dose adjustment
Other drug affecting NSAIDs			
Antacids	Indomethacin	Variable effects of different preparations: ●Aluminum-containing antacids reduce rate and extent of absorption of indomethacin ●Sodium bicarbonate increase rate and extent of absorption of indomethacin	No action required unless marked reduction in absorption results in poor response to NSAID; dose may need to be increased in this case

Table 1 Interactions with NSAIDS *continued*

Drug affected	NSAIDs implicated	Effect	Approach to management
Probenecid	Probably all NSAIDs	Reduction in metabolism and renal clearance of NSAIDs and acylglucuronide metabolites which are hydrolyzed back to parent drug	May be used therapeutically to increase the response to given dose of NSAID
Barbiturates	Phenylbutazone ? Other NSAIDs	Increased metabolic clearance of NSAID	May require higher doses of phenylbutazone
Caffeine	Aspirin	Increased rate of absorption of aspirin	No action
Cholestrramine	Naproxen and probably other NSAIDs	Anion exchange resin binds NSAIDs in gut reducing rate (?and extent) of absorption	Separate dosing times by 4 h; may need higher than expected dose of NSAID
Metaclopramide	Aspirin	Increased rate and extent of absorption of aspirin in patients with migraine	May be used therapeutically

B. PHARMACODYNAMIC

Antihypertensive agents — blockers, diuretics, ACE inhibitors, vasodilators	Indomethacin Other NSAIDs	Reduction in hypertensive effect, probably related to inhibition of renal prostaglandin synthesis (producing salt and water retention) and vascular prostagladin synthesis (producing increased vasoconstriction)	Avoid all NSAIDs in treated hypertensive patients is possible; if not, use sulindac preferentially. May need additional antihypertensive therapy

Table 1 Interactions with NSAIDS *continued*

Drug affected	NSAIDs implicated	Effect	Approach to management
Diuretics	Indomethacin Other NSAIDs	Reduction in natriuretic and diuretic effects; may exacerbate congestive cardiac failure	Avoid NSAIDs in patients with cardiac failure; use sulindac; monitor clinical signs of fluid retention
Anticoagulants	All NSAIDs	Gastrointestinal tract mucosal damage, together with inhibition of platelet aggregation, increasing risk of GI bleeding in patients on anticoagulants	Avoid all NSAIDs if possible
Hypoglycemic agents	Salicylate (high-dose)	Potentiation of hypoglycemic effects (mechanism unknown)	Monitor blood sugar level
Combination with increased risk of toxicity			
Diuretics,	All NSAIDs	Combination associated with increased risk of hemodynamic renal failure	Avoid combination if possible
Triamterene	Indomethacin	Potentiation of nephrotoxicity, including in subjects with normal renal function	Combination contraindicated
Potassium-sparing	All NSAIDs	Potassium retention and hyperkalemia	Avoid combination; monitor K

Adapted from Tonkin and Wing (1988)[444] with permission

icam[458], ketoprofen[459], naproxen[460], piroxicam[461] and tolmetin[462]. The effects of aspirin on plasma concentrations of indomethacin have been reported as showing either no effect[463] or reduction[455,464,465] in plasma concentrations: these differences might reflect differences in the sensitivities of the methods employed to determine the serum indomethacin levels. Although Hobbs and Twomey[466] initially reported no effect on the serum concentrations of piroxicam by aspirin, a lowering was noted by Bollet[467].

There is conflicting evidence in animal models that two NSAIDs are more effective than one[468,469] and there are few data to support such a view in humans[240,454,472]. Willkens and Segre[472] reported that aspirin and naproxen were better than either drug alone, but Furst et al.[473] were unable to confirm this with choline magnesium trisalicylate and naproxen. Although there is no evidence of an additive or synergistic effect of aspirin and NSAIDs, there is some evidence that side-effects are more common when two or more NSAIDs are taken concurrently[463,470].

Antacids and NSAIDs

Renal excretion is an important route of elimination of salicylates, especially when prescribed in doses of 3 g or more per day. Less than 10% of other NSAIDs are excreted unchanged in the urine, with the single exception of azapropazone, which is largely (approximately 75%) excreted unchanged. The renal excretion of salicylic acid is extremely sensitive to changes in pH: an increase due to ingestion of an alkali, e.g., magnesium hydroxide and aluminium hydroxide (Maalox®) will result in a marked increase in excretion[474]. This will cause a fall in salicylate plasma levels and a change in the patient's clinical status. If it is necessary to continue with antacid therapy, the dose of salicylate can be adjusted accordingly[474].

The effect of antacids administered at the same time as NSAIDs varies with the particular antacid and NSAID. Thus, the absorption of naproxen is not altered significantly by magnesium–aluminum hydroxide mixture[475] but is reduced by aluminum hydroxide alone[476]. Aspirin is widely formulated in a combination of antacids[477] but the only truly "buffered" aspirin is Alka-Seltzer®. Single doses of antacids do not significantly change the urinary pH. Antacids might alter the rate of absorption of NSAIDs, which is not of practical importance in the long-term management of chronic arthritis. Once again, considerable variation in the effect of different antacids is seen on different NSAIDs: thus, both the rate and extent of absorption of oxyphenbutazone are increased by combination with aluminum hydroxide and magnesium trisilicate[477].

The important clinical point is that variations in urinary pH as a result of ingestion of antacids should be considered when monitoring patients treated with high doses of salicylates, especially if no clinical response is being achieved despite ingestion of high doses of salicylates[477].

NSAIDs and anticoagulants

Aspirin depresses vitamin K-dependent synthesis of coagulation factors VII, IX, and X[264] but will only do this if the plasma salicylate concentration exceeds 2.2 mmol/l[479]. Aspirin, unlike nonacetylated salicylates, also causes prolongation of the bleeding time secondarily to impairment of platelet function. Aspirin might, therefore, cause increased bleeding if administered concurrently with oral anticoagulants[480,481]. However, of 363 patients on oral anticoagulants, of whom 59 were taking aspirin, only four demonstrated loss of control[482].

Phenylbutazone and oxyphenbutazone enhance the anticoagulant effect of warfarin in inhibiting the biotransformation of the S enantiomer, which is some five times more potent than the R enantiomer[483-486]. Originally the interaction was considered to be entirely due to protein-binding displacement[487] but this is only part of the explanation[488]. Stereoselective interactions with warfarin have been described with a number of other drugs with resulting augmentation of hypoprothrombinemic effect, e.g., sulfinpyrazone[489] and Distalgesic[490]. Azapropazone also enhances the anticoagulant effect of warfarin but the mechanism is not known[491]. None of the other NSAIDs appears to alter the effect of warfarin on prothrombin activity, at least to a degree to be of any clinical significance[492].

Patients who have a bleeding tendency, e.g., hemophilia, or who are receiving heparin or other anticoagulant therapy, should not be treated with aspirin or other NSAIDs but should be prescribed acetaminophen instead. Should an NSAID be necessary, then ibuprofen would appear to be the most suitable[492].

Although not definitively proven, there is a widely held belief that there is a synergism between ethanol and aspirin in causing gastrointestinal hemorrhage[493-495]. There is no evidence of such a synergism between nonacetylated salicylates and other NSAIDs and ethanol. The mechanism of the synergistic effect between aspirin and ethanol is not known, although both drugs are known to increase bleeding time[496] and inhibit platelet enzymes[497].

Antihypertensives, beta-adrenoreceptor blockers and diuretics and NSAIDs

Indomethacin inhibits the hypotensive actions of captopril[498], hydralazine[499], and prazosin[500].

Indomethacin has also been shown to attenuate angiotensin-converting enzyme inhibitors such as captopril, and beta-adrenergic blockers such as propranolol[501-503], probably by inhibition of vasodilatory prostaglandins[502] rather than by interfering with beta blockade[504,505]. Aspirin and other NSAIDs might have the same effect and, like indomethacin, cause acute renal failure[506].

Indomethacin, but not naproxen or sulindac, abrogate the antihypertensive action of hydrochlorothiazide[507] but there is controversy whether indomethacin inhibits the natriuretic effect of thiazide diuretics[508-510]. However, the diuretic, naturetic, and antihypertensive actions of furosemide are unequivocally decreased by indomethacin, aspirin, and ibuprofen[511-515], almost certainly owing to prostaglandin inhibition[516,517]. Favre et al.[518] showed that pretreatment with indomethacin and diflunisal reduced the naturetic effect of both furosemide and spironolactone but not hydrochlorothiazide and triamterene. The effects of spironolactone are competitively inhibited by salicylates[519]. Furosemide lowers indomethacin plasma concentrations but not to a degree which affects analgesic or anti-inflammatory effects[520]. Sulindac appears to be unique among the NSAIDs in not causing interference with diuretic or hypertensive control[521].

It must be appreciated that many of the studies on interactions of NSAIDs on antihypertensive and diuretic drugs are of an observational nature[522]. It is not clear whether indomethacin is more likely than others, with the exception of sulindac, to cause these interactions. The reversible renal impairment in normal subjects when prescribed a combination of indomethacin and triamterene might well be idiosyncratic[523]. There is no means of predicting a significant interaction between an NSAID and a diuretic, beta-adrenoreceptor blocker, or angiotensin-converting enzyme inhibitor. Wong et al.[521], however, calculated that about 1% of their patients attending a hospital hypertension clinic had interference with their blood pressure control in any one year. The actual rise in blood pressure was small, on average 4 mmHg, and certainly much smaller than that reported in observational studies[501,502,524].

Methotrexate and NSAIDs

Salicylates inhibit the renal clearance of methotrexate, which might cause an increase in the blood concentrations of methotrexate. This has resulted in death due to pancytopenia[525]. In addition salicylates displace methotrexate from its binding sites on serum albumin, but this does not appear to be of any clinical significance[526,527]. A clinically important interaction only occurs between salicylates and methotrexate when both are given in large doses: with the small pulse doses of methotrexate used to treat patients with rheumatoid or other inflammatory arthritis there is no interaction[528]. Phenylbutazone, indomethacin, naproxen, and diclofenac have also been described as interacting with methotrexate[529,530].

NSAIDs and lithium

Lithium accumulation might result from coadministration with diclofenac[531,532] and piroxicam[532]. Little information is available regarding other NSAIDs, which might well cause an interaction.

Corticosteroids and NSAIDs

Oral corticosteroid therapy results in an increased clearance of salicylate[474]. Whether this is the mechanism for the rise in plasma concentration of salicylate when corticosteroids are withdrawn[533,534] is unclear. A transient fall in serum salicylate has been recorded following intra-articular corticosteroids[535]. Prospective crossover studies[536] have failed to demonstrate any interaction between salicylates and corticosteroids.

Antidiabetic drugs and NSAIDs

The effects of salicylates on glucose metabolism are complex[537] and have been shown to include, in addition to a lowering of blood sugar, improved glucose tolerance and increased insulin secretion. It is, therefore, not surprising that salicylates have been shown to potentiate the effects of sulfonylurea antidiabetic drugs[538]. Salicylates might also displace the sulfonylureas from protein-binding sites and increase their clearance but the exact mechanism remains to be elucidated. Phenylbutazone and oxyphenbutazone inhibit the biotransformation of acetohexamide[539] and tolbutamide[540] so causing hypoglycemia. These drugs should, therefore, not be prescribed with sulfonylureas. Interactions have not been reported with other NSAIDs.

Digoxin and NSAIDs

Aspirin and ibuprofen have been found to increase serum digoxin levels but without digoxin toxicity. Aspirin has been reported to potentiate the cardiac toxicity of ouabain[541].

Phenytoin and NSAIDs

Phenylbutazone inhibits the biotransformation of phenytoin[542]. Salicylates displace phenytoin from its protein-binding sites but do not necessitate a change in dose[543-545]. However, free phenytoin appears to cause depletion of serum folate, which is essential for metabolic clearance of phenytoin[546]. Folate supplementation immediately corrects this.

Cimetidine and NSAIDs

Cimetidine has been called the "universal" inhibitor. It has earned this reputation as a result of its inhibition of the cytochrome P450-dependent mixed oxidases. A lowering of plasma indomethacin levels has been reported with the use of cimetidine[547] but does not appear to have clinical consequence. Cimetidine does not interact with naproxen[548]. The effects on other NSAIDs are not known.

Probenecid and NSAIDs

Probenecid inhibits the renal secretion of salicylate but this interaction is of little clinical significance unless the urine is alkaline[549]. Probenecid inhibits the glucuronidation of carprofen[550], diflunisal[551], indomethacin[552,553], ketoprofen[554], and naproxen[555], all of which form acyl-glucuronides that can be hydrolyzed back to the parent drug. The clinical significance has only been studied with indomethacin. The plasma concentrations are increased by probenecid with enhancement of analgesic and anti-inflammatory effect[552,553].

Glucocorticoids

The biotransformation of orally administered glucocorticoids has been shown to be enhanced by inducing agents such as phenobarbitone, phenytoin, and rifampicin[556-558]. These interactions have been shown to have clinical consequences[559] but can be easily overcome by adjusting the dose of corticosteroid.

In contrast, corticosteroids have only a minor, if indeed any, effect on the biotransformation of other drugs. Oral corticosteroids diminish the side-effects of cyclophosphamide[559]. Initially, when administered, they appear to inhibit the biotransformation but only by a factor of 25%[560].

SAARDs

Although D-penicillamine is a hydrolyzate of penicillin, previous penicillin allergy is not a contraindication to its use. A previous history of prior gold therapy does not appear to influence either efficacy or toxicity to D-penicillamine[561,562]. Combination therapy in rheumatoid arthritis with sulfasalazine and D-penicillamine or gold has not been associated with an increase in toxicity[563]. Food antacids[564,565] and oral iron[566] inhibit the absorption of D-penicillamine. Patients have been observed to develop D-penicillamine-induced proteinuria on cessation of iron therapy[565]. Trimethoprim–sulfamethoxazole has recently been reported to be associated with bone-marrow hypoplasia in patients receiving methotrexate[567,568]. Theoretically, interactions could arise from protein displacement, competition for renal tubular excretion or by an action on dihydrofolate reductase, since both drugs inhibit this enzyme. We have also observed severe leukopenia developing in a patient prescribed trimethroprim–sulfamethoxazole who was receiving levamisole[569].

Urate-lowering drugs

The efficacy and toxicity of azathioprine and t-mercaptopurine are both potentiated by allopurinol[570,571] and the dose of both purine analogs should be reduced to a quarter of the normal dose[572]. Allopurinol prolongs the plasma half-life of cyclophosphamide but leaves unchanged the alkylating activity of the plasma[573] and there is a suspicion that the combination of the two drugs might be associated with an increased incidence of bone-marrow depression[574] although this has been disputed[575].

Allopurinol does not affect the biotransformation of warfarin[576] but does so with dicoumarol in some individuals[540]. High doses of allopurinol, 600 mg daily, cause an increase in the plasma half-life of theophylline[577] but a lower dose, 300 mg/day, has no such effect[578]. The effects of allopurinol on the half-life of phenylbutazone are clinically insignificant[579]. Rashes commonly result from concurrent administration of allopurinol and ampicillin, the estimate being of a threefold increase[580].

Probenecid inhibits the renal excretion of salicylates and certain NSAIDs, allopurinol, and antibiotics such as penicillin and cephalosporins[447]. Probenecid also increases the plasma concentration of methotrexate by inhibiting the renal excretion of the latter[581]. Probenecid increases the natriuresis of chlorthiazide[582] but not furosemide[583].

The interaction between probenecid and allopurinol is complex. In approximately 50% of people the half-life of probenecid will be increased by up to two-thirds by allopurinol, the remaining 50% being unaffected[571,584]. Unfortunately it is not possible to identify how a patient will respond. Both drugs can be used concurrently provided care is taken. Probenecid and sulfinpyrazone are not additive in their uricosuric effect because probenecid inhibits the renal secretion of sulfinpyrazone[585].

Salicylates decrease the uricosuric effect of probenecid[586] and sulfinpyrazone[587] at plasma concentrations of salicylate greater than 50 μg/ml[586] but neither acetaminophen nor ibuprofen has this effect[588]. Sulfinpyrazone inhibits the biotransformation of warfarin[589,590] and tolbutamide[588]. However, the biotransformation of theophylline might be enhanced[591].

Patients with connective-tissue disorders commonly take a multiplicity of agents in an attempt to control disease. It is important to anticipate adverse reactions and interactions and to appreciate the therapeutic end-points one is attempting to achieve. By doing this on an individual basis, therapy in the rheumatic diseases can be optimized.

References

1. Rainford, K. D. (1987). Introduction and historical aspects of the side effects of anti-inflammatory analgesic drugs. In Brown, P. J. and Velo, A. P. (eds.) *Side-effects of Anti-Inflammatory Drugs*, Part I, Clinical and Epidemiological Aspects, pp. 3-26 (Lancaster: MTP).
2. Baum, C., Kennedy, D. L. and Forbes, M. B. (1985). Utilization of nonsteroidal anti-inflammatory drugs. *Arthritis Rheum.*, **28**, 686-692
3. Roth, S. H. (1988). NSAID and gastropathy: a rheumatologist's review. *J. Rheumatol.*, **15**, 912-919
4. Steinberg, A. D. (1983). On the therapy of rheumatoid arthritis. *Clin. Exp. Rheumatol.*, **1**, 85-86
5. Bitter, T. (1984). Combined disease-modifying chemotherapy for intractable rheumatoid arthritis. *Clin. Rheum. Dis.*, **10**, 417-428

6. Byron, M. A. and Mowat, A. G. (1985). Corticosteroid prescribing in rheumatoid arthritis — the fiction and the fact. *Br. J. Rheumatol.*, **25**, 164-166
7. Binder, A. I., Paice, E. W. and White, A. G. (1985). Corticosteroid treatment in rheumatoid arthritis. Letter to the Editor. *Br. J. Rheumatol.*, **24**, 380-381
8. Friesen, W. T., Hekster, Y. A., van de Putte, L. B. A. and Gribnau, F. W. J. (1985). Cross-sectional study of rheumatoid arthritis treatment in a university hospital. *Ann. Rheum. Dis.*, **44**, 372-378
9. van Saase, J., Vandenbroucke, J., Valkenburg, H., Boersma, J., Cats, A., Festen, J., Hartman, A., Huber-Bruning, O., Rasker, J. and Weber, J. (1987). Changing pattern of drug use in relation to disease duration of rheumatoid arthritis. *J. Rheumatol.*, **14**, 476-478
10. Brown, M. R. (1985). Corticosteroid treatment in rheumatoid arthritis. Letter to the Editor. *Br. J. Rheumatol.*, **24**, 378-382
11. Myles, A. (1985). Corticosteroid treatment in rheumatoid arthritis. Editorial. *Br. J. Rheumatol.*, **24**, 125-127
12. Harris, E. D. Jr., Emkey, R. D., Nichols, J. E. and Newberg, A. (1983). Low dose prednisone therapy in rheumatoid arthritis: a double blind study. *J. Rheumatol.*, **10**, 713-721
13. Lockie, L. M., Gomez, E. and Smith, D. M. (1983). Low dose adrenocorticosteroids in the management of elderly patients with rheumatoid arthritis: selected examples and summary of efficacy in the long-term treatment of 97 patients. *Semin. Arthritis Rheum.*, **12**, 373-381
14. Radia, M. and Furst, D. E. (1988). Comparison of three pulse methylprednisolone regimens in the treatment of rheumatoid arthritis. *J. Rheumatol.*, **15**, 242-246
15. Shipley, M. E., Bacon, P. A., Berry, H., Hazleman, B. L., Sturrock, R. D., Swinson, D. R. and Williams, I. A. (1988). Pulsed methylprednisolone in active early rheumatoid disease: a dose-ranging study. *Br. J. Rheumatol.*, **27**, 211-214
16. Needs, C. J., Smith, M., Boutagy, J., Donovan, S., Cosh, D., McCredie, M. and Brooks, P. M. (1988). Comparison of methylprednisolone (1g IV) with prednisolone (1g orally) in rheumatoid arthritis: a pharmacokinetic and clinical study. *J. Rheumatol.*, **15**, 224-228
17. Smith, M. D., Bertouch, J. V., Smith, A. M., Weatherall, M., Ahern, M. J., Brooks, P. M. and Roberts-Thomson, P. J. (1988). The clinical and immunological effects of pulse methylprednisolone therapy in rheumatoid arthritis: clinical effects. *J. Rheumatol.*, **15**, 229-232
18. Smith, M. D., Ahern, M. J., Brooks, P. M. and Roberts-Thomson, P. J. (1988). The clinical and immunological effects of pulse methylprednisolone therapy on rheumatoid arthritis. II. Effects on immune and inflammatory indices in peripheral blood. *J. Rheumatol.*, **15**, 233-237
19. Smith, M. D., Ahern, M. J., Brooks, P. M. and Roberts-Thomson, P. J. (1988). The clinical and immunological effects of pulse methylprednisolone therapy in rheumatoid arthritis. III. Effects on immune and inflammatory indices in synovial fluid. *J. Rheumatol.*, **15**, 238-241
20. Rynes, R. I., Krohel, G., Falbo, A., Reinecke, R. D., Wolfe, B. and Bartholomew, L. E. (1979). Ophthalmic safety of long-term hydroxychloroquine treatment. *Arthritis Rheum.*, **22**, 832-836
21. Mackenzie, A. H. and Sherbal, A. L. (1980). Chloroquine and hydroxychloroquine in rheumatological therapy. *Clin. Rheum. Dis.*, **6**, 545-566
22. Bellamy, N. and Brooks, P. M. (1986). Current practice in antimalarial drug prescribing in rheumatoid arthritis. *J. Rheumatol.*, **13**, 551-555
23. Svartz, M. (1948). The treatment of rheumatic polyarthritis with acid azo compounds. *Rheumatism*, **4**, 56-60
24. Sinclair, R. J. G. and Duthie, J. J. R. (1948). Salazopyrin in the treatment of rheumatoid arthritis. *Ann. Rheum. Dis.*, **8**, 226-231
25. Neumann, V. C., Grindulis, K. A., Hubbal, S., *et al.* (1983). Comparison between penicillamine and sulphasalazine in rheumatoid arthritis. Leeds-Birmingham trial. *Br. Med. J.*, **287**, 1099-1102
26. Pullar, T., Hunter, J. A. and Capell, H. A. (1983). Sulphasalazine in rheumatoid

arthritis: a double blind comparison of sulphasalazine with placebo and sodium aurothiomalate. *Br. Med. J.*, **287**, 1102–1104
27. Pinals, R. S., Kaplan, S. B., Lawson, J. G. et al. (1986). Sulfasalazine in rheumatoid arthritis. A double-blind, placebo-controlled trial. *Arthritis Rheum.*, **29**, 1427–1434
28. Pinals, R. S. (1988). Sulfasalazine in the rheumatic diseases. *Semin. Arthritis Rheum.*, **17**, 246–259
29. Black, R. L., O'Brien, W. M., Van Scott, E. J., Auerbach, R., Eisen, A. Z. and Bunim, J. J. (1964). Methotrexate therapy in psoriatic arthritis. *J. Am. Med. Assoc.*, **189**, 743–747
30. Tugwell, P., Bennett, K. and Gent, M. (1987). Methotrexate in rheumatoid arthritis: indications, contraindications, efficacy, safety. *Ann. Intern. Med.*, **107**, 358–366
31. Furst, D. E. and Kremer, J. M. (1988). Methotrexate in rheumatoid arthritis. *Arthritis Rheum.*, **31**, 305–314
32. De Ceulaer, K. et al. (1978). Dermatomyositis: observations on the use of immunosuppressive therapy and review of the literature. *Postgrad. Med. J.*, **54**, 516–527
33. Mason, M., Currey, H. L. F., Barnes, C. G. et al. (1969). Azathioprine in rheumatoid arthritis. *Br. Med. J.*, **1**, 420–422
34. Co-operating Clinics Committee of the American Rheumatism Association. (1970). A controlled trial of cyclophosphamide in rheumatoid arthritis. *N. Engl. J. Med.*, **282**, 883–889
35. De Silva, M. and Hazelman, B. L. (1981). Long-term azathioprine in rheumatoid arthritis: a double-blind study. *Ann. Rheum. Dis.*, **40**, 560–563
36. Huskisson, E. C. (1984). Azathioprine. *Clin. Rheum. Dis.*, **10**, 325–332
37. Cameron, J. S. (1979). Lupus nephritis. *Eur. J. Rheumatol. Inflamm.*, **3**, 100–111
38. Dinant, H., Decker, J. L., Klippel, J. H. et al. (1982). Alternative modes of cyclophosphamide and azathioprine therapy in lupus nephritis. *Ann. Intern. Med.*, **96**, 728–736
39. Carette, S., Klippel, J. H., Decker, J. L. et al. (1983). Controlled studies of oral immunosuppressive drugs in lupus nephritis. A long-term follow-up. *Ann. Intern. Med.*, **99** 1–8
40. Klippel, J. H., Austin, H. A., III, Balow, J. E., LeRiche, N. G. H., Steinberg, A. D., Plotz, P. H. and Decker, J. L. (1987). Studies of immunosuppressive drugs in the treatment of lupus nephritis. *Rheum. Dis. Clin. N. Am.*, **13**, 47–56
41. Kovarsky, J. (1983). Clinical pharmacology and toxicology of cyclophosphamide: emphasis on use in rheumatic diseases. *Semin. Arthritis Rheum.*, **12**, 359–372
42. Fauci, A. S. and Wolff, S. M. (1973). Wegener's granulomatosis: studies in eighteen patients and a review of the literature. *Medicine (Baltimore)*, **52**, 535–561
43. Reza, M. J., Dornfeld, L., Goldberg, L. S. et al. (1975). Wegener's granulomatosis: long-term follow-up of patients treated with cyclophosphamide. *Arthritis Rheum.*, **18**, 501–506
44. Fauci, A. S., Haynes, B. F. and Katz, P. (1978). The spectrum of vasculitis: clinical, pathologic, immunologic and therapeutic considerations. *Ann. Intern. Med.*, **89**, 660–676
45. Abel, T., Andrews, B. S., Cunningham, P. H. et al. (1980). Rheumatoid vasculitis: effect of cyclophosphamide on the clinical course and levels of circulating immune complexes. *Ann. Intern. Med.*, **93**, 407–413
46. Clements, P. J. and Davis, J. (1986). Cytotoxic drugs: their clinical application to the rheumatic diseases. *Semin. Arthritis Rheum.*, **15**, 231–254
47. Steinberg, A. D. (1986). The treatment of lupus nephritis. *Kidney Int.*, **30**, 769–787
48. Kirwan, J. and Currey, H. L. F. (1984). Rheumatoid arthritis: Disease modifying antirheumatic drugs. *Clin. Rheum. Dis.*, **9**, 581–588
49. van Rijthoven, A. W., Dijkmans, B. A., Goei, H. S. et al. (1986). Cyclosporin treatment for rheumatoid arthritis: a placebo-controlled double-blind multicentre study. *Ann. Rheum. Dis.*, **45**, 726–731
50. Weinblatt, M. E., Coblyn, J. S., Fraser, P. A., Anderson, R. J., Spraag, J., Trentham, D. E. and Austen, K. F. (1987). Cyclosporin: A treatment of refractory rheumatoid arthritis. *Arthritis Rheum.*, **30**, 11–17
51. Yocum, D. E., Klippel, J. H., Wilder, R. L., Gerber, N. L., Austin, H. A., III, Wahl,

S. M., Lesko L., Minor, J. R., Preuss, H. G., Yarboro, C., Berkebile, C. and Dougherty, S. (1988). Cyclosporin A in severe, treatment-refractory rheumatoid arthritis: a randomized study. *Ann. Intern. Med.*, **109**, 863-869
52. Martin, M. F. R., Surrall, K., McKenna, F., Dixon, J. S., Bird, V. A. and Wright, V. (1984). Captopril: A new treatment for rheumatoid arthritis. *Lancet*, **1**, 1325-1327
53. Fowler, P. D., Shadforth, M. F., Crook, P. R. and Lawton, A. (1984). Report on chloroquine and dapsone in the treatment of rheumatoid arthritis: a 6-month comparative study. *Ann. Rheum. Dis.*, **43**, 200-204
54. Grindulis, K. A. and McConkey, B. (1984). Outcome of attempts to treat rheumatoid arthritis with gold, penicillamine, sulphasalazine or dapsone. *Ann. Rheum. Dis.*, **43**, 398-401
55. Grindulis, K. A., Nichol, F. E. and Oldham, R. (1986). Phenytoin in rheumatoid arthritis. *J. Rheumatol.*, **13**, 1035-1039
56. MacFarlane, D. G., Clark, B. and Panayi, G. S. (1986). Pilot study of phenytoin in rheumatoid arthritis. *Ann. Rheum. Dis.*, **45**, 954-956
57. Symoens, J. and Schuemans, Y. (1979). Levamisole. *Clin. Rheum. Dis.*, **5**, 603-629
58. Capell, H. A., Hunter, J. A., Rennie, J. A. N. et al. (1981). Levamisole — a possible alternative to gold and penicillamine in the long term treatment of rheumatoid arthritis? *J. Rheumatol.*, **8**, 730-740
59. Runge, L. A. and Rynes, R. I. (1983). Balancing effectiveness and toxicity of levamisole in the treatment of rheumatoid arthritis. *Clin. Exp. Rheumatol.*, **1**, 125-131
60. Gutierrez-Rodriguez, O. (1984). Thalidomide: a promising new treatment for rheumatoid arthritis. *Arthritis Rheum.*, **27**, 1118-1121
61. Hadidi, T., Decker, J. L., El-Nagdy, L. and Samy, M. (1981). Ineffectiveness of levamisole in systemic lupus erythematosus. A controlled trial. *Arthritis Rheum.*, **24**, 60-63
62. Hopkins, R., Bird, H. A., Jones, H., Hill, J., Surrall, K. E., Astbury, C., Miller, A. and Wright, V. (1985). A double-blind controlled trial of etretinate (Tigason) and ibuprofen in psoriatic arthritis. *Ann. Rheum. Dis.*, **44**, 189-193
63. Ward, J. H., Williams, H. J., Egger, M. J. et al. (1983). Comparison of auranofin, gold sodium thiomalate and placebo in the treatment of rheumatoid arthritis. *Arthritis Rheum.*, **26**, 1303-1315
64. Chaffman, M., Brogden, R. N., Heel, R. C., Speight, T. M. and Avery, G. S. (1984). Auranofin; A preliminary review of its pharmacological properties and therapeutic use in rheumatoid arthritis. *Drugs*, **27**, 378-424
65. Davis, P. (1984). Auranofin. *Clin. Rheum. Dis.*, **10**, 369-383
66. Davis, P., Menard, H., Thompson, J. et al. (1985). One-year comparative study of gold sodium thiomalate and auranofin in the treatment of rheumatoid arthritis. *J. Rheumatol.*, **12**, 60-67
67. Williams, H. J., Dahl, S. L., Ward, J. R. et al. (1988). One year experience in patients treated with auranofin following completion of a parallel controlled trial comparing auranofin, gold sodium thiomalate and placebo. *Arthritis Rheum.*, **31**, 9-14
68. Kremer, J. M., Jubiz, W., Michalek, A. et al. (1987). Fish oil fatty acid supplementation in active rheumatoid arthritis: a double-blinded, controlled, crossover study. *Ann. Intern. Med.*, **106**, 497-503
69. Belch, J. I. F., Ansell, D., Madhouk, R., O'Dowd, A. and Sturrock, R. D. (1988). Effects of altering dietary essential fatty acids in requirements for non-steroidal anti-inflammatory drugs in patients with rheumatoid arthritis: a double blind placebo controlled study. *Ann. Rheum. Dis.*, **47**, 96-104
70. Magaro, M., Altomonte, L., Zoli, A., Mirone, L., De Sole, P., Di Mario, G., Lippa, S. and Oradei, A. (1988). Influence of diet with different lipid composition on neutrophil chemiluminescence and disease activity in patients with rheumatoid arthritis. *Ann. Rheum. Dis.*, **47**, 793-796
71. Ben-Yehuda, O., Tomer, Y. and Schoenfeld Y. (1988). Advances in therapy of autoimmune diseases. *Semin. Arthritis Rheum.*, **17**, 206-220
72. Veys, E. M., Mielants, H., Verbruggen, G., Crosclaude, J. P., Meyer, W., Gacazka, A. and Schindler, J. (1988). Interferon gamma in rheumatoid arthritis — a double

blind study comparing human recombinant interferon gamma with placebo. *J. Rheumatol.*, **15**, 570-574
73. Vrys, E. M. *et al.* (1982). Clinical response to therapy with Thymopoietin Pentapeptide (TP-5) in rheumatoid arthritis. *Ann. Rheum. Dis.*, **41**, 441-443
74. Thrower, P. A., Doyle, D. V., Scott, J. and Huskisson, E. C. (1982). Thymopoietin in rheumatoid arthritis. *Rheumatol. Rehabil.*, **21**, 72-77
75. Klippel, J. H. (1984). Apheresis biotechnology and the rheumatic diseases. *Arthritis Rheum.*, **27**, 1081-1085
76. Vaughan, J. H., Fox, R. I., Abresch, R. J. *et al.* (1984). Thoracic duct drainage in rheumatoid arthritis. *Clin. Exp. Immunol.*, **58**, 645-653
77. Zvaifler, N. J. (1987). Fractionated total lymphoid irradiation: a promising new treatment for rheumatoid arthritis? Yes, No, Maybe. Editorial. *Arthritis Rheum.*, **30**, 109-114
78. Yunus, M. B. (1988). Investigational therapy in rheumatoid arthritis. *Semin. Arthritis Rheum.*, **17**, 163-164
79. Wei, N., Klippel, J. H., Huston, D. P., Hall, R. P., Lawley, T. J., Balow, J. E., Steinberg, A. D. and Decker, J. L. (1983). Randomised trial of plasma exchange in mild systemic lupus erythematosus. *Lancet*, **1**, 17-22
80. Scheinberg, M. A. (1988). Clinical trials with biological response modifers in rheumatic diseases. *J. Rheumatol.*, **15**, 1056-1057
81. Dibner, M. D. and Ackerman, N. R. (1986). Biotechnology and new therapies for arthritis. *J. Rheumatol.*, **13**, 997-998
82. Kelley, W. M. and Fox, I. H. (1985). Gout and related disorders of purine metabolism. In Kelley, W. M., Harris, E. D., Ruddy, S. and Sledge, C. B. (eds.) *Textbook of Rheumatology*, pp. 1359-1398. (Philadelphia; W. B. Saunders)
83. Murrell, G. A. C. and Rapeport, W. G. (1986). Clinical pharmacokinetics of allopurinol. *Clin. Pharmacokin.*, **11**, 343-353
84. Hernandez, L. A., Dick, W. C., Mavrikakis, M. E. and Buchanan, W. W. (1978). The treatment of gout: a case for medical audit? *Scot. Med. J.*, **23**, 9-11
85. Famaey, J. P. (1988). Colchicine in therapy. State of the art and new perspectives for an old drug. *Clin. Exp. Rheumatol.*, **6**, 305-317
86. Ferrannini, E. and Pentimone, F. (1984). Marrow aplasia following colchicine treatment for gouty arthritis. *Clin. Exp. Rheumatol.*, **2**, 173-175
87. Stanley, M. W., Taurog, J. D. and Snover, D. C. (1984). Fatal colchicine toxicity: report of a case. *Clin. Exp. Rheumatol.*, **2**, 167-171
88. Pasero, G. (1984). Colchicine: should we still use it? *Clin. Exp. Rheumatol.*, **2**, 103-104
89. Huskisson, E. C. and Hart, F. D. (1982). Pain threshold and arthritis. *Br. Med. J.*, **4**, 193-195
90. Lee, P., Ahola, S. J., Grennan, D., Brooks, P. and Buchanan, W. W. (1974). Observations on drug prescribing in rheumatoid arthritis. *Br. Med. J.*, **1**, 424-426
91. Mason, D. I., Brooks, P. M., Lee, P., Kennedy, A. C. and Buchanan, W. W. (1975). Inpatient prescribing in a rheumatic diseases centre. A study of self-abasement. *Health Bull. (SHHD)*, **33**, 72-75
92. Rosenbloom, D. and Buchanan, W. W. (1983). Observations on written communications between physicians regarding patients' drug treatment compared to patients' recall. *Drug Intell. Clin. Pharmacol.*, **17**, 288-289
93. Gibson, T. and Clark, B. (1985). Use of simple analgesics in rheumatoid arthritis. *Ann. Rheum. Dis.*, **4U**, 27-29
94. Rennie, J. A. N., Mason, D. I. R. and Capell, H. A. (1977). Simple analgesics in rheumatoid arthritis. Editorial. *Scot. Med. J.*, **22**, 253-254
95. Pfeiffer, R. F. (1982). Drugs for pain in the elderly. *Geriatrics*, **37**, 67-76
96. Nuki, G. (1983). Non-steroidal analgesic and anti-inflammatory agents. *Br. Med. J.*, **287**, 39-43
97. Huskisson, E. C. (1974). Simple analgesics for arthritis. *Br. Med. J.*, **4**, 196-200
98. Kantor, T. G. (1980). Analgesics for arthritis. *Clin. Rheum. Dis.*, **6**, 525-531
99. Hart, F. D. (1987). Rational use of analgesics in the treatment of rheumatic disorders. *Drugs*, **33**, 85-93

100. Fremont-Smith, P. and Bayles, T. B. Salicylate therapy in rheumatoid arthritis. *J. Am. Med. Assoc.*, **192**, 103-106
101. Lee, P., Watson, M., Webb, J., Anderson, J. and Buchanan, W. W. (1975). Therapeutic effectiveness of paracetamol in rheumatoid arthritis. *Int. J. Clin. Pharmacol. Biopharm.*, **11**, 68-75
102. Lee, P., Anderson, J. A., Miller, J., Webb, J. and Buchanan, W. W. (1976). Evaluation of analgesic action and efficacy of antirheumatic drugs. Study of 10 drugs in 684 patients with rheumatoid arthritis. *J. Rheumatol.*, **3**, 283-295
103. Brooks, P. M., Walker, J. J., Lee, P., Bell, M. A., Buchanan, W. W., Fowler, P. D. and Anderson, J. A. (1975). Erprobung eines neuen acetylsalicysaure — Paracetamol — Praparates mit magensafttresistentem Uberzug (Safapryn) und zwei verschiedenen. Dosierungen von Phenylbutazon bei patienten mit primar chronischer polyarthritis auhaud eines neuen Bewertungsverfahrens. *Z. Rheumatol.*, **34**, 350-365
104. Nuki, G., Downie, W. W., Dick, W. C., Whaley, K., Spooner, J. B., Darby-Dowman, M. A. and Buchanan, W. W. (1973). Clinical trial of pentazocine in rheumatoid arthritis. Observations in the values of patent analgesics and placebos. *Ann. Rheum. Dis.*, **32**, 436-443
105. Brooks, P. M., Dougan, M. A., Mugford, A. and Meffin, E. (1982). Comparative effectiveness of five analgesics in patients with rheumatoid arthritis and osteoarthritis. *J. Rheumatol.*, **9**, 732-736
106. Hardin, J. G. and Kirk, K. A. (1979). Comparative effectiveness of five analgesics for the pain of rheumatoid arthritis. *J. Rheumatol.*, **6**, 405-442
107. Seideman, P. and Melander, A. (1988). Equianalgesic effects of paracetamol and indomethacin in rheumatoid arthritis. *Br. J. Rheumatol.*, **27**, 117-122
108. Emery, P. and Gibson, T. (1986). A double-blind study of the simple analgesic nefopam in rheumatoid arthritis. *Br. J. Rheumatol.*, **25**, 72-76
109. Nolan, L. and O'Malley, K. (1988). Prescribing for the elderly: Part II. Prescribing patterns: differences due to age. *J. Am. Geriatr. Soc.*, **36**, 245-254
110. Bellville, J. W., Forrest, W. H., Miller, E. and Brown, B. W. (1971). Influence of age on pain relief from analgesics. *J. Am. Med. Assoc.*, **217**, 1835-1841
111. Berkowitz, B. A., Ngai, S. H., Yang, J. C., Hempstead, J. and Spector, S. (1975). The disposition of morphine in surgical patients. *Clin. Pharmacol. Ther.*, **17**, 629-634
112. Mather, L. E., Tucker, G. T., Pflug, A. E., Lindop, M. J. and Wilderson, C. (1975). Meperidine kinetics in man. *Clin. Pharmacol. Ther.*, **17**, 21-31
113. Vestal, R. E. (1978). Drug use in the elderly: a review of the problems and special considerations. *Drugs*, **16**, 358-382
114. Preston, S. J., Arnold, M. H., Beller, E. M., Brooks, P. M. and Buchanan, W. W. (1989). Comparative analgesic and anti-inflammatory properties of sodium salicylate and acetyl salicylic acid (aspirin) in rheumatoid arthritis. *Br. J. Clin. Pharmacol.*, **27**, 607-611
115. Lee, P., Webb, J., Anderson, J. and Buchanan, W. W. (1973). Method of assessing therapeutic potential of anti-inflammatory anti-rheumatic drugs in rheumatoid arthritis. *Br. Med. J.*, **2**, 685-688
116. Maclagan, T. J. (1876). The treatment of acute rheumatism by salicin. *Lancet*, **1**, 342-343
117. Huskisson, E. C., Woolf, D. L., Balme, H. W., Scott, J. and Franklyn, S. (1976). Four new anti-inflammatory drugs: responses and variations. *Br. Med. J.*, **1**, 1048-1049
118. Scott, D. L., Roden, S., Marshall, T. and Kendall, M. J. (1982). Variations in response to non-steroidal anti-inflammatory drugs. *Br. J. Clin. Pharmacol.*, **14**, 691-694
119. Capell, H. A., Konetschnik, B. and Glass, R. C. (1977). Anti-inflammatory analgesic drug responders and non-responders: a clinico-pharmacological study of ibuprofen. *Br. J. Clin. Pharmacol.*, **15**, 311-316
120. Baber, N., Halliday, L. D. C., Van Den Heuvel, W. J. A., Walker, R. W., Sibeon, R., Keenan, J. P., Littler, T. and Orme, M.'le (1979). Indomethacin in rheumatoid arthritis: clinical effects pharmacokinetics and platelet studies in responders and non-responders. *Ann. Rheum. Dis.*, **38**, 128-140
121. Ekstrand, R., Alvan, G., Orme, M.'le, Lewander, R., Palmer, L. and Sarby, B. (1980).

Double-blind dose response study of indomethacin in rheumatoid arthritis. *Eur. J. Clin. Pharmacol.*, **17**, 437-442
122. Orme, M., Baber, N., Keenan, J., Halliday, L., Sibeon, R. and Littler, T. (1981). Pharmacokinetics and biochemical effects in responders and non-responders to non-steroidal anti-inflammatory drugs. *Scand. J. Rheumatol.*, **39** (suppl.), 19-27
123. Preston, S. J., Arnold, M. H., Beller, E. M., Brooks, P. M. and Buchanan, W. W. (1988). Variability in response to non-steroidal anti-inflammatory analgesics. Evidence from controlled clinical therapeutic trials of flurbiprofen in rheumatoid arthritis. *Br. J. Clin. Pharmacol.*, **26**, 759-764
124. Spector, R. and Park, G. D. (1985). Regression to the mean: a potential source of error in clinical pharmacological studies. *Drug Intell. Clin. Pharm.*, **19**, 916-919
125. Furst, D. E., Tozer, T. N. and Melmon, K. L. (1979). Salicylate clearance, the resultant of protein binding and metabolism. *Clin. Pharmacol. Ther.*, **26**, 380-389
126. Muller, F. U., Hundt, H. K. L. and de Kock, A. C. (1975). Decreased steady-state salicylic acid plasma levels associated with aspiring ingestion. *Curr. Med. Res. Opin.*, **3**, 417-422
127. Furst, D. E., Gupta, N. and Paulus, H. E. (1977). Salicylate metabolism in twins. *Clin. Invest.*, **60**, 32-38
128. Graham, G. G., Day, R. O., Champion, G. D., Lee, E. and Newton, K. (1984). Aspects of the clinical pharmacology of non-steroidal anti-inflammatory drugs. *Clin. Rheum. Dis.*, **10**, 229-249
129. Bruck, E., Fearnley, M. E., Meanock, I. and Patley, H. (1954). Phenylbutazone therapy. Relation between the toxic and therapeutic effects and the blood level. *Lancet*, **1**, 225-228
130. Orme, M., Holt, P. J. L., Hughes, G. R. V., Bulpitt, C. J., Draffan, G. H., Thorgiersson, S. S., Williams, F. and Davies, D. S. (1976). Plasma concentration of phenylbutazone and its therapeutic effect — studies in patients with rheumatoid arthritis. *Br. J. Clin. Pharmacol.*, **3**, 185-191
131. Brooks, P. M., Walker, J. J., Dick, W. C., Anderson, J. J. and Fowler, P. D. (1975). Phenlybutazone: A clinicopharmacological study in rheumatoid arthritis. *Br. J. Clin. Pharmacol.*, **2**, 437-442
132. Grennan, D. M., Aarons, L., Siddiqui, M. *et al.* (1983). Dose-response study with ibuprofen in rheumatoid arthritis: clinical and pharmacokinetic findings. *Br. J. Clin. Pharmacol.*, **15**, 311-316
133. Day, R. O., Furst, D. E., Dromgoole, S. H., Kamm, B., Roe, R. and Paulus, H. E. (1982). Relation of serum naproxen concentration to efficacy in rheumatoid arthritis. *Clin. Pharmacol. Ther.*, **31**, 733-740
134. Dunagan, F. M., McGill, P. E., Kelman, A. W. and Whiting, B. (1988). Naproxen dose and concentration : response relationship in rheumatoid arthritis. *Br. J. Rheumatol.*, **27**, 48-53
135. Dunagan, F. M., McGill, P. E., Kelman, A. W. and Whiting, B. (1986). Quantitation of dose and concentration effects relationships for fenclofenac in rheumatoid arthritis. *Br. J. Clin. Pharmacol.*, **21**, 409-416
136. Furst, D. E., Caldwell, J. R., Klugman, M. P., Enthoven, D., Rittweger, K., Scheer, R., Sarkissian, E. and Dromgoole, S. (1988). Serum concentration and dose-response relationships for carprofen in rheumatoid arthritis. *Clin. Pharmacol. Ther.*, **44**, 186-194
137. Boardman, P. L. and Hart, F. D. (1967). Clinical measurement of the anti-inflammatory effects of salicylates in rheumatoid arthritis. *Br. Med. J.*, **2**, 264-268
138. Capell, H. A., Rennie, J. A. N., Rooney, P. J. *et al.* (1979). Patient compliance: a novel method of testing non-steroidal anti-inflammatory analgesics in rheumatoid arthritis. *J. Rheumatol.*, **6**, 584-593
139. Pullar, T., Zoma, A. A., Madhok, R., Hunter, J. A. and Capell, H. A. (1985). Have the new NSAIDs contributed to the management of rheumatoid arthritis? *Scott. Med. J.*, **30**, 161-163
140. Reese, R. W. (1985). Long-term studies of isoxicam in the treatment of rheumatoid arthritis. *Am. J. Med.*, **79** (suppl. 4B), 12-16
141. Fries, J. F., Spitz, P. W., Mitchell, D. M., Roth, S. H., Wolfe, F. and Bloch, D. A.

(1986). Impact of specific therapy upon rheumatoid arthritis. *Arthritis Rheum.*, **29**, 620-627
142. Nagaya, T., Niwa, S., Harada, S. and Konishi, Y. (1988). Efficacy and tolerance of tiaprofenic acid during long-term administration to rheumatoid arthritis patients. *Drugs*, **35** (suppl. 1), 101-106
143. Deyo, R. A., Inui, T. S. and Sullivan, B. (1981). Non-compliance with arthritis drugs: magnitude, correlates and clinical implications *J. Rheumatol.*, **8**, 931-936
144. Beck, N. C., Parker, J. C., Frank, R. G., Geden, E. A., Kay, D. R., Gamache, M., Shivvers, M., Smith, E. and Anderson, S. (1988). Patients with rheumatoid arthritis at high risk for non-compliance with salicylate treatment regimens. *J. Rheumatol.*, **15**, 1081-1084
145. Pullar, T., Birtwell, A. J., Wiles, P. G., Hay, A. and Feely, M. P. (1988). Use of a pharmacologic indicator to compare compliance with tablets prescribed to be taken once, twice and three times daily. *Clin. Pharmacol. Ther.*, **44**, 540-555
146. Schapira, K., McClelland, H. A., Griffiths, N. R. and Newell, D. J. (1970). Study on the effects of tablet colour on the treatment of anxiety states. *Br. Med. J.*, **2**, 446-449
147. Max, M. B., Schafer, S. C., Culnane, M., Dubner, R. and Gracely, R. H. (1988). Association of pain relief with drug side effects in post hepatic neuralgia: a single-dose study of clonidine, codeine, ibuprofen and placebo. *Clin. Pharmacol. Ther.*, **43**, 363-371
148. Schapira, K., McClelland, H. A., Griffiths, N. R. and Newell, P. J. (1970). Study on the effects of tablet colour in the treatment of anxiety states. *Br. Med. J.*, **2**, 446-449
149. Scott, D. L. and Bacon, P. A. (1985). Joint damage in rheumatoid arthritis: radiological assessments and the effects of anti-rheumatic drugs. *Rheumatol Int.*, **5**, 193-199
150. Mikulaschek, W. M. (1982). An update on long-term efficacy and safety with benoxaprofen. *Eur. J. Rheumatol. Inflamm.*, **5**, 206-215
151. Gosh, P. (1988). Anti-rheumatic drugs and cartilage. *Baillières Clin. Rheumatol.*, **2**, 309-338
152. Herman, J. H., Appel, A. M. and Hess, E. V. (1987). Modulation of cartilage destruction by select non-steroidal anti-inflammatory drugs. *Arthritis Rheum.*, **30**, 257-265
153. Spector, R., Park, G. D., Johnson, G. F. and Vesell, E. S. (1988). Therapeutic drug monitoring. *Clin. Pharmacol. Ther.*, **43**, 345-353
154. Day, R. O., Furst, D. E., Dromgoole, S. H., Kamm, B., Roe, R. and Paulus, H. E. (1982). Relationship of serum naproxen concentration to efficacy in rheumatoid arthritis. *Clin. Pharmacol. Ther.*, **31**, 733-740
155. Orme, M.'le. (1982). Plasma concentrations and therapeutic effect of anti-inflammatory and anti-rheumatic drugs. *Pharmacol. Ther.*, **16**, 167-180
156. Porter, R. S. (1984). Factors determining efficacy of NSAIDs. *Drug Intell. Clin. Pharm.*, **18**, 42-51
157. Perucca, E., Grimaldi, R. and Crema, A. (1985). Interpretation of drug levels in acute and chronic states. *Clin. Pharmacokin.*, **10**, 498-513
158. Day, R. O., Graham, G. G. and Williams, K. M. (1988). Pharmacokinetics of non-steroidal anti-inflammatory drugs. *Baillières Clin. Rheumatol.*, **2**, 363-393
159. Vozeh, S. (1987). Cost effectiveness of therapeutic drug monitoring. *Clin. Pharmacokin.*, **13**, 131-140
160. Helleberg, L. (1981). Clinical pharmacokinetics of indomethacin. *Clin. Pharmacokin.*, **6**, 245-258
161. Orozco-Alcala, J. J. and Baum, J. (1974). Treatment of juvenile rheumatoid arthritis — a world survey. *J. Rheumatol.*, **1**, 187
162. Lindsley, C. B. (1981). Pharmacotherapy of juvenile rheumatoid arthritis. *Pediatr. Clin. North Am.*, **28**, 161-177
163. Cassidy, J. T. (1980). Rheumatic diseases in childhood. In: Kelley, W. N., Harris, E. D., Ruddy, S. and Sledge, C. B. (eds.) *Textbook of Rheumatology*, vol. 2, 2nd edn. pp. 1247-1277. (Philadelphia: W. B. Saunders)
164. Makela, A. L., Yrjana, T. and Mattila, M. (1979). Dosage of salicylates for children

with juvenile rheumatoid arthritis. A prospective clinical trial with three different preparations of acetyl salicylic acid. *Acta Paediatr. Scand.*, **68**, 423-430
165. Pachman, L. M., Olufs, R., Procknal, J. A. and Levy, G. (1979). Pharmacokinetic monitoring of salicylate therapy in children with juvenile rheumatoid arthritis. *Arthritis Rheum.*, **22**, 826-831
166. O'Malley, K., Crooks, J., Duke, E. and Stevenson, I. H. (1971). Effect of age and sex on human drug metabolism. *Br. Med. J.*, **3**, 607-609
167. Paulus, H. E., Siegel, M., Mongan, E., Okun, R. and Calabro, J. J. (1971). Variations of serum concentrations and half-life of salicylate in patients with rheumatoid arthritis. *Arthritis Rheum.*, **14**, 527-531
168. Champion, G. D., Day, R. O. and Graham, G. G. (1975). Salicylates in rheumatoid arthritis. *Clin. Rheumatol.*, **1**, 245-265
169. Mandelli, M. and Tognoni, G. (1980). Monitoring plasma concentrations of salicylate. *Clin. Pharmacokinet.*, **5**, 424-440
170. Tugwell, P., Hart, L., Kraag, G., Park, A., Dok, C., Bianchi, F., Goldsmith, C. and Buchanan, W. W. (1984). Controlled trial of clinical utility of serum salicylate monitoring in rheumatoid arthritis. *J. Rheumatol.*, **11**, 457-461
171. Mongan, E., Kelly, P., Nies, K., Porter, W. W. *et al.* (1973). Tinnitus as an indication of therapeutic serum salicylate levels. *J. Am. Med. Assoc.*, **226**, 142-145
172. Dromgoole, S. H., Furst, D. E. and Paulus, H. E. (1982). Rational approaches to the use of salicylates in the treatment of rheumatoid arthritis. *Semin. Arthritis Rheum.*, **11**, 257-283
173. Halla, J. T. and Hardin, J. G. (1988). Salicylate ototoxicity in patients with rheumatoid arthritis: a controlled study. *Ann. Rheum. Dis.*, **47**, 134-137
174. Furst, D. E., Tozer, R. N. and Melmon, K. L. (1979). Salicylate clearance, the resultant of protein binding and metabolism. *Clin. Pharmacol. Ther.*, **26**, 380-389
175. Friesen, A. J. D. (1983). Adverse drug reactions in the geriatric client. In Pagliaro, L. A. and Pagliaro, A. M. (eds.) *Pharmacologic Aspects of Aging.* pp. 257-293. (St. Louis: C. V. Mosby)
176. Roberts, M. S., Rumble, R. H., Wainwimolruk, S. *et al.* (1983). Pharmacokinetics of aspirin and salicylate in elderly subjects and in patients with alcoholic liver disease. *Eur. J. Clin. Pharmacol.*, **25**, 253-261
177. Grigor, R. R., Spitz, P. W. and Furst, D. E. (1987). Salicylate toxicity in elderly patients with rheumatoid arthritis. *J. Rheumatol.*, **14**, 60-66
178. Vincent, P. C. (1986). Drug-induced aplastic anaemia and agranulocytosis. Incidence and mechanisms. *Drugs*, **31**, 52-63
179. Inman, W. H. W. (1977). Study of fatal bone marrow depression with special reference to phenylbutazone and oxyphenbutazone. *Br. Med. J.*, **1**, 1500-1505
180. O'Malley, K., Crooks, J., Duke, E. and Stevenson, I. H. (1971). Effect of age and sex on human drug metabolism. *Br. Med. J.*, **3**, 607-609
181. Cunningham, J. L., Leyland, M. J., Delamore, I. W. and Price-Evans, D. A. (1974). Acetanilide oxidation in phenylbutazone-associated hypoplastic anaemia. *Br. Med. J.*, **3**, 313-317
182. Fauci, A. S., Dale, D. C. and Balow, J. E. (1976). Glucocorticoid therapy: Mechanisms of action and clinical considerations. *Ann. Intern. Med.*, **84**, 304-315
183. Champion, G. D., Cairns, D. R., Bieri, D., Adena, M. A., Browne, C. D., Cohen, M. L., Day, R. O., Edmonds, J. P., Graham, G. G., de Jager, J. and Sambrook, P. N. (1988). Dose-response studies and longterm evaluation of auranofin in rheumatoid arthritis. *J. Rheumatol.*, **15**, 28-34
184. Dahl, S., Coleman, M. L., Williams, J. H. *et al.* (1985). Lack of correlation between blood gold concentrations and clinical response in patients with definite or classic rheumatoid arthritis receiving auranofin or gold sodium thiomalate. *Arthritis Rheum.*, **28**, 1211-1218
185. Kremer, J. M., Galivan, J., Streckfuss, A. and Kamen, B. (1986). Methotrexate metabolism analysis in blood and liver of rheumatoid arthritis patients. Association with hepatic folate deficiency and formation of polyglutamates. *Arthritis Rheum.*, **29**, 832-835
186. Edelman, J., Russell, A. S., Biggs, D. F., Rothwell, R. S. and Coates, J. (1983). Methotrexate levels, a guide to therapy? *Clin. Exp. Rheumatol.*, **1**, 153-156

187. Levy, R. H. and Moreland, T. E. (1984). Rationale for monitoring free drug levels. *Clin. Pharmacokin*, **9** (suppl. 1), 1–9
188. Svensson, C. K., Woodruff, M. N., Baxter, J. G. and Lalka, D. (1986). Free drug concentration monitoring in clinical practice. Rationale and current status. *Clin. Pharmacokin.*, **11**, 450–469
189. Lin, J. H., Cocchetto, D. M. and Duggan, D. E. (1987). Protein binding as a primary determinant of the clinical pharmacokinetic properties of non-steroidal anti-inflammatory drugs. *Clin. Pharmacokin.*, **12**, 402–432
190. Wallace, S. M. and Verbeeck, R. K. (1987). Plasma protein binding of drugs in the elderly. *Clin. Pharmacokin.*, **12**, 41–72
191. Borga, O., Oda-Cederlof, I. and Ringberger, V. (1976). Protein binding of salicylate in uremic and normal plasma. *Clin. Pharmacol. Ther.*, **20**, 464–475
192. Gurwich, E. L., Raees, S. M., Skosey, J. and Niazi, S. (1984). Unbound plasma salicylate concentration in rheumatoid arthritis patients. *Br. J. Rheumatol.*, **23**, 66–73
193. Rudge, S. R., Perrett, D. and Swannell, A. J. (1984). Free thiomalate levels in patients with rheumatoid arthritis treated with disodium aurothiomalate therapy: relationship to clinical outcome of therapy. *Ann. Rheum. Dis.*, **43**, 698–702
194. Heath, M. J. (1988). Measurement of "free" gold in patients receiving disodium aurothiomalate and the association of high free to total gold levels with toxicity. *Ann. Rheum. Dis.*, **47**, 18–21
195. Lam, Y. W. F. (1988). Stereoselectivity: an issue of significant importance in clinical pharmacology. *Pharmacotherapy*, **8**, 147–157
196. Caldwell, J., Hutt, A. J. and Fournel-Gigleux, S. (1988). The metabolic chiral inversion and dispositional enantioselectivity of the 2-arylpropionic acids and their biological consequences. *Biochem. Pharmacol.*, **37**, 105–114
197. Jamali, F. (1988). Pharmacokinetics of enantiomers of chiral non-steroidal anti-inflammatory drugs. *Eur. J. Drug. Metab. Pharmacokin.*, **13**, 1–9
198. Caldwell, J. and Marsh, M. V. (1983). Interrelationships between xenobiotic metabolism and lipid biosynthesis. *Biochem. Pharmacol.*, **32**, 1667–1672
199. Williams, K., Day, R., Knihinicki, R. and Duffield, A. (1986). The stereoselective uptake of ibuprofen enantiomers into adipose tissue. *Biochem. Pharmacol.*, **35**, 3403–3405
200. Giansiracusa, D. F., Blumberg, S. and Kantrowitz, F. G. (1980). Aseptic meningitis associated with ibuprofen. *Arch. Intern. Med.*, **140**, 1553
201. Ballas, Z. K. and Donta, S. T. (1982). Sulindac-induced aseptic meningitis. *Arch. Intern. Med.*, **142**, 165–166
202. Ruppert, G. B. and Barth, W. F. (1981). Tolmetin-induced aseptic meningitis. *J. Am. Med. Assoc.*, **245**, 67–68
203. Kremer, I., Ritz, R. and Brummer, F. (1983). Aseptic meningitis as an adverse effect of co-trimoxazole. *N. Engl. J. Med.*, **308**, 1481
204. Kalow, W. (1987). Genetic variation in the human hepatic cytochrome P-450 system. *Eur. J. Clin. Pharmacol.*, **31**, 633–641
205. Swift, C. G. and Triggs, E. J. (1987). Clinical pharmaco-kinetics in the elderly. In Swift, C. G. (ed.) *Clinical Pharmacology in the Elderly*, pp. 31–82. (New York: Marcel Dekker)
206. Triggs, E. J., Nation, R. L., Long, A. and Ashley, J. J. (1975). Pharmacokinetics in the elderly. *Eur. J. Clin. Pharmacol.*, **8**, 55–62
207. Greenblatt, D. J., Abernethy, D. R., Matlis, R., Harmatz, J. S. and Shader, R. I. (1984). Absorption and disposition of ibuprofen in the elderly. *Arthritis Rheum.*, **27**, 1066–1069
208. Advenier, C., Roux, A., Gobert, C., Massias, P., Varoquaux, O. and Slouvat, B. (1983). Pharmacokinetics of ketoprofen in the elderly. *Br. J. Clin. Pharmacol.*, **16**, 65–70
209. Richardson, C. J., Blocka, K. L., Ross, S. G. and Verbeeck, R. K. (1985). Effects of age and sex on piroxicam disposition. *Clin. Pharmacol. Ther.*, **37**, 13–18
210. Verbeeck, R. K., Richardson, C. J. and Blocka, K. L. N. (1986). Clinical pharmaco-kinetics of piroxicam. *J. Rheumatol.*, **13**, 789–796
211. Blocka, K. L. N., Richardson, C. J., Wallace, S. M., Ross, S. G. and Verbeeck, R. K.

(1988). The effect of age on piroxicam disposition in rheumatoid arthritis. *J. Rheumatol.*, **15**, 757-763
212. Rugstad, H. E., Hundal, O., Holme, I., Herland, O. B., Husby, G. and Giercksky, K. E. (1986). Piroxicam and naproxen plasma concentrations in patients with osteoarthritis: relation to age, sex, efficacy and adverse events. *Clin. Rheumatol.*, **5**, 389-398
213. Woolf, A. D., Rogers, H. J., Bradbrook, I. D. and Corless, D. (1983). Pharmacokinetic observations on piroxicam in young adult, middle-aged and elderly patients. *Br. J. Clin. Pharmacol.*, **16**, 433-437
214. Hobbs, D. C. and Gordon, A. J. (1984). Absence of an effect of age in the pharmacokinetics of piroxicam. *Int. Congr. Symp. Ser. Roy. Soc. Med.*, **67**, 91-94
215. Darragh, A., Gordon, A. J., O'Byrne, H., Hobbs, D. and Casey, E. (1985). Single-dose and steady-state pharmaco-kinetics of piroxicam in elderly vs. young adults. *Eur. J. Clin. Pharmacol.*, **28**, 305-309
216. Woodhouse, K. W. and Wynne, H. (1987). The pharmacokinetics of non-steroidal anti-inflammatory drugs in the elderly. *Clin. Pharmacokin.*, **12**, 111-121
217. Vesell, E. S. (1982). On the significance of host factors that affect drug disposition. *Clin. Pharmacol. Ther.*, **31**, 1-7
218. Davies, D. S., Kahn, G. C., Murray, S., Brodie, M. J. and Boobis, A. R. (1981). Evidence for an enzymatic defect in the 4-hydroxylation of debrisoquine by human liver. *Br. J. Clin. Pharmacol.*, **11**, 89-91
219. Jurima, M., Imaba, T. and Kalow, W. (1984). Sparteine oxidation by the human liver: absence of inhibition by mephenytoin. *Clin. Pharmacol. Ther.*, **35**, 426-428
220. Meffin, P. J. (1985). The effect of renal dysfunction on the disposition of non-steroidal anti-inflammatory drugs forming acyl glucuronides. *Agents Actions*, suppl. 17, 85-89
221. Meffin, P. J., Zilm, D. M. and Veenendaal, J. R. (1983). Reduced clofibric acid clearance in renal dysfunction is due to a futile cycle. *J. Pharmacol. Exp. Ther.*, **227**, 732-738
222. Verbeeck, R. K., Wallace, S. M. and Loewen, G. R. (1984). Reduced elimination of ketoprofen in the elderly is not necessarily due to impaired glucuronidation. *Br. J. Clin. Pharmacol.*, **17**, 783-784
223. Taggart, H., McA. and Alderdice, J. M. (1982). Fatal cholestatic jaundice in elderly patients taking benoxaprofen. *Br. Med. J.*, **284**, 1372
224. Singer, J. Z. and Wallace, S. L. (1986). The allopurinol hypersensitivity syndrome. Unnecessary morbidity and mortality. *Arthritis Rheum.*, **29**, 82-86
225. Wood, M. H., Sebel, E. and O'Sullivan, W. J. (1972). Allopurinol and thiazides (Letter). *Lancet*, **1**, 751
226. Young, J. L., Boswell, R. B. and Nies, A. S. (1974). Severe allopurinol sensitivity. *Arch. Intern. Med.*, **134**, 553-558
227. Hande, K. R., Noone, R. M. and Store, W. J. (1984). Severe allopurinol toxicity. *Am. J. Med.*, **76**, 47-56
228. Rosenbloom, D., Brooks, P., Bellamy, N. and Buchanan, W. W. (1985). *Clinical Trials in the Rheumatic Diseases*, (New York: Praeger), pp. 280-292
229. Bird, H. A. (1987). Disease modifying drugs for rheumatoid arthritis: asset or liability? Editorial. *Clin. Rheumatol.*, **6**, 486-488
230. Kirwan, J. R. and Currey, H. L. F. (1983). Rheumatoid arthritis — disease modifying drugs. *Clin. Rheum. Dis.*, **9**, 581-600
231. Iannauzzi, L., Dawson, N., Zein, N. and Kushner, I. (1983). Does any therapy slow radiographic deterioration in rheumatoid arthritis? *N. Engl. J. Med.*, **309**, 1023-1027
232. Scott, D. L., Grindulis, K. A., Struthers, G. R., Coulton, B. L., Popert, A. J. and Bacon, P. A. (1984). Progression of radiological changes in rheumatoid arthritis. *Ann. Rheum. Dis.*, **43**, 8-17
233. Scott, D. L., Dawes, P. T., Fowler, P. D., Grindulis, K. A., Shadforth, M. and Bacon, P. A. (1985). Antirheumatic drugs and joint damage in rheumatoid arthritis. *Q.J. Med.*, **54**, 49-59
234. Scott, D. L. and Bacon, P. A. (1985). Joint damage in rheumatoid arthritis: radiological assessments and the effects of antirheumatic drugs. *Rheumatol. Int.*, **5**, 193-199

235. Pullar, T., Hunter, J. A. and Capell, H. A. (1984). Does second-line therapy affect the radiological progression of rheumatoid arthritis? *Ann. Rheum. Dis.*, **43**, 18-23
236. Pullar, T. and Capell, H. A. (1985). A rheumatological dilemma: is it possible to modify the course of rheumatoid arthritis? Can we answer the question? *Ann. Rheum. Dis.*, **44**, 134-140
237. Pullar, T., Hunter, J. A. and Capell, H. A. (1987). Effect of sulphasalazine on the radiological progression of rheumatoid arthritis. *Ann. Rheum. Dis.*, **46**, 398-402
238. Amos, R. S., Constable, T. J., Crockson, R. A., Crockson, A. P. and McConkey, B. (1977). Rheumatoid arthritis: relation of serum C-reactive protein and erythrocyte sedimentation rates to radiographic changes. *Br. Med. J.*, **1**, 195-197
239. Wright, V. and Amos, R. (1980). Do drugs change the course of rheumatoid arthritis? *Br. Med. J.*, **1**, 193-194
240. Anonymous. (1981). Inducing remission in rheumatoid arthritis. *Lancet*, **1**, 193-194
241. Co-operating Clinics Committee of the American Rheumatism Association. (1973). A controlled trial of gold salt therapy in rheumatoid arthritis. *Arthritis Rheum.*, **16**, 353-358
242. Sigler, J. W., Bluhm, G. B., Duncan, H., Sharp, J. T., Ensign, D. C. and McCrann, W. R. (1974). Gold salts in the treatment of rheumatoid arthritis. A double-blind study. *Ann. Intern. Med.*, **80**, 21-26
243. Co-operating Clinics Committee of the American Rheumatism Association. (1970). A controlled trial of cyclophosphamide in rheumatoid arthritis. *N. Engl. J. Med.*, **283**, 883-889
244. Luukkainen, R., Isomaki, H. and Kajander, A. (1977). Effect of gold treatment on the progression of erosions in RA patients. *Scand. J. Rheumatol.*, **6**, 123-127
245. Luukkainen, R., Kajander, A. and Isomaki, H. (1977). Effects of gold on the progression of erosions in rheumatoid arthritis. *Scand. J. Rheumatol.*, **6**, 189-192
246. Larsen, A., Dale, K. and Eck, M. (1977). Radiographic evaluation of rheumatoid arthritis and related conditions by standard reference films. *Acta Radiol. [Diagn]. (Stockh).*, **18**, 481-491
247. Sharp, J. T., Young, D. Y., Bluhm, G. B., Brook, A., Brower, A. C., Corbett, M., Decker, J. L., Genant, H. K., Gofton, J. P., Goodman, N., Larsen, A., Lidsky, M. D., Pussila, P., Weinstein, A. S. and Weissman, B. N. (1985). How many joints in the hands and wrists should be included in a score of radiologic abnormalities used to assess rheumatoid arthritis? *Arthritis Rheum.*, **28**, 1326-1335
248. Buckland-Wright, J. C. (1983). X-ray assessment of activity in rheumatoid disease. *Br. J. Rheumatol.*, **22**, 3-10
249. Mewa, A. M., Pui, M., Cockshott, W. P. and Buchanan, W. W. (1983). Observer differences in detecting erosions in radiographs of rheumatoid arthritis. A comparison of postero-anterior, Norgaard and Brewerton views. *J. Rheumatol.*, **10**, 216-221
250. Fries, J. F., Bloch, D. A., Sharp, J. T., McShane, D. J., Spitz, P., Bluhm, G. B., Forrester, D., Genant, H., Goftin, P., Richman, S., Weissman, B. and Wolfe, F. (1986). Assessment of radiologic progression in rheumatoid arthritis. A randomized, controlled trial. *Arthritis Rheum.*, **29**, 1-9
251. Gaydecki, P. A., Browne, M., Mamtora, H. and Grennan, D. M. (1987). Measurement of radiographic changes occurring in rheumatoid arthritis by image analysis techniques. *Ann. Rheum. Dis.*, **46**, 296-301
252. Buckland-Wright, J. C. (1984). Microfocal radiographic examinations of erosions in the wrist and hand of patients with rheumatoid arthritis. *Ann. Rheum. Dis.*, **43**, 150-170
253. Pullar, T., Peaker, S., Martin, M. F. R., Bird, H. A. and Feely, M. P. (1988). The use of a pharmacological indicator to investigate compliance in patients with a poor response to antirheumatic therapy. *Br. J. Rheumatol.*, **27**, 381-384
254. Mottonen, T. J. (1988). Prediction of erosiveness and rate of development of new erosions in early rheumatoid arthritis. *Ann. Rheum. Dis.*, **47**, 648-653
255. van der Heijde, D. M. F. M., van Riel, P. L. C. M., van Rijswijk, M. H. and van de Putte, L. B. A. (1988). Influence of prognostic features on the final outcome in rheumatoid arthritis: a review of the literature. *Semin. Arthritis Rheum.*, **17**, 284-292
256. Tishler, M., Caspi, D., Rosenbach, T. O., Fishel, B., Wigler, I., Segal, R., Gazt, E. and

Yarom, M. (1988). Methotrexate in rheumatoid arthritis: a prospective study in Israeli patients with immunogenetic correlations. *Ann. Rheum. Dis.*, **47**, 654-659
257. Weinblatt, M. E., Coblyn, J. S., Fox, D. A., Fraser, P. A., Holdsworth, D. E., Glass, D. N. and Trentham, D. E. (1985). Efficacy of low dose methotrexate in rheumatoid arthritis. *N. Engl. J. Med.*, **312**, 818-822
258. Alarcon, G. S., Guyton, J. M., Acton, R. T., Barger, B. O. and Koopman, W. J. (1986). DR2 positivity and response to methotrexate in rheumatoid arthritis. Letter to the Editor. *Arthritis Rheum.*, **29**, 151
259. van de Putte, L. B. A., Speerstra, F., van Riel, P. L. C. M., Boerbooms, A. M. U., Bosch, P. J. I., Van'T, P. and Reekers, P. (1986). Remarkably similar response to gold 001therapy in HLA identical sibs with rheumatoid arthritis. *Ann. Rheum. Dis.*, **45**, 1004-1006
260. O'Duffy, J. D., O'Fallon, W. M., Hunder, G. G., McDuffie, F. C., and Moore, S. B. (1984). An attempt to predict the response to gold therapy in rheumatoid arthritis. *Arthritis Rheum.*, **27**, 1210-1217
261. Carette, S., Lang, J. Y., Mathieu, J. P., Roy, R. and Morisette, J. (1985). HLA and the response to gold therapy in rheumatoid arthritis. Letter to the Editor. *Arthritis Rheum.*, **25**, 233
262. Giannini, E. H., Brewer, E. J., Person, D. A., and He, X. (1986). Longterm auranofin therapy in patients with juvenile rheumatoid arthritis. *J. Rheumatol.*, **13**, 768-770
263. Champion, G. D., Cairns, D. R., Bieri, D., Adena, M. A., Browne, C. D., Cohen, M. L., Day, R. O., Edmonds, J. P., Graham, G., de Jager, J. and Sambrook, P. N. (1988). Dose response studies and longterm evaluation of auranofin in rheumatoid arthritis. *J. Rheumatol.*, **15**, 28-34
264. Pinals, R. S. (1988). Sulfasalazine in the rheumatic disease. *Semin. Arthritis Rheum.*, **17**, 246-259
265. Martin, L., Sitar, D. S., Chalmers, I. M. and Hunter, T. (1985). Sulfasalazine in severe rheumatoid arthritis: a study to assess potential correlates of efficacy and toxicity. *J. Rheumatol.*, **12**, 270-273
266. Pullar, T., Hunter, J. A. and Capell, H. A. (1988). Effect of acetylator phenotype on efficacy and toxicity of sulphasalazine in rheumatoid arthritis. *Ann. Rheum. Dis.*, **44**, 831-837.
267. Bax, D. E., Greaves, M. S. and Amos, R. S. (1986). Sulphasalazine for rheumatoid arthritis: relationship between dose, acetylator phenotype and response to treatment. *Br. J. Rheumatol.*, **25**, 282-284
268. Richter, J. A., Runge, L. A., Pinals, R. S. and Oates, R. P. (1980). Analysis of treatment terminators with gold and antimalarial compounds in RA. *J. Rheumatol.*, **7**, 153-159
269. Situnayake, R. D., Grindulis, K. A. and McConkey, B. (1987). Long term treatment of rheumatoid arthritis with sulphasalazine, gold, or penicillamine: a comparison using life-table methods. *Ann. Rheum. Dis.*, **46**, 177-183
270. Paulus, H. E. (1982). An overview of benefit/risk of disease modifying treatment of RA as of today. *Ann. Rheum. Dis.*, **41** (suppl.), 26-60
271. Thompson, P. W., Kirwan, J. R. and Barnes, G. G. (1985). Practical results of treatment with disease modifying anti-rheumatic drugs. *Br. J. Rheumatol.*, **24**, 167-175
272. Ahern, M. J., Hall, N. D., Case, K. and Maddison, P. J. (1984). D-Penicillamine withdrawal in rheumatoid arthritis. *Ann. Rheum. Dis.*, **43**, 213-217
273. Rae, K. J., MacKay, C. N. N., McNeil, C. J., Brown, D. H., Smith, W. E., Lewis, D. and Capell, H. A. (1986). Early and late changes in sulphydryl group and copper protein concentrations and activities during drug treatment with aurothiomalate and auranofin. *Ann. Rheum. Dis.*, **45**, 839-846
274. Joint Committee of the Medical Research Council and the Nuffield Foundation. (1959). A comparison of prednisolone with aspirin or other analgesics in the treatment of rheumatoid arthritis. *Ann. Rheum. Dis.*, **18**, 173-187
275. Joint Committee of the Medical Research Council and the Nuffield Foundation. (1960). A comparison of prednisolone with aspirin or other analgesics in the treatment of rheumatoid arthritis. *Ann. Rheum. Dis.*, **19**, 331-337

276. Bernsten, C. and Freyberg, R. H. (1961). Rheumatoid patients after five or more years of corticosteroid treatment: a comparative analysis of 183 cases. *Ann. Intern. Med.*, **54**, 938-953
277. West, H. F. (1967). Rheumatoid arthritis: the relevance of clinical knowledge to research activities. *Abstracts World Med.*, **41**, 401-417
278. Byron, M. A. and Kirwan, J. R. (1986). Corticosteroids in rheumatoid arthritis: is a trial of their 'disease modifying' potential feasible? *Ann. Rheum. Dis.*, **46**, 171-173
279. Steinberg, A. D. (1988). The treatment of lupus nephritis. *Kidney Int.*, **30**, 769-787
280. Pollak, V. E., Pirani, C. L. and Schwartz, F. (1964). Natural history of the renal manifestations of systemic lupus erythematosus. *J. Lab. Clin. Med.*, **63**, 537-550
281. Baldwin, D. S., Lowenstein, J., Rothfield, N. F., Gallo, G. and McCluskey, R. T. (1970). The clinical course of the proliferative and membranous forms of lupus nephritis. *Ann. Intern. Med.*, **73**, 929-942
282. Ginzler, E. M., Nicastri, A. D., Chen, C. K., Friedman, E. A., Diamond, H. S. and Kaplan, D. (1974). Progression of mesangial and focal diffuse nephritis. *N. Engl. J. Med.*, **291**, 693-696
283. Appel, G. B., Silva, F. G., Pirani, C. L., Meltzer, J. I. and Estes, D. (1978). Renal involvement in systemic lupus erythematosus (SLE): a study of 56 patient emphasizing histologic classification. *Medicine (Baltimore)*, **57**, 371-410
284. Cameron, J. S., Turner, D. R. and Ogg, L. S. (1979). Systemic lupus with nephritis. A long term study. *Q. J. Med.*, **48**, 1-24
285. Lee, H. S., Mujaia, S. K., Kasinath, B. S., Spargo, B. H. and Katz, A. I. (1984). Cause of renal pathology in patients with systemic lupus erythematosus. *Am. J. Med.*, **77**, 612-620
286. Gershwin, M. E. and Steinberg, A. D. (1974). Qualitative characteristics of anti-DNA antibodies in lupus nephritis. *Arthritis Rheum.*, **17**, 947-952
287. Pollak, V. E., Pirani, C. L. and Kark, R. M. (1961). Effect of large dose of prednisone on the renal lesions and life span of patents with lupus glomerulonephritis. *J. Lab. Clin. Med.*, **57**, 495-511
288. Henriksson, K. G. and Sandstedt, P. (1982). Polymyositis — treatment and prognosis. A study of 107 patients. *Acta Neurol. Scand.*, **65**, 280-300
289. Winkelmann, R. K., Mulder, D. W., Lambert, E. H., Howard, F. M. and Diessner, G. R. (1968). Course of dermatomyositis-polymyositis: comparison of untreated and cortisone-treated patients. *Mayo Clin. Proc.*, **43**, 545-556
290. Carpenter, J. R., Burch, T. W., Engel, A. G. and O'Brien, P. C. (1977). Survival in polymyositis: corticosteroids and risk factors. *J. Rheumatol.*, **4**, 207-214
291. Hudson, P. (1984). Polymyositis and dermatomyositis in adults. *Clin. Rheum. Dis.*, **10**, 85-93
292. Vignos, P. J., Bowling, G. F. and Watkins, M. P. (1964). Polymyositis effect of corticosteroids on final results. *Arch. Intern. Med.*, **114**, 263-277
293. Bunch, T. W., (1981). Worthington, J. W., Combs, J. J., Ilstrup, D. M. and Engel, A. G. (1980). Azathioprine with prednisone for polymyositis: a controlled, clinical trial. *Ann. Intern. Med.*, **92**, 365-369
294. Bunch, T. W. (1981). Prednisone and azathioprine for polymyositis: long-term followup. *Arthritis Rheum.*, **24**, 45-48
295. Woo, T. Y., Callen, J. P., Voorhees, J. J., Bickers, D. R., Hanno, R. and Hawkins, C. (1984). Cutaneous lesions of dermatomyositis are improved by hydroxychloroquine. *J. Am. Acad. Dermatol.*, **10**, 592-600
296. Carpenter, S., Karpati, G., Heller, I. and Eisen, A. (1978). Inclusion body myositis: a distinct variety of idiopathic inflammatory myopathy. *Neurology*, **28**, 8-17
297. Girdwood, R. H. (1974). Death after taking medicaments. *Br. Med. J.*, **1**, 501-504
298. Lee, P., McCusker, S., Allison, A. and Nuki, G. (1973). Adverse reactions in patients with rheumatic diseases. *Ann. Rheum. Dis.*, **32**, 565-573
299. Brooks, P. M., Stephens, W. H., Stephens, M. E. B. and Buchanan, W. W. (1975). How safe are anti-rheumatic drugs? A study of possible iatrogenic deaths in patients with rheumatoid arthritis. *Health Bull. (SHHD)*, **33**, 108-111
300. Reed, W. B. and Wright, V. (1966). Psoriatic arthritis. In Hill, A. G. S. (ed.) *Modern Trends in Rheumatology*, pp. 375-383. (London: Butterworths)

301. Mutru, O., Koota, K. and Isomaki, H. (1976). Cause of death in autopsied rheumatoid arthritis patients. *Scand. J. Rheumatol.*, **5**, 239-240
302. Constable, T. J., McConkey, B. and Paton, A. (1978). The cause of death in rheumatoid arthritis. *Ann. Rheum. Dis.*, **37**, 569
303. Vandenbroucke, J. P., Hazevoet, H. M. and Cats, A. (1984). Survival and cause of death in rheumatoid arthritis: a 25 year prospective followup. *J. Rheumatol.*, **11**, 158-161
304. Mitchell, D. M., Spitz, P. W., Young, D. Y., Bloch, D. A., McShane, D. J. and Fries, J. F. (1986). Survival, prognosis and causes of death in rheumatoid arthritis. *Arthritis Rheum.*, **29**, 706-714
305. Pincus, T. and Callahan, L. F. (1985). Formal education as a marker for increased mortality and morbidity in rheumatoid arthritis. *J. Chronic Dis.*, **38**, 973-984
306. Prior, P., Symmons, D. P. M., Scott, D. L., Brown, R. and Hawkins, C. F. (1984). Cause of death in rheumatoid arthritis. *Br. J. Rheumatol.*, **23**, 92-99
307. Atwater, E. C. and Jacox, R. F. (1967). The death certificate in rheumatoid arthritis. *Arthritis Rheum.*, **10**, 259
308. Allebeck, P., Ahlbom, A. and Allander, E. (1981). Increased mortality among persons with rheumatoid arthritis, but where RA does not appear on the death certificate. *Scand. J. Rheumatol.*, **10**, 301-306
309. Wicks, I. P., Moore, J. and Fleming, A. (1988). Australian mortality statistics for rheumatoid arthritis 1950-81: analysis of death certificate data. *Ann. Rheum. Dis.*, **47**, 563-569
310. Taggart, H. Mc. and Alderidge, J. M. (1982). Fatal cholestatic jaundice in elderly patients taking benoxaprofen. *Br. Med. J.*, **284**, 1372
311. Anonymous. Benoxaprofen. Editorial. *Br. Med. J.*, **285**, 459-460
312. Venulet, J. (ed.) *Assessing Causes of Adverse Drug Reactions* (New York: Academic Press)
313. Huskisson, E. C. and Wojtulewski, J. A. (1974). Measurement of side effects of drugs. *Br. Med. J.*, **2**, 698-699
314. Coles, L. S., Fries, J. F., Kraines, R. G. *et al.* (1983). From experiment to experience: side effects of nonsteroidal anti-inflammatory drugs. *Am. J. Med.*, **74**, 820-828
315. Steel, K., Gertman, P. M., Crescenzi, C. *et al.* (1981). Iatrogenic illness on a general medical service at a university hospital. *N. Engl. J. Med.*, **304**, 638-642
316. Strand, L. J. (1982). Upper gastrointestinal effects of newer nonsteroidal anti-inflammatory agents. In: *Drugs and Peptic Ulcer: Pathogenesis of Ulcer Induction Revealed by Drug Studies in Humans and Animals*, vol. III, pp. 8-24. (Boca Raton, Fla.: CRC Press)
317. Naranjo, L. A., Busto, U., Sellers, E. M. *et al.* (1980). A method for estimating the probability of adverse drug reactions. *Clin. Pharmacol. Ther.*, **30**, 239-245
318. Girard, M. (1984). Testing the methods of assessment for adverse drug reactions. *Adverse Drug React. Acute Poison. Rev.*, **4**, 237-244
319. Capell, H. A., Rennie, J. A. N. and Rooney, P. J. (1979). Patient compliance: a novel method of testing non-steroidal anti-inflammatory analgesics in rheumatoid arthritis. *J. Rheumatol.*, **6**, 584-593
320. Situnayake, R. D., Grindulis, K. A. and McConkey, B. (1987). Remarkably similar response to gold therapy in HLA identical sibs with rheumatoid arthritis. *Ann. Rheum. Dis.*, **45**, 1004-1006
321. Barr, D. P. (1955). Hazards of modern diagnosis and therapy — the price we pay. *J. Am. Med. Assoc.*, **129**, 1452
322. Venulet, J., Blattner, R., von Bulow, J. and Berneker, G. C. (1982). How good are articles on adverse drug reactions? *Br. Med. J.*, **284**, 252-254
323. Griffin, J. P. and Weber, J. C. P. (1986). Voluntary systems of adverse reaction reporting — part II. *Adverse Drug React. Acute Poison. Rev.*, **1**, 23-55
324. Rogers, A. S. (1987). Adverse drug events: identification and attribution. *Drug Intell. Clin. Pharm.*, **21**, 915-920
325. Gordon, A. J. and Sachs, R. (1987). Potential biases influencing interpretation of data from worldwide spontaneous ADR reports. In Rainsford, K. D. and Velo, G. P. (eds.) *Side-Effects of Anti-Inflammatory Drugs, Part I. Clinical and Epidemiological Aspects*, pp. 105-110. (Lancaster: MTP)

326. Weber, J. C. P. (1984). Epidemiology of adverse drug reactions to non-steroidal anti-inflammatory drugs. *Adv. Inflam. Res.*, **6**, 1–7
327. Fries, J. F. (1988). Postmarketing drug surveillance: are our priorities right? *J. Rheumatol.*, **15**, 389–390
328. Inman, W. H. W. (1984). Risks in medical intervention. *PEM News*, **2**, 16–36
329. Bell, R. L. and Smith, E. O. (1982). Clinical trials in post-marketing surveillance of drugs. *Controlled Clin. Trials*, **3**, 61–68
330. Porta, M. S. and Hartzema, A. G. (1987). The contribution of epidemiology to the study of drugs. *Drug Intell. Clin. Pharm.*, **21**, 741–747
331. Lasagna, L. (1983). Discovering adverse drug reactions. *J. Am. Med. Assoc.*, **249**, 2224–2225
332. Rossi, A. C. and Knapp, D. E. (1984). Discovery of new adverse drug reactions — a review of the Food and Drug Administration's reporting system. *J. Am. Med. Assoc.*, **252**, 1030–1033
333. Fries, J. F., Bloch, D. A., Segal, M. R., Spitz, P. W., Williams, C. and Lane, N. E. (1988). Postmarketing surveillance in rheumatology: analysis of purpura and upper abdominal pain. *J. Rheumatol.*, **15**, 348–355
334. Sackett, D. L., Haynes, R. B., Gent, M. and Taylor, D. W. (1986). Compliance. In Inman, W. H. W. (ed.) *Monitoring for Drug Safety*, 2nd edn. pp. 471–483. (Lancaster: MTP)
335. Lawson, D. H. (1984). Pharmaco-epidemiology: a new discipline. *Br. Med. J.*, **289**, 940–941
336. Nelson, R. C. (1988). Drug safety, pharmacoepidemiology and regulatory decision making. *Drug Intell. Clin. Pharm.*, **22**, 336–344
337. Tilson, H. H. (1988). Pharmacoepidemiology: the future. *Drug Intell. Clin. Pharm.*, **22**, 416–421
338. Stergachis, A. S. (1988). Record linkage studies for postmarketing drug surveillance: data quality and validity considerations. *Drug Intell. Clin. Pharm.*, **22**, 157–161
339. Cohen, M. R. (1977). A compilation of abstracts and index of articles published by the Boston Collaborative Drug Surveillance Program. *Hosp. Pharm.*, **12**, 455–492
340. Fox, D. A. and Jick, H. (1984). Nonsteroidal anti-inflammatory drugs and renal disease. *J. Am. Med. Assoc.*, **251**, 1299–1300
341. Danielson, D. A., Douglas, S. W., III, Herzog, P., Jick, H. and Porter, J. B. (1984). Drug-induced blood disorders. *J. Am. Med. Assoc.*, **252**, 3257–3260
342. Inman, W. H. W. and Rawson, N. S. B. (1987). Prescription-event monitoring of five non-steroidal anti-inflammatory drugs. In Rainsford, K. D. and Velo, G. P. (eds.) *Side-effects of Anti-inflammatory Drugs*, Part I, pp. 111–124. (Lancaster: MTP)
343. Inman, W. H. M. (1981). Postmarketing surveillance of adverse drug reactions in general practice. 1. Search for new methods. *Br. Med. J.*, **282**, 1131–1132
344. Newrick, P. G. and Bainton, D. (1987). Benoxaprofen — adverse reactions and monitoring in general practice. *Br. J. Clin. Pharmacol.*, **23**, 195–198
345. Rossi, A. C., Knapp, D. E., Anello, C. *et al.* (1983). Discovery of adverse drug reactions: a comparison of selected phase IV studies with spontaneous reporting methods. *J. Am. Med. Assoc.*, **249**, 2226–2228
346. Venning, G. R. (1983). Identification of adverse drug reactions to new drugs. IV — Verification of suspected adverse reactions. *Br. Med. J.*, **286**, 544–547
347. O'Brien, W. M. (1987). Rare adverse reactions to non-steroidal anti-inflammatory drugs. In Rainsford, K. D. and Velo, G. P. (eds.) *Side-Effects of Anti-Inflammatory Drugs*, Part I Clinical and Epidemiological Aspects, pp. 73–98. (Lancaster: MTP)
348. Lamy, P. P. (1985). New dimensions and opportunities. *Drug Intell. Clin. Pharm.*, **19**, 399–402
349. Nolan, L. and O'Malley, K. (1988). Prescribing for the elderly. Part I. Sensitivity of the elderly to adverse drug reactions. *J. Am. Geriatr. Soc.*, **36**, 142–149
350. McDermott, F. T. (1985). Mortality from bleeding peptic ulcer. Alfred Hospital Melbourne, 1976–1980. *Med. J. Aust.*, **142**, 11–14
351. A report of the Royal College of Physicians. (1984). *Medication for the Elderly. J. R. Coll. Physicians. (Lond).*, **18**, 7–9

352. Gosney, M. and Tallis, R. (1984). Prescription of contra indicated and interacting drug in elderly patients admitted to hospital. *Lancet*, **2**, 564–567
353. Shimp, L. A., Ascione, F. J., Glazer, H. M. and Atwood, B. F. (1985). Potential medication-related problems in noninstitutionalized elderly. *Drug Intell. Clin. Pharm.*, **19**, 766–772
354. Steele, K., Mills, K. A., Gilliland, A. E., Irwin, W. and Taggart, A. (1987). Repeat prescribing of non-steroidal anti-inflammatory drugs excluding aspirin: how careful are we? *Br. Med. J.*, **295**, 962–964
355. Nicol, F. and Gebbie, H. (1984). Repeat prescribing in the elderly. A case for audit? *Scott. Med. J.*, **29**, 21–24
356. Francke, D. E. (1967). The clinical pharmacist. Editorial. *Drug Intell. Clin. Pharm.*, **1**, 243
357. Eriksen, I. L. and Andrew, E. (1986). Pharmacist involvement in Norweigian clinical drug trials: a questionnaire study. *Drug Intell. Clin. Pharm.*, **20**, 391–395
358. Ascione, F. J. and Shimp, L. A. (1984). The effectiveness of four education strategies in the elderly. *Drug Intell. Clin. Pharm.*, **18**, 926–931
359. Smith, M. C. and Sharpe, T. R. (1984). A study of pharmacists' involvement in drug use by the elderly. *Drug Intell. Clin. Pharm.*, **18**, 525–529
360. Kean, W. F. and Buchanan, W. W. (1987). Antirheumatic drug therapy in the elderly: a case of failure to identify the correct issues? *J. Am. Geriatr. Soc.*, **35**, 363–364
361. MacLennan, W. J. (1988). The ageing society. *Br. J. Hosp. Med.*, **39**, 112–120
362. Horrocks, P. The case for geriatric medicine as an age related specialty. In Isaacs, B. (ed.) *Recent Advances in Geriatric Medicine*, vol. 2, pp. 259–277. (Edinburgh: Churchill Livingstone)
363. Sheldrake, F. E., Webber, J. M. and Marsh, B. D. (1977). A long-term assessment of flurbiprofen. *Curr. Med. Res. Opin.*, **5**, 106–116
364. Rainsford, K. D. (1987). Mechanisms of gastric contrasted with intestinal damage by non-steroidal anti-inflammatory drugs. In Rainsford, K. D. and Velo, G. P. (eds.) *Side-effects of Anti-Inflammatory Drugs, Part 2, Studies in Major Organ Systems*, pp. 3–28. (Lancaster: MTP)
365. Hort, J. F. (1975). Adverse reactions to alclofenac. *Curr. Med. Res. Opin.*, **3**, 333
366. O'Brien, W. M. (1968). Indomethacin: a survey of clinical trials. *Clin. Pharmacol. Ther.*, **9**, 94–107
367. Williams, K. and Lee, E. (1985). Importance of drug enantiomers in clinical pharmacology. *Drugs*, **30**, 333–354
368. Lam, Y. W. F. (1988). Stereoselectivity: an issue of significant importance in clinical pharmacology. *Pharmacotherapy*, **8**, 147–157
369. Stastny, P. (1978). Association of the B cell alloantigen DRW4 with rheumatoid arthritis. *N. Engl. J. Med.*, **298**, 869–871
370. Panayi, G. S., Wooley, P. and Batchelor, J. R. (1978). Genetic basis of rheumatoid disease: HLA antigens, disease manifestations, and toxic reactions to drugs. *Br. Med. J.*, **2**, 1326–1238
371. Ford, P. M. (1984). HLA antigens and drug toxicity in rheumatoid arthritis. *J. Rheumatol.*, **11**, 259–261
372. McMichael, A. J., Sasazuki, T., McDevitt, H. O. and Payne, R. O. (1977). Increased frequency of HLA-CW3 and HLA-DW4 in rheumatoid arthritis. *Arthritis Rheum.*, **20**, 1037–1042
373. Wooley, P. H., Griffin, J., Panayi, G. S., Batchelor, J. R., Welsh, K. I. and Gibson, J. J. (1980). HLA-DR antigens and toxic reaction to sodium gold aurothiomalate and D-Penicillamine in patients with rheumatoid arthritis. *N. Engl. J. Med.*, **303**, 300–302
374. Bardin, T., Dryll, A., Debeyre, N., Ryckewaert, A., Legrand, L., Marcelli, A. and Daussett, J. (1982). HLA system and side effects of gold salts and D-Penicillamine treatment of rheumatoid arthritis. *Ann. Rheum. Dis.*, **41**, 599–601
375. Gran, J. T., Husby, G. and Thorsby, E. (1983). HLA-DR antigens and gold toxicity. *Ann. Rheum. Dis.*, **42**, 63–66
376. Speerstra, F., Reekers, P., van de Putte, L. B. A., Vandenbroucke, J. P., Rasker, J. J. and de Rooij, D. (1983). HLA-DR antigens and proteinuria induced by auro-

thioglucose and D-Penicillamine in patients with rheumatoid arthritis. *J. Rheumatol.*, **10**, 948–953
377. Bensen, W. G., Moore, N., Tugwell, P., D'Souza, M. and Singal, D. P. (1984). HLA antigens and toxic reactions to sodium aurothiomalate in patients with rheumatoid arthritis. *J. Rheumatol.*, **11**, 358–361
378. Scherak, O., Smolen, J. S. and Mayr, W. R. (1984). HLA antigens and toxicity to gold and penicillamine in rheumatoid arthritis. *J. Rheumatol.*, **11**, 610–614
379. Hakala, M., van Assendelft, A. H. W., Ilonen, J., Jalava, S. and Tiilikainen, A. (1986). Association of different HLA antigens with various toxic effects of gold salts in rheumatoid arthritis. *Ann. Rheum. Dis.*, **45**, 177–182
380. Tishler, M., Caspi, D., Gazit, E. and Yarom, M. (1988). Association of HLA-B35 with mucocutaneous lesions in Israeli patients with rheumatoid arthritis receiving gold treatment. *Ann. Rheum. Dis.*, **47**, 215–217
381. Billingsley, L. M. and Stevens, M. B. (1981). The relationship between D-Penicillamine-induced proteinuria and prior gold nephropathy. *Johns Hopkins Med. J.*, **148**, 64–67
382. Stein, H. B., Schroeder, M. L. and Dillon, A. M. (1986). Penicillamine induced proteinuria: risk factors. *Semin. Arthritis Rheum.*, **15**, 282–287
383. Stockman, A., Zilko, P. J., Major, G. A. C., Tait, B. D., Property, D. N., Mathews, J. D., Hannah, M. C., McCluskey, J. and Muirden, K. D. (1986). Genetic markers in rheumatoid arthritis. Relationship to toxicity from D-Penicillamine. *J. Rheumatol.*, **13**, 269–273
384. Barger, B. O., Acton, R. T., Koopman, W. J. and Alarcon, G. S. (1984). DR antigens and gold toxicity in white rheumatoid arthritis patients. *Arthritis Rheum.*, **27**, 601–605
385. Dequeker, J., Wanghe, P. V. and Verdickt, W. (1984). A systematic survey of HLA A, B, C and D antigens and drug toxicity in rheumatoid arthritis. *J. Rheumatol.*, **11**, 282–286
386. Gladman, D. D. and Anhorn, K. A. B. (1986). HLA and disease manifestations in rheumatoid arthritis: a Canadian experience. *J. Rheumatol.*, **13**, 274–276
387. Chales, G., Fauchet, R. and Pawlotsky, Y. (1983). Les determinants HLA-DR dans les rhumatismes inflammatoires croniques. *Rev. Rheum. Mal. Osteoartic.*, **50**, 525–531
388. Perrier, P., Raffoux, C., Thomas, Ph, Tamasier, J. N., Busson, M., Gaucher, A. and Streiff, F. (1985). HLA antigens and toxic reactions to sodium aurothio propanol sulphonate and D-Penicillamine in patients with rheumatoid arthritis. *Ann. Rheum. Dis.*, **44**, 621–624
389. Halla, J. T., Cassidy, J. and Hardin, J. G. (1982). Sequential gold and penicillamine therapy in rheumatoid arthritis. *Am. J. Med.*, **72**, 423–426
390. Barin, P. A., Tribe, C. R. and Mackenzie, J. C. (1976). Penicillamine nephropathy in rheumatoid arthritis. A clinical, pathological and immunological study. *Q. J. Med.*, **45**, 661–684
391. Howard-Lock, H. E., Lock, C. J. L., Mewa, A. and Kean, W. F. (1986). D-Penicillamine: chemistry and clinical use in rheumatic disease. *Semin. Arthritis Rheum.*, **15**, 261–281
392. Klouda, P. T., Manos, J. and Acheson, E. J. (1979). Strong association between idiopathic membranous nephropathy and HLA-DRW3. *Lancet*, **2**, 770–771
393. Cunningham, T. J., Tait, B. D. and Mathews, J. D. (1982). Clinical rheumatoid vasculitis associated with the B8 DR3 phenotype. *Rheumatol. Int.*, **2**, 137–139
394. Whittingham, S., Mathews, J. D. and Schanfield, M. S. (1983). HLA and Gm genes in systemic lupus erythematosus tissue. *Antigens*, **21**, 50–70
395. Mellman, I. (1988). Relationships between structure and function in the Fc receptor family. *Curr. Opin. Immunol.*, **1**, 16–25
396. Lawley, T. J., Hall, R. P. and Fauci, A. S. (1981). Defective Fc receptor functions associated with HLA-B8/DRW3 haplotype studies on patients with dermatitis herpetiformis and normal subjects. *N. Engl. J. Med.*, **304**, 185–192
397. Legrand, L., Rivat-Perran, L. and Huttin, C. (1982). HLA and Gm linked genes affecting the degradation rate of antigens (sheep red blood cells) endocytized by macrophages. *Human Immunol.*, **4**, 1–13

398. Saphir, J. R. and Ney, R. G. (1966). Delayed thrombocytopenic purpura after diminutive gold therapy. *J. Am. Med. Assoc.*, **195**, 782–784
399. Kay, A. C. L. (1976). Myelotoxicity of gold. *Br. Med. J.*, **1**, 266–268
400. Coblyn, J. S., Weinblatt, M., Hodsworth, D. and Glass, D. (1981). Gold-induced thrombocytopenia: a clinical and immunogenetic study of twenty-three patients. *Ann. Intern. Med.*, **95**, 178–181
401. Adachi, J. D., Benson, W. G., Singal, D. P. and Powers, P. J. (1984). Gold induced thrombocytopenia: platelet associated IgG and HLA typing in three patients. *J. Rheumatol.*, **11**, 355–357
402. Madhok, R., Pullar, T., Capell, H. A., Dawood, F., Sturrock, R. D. and Dick, H. M. (1985). Chrysotherapy and thrombocytopenia. *Ann. Rheum. Dis.*, **44**, 289–591
403. Adachi, J. D., Bensen, W. G., Kassam, Y., Powers, P. J., Bianchi, F. A., Cividino, A., Kean, W. F., Rooney, P. J., Craig, G. L., Buchanan, W. W., Tugwell, P. X., Gordon, D. A., Lucarelli, A. and Singal, D. P. (1987). Gold induced thrombocytopenia: 12 cases and a review of the literature. *Semin. Arthritis Rheum.*, **16**, 287–293
404. Moens, H. J. B., Ament, B. J. W., Feltkamp, B. W. and van der Korst, J. K. (1987). Longterm followup of treatment with D-Penicillamine for rheumatoid arthritis: effectivity and toxicity in relation to HLA antigens. *J. Rheumatol.*, **14**, 1115–1119
405. Camp, A. V. (1981). Hematologic toxicity from penicillamine in rheumatoid arthritis. *J. Rheumatol.*, **8** (suppl.), 164–165
406. Nusslein, H. G., Jahn, H., Losch, G., Guggenmoos-Holzmann, I., Leibold, W. and Kalden, J. R. (1984). Association of HLA-BW35 with mucocutaneous lesions in rheumatoid arthritis patients undergoing sodium aurothiomalate therapy. *Arthritis Rheum.*, **27**, 833–836
407. Tishler, M., Caspi, D., Rosenbach, T. O., Fishel, B., Wigler, I., Segal, R., Gazit, E. and Yaron, M. (1988). Methotrexate in rheumatoid arthritis: a prospective study in Israeli patients with immunogenetic correlations. *Ann. Rheum. Dis.*, **47**, 654–659
408. Alarcon, G. S., Koopman, W. J., Acton, R. T. and Barger, B. O. (1985). HLA-BW35 and gold toxicity in rheumatoid arthritis. *Arthritis Rheum.*, **28**, 236–237
409. Gran, J. T. and Husby, G. (1986). HLA-BW35 and mucocutaneous toxicity in rheumatoid arthritis treated with gold. (Letter). *Arthritis Rheum.*, **29**, 303
410. Aaron, S., Davis, P. and Bertouch, J. (1986). HLA-DR antigens in gold-induced neutropenia. *Arthritis Rheum.*, **29**, 1515–1517
411. Dinant, H. J., Muller, W. H., van den Berg-Loonen, E. M., Nijenhuis, L. E. and Engelfriet, C. O. (1980). HLA-DRW4 in Felty's syndrome. (Letter). *Arthritis Rheum.*, **23**, 1336
412. Friman, C., Schlaut, J. and Davis, P. (1985). HLA-DR4 in Felty's syndrome (Letter). *J. Rheumatol.*, **12**, 628–629
413. Garlepp, M. J., Dawkins, R. L. and Christiansen, F. T. (1983). HLA antigens and acetylcholine receptor antibodies in penicillamine induced myasthenia gravis. *Br. Med. J.*, **286**, 338–340
414. Pinals, R. S. (1988). Sulfasalazine in the rheumatic diseases. *Semin. Arthritis Rheum.*, **17**, 246–259
415. Tishler, M., Caspi, D., Rosenbach, T. O. *et al.* (1988). Methotrexate in rheumatoid arthritis: a prospective study in Israeli patents with immunogenetic correlations. *Ann. Rheum. Dis.*, **47**, 654–659
416. Gispen, J. G., Alarcon, G. S., Johnson, J. J., Acton, R. T., Barger, B. O. and Koopman, W. J. (1987). Toxicity to methotrexate in rheumatoid arthritis. *J. Rheumatol.*, **14**, 74–79
417. Schiff, B., Mizrahi, Y., Orgad, S., Yaron, M. and Gazit, E. (1982). Association of HLA-AW31 and HLA-DR1 with adult rheumatoid arthritis. *Ann. Rheum. Dis.*, **41**, 403–404
418. Karr, R. W., Rodey, G. E., Lee, T. and Schwartz, B. D. (1980). Association of HLA-DRW4 with rheumatoid arthritis in black and white patients. *Arthritis Rheum.*, **23**, 1241–1245
419. Drayer, D. E. and Reidenberg, M. M. (1977). Clinical consequences of polymorphic acetylation of basic drugs. *Clin. Pharmacol. Ther.*, **22**, 251–258

420. Clark, D. W. J. (1985). Genetically determined variability in acetylation and oxidation; therapeutic implications. *Drugs*, **29**, 342-375
421. Grant, D. M., Tang, B. K. and Kalow, W. (1984). A simple test for acetylator phenotype using caffeine. *Br. J. Clin. Pharmacol.*, **17**, 459-464
422. Perry, H. M. Jr, Tan, E. M., Cordody, S. and Sahamato, A. (1970). Relationship of acetyl transferase activity to antinuclear antibodies and toxic symptoms on hypertensive patients treated with hydralazine. *J. Lab. Clin. Med.*, **76**, 114-125
423. Perry, H. M., Jr. (1973). Late toxicity to hydralazine resembling systemic lupus erythematosus or rheumatoid arthritis. *Am. J. Med.*, **54**, 58-71
424. Harland, S. J., Facchini, V. and Timbrell, J. A. (1980). Hydralazine-induced systemic lupus-like syndrome in a patient of the rapid acetylator phenotype. *Br. Med. J.*, **281**, 273-274
425. Vandenberg, M. J., Wright, P., Holmes, J., Rogers, H. J. and Ahmad, R. A. (1982). The hypotensive response to hydralazine in triple therapy is not related to acetylator phenotype. *Br. J. Clin. Pharmacol.*, **13**, 747-750
426. Mansilla-Tinoco, R., Harland, S. J., Ryan, P. J. *et al.* (1982). Hydralazine antinuclear antibodies and the lupus syndrome. *Br. Med. J.*, **284**, 936-939
427. Batchelor, J. R., Welsh, K. J., Mansilla-Tinoco, R. *et al.* (1982). Hydralazine-induced systemic lupus erythematosus: influence of HLA-DR and sex on susceptibility. *Lancet*, **1**, 1107-1109
428. Woosley, R. L., Drayer, D. E., Reidenberg, M. M. *et al.* (1978). Effect of acetylator phenotype on the rate at which procainamide induced antinuclear antibodies and the lupus syndrome. *N. Engl. J. Med.*, **298**, 1157-1159
429. Sonnhag, C., Karlsson, E. and Hed, J. (1979). Procainamide-induced lupus erythematosus-like syndrome in relation to acetylator phenotype and plasma levels of procainamide. *Acta Med. Scand.*, **206**, 245-251
430. Lahita, R., Kluger, J., Dryer, D. E., Koffler, D. and Reidenberg, M. M. (1979). Antibodies to nuclear antigens in patients treated with procainamide or acetylprocainamide. *N. Engl. J. Med.*, **301**, 1382-1385
431. Farr, M., Scott, D. G. I. and Bacon, P. A. (1986). Side effect profile of 200 patients with inflammatory arthritis treated with sulphasalazine. *Drugs*, **32** (suppl. 1), 49-53
432. Martin, L., Sitar, D. S., Chalmers, I. M. and Hunter, T. (1985). Sulfasalazine in severe rheumatoid arthritis. A study to assess potential correlates of efficacy and toxicity. *J. Rheumatol.*, **12**, 270-273
433. Pullar, T., Hunter, J. A. and Capell, H. A. (1985). Effect of acetylator phenotype on efficacy and toxicity of sulphasalazine in rheumatoid arthritis. *Ann. Rheum. Dis.*, **44**, 831-837
434. Sharp, M. E., Wallace, S., Hindmarsh, K. W. and Brown, M. A. (1981). Acetylator phenotype and serum levels of sulphapyridine in patients with inflammatory bowel disease. *Eur. J. Clin. Pharmacol.*, **21**, 243-250
435. Bax, D. E., Greaves, M. S. and Amos, R. S. (1986). Sulphasalazine for rheumatoid arthritis: relationship between dose, acetylator phenotype and response to treatment. *Br. J. Rheumatol.*, **25**, 282-284
436. Chan, T. K., Todd, D. and Tso, S. C. (1976). Drug-induced hemolysis in glucose 6-phosphate dehydrogenase deficiency. *Br. Med. J.*, **2**, 1227
437. Glader, B. E. (1976). Evaluation of the hemolytic role of aspirin in glucose 6-phosphate dehydrogenase deficiency. *J. Pediatr.*, **89**, 1027
438. Sanford-Driscoll, M. and Knodel, L. C. (1986). Induction of hemolytic anemia by non-steroidal anti-inflammatory drugs. *Drug Intell. Clin. Pharm.*, **20**, 925-934
439. Colonna, P. (1981). Aspirin and glucose-6-phosphate dehydrogenase deficiency. Letter to the Editor. *Br. Med. J.*, **283**, 1189
440. Ayesh, R., Mitchell, S. C., Waring, R. H., Withrington, R. H., Seifert, M. H. and Smith, L. (1987). Sodium aurothiomalate toxicity and sulphoxidation capacity in rheumatoid arthritis patients. *Br. J. Rheumatol.*, **26**, 197-201
441. Roe, C. R. Metabolic disorders producing a Reye-like syndrome in *Reye's Syndrome. Round Table Symposium No. 8*. (London: Royal Society of Medicine)
442. Boston Collaborative Drug Surveillance Programme Adverse Drug Interactions. (1972). *J. Am. Med. Assoc.*, **220**, 1238-1239

443. Puckett, W. H. and Visconti, J. A. (1971). An epidemiologic study of the clinical significance of drug-drug interaction in a private community hospital. *Am. J. Hosp. Pharm.*, **28**, 247-253
444. Tonkin, A. L. and Wing, L. M. H. (1988). Interactions of non-steroidal anti-inflammatory drugs. *Baillière's Clin. Rheumatol.*, **2**, 455-483
445. Abramowicz, M. (ed.) (1981). Clinically established interactions with antirheumatic drugs. *Med. Lett.*, **23**, 17-28
446. Abramowicz, M. (ed.) (1984). Clinically established interactions with antirheumatic drugs. *Med. Lett.*, **26**, 11-14
447. Day, R. O., Graham, G. G., Champion, G. D. and Lee, E. (1984). Anti-rheumatic drug interactions. *Clin. Rheum. Dis.*, **10**, 251-257
448. McInnes, G. T. and Brodie, M. J. (1988). Drug interactions that matter. A critical reappraisal. *Drugs*, **36**, 83-110
449. Lee, P., Ahola, S. J., Grennan, D., Brooks, P. and Buchanan, W. W. (1974). Observations on drug prescribing in rheumatoid arthritis. *Br. Med. J.*, **1**, 424-426
450. Grennan, D. M., Karetai, M. and Palmer, D. G. (1977). Drug prescribing in rheumatoid arthritis in Otago. *N.Z. Med. J.*, **86**, 130-132
451. Rosenbloom, D. and Buchanan, W. W. (1983). Observations on written communications between physicians regarding patients' drug treatment compared to patients' recall. *Drug Intell. Clin. Pharm.*, **17**, 288-289
452. Muller, F. O., Fundt, H. K. L. and Muller, D. G. Pharmacokinetic and pharmacodynamic implications of long-term administration of non-steroidal anti-inflammatory agents. *Int. J. Clin. Pharmacol.*, **15**, 397-402
453. Tempero, K. F., Cirillo, V. J. and Steelman, S. L. (1978). Diflunisal: chemistry, toxicology, experimental and human pharmacology. In Huskisson, E. C. and Caldwell, A. S. D. (eds.) *Diflunisal, Royal Society of Medicine International Congress and Symposium Series No. 6*. pp. 1-18 (London: Academic Press and the Royal Society of Medicine)
454. Sloboda, A. E., Tolman, E. L., Osterberg, A. C. and Panagides, J. (1980). The pharmacological properties of fenbufen: a review. *Arzneimittel Forschung/Drug Res.*, **30**, 716-721
455. Rubin, A., Rodda, B. E., Warwick, P., Gruber, C. M., Jr. and Ridolfo, A. S. (1973). Interactions of aspirin with non-steroidal anti-inflammatory drugs in man. *Arthritis Rheum.*, **16**, 635-645
456. Brooks, P. M. and Khong, T. K. (1977). Flublindprofen-aspirin interaction: a double crossover study. *Curr. Med. Res. Opin.*, **5**, 53-57
457. Grennan, D. M., Ferry, D. G., Ashworth, M. E., Kenny, R. E. and MacKinnon, M. (1979). The aspirin-ibuprofen interaction in rheumatoid arthritis. *Br. J. Clin. Pharmacol.*, **8**, 497-503
458. Grace, E. M., Mewa, A. A. M., Sweeney, G. D., Rosenfeld, J. M., Darke, A. C. and Buchanan, W. W. (1986). Lowering of plasma isoxicam concentrations with acetylsalicylic acid. *J. Rheumatol.*, **13**, 1119-1121
459. Williams, R. L., Upton, R. A., Buskin, J. M. and Jones, R. M. (1981). Ketoprofen-aspirin interactions. *Clin. Pharmacol. Ther.*, **30**, 226-231
460. Segre, E. J., Chaplin, M., Forchelli, Runkel, R. and Sevelius, H. (1974). Naproxen-aspirin interactions in man. *Clin. Pharmacol. Ther.*, **15**, 374-379
461. Miller, D. R. (1981). Combination use of nonsteroidal anti-inflammatory drugs. *Drug Intell. Clin. Pharm.*, **15**, 3-7
462. Cressman, W. A., Wortham, G. F. and Plostnicks, J. (1976). Absorption and excretion of tolmetin in man. *Clin. Pharmacol. Ther.*, **19**, 224-233
463. Brooks, P. M., Walker, J. J., Bell, M. A., Buchanan, W. W. and Rhymer, A. R. (1975). Indomethacin-aspirin interaction: A clinical appraisal. *Br. Med. J.*, **3**, 69-71
464. Champion, G. D., Paulus, H. E. *et al.* (1972). The effect of aspirin in serum indomethacin. *Clin. Pharmacol. Ther.*, **13**, 239-244
465. Kwan, K. C., Breault, C. O., Davis, R. L. *et al.* (1978). Effects of concomitant aspirin administration on the pharmacokinetics of indomethacin in man. *J. Pharmacokin. Biopharm.*, **6**, 451-476

466. Hobbs, D. C. and Twomey, T. M. (1979). Piroxicam pharmacokinetics in man: aspirin and antacid interaction studies. *J. Clin. Pharmacol.*, **19**, 270-281
467. Bollet, A. J. (1985). Piroxicam serum levels in patients treated for rheumatic diseases. *Semin. Arthritis Rheum.*, **14**, 25-28
468. Garrett, R., Manthey, B., Vernon-Roberts, B. and Brooks, P. M. (1983). Assessment of non-steroidal anti-inflammatory drug combinations by the polyurethane sponge implantation model in the rat. *Ann. Rheum. Dis.*, **42**, 439-442
469. Palmer, D. R., Highton, J., Mackinnon, M. J. and Myers, D. B. (1985). Non-steroidal anti-inflammatory drugs in combination. Experimental observations. *Clin. Exp. Rheumatol.*, **3**, 111-116
470. Huskisson, E. C. (1979). Routine drug treatment of rheumatoid arthritis and other rheumatic diseases. *Clin. Rheum. Dis.*, **5**, 697-706
471. Morgan, J. and Furst, D. E. (1986). Implications of drug therapy in the elderly. *Clin. Rheum. Dis.*, **12**, 227-244
472. Wilkens, R. F. and Segre, E. J. (1976). Combination therapy with naproxen and aspirin in rheumatoid arthritis. *Arthritis Rheum.*, **19**, 677-682
473. Furst, D. E., Blocka, K., Cassell, S., Harris, E. R., Hirschberg, J. M., Josephson, N., Lachenbruch, P. A., Trimble, R. B. and Paulus, H. E. (1987). A controlled study of concurrent therapy with a nonacetylated salicylate and naproxen in rheumatoid arthritis. *Arthritis Rheum.*, **30**, 146-153
474. Graham, G. G., Champion, G. D., Day, R. O. and Paull, P. D. (1977). Patterns of plasma concentrations and urinary excretion of salicylate in rheumatoid arthritis. *Clin. Pharmacol. Ther.*, **22**, 410-420
475. Segre, E. J., Sevelius, H. and Varady, J. (1974). Effects of antacids on naproxen absorption. *N. Engl. J. Med.*, **291**, 582-583
476. Segre, E. J. Naprosyn metabolism in man. In Christie, E. A. (ed.) *Naprosyn in the Treatment of Rheumatic Diseases*. Proceedings of a Symposium; Maidenhead: Syntex, p. 11.
477. Dugal, R., Dupuis, C., Bertrand, M. and Gagnon, M. A. (1980). The effect of buffering on oxyphenbutazone absorption kinetics and systemic availability. *Biopharm. Drug Disp.*, **1**, 307-321
478. Loew, D. and Vinazzer, H. (1976). Dose dependent influence of acetylsalicylic acid on platelet functions and plasmatic coagulation factors. *Haemostasis*, **5**, 239-249
479. Rothschild, B. M. (1979). Hematologic perturbations associated with salicylate. *Clin. Pharmacol. Ther.*, **26**, 145-152
480. Dale, J., Myhre, E. and Loew, D. (1980). Bleeding during acetylsalicylic acid and anticoagulant therapy in patients with reduced platelet reactivity after aortic valve replacement. *Am. Heart J.*, **99**, 746-752
481. Chesebro, J. H. *et al.* (1983). Trial of combined warfarin plus dipyridamole or aspirin therapy in prosthetic heart valve replacement: Dangers of aspirin compared with dipyridamole. *Am. J. Cardiol.*, **51**, 1537-1541
482. Starr, K. J. and Petrie, J. C. (1972). Drug interactions in patients on long term anticoagulant and antihypertensive adrenergic neuron-blocking drugs. *Br. Med. J.*, **165**, 133-135
483. Breckenridge, A. M., Orme, M., Wesseling, H., Lewis, R. J. and Gibbons, R. (1974). Pharmacokinetics and pharmacodynamics of the enantiomers of warfarin in man. *Clin. Phamacol. Ther.*, **15**, 424-430
484. Lewis, R. J., Trager, W. F., Chan, K. C., Breckenridge, A. *et al.* (1974). Warfarin: stereochemical aspects of its metabolism and the interaction with phenylbutazone. *J. Clin. Invest.*, **53**, 1607-1617
485. O'Reilly, R. A., Trager, W. F., Motley, C. H., Howald, W. *et al.* (1980). Stereoselective interaction of phenyl-butazone with [^{12}C ^{13}C] warfarin pseudo racemates in man. *J. Clin. Invest.*, **65**, 746-753
486. Banefield, C., O'Reilly, R., Chan, S. M., Rowland, M. *et al.* (1983). Phenylbutazone-warfarin interactions in man: further stereochemical and metabolic considerations. *Br. J. Clin. Pharmacol.*, **16**, 669-675
487. Aggeler, P. M., O'Reilly, R. A., Leong, L. and Kowitz, P. E. (1967). Potentiation of anticoagulant effect of warfarin by phenylbutazone. *N. Engl. J. Med.*, **276**, 496-501

488. Toon, S. and Trager, W. F. (1984). Pharmacokinetic implications of stereoselective changes in plasma-protein binding: warfarin-sulfinpyrazone. *J. Pharm. Sci.*, **73**, 1671–1673
489. O'Reilly, R. A. (1982). Stereoselective interaction of sulphinpyrazone with racemic warfarin and its separated enantiomorphs in man. *Circulation*, **65**, 202–207
490. Orme, M., Breckenridge, A. and Coop, P. (1976). Warfarin and distalgesic interaction. *Br. Med. J.*, **1**, 200
491. Green, A. E., Hort, J. F. and Korn, H. E. T. (1977). Potentiation of warfarin by azapropazone. *Br. Med. J.*, **1**, 1532
492. Pullar, T. and Capell, H. A. (1983). Interaction between oral anticoagulant drugs and nonsteroidal anti-inflammatory agents: a review. *Scott. Med. J.*, **28**, 42–47
493. Goulston, N. K. and Cooke, A. R. (1968). Alcohol, aspirin and gastrointestinal bleeding. *Br. Med. J.*, **4**, 664–665
494. Needham, C. D., Kyle, J., Jones, P. F., Johnson, S. J. and Kerridge, D. F. (1971). Aspirin and alcohol in gastrointestinal haemorrhage. *Gut*, **12**, 819–821
495. Falaye, J. M. and Odutola, T. A. (1978). The economic potential and the role of aspirin and alcohol ingestion in relation to haematemesis and malaena. *Niger. Med. J.*, **8**, 526–530
496. Deykin, D., Janson, P. and McMahon, L. (1982). Ethanol potentiation of aspirin induced prolongation of bleeding time. *N. Engl. J. Med.*, **306**, 852–854
497. Tabakoff, B., Hoffman, P. L., Lee, J. M., Saito, T., Willard, B. and DeLeon-Jones, F. (1988). Differences in platelet enzyme activity between alcoholics and nonalcoholics. *N. Engl. J. Med.*, **318**, 134–139
498. Witzgall, H., Hirsch, F., Scherer, B. and Weber, P. C. (1982). Acute haemodynamic and hormonal effects of captopril are diminished by indomethacin. *Clin. Sci.*, **62**, 611–615
499. Slack, B. L., Warmer, M. E. and Keiser, H. R. (1978). The effect of prostaglandin synthetase inhibition on the action of hydralazine. *Circulation*, **58** (suppl. II), 21
500. Rubin, P., Jackson, G. and Blaschke, T. (1980). Studies on the clinical pharmacology of prazosin. II. The influence of indomethacin and of propranolol on the action and disposition of prazosin. *Br. J. Clin. Pharmacol.*, **10**, 33–39
501. Durao, V., Martins-Prata, M. and Goncalves, L. M. P. (1977). Modification of antihypertensive effect of β-adrenoreceptor-blocking agents by inhibition of endogenous prostaglandin synthesis. *Lancet*, **2**, 1005–1007
502. Watkins, J., Abbot, E. C., Hensby, C. N. *et al.* (1980). Attenuation of hypotensive effect of propranolal and thiazide diuretics by indomethacin. *Br. Med. J.*, **281**, 702–705
503. Salvetti, A. and Arzilli, F. (1982). Interaction between oxprenolol and indomethacin on blood pressure in essential hypertensive patients. *Eur. J. Clin. Pharmacol.*, **22**, 197–201
504. Sziegoleit, W., Rausch, J., Polak, G. Y. *et al.* (1982). Influence of acetylsalicylic acid on acute circulatory effects of the beta blocking agents pindolol and propranolol in humans. *Int. J. Clin. Ther. Toxicol.*, **20**, 423–430
505. Smith, S. R., Gibson, R., Bradley, D. and Kendall, M. J. (1983). Failure of indomethacin to modify β-adrenoceptor blockade. *Br. J. Clin. Pharmacol.*, **15**, 267–268
506. James, D. W., Cleland, L. G., Robinson, C. W. and Leonello, P. P. (1982). Reversible renal failure associated with treatment with a beta-adrenergic receptor blocking drug and nonsteroidal anti-inflammatory drugs. *Med. J. Aust.*, **1**, 232–235
507. Koopmans, P. P., Thien, T. H. and Gribnau, F. W. J. (1984). Influence of nonsteroidal anti-inflammatory drugs on diuretic treatment of mild to moderate essential hypertension. *Br. Med. J.*, **289**, 1492–1494
508. Brater, D. (1977). Interactions of probenecid and indomethacin on the diuretic effects of chlorothiazide in human volunteers. (Abstract). *Clin. Res.*, **25**, 268
509. Fanelli, G. M., Bohn, D. L., Camp, A. E. and Shun, W. K. (1980). Ability of indomethacin to modify hydro-chlorothiazide diuresis and natriuresis by the chimpanzee kidney. *J. Pharmacol. Exp. Ther.*, **213**, 596–599
510. Williams, R. L., Davies, R. O., Berman, R. S. *et al.* (1982). Hydro-chlorothiazide

pharmacokinetics and pharmacologic effect: the influence of indomethacin. *J. Clin. Pharmacol.*, **22**, 32–41
511. Patak, R., Mookerjee, B. K., Bentzel, D. J. et al. (1975). Antagonism of the effects of furosemide by indomethacin in normal and hypertensive man. *Prostaglandins*, **10**, 649–659
512. Planas, R., Arroyo, V., Rimolo, A. et al. (1983). Acetyl-salicylic acid suppresses the renal haemo-dipromine effect and reduces the diuretic action of furosemide in cirrhosis with ascites. *Gastroenterology*, **84**, 247–252
513. Frolich, J. C., Hollifield, J. W., Dormois, J. C. et al. (1976). Suppression of plasma renin activity by indomethacin in man. *Circulation Res.*, **39**, 447–452
514. Bartoli, E., Arras, S., Faedda, R. et al. (1980). Blunting of furosemide diuresis by aspirin in man. *J. Clin. Pharmacol.*, **20**, 452–458
515. Yeung-Laiwah, A. C. and Mactier, R. A. (1981). Antagonistic effect of non-steroidal anti-inflammatory drugs on frusemide-induced diuresis in cardiac failure. *Br. Med. J.*, **283**, 714
516. Chennavasin, T., Seiwell, R. and Brater, D. C. (1980). Pharmacokinetic-dynamic analysis of the indomethacin-furosemide interaction in man. *J. Pharmacol. Exp. Ther.*, **215**, 77–81
517. Tan, S. Y. and Mulrow, P. J. (1977). Inhibition of the renin-aldosterone response to furosemide by indomethacin. *J. Clin. Endocrinol. Metab.*, **45**, 174–176
518. Favre, L., Glasson, P. H., Riondel, A. and Vallotton, M. B. (1983). Interaction of diuretics and non-steroidal anti-inflammatory drugs in man. *Clin. Sci.*, **64**, 407–415
519. Hofman, L. M., Krupnick, M. I. and Garcia, H. A. (1972). Interactions of spironolactone and hydro-cholorothiazide with aspirin in the rat and dog. *J. Pharmacol. Exp. Ther.*, **180**, 1–5
520. Brooks, P. M., Bell, M. A., Lee, P. et al. (1974). The effect of frusemide and indomethacin plasma levels. *Br. J. Clin. Pharmacol.*, **1**, 485–489
521. Wong, D. G., Spence, J. D. and Lamki, L. (1986). Effect of non-steroidal anti-inflammatory drugs on control of hypertension by beta-blockers and diuretics. *Lancet*, **1**, 997–1001
522. Radack, K. and Deck, C. (1987). Do non-steroidal anti-inflammatory drugs interfere with blood pressure control in hypertensive patients? *J. Gen. Intern. Med.*, **2**, 108–112
523. Favre, L., Glasson, P. and Vallotton, M. B. (1982). Reversible acute renal failure from combined triamterene and indomethacin. *Ann. Intern. Med.*, **96**, 317–320
524. Webster, J. (1985). Interactions of NSAIDs with diuretic and β-blockers: mechanisms and clinical implications. *Drugs*, **30**, 32–41
525. Mandel, M. A. (1976). The synergistic effect of salicylates on methotrexate toxicity. *Plastic Reconstr. Surg.*, **57**, 733–737
526. Liegler, D. G., Henderson, E. S., Hahn, M. A. and Oliverio, V. T. (1969). The effect of organic acids on renal clearance of methotrexate in man. *Clin. Pharmacol. Ther.*, **10**, 849–857
527. Shen, D. D. and Azarnoff, D. L. (1978). Clinical pharmacokinetics of methotrexate. *Clin. Pharmacokin.*, **3**, 1–13
528. Ahern, M., Booth, M., Loxton, A. et al. (1988). Methotrexate kinetics in rheumatoid arthritis: is there an interaction with nonsteroidal anti-inflammatory drugs? *J. Rheumatol.*, **15**, 1356–1360
529. Adams, J. D. and Hunter, G. A. (1976). Drug interactions in psoriasis. *Aust. J., Dermatol.*, **17**, 39–40
530. Stockley, I. H. (1987). Methotrexate-NSAID interactions. *Drug Intell. Clin. Pharm.*, **21**, 546
531. Reiman, J. W. and Frolich, J. C. (1981). Effects of diclofenac on lithium kinetics. *Clin. Pharmacol. Ther.*, **30**, 348–352
532. Frolich, J. C., Leftwich, R., Ragheb, M., Oates, J. A., Reimann, I. and Buchanan, D. (1979). Indomethacin increases plasma lithium. *Br. Med. J.*, **1**, 1115–1116
533. Klinenberg, J. R. and Miller, F. (1965). Effects of corticosteroids on blood salicylate concentrations. *J. Am. Med. Assoc.*, **194**, 131–134
534. Muirden, K. D. and Barraclough, D. R. E. (1976). Drug interaction in the

management of rheumatoid arthritis. *Aust. N. Z. J. Med.*, **6** (suppl. 2), 14-17
535. Baer, P. A., Shore, A. and Ikeman, R. L. (1987). Transient fall in serum salicylate levels following intra-articular injection of steroid in patients with rheumatoid arthritis. *Arthritis Rheum.*, **30**, 345-347
536. Day, R. O., Harris, G., Brown, M. and Graham, G. (1983). Aspirin-glucocorticosteroid interaction in man. *Clin. Exp. Physiol. Pharmacol.*, **10**, 717 (Abstract)
537. Seino, Y., Usami, M., Nakahara, H., Takemura, J., Nishi, S., Ishida, H., Ideda, M. and Imura, H. (1982). Effect of acetyl salicylic acid on blood glucose and glucose regulatory hormones in mild diabetes. *Prostaglandins Leukotrienes Med.*, **8**, 49-53
538. Stowers, J. M., Constable, L. W. and Hunter, R. B. (1959). Clinical and pharmacological comparisons of chlorpropamide and other sulphonylureas. *Ann. N.Y. Acad. Sci.*, **74**, 698-695
539. Field, J. B., Ohta, M., Boyle, C. and Remer, A. (1967). Potentiation of acetohexamide hypoglycaemia by phenylbutazone. *N. Engl. J. Med.*, **277**, 407-415
540. Pond, S. M., Birkett, D. J. and Wade, D. N. (1977). Mechanisms of inhibitions of tolbutamide metabolism: phenylbutazone, oxyphenbutazone, sulphenazole. *Clin. Pharmacol. Ther.*, **22**, 573-579
541. Wilkerson, R. D. and Glenn, T. M. (1977). Influence of non-steroidal antiinflammatory drugs on ouabain toxicity. *Am. Heart. J.*, **9U**, 454-459
542. Andreasan, P. B., Froland, A., Skovsted, L. *et al.* (1973). Diphenylhydantoin half-life in man and its inhibition by phenylbutazone: the role of genetic factors. *Acta Med. Scand.*, **193**, 561-564
543. Fraser, D. G., Ludden, T. M., Evens, R. P. and Sutherland, E. W. (1980). Displacement of phenytoin from plasma binding sites by salicylate. *Clin. Pharmacol. Ther.*, **27**, 165-169
544. Leonard, R. F., Knott, P. J., Rankin, G. O. *et al.* (1981). Phenytoin-salicylate interaction. *Clin. Pharmacol. Ther.*, **29**, 56-60
545. Paxton, J. W. (1980). Effects of aspirin on salivary and serum phenytoin kinetics in healthy subjects. *Clin. Pharmacol. Ther.*, **27**, 170-178
546. Inoue, F. and Walsh, R. J. (1983). Folate supplements and phenytoin-salicylate interactions. *Neurology*, **33**, 115-116
547. Howes, C. A., Pullar, T. and Sourindhrin, I. (1983). Reduced steady-state plasma concentrations of chlorpromazine and indomethacin in patients receiving cimetidine. *Eur. J. Clin. Pharmacol.*, **24**, 99-102
548. Holford, N. H. G., Altman, D., Riegelman, S. *et al.* (1981). Pharmacokinetic and pharmacodynamic study of cimetidine administered with naproxen. (Abstract). *Clin. Pharmacol. Ther.*, **29**, 251-252
549. Gutman, A. B., Yu, T. F. and Sirota, J. H. (1955). A study by simultaneous clearance techniques of salicylate excretion in man. Effect of alkalinization of the urine by bicarbonate administration: effect of probenecid. *J. Clin. Invest.*, **34**, 711-721
550. Yu, T. F. and Perel, J. (1980). Pharmacokinetic and clinical studies of carprofen in gout. *J. Clin. Pharmacol.*, **20**, 347-351
551. Meffin, P. J., Veenendahl, J. R. and Brooks, P. M. (1981). Diflunisal-probenecid interaction: Michaelis-Menten kinetics with competitive inhibition. *Int. Congr. Pharmacol. Tokyo*, Abstract 0-8
552. Brooks, P. M., Bell, M. A., Sturrock, R. D., Famaey, J. P. and Dick, W. C. (1974). The clinical significance of indomethacin-probenecid interaction. *Br. J. Clin. Pharmacol.*, **1**, 287-290
553. Baber, N., Halliday, L., Sibeon, R. *et al.* (1978). The interaction between indomethacin and probenecid: a clinical and pharmacokinetic study. *Clin. Pharmacol. Ther.*, **24**, 298-306
554. Upton, R. A., Williams, R. L., Buskin, N. H. and Jones, R. M. (1980). Effects of probenecid on ketoprofen kinetics. *Clin. Pharmacol. Ther.*, **31**, 705-712
555. Runkel, R., Mroszczak, E., Chaplin, M., Sevelius, H. and Segre, E. (1978). Naproxen-probenecid interaction. *Clin. Pharmacol. Ther.*, **25**, 706-713
556. Brooks, P. M., Buchanan, W. W., Grove, M. and Downie, W. W. (1976). Effects of enzyme induction on the metabolism of prednisolone. *Ann. Rheum. Dis.*, **35**, 339-343

557. Petereit, M. S. and Meikle, A. W. (1977). Effectiveness of prednisolone during phenytoin therapy. *Clin. Pharmacol. Ther.*, **22**, 912–916
558. Jubiz, W. and Meikle, A. W. (1979). Alterations of glucocorticoid actions by other drugs and disease states. *Drugs*, **18**, 113–121
559. Steinberg, A. D. (1986). The treatment of lupus nephritis. *Kidney Int.*, **30**, 769–787
560. Faber, O. K., Mouridsen, H. T. and Skovstein, L. (1974). The biotransformation of cyclophosphamide in man: influence of prednisone. *Acta Pharm. Toxicol.*, **35**, 195–200
561. Kean, W. F., Lock, C. J. L., Howard-Locke, H. E. and Buchanan, W. W. (1982). Prior gold therapy does not influence the adverse effects of D-Penicillamine in rheumatoid arthritis. *Arthritis Rheum.*, **25**, 917–922
562. Champion, G. D., Sambrook, P. N., Brown, C. D. *et al.* Influence of previous gold on D-Penicillamine toxicity. In Dawkins, R. L., Christiansen, F. T. and Zilko, P. J. (eds.) *Immunogenetics in Rheumatology: Musculoskeletal Disease and D-Penicillamine*, pp. 311–315. (Amsterdam: Excerpta Medica)
563. Farr, M., Kitas, G. and Bacon, P. A. (1988). Sulphasalazine in rheumatoid arthritis: combination therapy with D-Penicillamine or sodium aurothiomalate. *Clin. Rheumatol.*, **7**, 242–248
564. Osman, M. A., Patel, R. B., Schuna, A. *et al.* (1983). Reduction in oral penicillamine absorption by food, antacid and ferrous sulphate. *Clin. Pharmacol. Ther.*, **33**, 465–470
565. Harkness, J. A. L. and Blake, D. R. (1982). Penicillamine nephropathy and iron. *Lancet*, **2**, 1368–1369
566. Lyle, W. H., Pearcey, D. F. and Jui, M. (1977). Inhibition of penicillamine-induced cupruresis by oral iron. *Proc. Roy. Soc. Med.*, **70** (suppl. 3), 48–49
567. Maricic, M., Davis, M. and Gall, E. P. (1986). Megaloblastic pancytopenia in a patient receiving concurrent methotrexate and trimethoprim-sulfamethoxazole treatment. *Arthritis Rheum.*, **29**, 133–135
568. Thomas, M. H. and Gutterman, L. A. (1986). Methotrexate toxicity in a patient receiving trimethoprim-sulfamethoxazole. *Arthritis Rheum.*, **13**, 440–441
569. El-Ghobarey, A. F., Mavrikakis, M. E., Macleod, M. E. *et al.* (1978). Clinical and laboratory studies of levamisole in patients with rheumatoid arthritis. *Q. J. Med.*, **67**, 385–400
570. Kelley, W. N. (1975). Effects of drugs on uric acid in man. *Ann. Rev. Pharmacol. Toxicol.*, **15**, 327–350
571. Elion, G. B. Allopurinol and other inhibitors of urate synthesis. In Kelly, W. N. and Weiner, I. M. (eds.) *Handbook of Experimental Pharmacology*, pp. 485–514 (Berlin: Springer-Verlag)
572. Calabresi, P. and Parks, R. E. Chemotherapy of neoplastic diseases. In Gilman, A. G., Goodman, L. S. and Gilman, A. (eds.) *The Pharmacological Basis of Therapeutics*, pp. 1249–1313 (New York: Macmillan)
573. Bagley, C. M., Bostick, F. W. and De Vita, V. T. (1973). Clinical pharmacology of cyclophosphamide. *Cancer Res.*, **33**, 226–233
574. Boston Collaborative Drug Surveillance Program. (1974). Allopurinol and cytotoxic drugs. Interaction in relation to bone marrow suppression. *J. Am. Med. Assoc.*, **227**, 1036–1040
575. Lyon, G. M. (1974). Allopurinol and cytotoxic agents. *J. Am. Med. Assoc.*, **228**, 1371–?
576. Rawlins, M. S. and Smith, S. E. (1973). Influence of allopurinol on drug metabolism in man. *Br. J. Pharmacol.*, **48**, 693–698
577. Manfredi, R. and Vesell, E. S. (1981). Inhibition of theophylline metabolism by long term allopurinol administration. *Clin. Pharmacol. Ther.*, **29**, 224–229
578. Vozeh, S., Powell, J. R. and Cupit, G. C. (1980). Influence of allopurinol on theophylline disposition in adults. *Clin. Pharmacol. Ther.*, **27**, 194–197
579. Horwitz, D., Thorgeirsson, S. S. and Mitchell, J. R. (1977). The influence of allopurinol and size of dose on the metabolism of phenylbutazone in patients with gout. *Eur. J. Clin. Pharmacol.*, **12**, 133–136
580. Boston Collaborative Drug Surveillance Program (1972). Excess of ampicillin rashes associated with allopurinol on hyperuricemia. *N. Engl. J. Med.*, **286**, 505–507
581. Aherne, G. W., Piall, E. M., Marks, V. *et al.* (1978), Prolongation and enhancement of serum methotrexate concentrations by probenecid. *Br. Med. J.*, **1**, 1097–1099

582. Brater, D. C. (1978). Increase in diuretic effect of chlorothiazide by probenecid. *Clin. Pharmacol. Ther.*, **23**, 259-265
583. Homeida, M., Roberts, C. and Branch, R. A. (1977). Influence of probenecid kinetics and dynamics in man. *Clin. Pharmacol. Ther.*, **22**, 402-409
584. Tjandramarga, T. B., Cucinell, S. A., Israil, Z. H. *et al.* (1972). Observations in the disposition of probenecid in patients receiving allopurinol. *Pharmacology*, **8**, 259-272
585. Perel, J. M., Dayton, P. G., Snell, M. M. *et al.* (1969). Studies of interactions among drugs in man at the renal level: probenecid and sulfinpyrazone. *Clin. Pharmacol. Ther.*, **10**, 834-840
586. Pascale, L. R., Dubin, A., Bronsky, D. and Hoffman, W. S. (1955). Inhibition of the uricosuric action of Benemid by salicylate. *J. Lab. Clin. Med.*, **45**, 771-777
587. Yu, T. F., Dayton, P. G. and Gutman, A. B. (1963). Mutual suppression of the uricosuric effects of sulfinpyrazone and salicylate. A study in interactions between drugs. *J. Clin. Invest.*, **42**, 1330-1339
588. Brooks, C. D. and Ulrich, J. E. (1980). Effect of ibuprofen or aspirin on probenecid-induced uricosuria. *J. Int. Med. Res.*, **8**, 283-285
589. Thompson, P. L. and Serjeant, C. (1981). Potentially serious interaction of warfarin with sulphinpyrazone. *Med. J. Aust.*, **1**, 41
590. Miners, J. O., Foenander, T., Wanwimolruk, S. *et al.* (1982). Interactions of sulphinpyrazone with warfarin. *Eur. J. Clin. Pharmacol.*, **22**, 327-331
591. Miners, J. O., Foenander, T., Wanwimolruk, S. *et al.* (1982). The effect of sulphinpyrazone on oxidative drug metabolism in man: inhibition of tolbutamide elimination. *Eur. J. Clin. Pharmacol.*, **22**, 321-326

18
Prediction of organ system toxicity with antirheumatic drug therapy

W. W. BUCHANAN and P. M. BROOKS

"Tripas llevan, que no pies a Tripas"
Cervantes (1547-1616), *Don Quixote*, Part II, Chapter IV.

Adverse reactions to antirheumatic drugs occur in every organ system in the body, especially common being those affecting the gastrointestinal tract and skin[1]. In recent years, there has been enormous interest in the effects of NSAIDs on the gastrointestinal tract[2] and a whole industry of cytoprotection has evolved to combat these effects[3,4]. The purpose of this chapter is to critically review the evidence of adverse drug reactions on the gastrointestinal tract, liver, and kidneys and to attempt to determine whether such side-effects can be predicted.

GASTROINTESTINAL SYSTEM

The effects of antirheumatic drugs on the gastrointestinal tract can be broadly classified into four main groups.

1. Dyspepsia
2. Microbleeding
3. Acute gastrointestinal haemorrhage and perforation
4. Miscellaneous

Dyspepsia

Of these, dyspepsia is by far the most common if not the most serious. The incidence of dyspepsia varies in different series but can be as high as 60% depending on whether the symptoms are elicited specifically or whether general questions are asked[5-11]. Some 5-15% of patients with rheumatoid arthritis can be expected to discontinue

NSAID therapy because of dyspepsia within a 6-month period[12-16]. Dyspepsia, due to salicylate therapy, is dose-related[17], but does not correlate with salicylate blood concentrations[18]. Dyspepsia is not a reliable predictor of mucosal damage at endoscopy or of microbleeding[4,7,9,19-29] and is not related to the presence of *Helicobacter pylori*[26,29]. Patients who are elderly[30] and have a past history of peptic ulcer[31] appear, however, to have an increased incidence of dyspepsia. Suggestion may also play an important role, since dyspepsia can occur with placebo[32,33]. No clinically significant differences appear to exist in the incidence of dyspepsia with different chemical classes of NSAIDs[24]. Enteric-coated preparations and suppositories have been claimed to reduce dyspepsia[34] but this is not always the case as indomethacin suppositories[35] still produce this symptom, perhaps because of a central effect[36]. Sustained release preparations of indomethacin similarly do not decrease dyspepsia[37], perhaps owing to the enterohepatic circulation of the drug[38]. Buffered aspirin is associated with the same incidence of dyspepsia as occurs with plain tablets[39,40]. Choline magnesium trisalicylate and choline salicylate are associated with less dyspepsia[41], but many patients find the taste of the latter unacceptable for long-term use[42]. It should be noted that enteric-coated preparations have in general a lower peak plasma concentration (CMax) than plain tablets, although a similar area under concentration curve (AUC)[43], but appear just as effective in the treatment of chronic inflammatory joint disease. Enteric-coated preparations need to be used carefully in elderly patients, where gastric stasis may lead to delayed passage of tablets from the stomach with subsequent release of toxic doses of the drug[44]. Taking medication with food or alkali is often recommended to reduce dyspepsia, but there is no published evidence to support this[32].

Recent studies have shown that cimetidine[45,46], misoprostol[17] and sucralfate[47] relieve NSAID-induced dyspepsia, but more extensive studies over longer periods of time will be required to show whether this is cost-effective. It is not possible to predict which patients will develop dyspepsia when prescribed salicylates or other NSAIDs. Although there is no proof that acetylsalicylic acid causes any more dyspepsia than any of the newer NSAIDs, there is an increasing move away from aspirin as the NSAID of choice for patients with rheumatoid arthritis[48].

Dyspepsia is common in patients on oral corticosteroids, especially when high doses are used[49]. This dyspepsia is associated with very little or no gastric mucosal abnormalities as demonstrated by endoscopy[7,50-52] and no increase in gastric microbleeding[53]. Lockie *et al.*[54] observed that only 1 of 97 patients with rheumatoid arthritis over 60 years of age treated with low-dose prednisolone (average 5–7.5 mg/day) had to stop therapy because of gastric symptoms.

D-Penicillamine has been reported to cause a high incidence of gastrointestinal complaints, especially at the beginning of therapy[55,56], although these symptoms may also occur later[57]. It should, however, be noted that patients on clinical trials treated with placebo also develop a high incidence of dyspepsia, making the findings with D-penicillamine difficult to evaluate[58,59]. Dyspepsia rarely requires D-penicillamine therapy to be discontinued, and usually responds to reduction in dose, taking the tablets with meals, or administering them with alkali[57,60]. Chrysotherapy is seldom stopped because of dyspepsia[60] but between 10% and 20% of patients on sulfasalazine cease the drug because of gastrointestinal symptoms[60-64]. Hydroxychloroquine is associated with gastrointestinal symptoms in approximately 10% of patients, which is significantly less than with chloroquine[65,66]. Anorexia, nausea, and vomiting are common side-effects, occurring in approximately one-third to two-thirds of patients with rheumatoid arthritis treated with methotrexate, but usually respond to manipulation of the dosing regimen or to adding antacids[67]. The same symptoms are occasionally problems in patients with rheumatoid arthritis treated with azathioprine[68]. These symptoms usually occur within the first few weeks of beginning therapy and are not dose-related. Nausea and vomiting are common in cyclophosphamide-treated patients and are not influenced by the route of administration[69]. The onset of nausea coincides with the peak of plasma concentration of phosphoramide mustard[70]. Cyclosporin, a relatively recent treatment for rheumatoid arthritis, also produces a significant incidence of nausea and other gastrointestinal side-effects.

But the question is, can dyspepsia as a result of these drug therapies be predicted? Certainly, the choice of drug is an important determinant — a low incidence of dyspepsia with chrysotherapy, but a relatively high incidence with Salazopyrin. A patient with a past history or with an active peptic ulcer certainly can be expected to have an increased likelihood of dyspepsia when treated with salicylates or with other NSAIDs[31]. Patients with rheumatoid arthritis who are slow acetylators are more prone to develop anorexia, nausea, and vomiting, but the association is not strong enough to allow prediction in individual patients. There is no evidence that patients with different rheumatic diseases have a different incidence of dyspepsia[11].

Gastric mucosal damage and microbleeding

The ability of the gastric mucosa to defend itself against acid injury is still incompletely understood[4,11,71-72], although a number of different mechanisms have been identified, including a mucous bicarbonate layer and absorbed layer of phospholipids covering the epithelial surface and a rich blood supply[73-79]. The role of prostaglandins as cytoprotective agents, first suggested by Sir John Vane[80], has been amply demonstrated. The prostaglandins of the 'E' series have been shown to increase the synthesis of mucus and bicarbonates, increase the thickness of mucous gel, increase the surface hydrophilicity of the gastric mucosa by increasing surface active phospholipids, and increase mucosal blood flow while diminishing acid and pepsin[81,82,98]. Since prostaglandins are inhibited by salicylates and other NSAIDs[96-99] it is not difficult to see why the latter may have the opposite effect, and why misoprostol, a prostaglandin 'E' analog, has been found to protect the gastric mucosa against these drugs[17,100-109]. However, several workers have noted no correlation between suppression of mucosal concentrations of prostaglandins and gastric lesions induced by NSAIDs[79,95,110-113]. This has led to the suggestion that the consequences of NSAID therapy may divert arachidonate through the lipoxygenase pathway[114,115] or that prostaglandins may act largely by facilitating repair of the damaged mucosa[116-118]. Administration of prostaglandin analogs is complicated by a high incidence of diarrhea and gastric hyperplasia[119] with the potential for neoplastic change[4]. The concept that gastric mucosal damage by NSAIDs is solely due to inhibition of cyclooxygenase is too simple[72,79,113] and other factors need to be taken into account.

Hydrochloric acid is important in the pathogenesis of gastric damage by back-diffusion of hydrogen irons into the mucosal cells. For example, patients who suffer from achlorhydria have less microbleeding when exposed to acetylsalicylic acid[120,121]. It might, therefore, be expected that cimetidine and ranitidine would prevent NSAID-induced gastric erosions and this indeed appears to be so[26,45,46,122-133], although Roth et al.[134] found little evidence for this in a double-blind trial of cimetidine, and Lanza et al.[106] found protection only for duodenal lesions with ranitidine. Bijlsma[45], however, found in his study that 12% of patients had a relapse of gastric ulceration when cimetidine was discontinued, which is approximately the same as with uncomplicated peptic ulcer. Sucralfate, a nonabsorbable basic aluminum salt of sucrose octasulfate, has also been found to be effective in treating aspirin-induced gastric lesions[47,135,137], although Lanza et al.[107] found it less effective than misoprostol. Concern has been raised regarding aluminum toxicity with long-term use of sucralfate[4] but to date none has been reported.

Acute gastric mucosal lesions have been reported in nearly 100% of patients who are administered acetylsalicylic acid (ASA) orally[138-141]. These lesions consist of erythema, hemorrhage, shallow erosions 1–2 mm in diameter, and ulcers greater than 0.5 cm in diameter that penetrate the mucosal layer. These lesions, especially hemorrhages, may occur within minutes of ingestion, especially if the patient is fasting, although erosions and ulcers usually take several hours to develop[139]. If no further ASA is administered, the gastric mucosa returns to normal within a week, while erosions and ulcers may take longer to heal[2,23,139,141,142]. Patients who are receiving long-term salicylate therapy have been found to have a high incidence of gastric erosions and ulcers[7,19,143]. However, approximately 20% of normal subjects not receiving salicylates or other NSAIDs have gastric mucosal lesions on endoscopy[19,144,145]. ASA appears to cause more severe and extensive lesions than other NSAIDs[7,9,32,146-150], although Larkai et al.[27] did not confirm this. The greater the dose of ASA or NSAID the more the mucosal damage[23,148,149,151], although again some groups[11] would dispute this. There is some evidence for an additive effect on gastric mucosal damage where two or more NSAIDs are administered concurrently[7,124,152,153]. All NSAIDs produce gastric mucosal lesions[7,9,11,19,146,147,154-161], no one chemical class has been shown clearly to be less injurious[24]. Acetaminophen does not, however, cause gastric mucosal damage[162] despite the fact that it reduces mucosal prostaglandins[88,163] and is frequently taken by patients who have gastrointestinal haemorrhage[164]. Acetaminophen does not have an additive effect with ASA[165] and indeed has been claimed by at least one group[166] to be cytoprotective against ASA.

Enteric-coated ASA, and buffered or nonacetylated salicylates have been reported to cause less gastric mucosal damage[7,19,167-175], although Mitchell et al.[176] found gastric mucosal cell exfoliation greater with choline magnesium trisalicylate than plain ASA. Toxicity with enteric-coated and slow-release preparations of newer NSAIDs has also been claimed to be less in terms of gastric mucosal damage[9,10,35,74,148,149,156,157,176-181]. The prodrug, sulindac, was found by Graham et al.[10] not to produce mucosal injury, but studies in patients with arthritis treated over a period of time indicate significant degrees of ulceration similar to other NSAIDs[7,85,182]. Whether the same will hold true for etodolac and carprofen, which have also been found to be free from gastric toxicity in the short term[179,181], remains to be seen. Although in general newer slow-release preparations of NSAIDs have proven less toxic to the gastric mucosa than standard preparations, exceptions have been noted. Thus, a controlled-release preparation of indomethacin produced more microbleeding than the standard preparation[150] and a slow-release formulation of ketoprofen produced more gastric mucosal damage as detected by endoscopy than standard ketoprofen[183]. Intravenous ASA has been reported to have little or no effect on gastric mucosa[184]. Indomethacin suppositories have been reported to produce less gastric injury than the same dose given orally and with essentially similar blood concentrations[35], but a study by Hansen et al.[185] using a higher dose of indomethacin failed to support this finding.

Although ASA and other NSAIDs have been reported to cause gastric ulceration, small duodenal ulcers have also been observed at endoscopy[27,102,139,167,186] even after 24 hours[162]. It is interesting to speculate whether these drugs, especially ASA, might cause duodenal ulcer. ASA has been implicated particularly in eastern Australia, as a cause of gastric ulcer, especially in females[118,143,144,187-198], perhaps due to a failure of mucosal adaptation[199-203]. This refers to the phenomenon whereby mucosal repair occurs despite continuation of ASA or NSAID therapy. This process may be due to mucosal cells being replaced by a younger and more resistant population of cells[200], an event similar to the shedding of renal tubular cells lasting 10–14 days after ASA ingestion[204]. It should be noted that not all workers have found evidence of this phenomenon[175]. Gastric ulcers induced by salicylates or NSAIDs are usually situated at the antrum and surrounded by normal mucosa, whereas benign gastric ulcers arising de novo are usually present in the body of the stomach and surrounded by mucosa affected with chronic gastritis[165,190,192]. Peptic ulcers, both gastric and duodenal, in patients receiving salicylates and NSAIDs and even oral corticosteroids do not have any significant delay in healing[123,198,205-210], nor indeed in the recurrence rate[211].

Whether oral corticosteroid therapy causes gastric mucosal damage, and in particular peptic ulcers, remains a matter of debate[190,212-215]. In an extensive and critical review, Conn and Blitzer[212] came to the conclusion that oral corticosteroids did not cause peptic ulcer unless prescribed for longer than 30 days or in a total dose exceeding 1 g of prednisolone or equivalent. Messer et al.[213], on the other hand, concluded that oral corticosteroid therapy in those doses did increase the risk of peptic ulceration and hemorrhage. Gastroscopy after 6 days of 1 g/day prednisolone intravenously revealed no mucosal damage[216] and Caruso and Porro[7] found gastric mucosal damage in only 3 of 21 patients (14%) with rheumatoid arthritis receiving oral corticosteroid therapy, compared to 13 of 26 (50%) who were receiving ASA. Oral corticosteroids do not increase gastric microbleeding[217] and some studies have even shown low-dose oral corticosteroid therapy to be cytoprotective in both animals and man. However, steroids do potentiate the toxic effects of ASA and NSAIDs[212,218,219]. If, indeed, oral corticosteroids do lead to gastric mucosal injury when taken with ASA or NSAIDs, the question remains as to the mechanism. Conceivably, oral corticosteroids may cause a reduction in gastric mucus production[216] or interfere with gastric membrane repair[11]. However, as previously mentioned, the rate of healing of peptic ulcers in patients receiving oral corticosteroid therapy is not impaired[206]. There is no evidence that slow-acting antirheumatic drugs either cause or exacerbate peptic ulcer disease[220].

Microbleeding as a result of aspirin or NSAID ingestion has been determined both by tests for occult blood in the stools and by the amount of radioactive chromium-51 labeled red cells in stool samples[221]. Using the latter technique, normal subjects have been found to lose between 0.5 and 2 ml of blood per day in their stools[222]. Up to 3 ml/day is regarded as being clinically insignificant, since the gastrointestinal tract can compensate by increasing the normal uptake of iron beyond 1-2 mg per day. However, when blood loss is of the order of 10 ml/day or more, iron deficiency anemia will occur[223]. High doses of ASA frequently lead to more than 4 ml of blood loss per day as determined by the chromium-51 labeled erythrocyte method[33], and some patients on chronic aspirin therapy may lose in excess of 10 ml/day. Although the intraindividual variation in the amount of blood loss is low[223-226] the interindividual variation is high, and it appears to be those patients who consistently lose excessive amounts of blood in their stools who are liable to develop anemia[227,245,246]. The amount of blood loss with aspirin is dose-related[228] and can be reduced by large doses of alkali[229,230], or by using enteric coated[231] or nonacetylated salicylates rather than plain aspirin[232-236]. All the NSAIDs are associated with less bleeding than aspirin[11,150,237,238].

Sustained-release formulations of NSAIDs have not always been found to cause less bleeding than standard preparations[237] although other workers have reported that they do[239]. More surprisingly, the elderly have been found to have less blood loss with aspirin than younger patients[228,240], which may be due to the high incidence of chronic atrophic gastritis and hypochlorhydria in elderly persons, including those with rheumatoid arthritis[241], since the lower the gastric intraluminal pH the higher the risk of bleeding[162]. The magnitude of microbleeding does not always correlate with dyspepsia[224] or endoscopic findings[237,241a] and is not predictive of acute gastrointestinal hemorrhage[241b]. Human gastric mucosal bleeding induced by ASA is not due to a defect in hemostasis, since the same does not occur with warfarin[242] and cannot be reduced by a hemostatic agent such as ethamsylate[243]. Patients with rheumatoid arthritis have recently been shown by Weber et al.[244] to have decreased iron absorption, especially when their disease is active. One might, therefore, expect iron deficiency to be common in patients with RA treated with aspirin therapy but, surprisingly, this is not so.

Fecal chromium loss can be augmented by hepatobiliary chromium transport, i.e., secretion into the bile[247,248], and salicylates, both acetylated and nonacetylated, have been shown to increase the flow rate of bile[249]. So far, these potentially confounding factors have not been taken into account in any of the studies on microbleeding.

Acute gastrointestinal hemorrhage and perforation

There is perhaps no more controversial area in medicine than the risk of acute gastrointestinal (GI) hemorrhage or perforation as a result of ASA or NSAID medication[2,11,164,197,250]. The incidence of major GI hemorrhage and perforation is low in comparison to the number of prescriptions issued[2,251-254] but nevertheless it has been reported with even small doses of ASA[255,256]. Faulkner et al.[254] considered that elderly patients who had taken ASA were between two and three times more likely to be admitted to hospital with acute GI hemorrhage. However, the true incidence of major GI hemorrhage is impossible to assess from anecdotal reports in uncontrolled studies[257-259] or even from spontaneous reporting systems[11,33,260]. The true incidence cannot be obtained from voluntary reporting systems, since only a small proportion of adverse effects are reported[115,260]. Furthermore, the "Weber" effect[261-263], whereby the number of adverse reactions reported spontaneously for the first two years after the release of a new drug is high, might bias the results, such as occurred with piroxicam[253,259,264]. Moreover, patients with dyspepsia or with peptic ulcer disease are more likely to be prescribed acetaminophen or one of the newer NSAIDs, so giving rise to the false conclusion that they are particularly prone to acute GI hemorrhage[164,195,210,211,265-268]. A number of pharmacoepidemiologic studies have been reported on the subject, including several prospective and retrospective cohort studies[269,273] and record linkage studies[182,252]. These studies have been critically reviewed[277,278] and the difficulties of interpretation discussed[280]. The conclusions reached have varied from finding no proof of any association[281,282] to cautious admission that such might exist[182,277], or unequivocal acceptance by the majority of authors[118,177,182,196,198,226,250,251,265,269,270,274,283-289]. Parry and Wood[226] observed that rechallenge with ASA did not lead to further hemorrhage. In a prospective study of 2400 patients with rheumatoid arthritis followed for an average of 3.5 years, Fries et al.[250] identified the following risk factors for acute gastrointestinal hemorrhage — age, female sex, history of previous upper abdominal pain requiring stopping NSAIDs or previous use of antacids or H2 receptor antagonists, and concurrent corticosteroid therapy. Fries and his colleagues[250] were careful to point out that their analysis was univariate, and as the variables were interdependent it was not possible to determine the relative importance of the risk factors. Their hazard ratio for "gastrointestinal" hospitalization was calculated at 6.45 times that of patients not on NSAIDs, which is certainly higher than that estimated by other workers[251-254,285]. There is a large corpus of evidence to confirm the opinion of Fries et al.[250] that the elderly are particularly prone to both acute gastrointestinal bleeding[7,11,118,144,177,182,195,226,254,261,269-272,276,280,285,290-302] and perforation[269,271,291,303]. Most authors agree with Fries et al.[250] that females are at greater risk, but Parry and Wood[226] and, more recently, Llewellyn and Pritchard[299] considered males more vulnerable to these complications. The mortality from both hemorrhage and perforation is considerable in the elderly[269,304,305] and these complications may not be preceded by any symptoms[182,268,269,271,272,295], which indeed Skander and Ryan[301] have emphasized may be masked by the NSAID. It should be noted, however, that not all authors have found age a hazard with ASA or NSAID therapy[251,275,306-308]. The problem is in the definition of the elderly — there is a considerable difference in healthy subjects who have reached their seventies and frail old ladies in long-care institutions[309].

Interestingly, saliva contains both mucus and bicarbonate as well as epidermal growth factor[310], which has been shown to protect against NSAID gastric mucosal damage[311]. There is a considerable reduction in salivary flow in elderly women[312] and it is interesting to speculate the influence this has on the occurrence of gastrointestinal complications.

The incidence of bleeding with different NSAIDs is difficult to obtain[198,308], but with few exceptions[253] most authors are of the opinion that there is little difference among the newer NSAIDs[313-316], which most agree[7,11,32] are less toxic than ASA. However, without properly controlled clinical trials it is impossible to draw any definite conclusions. As previously mentioned, there is evidence that nonacetylated salicylates are less likely to cause gastric injury[7,19,167-175], and, since there is evidence that in equivalent dosage they are equipotent with ASA as anti-inflammatory analgesics[317-319], there appears a prima facie case for their use in rheumatologic practice[320].

It is frequently forgotten in epidemiologic studies on gastrointestinal adverse reactions to ASA and NSAIDs that other drugs, such as oral potassium tablets, are also injurious[321], though toxicity may be reduced with liquid formulations[322,323]. It is still uncertain whether concomitant oral corticosteroid therapy is a risk factor in acute gastrointestinal bleeding and perforation[197,283,324]. Since the classic observations of Beaumont[325], the capacity of alcohol to disrupt the gastric mucosal barrier has been well recognized[326,327]. It is therefore not surprising that alcohol ingestion has been implicated as an additive factor in ASA and ulcerogenesis[328-332], but the estimation of the risk is difficult[332]. Similarly, the effects of smoking[24,198,250,331,333,334] on NSAID-induced peptic ulceration are unclear. Whether patients with preexisting gastric or duodenal ulcers are more prone to bleed when prescribed ASA or NSAIDs remains debatable[233,335,336]. There is a suspicion that the gastric mucosa in patients with rheumatoid arthritis may be more susceptible to injury with ASA and NSAIDs[7,11,22,50,196,198,336-339], but proof is difficult to obtain. Patients with esophageal varices are clearly more likely to bleed, as are those with a bleeding disorder or on anticoagulant therapy[333]. The bleeding time of the gastric mucosa is not prolonged in patients receiving ASA[340].

In addition to the stomach and duodenum, other areas of the gastrointestinal tract may be damaged with antirheumatic drugs. In elderly patients, especially those in long-care institutions, benign esophageal stricture and hemorrhage may result from ASA or NSAID tablets lodging in the esophagus[341-345]. This has also been described with other medications such as oral iron, vitamin C, tetracycline, and potassium[346,347]. Indium-111 labeled polymorphonuclear leukocyte scans in patients with rheumatoid arthritis receiving NSAIDs have shown increased accumulation of label in the cecum although no obvious mucosal damage was identified at ileocolonoscopy[350-353]. Intestinal probes have also indicated that NSAIDs may cause bowel damage[348,349,353-355]. Reports of ileal, duodenal and colonic hemorrhage, perforation, and stricture formation would appear to confirm this[356-375]. It has been suggested that drugs such as indomethacin and piroxicam that have high enterohepatic circulation may be more likely to cause such lesions, but this awaits confirmation[376-378]. Deaths from perforation of colonic diverticula have been observed, particularly in patients on long-standing oral corticosteroid therapy[379]. Benign gastrocolic fistula has been reported in patients receiving salicylates and oral corticosteroid therapy[380] and rectal bleeding[381] and rectovaginal fistula formation[382] has been observed as a result of indomethacin suppositories.

The fenemates have long been recognized as causing diarrhea but it is only relatively recently that steatorrhea has been reported with these drugs[383,384]. Acute necrotizing enterocolitis is associated with indomethacin use in infants[363], and several authors[374,385] have reported the induction and relapse of ulcerative colitis with the use of NSAIDs.

Auranofin frequently causes a dose-related diarrhea[385,386], probably due to a reversible defect in intestinal permeability[387] perhaps because the majority of the drug is excreted in the feces[388]. Both auranofin[389] and injectable gold complexes[390] have been reported to cause an enterocolitis. One patient has been reported with acute colitis while receiving D-penicillamine[391], and azathioprine may be associated with severe diarrhea mimicking gastroenteritis[392].

Perhaps the only potential benefit from a gastrointestinal point of view of the use of antirheumatic drugs is that NSAIDs may prevent gallstone recurrence after gallbladder surgery[393]. Unfortunately, it is not possible to predict that an individual patient may develop a GI adverse reaction with antirheumatic drug therapy. However, there is growing evidence that the elderly may be more prone to GI complications. Whether such patients should have routine cytoprotective therapy remains debatable[394]. All of the clinical therapeutic trials with cytoprotective drugs have been short-term, and there is potential for toxicity with their long-term use[4].

LIVER DISEASE

Many drugs damage the liver, either as a result of a direct toxic effect or idiosyncratic reaction. Two of the most obvious forms of liver cell injury produced by antirheumatic drugs are centrilobular necrosis resulting from acetaminophen overdose and acute or granulomatous hepatitis, secondary to phenylbutazone[395]. Hepatotoxicity has been described with many of the antirheumatic drugs, the most common being salicylates. Increased concentrations of plasma transaminases as a consequence of salicylate therapy have been reported in acute rheumatic fever[396], juvenile arthritis[397-401], rheumatoid arthritis[402,403], systemic lupus erythematosus[403-405], and Reiter's syndrome[406]. During prospective clinical trials involving 1252 patients with rheumatoid arthritis reported to the FDA in the United States, 67 (5.4%) developed one or more elevations of liver enzymes[407]. Paulus[408] considered that the elderly, decreased renal function, prolonged therapy especially with high doses, multiple drug use, and severe disease such as lupus erythematosus were all predisposing factors. One of the factors that might be relevant to salicylate transaminitis is "hypoalbuminemia," since this will result in an increased serum concentration of free salicylate[409,410]. In studies on rat liver cells cultured in monolayers, Tolman et al.[411] found that lactic dehydrogenase concentrations rose in the media with increasing doses of salicylate, and could be reduced if high concentrations of albumin were added to the media. Hypoalbuminemia is a feature of severe inflammatory disease and may be the common factor in the diseases in which elevated liver enzymes have been reported following salicylate therapy. However, it should be noted that "transaminitis" might also occur in normals[412]. It is not clear from the literature whether ASA is more prone to cause these effects than nonacetylated salicylate, although both are known to cause the condition. In the majority of patients, the biochemical abnormalities return to normal when salicylate therapy is discontinued, or even when it is continued[407]. In some patients, hepatic dysfunction may be severe enough to prolong the prothrombin time[401,403,413]. Hepatic biopsy studies have been infrequent, but changes include centrilobular hepatocellular degeneration with a periportal inflammatory infiltrate containing neutrophils, eosinophils, plasma cells, and lymphocytes[400,403,405]. One biopsy demonstrated changes of chronic active hepatitis that may have been coincidental, although attributed possibly to salicylate therapy by the authors[404]. It must be remembered that minor biochemical and pathologic abnormalities, including mitochondrial autoantibodies, are not infrequent in adult patients with rheumatoid arthritis, and are probably associated with immune disturbance of the disease rather than its treatment, since they are also found in patients with primary Sjögren's syndrome[414,415].

Reye's syndrome

In 1963 Reye et al.[416] and Johnson et al.[417] reported a syndrome in children consisting of encephalopathy and fatty metamorphosis of the liver. Subsequently, the syndrome was associated with outbreaks of influenza B and chickenpox, with a peak incidence between 5 and 15 years of age[418-420] and carrying a mortality between 20% and 40%[419,421,422]. The syndrome has also been described in adults[423]. The principal clinical features include an encephalopathy, varying in severity from drowsiness to deep coma and associated with severe vomiting and hepatomegaly. The serum transaminases and lactic dehydrogenase and blood ammonia concentrations are significantly elevated and in extremely severe cases hypoglycemia, acid–base disturbances, and coagulation abnormalities may ensue. Jaundice is, however, surprisingly absent. Findings on liver biopsy have been interpreted both as the same as[424], or distinct from[425-427], those seen in acute salicylate poisoning. Ultrastructural, histochemical, and biochemical changes in the mitochondria have been consistently observed in Reye's syndrome[425]. Influenza B virus infection[428] and salicylates[429,430] have both been shown to uncouple oxidative phosphorylation in liver mitochondria in vitro, which might explain the increase in free fatty acids, hyperammonemia[431], and the specific inhibition of mitochrondrial enzyme activity with preservation of cystosolic enzymes[432-435]. It has also been suggested that children who develop Reye's syndrome may have lower aspirin esterases[436], but this has not been confirmed.

Case control studies in the 1980s established an association between ingestion of aspirin and Reye's syndrome[418,419,437-440]. However, while some of the studies noted that patients with Reye's syndrome had received higher doses of aspirin than controls[418,437,438], others[441] noted that most patients had received doses well below the upper limit for antipyretic therapy (80 mg/kg per day). Furthermore, only 90% of patients with Reye's syndrome had received aspirin in the studies demonstrating an association[418,437,440] compared to 40-70% of the controls[442]. Nevertheless, there has been a demonstrable decline in the incidence of Reye's syndrome[443-446] by approximately 50% that has paralleled the decline in the use of aspirin. The syndrome has not, however, become an "endangered" disease as Sienko et al.[445] has suggested, since it continues to be reported in children with juvenile arthritis[447-449] where it certainly is not a random event[450]. In recent years there have been a growing number of metabolic disorders that mimic Reye's syndrome and are usually seen in children less than 5 years of age[446,451].

It is not possible to predict which child may develop Reye's syndrome if prescribed aspirin. Certainly, the drug should not be given as an antipyretic in a viral infection, especially influenza B or chickenpox, Acetaminophen is now the recommended antipyretic in children[452] but it is worth keeping in mind that impairment of mitochondrial oxidative energy metabolism has been demonstrated following acetaminophen-induced hepatic toxicity in animals[453].

Nonsteroidal anti-inflammatory analgesics

A small number of cases of acute hepatitis secondary to NSAIDs have been reported[454,455]. These have included dicoflenac, ketoprofen, ibuprofen, indomethacin, naproxen, niflumic acid, piroxicam, pirprofen, sulindac, and tolfenamic acid[454,455]. These have been of mixed immuno-allergic type, cytolytic as well as cholestatic. The complications appear to be more common in elderly women taking multiple medications[456]. Monitoring of routine liver function tests has been recommended with chronic medication, especially during the first 6 months of NSAID therapy, since several fatalities have been reported[454,455]. There appears at present no way of predicting which patients may develop this complication. Of the NSAIDs, sulindac and dicoflenac have been reported most commonly as producing this type of adverse reaction[457,458].

Of the disease-modifying agents, methotrexate is the most likely to result in hepatic damage[459-464]. There appears to be a correlation with dose and duration of therapy, alcohol consumption, and obesity and the development of hepatic fibrosis[464-466], although this has not been the experience of all workers[467]. After 2 years of therapy, Kremer et al.[464] found evidence of only a mild degree of fibrosis, although recently Bjorkman et al.[461] showed minor light-microscopic evidence of fibrosis after 10 years of therapy but increased collagen fibers could be found in the spaces of Disse. Transient elevations of liver enzymes frequently occurred during methotrexate therapy but whether it was due to methotrexate or other antirheumatic drugs is unknown[468-470]. A small amount of alcohol, more than 2-4 oz per week, appears not to be harmful to patients receiving methotrexate therapy[459] and there is some evidence that folic acid[471] and leucovorin[472] supplementation decreases long-term hepatotoxicity but this requires further study[462]. Obesity has been noted to be a definite risk factor in the development of cirrhosis in patients with psoriatic arthritis[465,473]. As in the study by Kremer et al.[464] in rheumatoid arthritis there does not appear to be a correlation between elevated serum transaminase levels and the development of cirrhosis in psoriatic arthritis[465,466,469,470]. However, the higher and the more persistently elevated the hepatic enzymes, the more likely the patient is to have liver damage[474]. Bromsulphthaline testing has also not proven useful as a predictor of hepatic fibrosis[475] but ultrasonography may be of more value[476]. Whether patients who are being treated with methotrexate should have liver biopsies remains a matter of debate[464] but there would seem no justification unless risk factors are involved or persistent enzyme elevation occurs.

Azathioprine may cause hepatic damage, but less commonly than methotrexate[477]. Elevation of liver enzymes, hypersensitivity hepatitis with cholestasis and jaundice, fibrosis, and frank cirrhosis have all been recorded[478-484] with an occasional fatality[478]. Likewise, it is not possible to predict those patients who will develop transient liver enzyme elevations or severe cholestatic jaundice with sulfasalazine[485-487]. Cyclophosphamide may also cause liver damage[488-491] as may D-penicillamine[492-494] but prediction is again not possible. Hepatotoxicity has been recorded with cyclosporin A therapy in transplant patients[495] but in this instance the complication is dose-dependent. Whaley and Webb[395], in a review of liver and kidney disease in patients with rheumatoid arthritis, observed that references to gold therapy causing hepatitis were all prior to 1936 but recently a case of reversible liver damage was reported by Lothian et al.[496]. Neither levamisole[497] nor chloroquine[498] appears to cause liver damage.

Acetaminophen (paracetamol) very rarely results in liver damage in healthy subjects at recommended daily dose[499,500], even when taken on a regular basis for many years[501,502]. However, several anecdotal reports of hepatic damage have been published with continuing daily use[503-508] even within the accepted therapeutic range[503-505,507,508]. Hepatic toxicity is due to a highly toxic reactive intermediate metabolite N-acetyl-p-benzoquinone imine[510], which is inactivated by liver glutathione[410,511,512]. There may be a deficiency of glutathione due to malnutrition or chronic alcoholism[410,503,506,511,513,514] and in this situation hepatocellular necrosis may occur[450]. Induction of the cytochrome-dependent P450 mixed function oxidase system predisposes to these complications[509,511] and may be another reason why the complication is common among alcoholics[401,503,511]. Another risk factor is preexisting liver disease[504,507]. In chronic liver disease the plasma half-life of acetaminophen is only slightly prolonged[513] but chronic administration of acetaminophen depletes liver glutathione stores[505], leading to an increased risk of hepatotoxicity. Acetaminophen may therefore not be as innocuous as previously thought[515] and should always be considered a potential cause of adverse drug reaction in elderly patients with unexplained liver dysfunction[516].

GENITOURINARY TRACT

Identification of patients at risk from renal toxicity syndromes with NSAIDs is now possible, the only exceptions being idiosyncratic reactions and analgesic nephropathy[517-523]. The renal syndromes that have been identified as resulting from NSAID include:

1. Hemodynamic or functional acute renal failure
2. Hyponatremia
3. Hyperkalemia
4. Interstitial nephritis
5. Analgesic nephropathy
6. Acute flank pain and diminished renal function[524]

The first three are clearly related to inhibition of renal prostaglandin production, while the relationship of inhibition of renal cyclooxygenase in interstitial nephritis or analgesic nephropathy remains uncertain[525-536]. In addition, both salicylates[537] and indomethacin[538,539] have been shown to depress plasma renin concentrations.

Hemodynamic or functional acute renal failure

This complication is most commonly seen in elderly patients who are receiving treatment for congestive cardiac failure and have renal insufficiency, or who are hypovolemic owing to diminished fluid intake or excessive loss. There is usually complete reversibility within 1-3 days, but if unrecognized it may prove fatal[521,541]. Patients with underlying renal disease[542] and hepatic cirrhosis[536,543] are also vulnerable to this complication. Blackshear et al.[521] concluded that advanced age, atherosclerotic cardiovascular disease, and concurrent diuretic therapy induced dependence on renal prostaglandin production for maintenance of renal function. Renal blood flow normally falls with age, especially in the presence of hypertension, and creatinine clearance at 80 years of age is approximately half that at 40[544,545]. It can readily be appreciated why an NSAID that inhibits prostaglandin production might lead to acute renal failure in such patients[540].

Hyponatremia

Reduction in extracellular volume is usually accompanied by hyponatremia. This causes release of vasopressin, which in turn stimulates the production of prostaglandins. Consequently, NSAIDs, by blocking prostaglandin synthesis, enhance the action of vasopressin, thus increasing water retention and consequently are effective in treating nephrogenic diabetes insipidus. Hyponatremia in the elderly might produce confusion, the cause of which can easily be overlooked in a long-term institutionalized patient.

Hyperkalemia

Volume depletion, especially if associated with sodium restriction, impairs the renal excretion of potassium. NSAIDs may cause hypokalemia and acute renal failure by inhibiting renal prostaglandin synthesis and by decreasing plasma renin activity[537,539,546]. Hyporeninemic hypoaldosteronism has been reported with and without renal insufficiency[547-549]. This condition is particularly likely to occur in patients with congestive cardiac failure and renal insufficiency who are receiving potassium-sparing diuretics[550a,551].

Patients who are prone to the above three complications of NSAID are usually elderly, with congestive cardiac failure, hypertension, and renal insufficiency. Patients with cirrhosis of the liver[530,536] and renal disease[533] are also prone to these complications. The risk is heightened by hypovolemia and diuretic therapy. NSAIDs blunt the action of diuretics[552,553] by a direct effect on the tubules[554] and also reduce the effectiveness of hypotensive drugs[552]. Sulindac, a prodrug, has been claimed to be renal sparing[555-563]. However, this has not been confirmed[564-570] and cases of acute renal failure induced by sulindac have been described[571]. Azapropazone has a long plasma half-life (18 hours) and is largely excreted unchanged in the urine (75%)[572]. Since azapropazone has been found to be retained in renal failure[573] it should be avoided in patients with risk factors for the renal complications described above. Oxypurinol is the active metabolite of allopurinol and its normal long plasma half-life, at 18–30 hours, is considerably extended in the presence of renal failure[574]. Patients with gout who have renal insufficiency should not be prescribed allopurinol, to avoid the so-called allopurinol hypersensitivity syndrome, which probably results from oxypurinol toxicity[575-580]. However, the syndrome can also occur with normal serum oxypurinol levels, suggesting that it might be immunologically mediated[581]. NSAIDs that form glucuronide conjugates, e.g., ketoprofen, indomethacin, diflunisal, and naproxen, may have their plasma half-lives prolonged in the presence of renal failure[582,583], as a result of the conjugates being hydrolyzed back to the parent compound (the so-called futile cycle)[584,585]. To date, none of these NSAIDs has been particularly implicated in causing the above-mentioned syndrome. However, it is quite possible that this was the mechanism of toxicity of the ill-fated benoxaprofen, which is biotransformed to an ester glucuronide. Since this drug was prescribed as a racemic mixture it is possible that stereoinversion also occurred, giving a disproportionate increase in the active S isomer. ASA and other NSAIDs have no detrimental effects in subjects with normal renal function[558,586,587] even when sodium depleted[588]. Only transient rises in serum creatinine have been observed in healthy subjects when prescribed ASA[589,590], which quickly returns to normal when the drug is discontinued[591]. A transient celluria occurs in normal subjects when ASA is first prescribed, but disappears after 10 days[204]. Depression of creatinine clearance and increased serum creatinine concentrations have only been reported with ASA in clinical settings of impaired renal function[592-596].

Interstitial nephritis

This is a rare complication of NSAID therapy that cannot be predicted[518,597-612]. The complication usually occurs after 6 months of therapy with a range of 2 weeks to 18 months[521,550,606]. The majority of patients have been 60 years of age or older and approximately 75% of cases have been reported following fenoprofen[521,601,606,609,613,614]. The complication is characterized by an acute infiltration of T lymphocytes of the cytotoxic-suppressor subset[606,610,612] or eosinophils[615] in the interstitial tissues of the kidney. Eosinophiluria may be present[615]. Proteinuria is not infrequently in the nephrotic range and associated with renal failure[518,519]. Only a small number of patients have features of a hypersensitivity reaction such as fever, rash, or eosinophilia[521]. The condition is usually reversible when the drug is discontinued[615]. Occasionally, however, high-dose corticosteroid therapy and dialysis may be necessary to assist recovery[516]. To date, no case of interstitial nephritis has been reported with salicylates.

Analgesic nephropathy

Although phenacetin was the initial component of analgesic mixtures implicated as a cause of analgesic nephropathy[616-623] it is now clear that the syndrome can occur with ASA and other NSAIDs[622,624-634]. The mean age of patients who develop this complication was 62 years in the review by Nanra and Kincaid-Smith[625]. The pathogenesis is currently believed to be due to the antiprostaglandin effects of the NSAIDs[518,521,615,628,630,635], and in this connection it is of interest that the prostaglandin analog PGE_2 has been shown capable of preventing mefenamic acid-induced renal capillary necrosis in rats[636]. Volume depletion may be important also in the pathogenesis[630]. However, it is not possible to predict which patients will develop this complication and several long-term studies of ASA have failed to identify even a single case[637-639]. It is also not possible to predict which patient with analgesic nephropathy will later develop a transitional cell carcinoma of the ureter and bladder[640-642].

Slow-acting and immunoregulatory agents

Gold nephropathy is perhaps the best known side-effect of drugs in this class. It is heralded by proteinuria that has been reported to occur in up to 10% of patients[643]. Renal biopsy shows a membranous glomerulonephritis with immune complexes in the glomerular basement membrane[643]. It has been suggested that the initial damage occurs in the renal tubules, which release antigens to complex with autoantibodies and cause the glomerulonephritis[644,645]. Some 10-30% of patients develop the nephrotic syndrome, but rarely renal failure, and the condition responds to discontinuation of therapy[643,646,647]. Gold nephropathy has been reported in a patient with renal amyloidosis that responded to combination therapy of corticosteroids and azathioprine[648].

D-Penicillamine can also be complicated by renal toxicity. As with gold, proteinuria is the usual clinical outcome and histologic examination discloses either minimal change, mesangioproliferative, or membranous nephropathy[649-652]. The prognosis is generally good[652]. However, rapidly progressive glomerulonephritis with epithelial crescents necessitating hemodialysis or leading to death has been reported with the use of D-penicillamine in patients with rheumatoid arthritis, progressive systemic sclerosis, primary biliary cirrhosis, and Wilson's disease[653-660]. Many of these patients were described as having Goodpasture's syndrome as they had hemoptysis[653-657]. However, antiglomerular basement membrane antibodies were detected[653-656,658,660] and two patients typed for HLA-DR2 were negative[657,660]. There is thus no means of identifying which patients may be at risk of developing this life-threatening condition.

The most troublesome adverse effect of cyclosporin A is a dose-related nephrotoxicity, which usually leads to asymptomatic elevations in serum creatinine concentrations[661,662]. Fulminant acute renal failure has been reported in patients receiving high doses of the drug for bone marrow transplantation[663]. The mechanism of cyclosporin-induced nephrotoxicity remains uncertain, but may involve vasoconstriction rather than direct tubular toxicity[662]. Studies are now in progress to determine whether the prostaglandin E_2 analog misoprostol may reduce renal toxicity. Hypertension may accompany rising serum creatinine levels and may be aggravated by accompanying use of cyclooxygenase inhibitors such as NSAIDs. There is preliminary evidence that the use of low doses of cyclosporin A (5 mg/kg) may reduce the incidence of nephrotoxicity and hypertension[664]. In general, these complications are reversed on discontinuation of therapy[664-668].

Renal complications do not occur with levamisole[663] or sulfasalazine[64] but have been reported with azathioprine[669] and methotrexate[670]. However, hematuria has only been reported with azathioprine as part of a hypersensitivity reaction[669] and low doses of methotrexate such as are used in the treatment of rheumatoid arthritis appear to be free from nephrotoxicity[671].

Bladder complications are particularly troublesome with cyclophosphamide. These include hemorrhagic cystitis, bladder fibrosis, and bladder carcinoma[672-677]. Both unmetabolized drug and active metabolites are excreted by the kidney[678] and it is the latter (especially the metabolite acrolein) that are believed to cause damage to the transitional epithelium[679]. The risk of these complications can be minimized by concurrent administration of large volumes of fluid and protective reducing agents[670]. Bladder irrigation may be used in patients with limitations of bladder emptying[670] and administration of saline may be useful in preventing water intoxication from inappropriate ADH syndrome caused by the drug[680]. Plotz and his colleagues[676,677] have published on bladder complications in 43 patients with systemic lupus erythematosus and 11 patients with rheumatoid arthritis who had received treatment with cyclophosphamide administered either orally or intravenously. During the observation period of 241 patient-years, 7 patients developed hemorrhagic cystitis and 2 bladder carcinoma. Interestingly, these complications did not occur in 12 patients with systemic lupus erythematosus who received intravenous cyclophosphamide, a finding that was subsequently upheld in a larger number of patients by the same authors[681]. McCune and his colleagues[682] also reported no hemorrhagic cystitis in 9 patients treated with monthly intravenous pulse cyclophosphamide over a 6-month period. A worrying feature of the study of Plotz et al.[677] was that 2 patients developed bladder carcinoma 28 and 60 months after withdrawal from the drug. The risks of bladder neoplasm appear to be increased by a history of cystitis but, as Plotz et al.[677] point out, its absence does not preclude development of neoplasm. Bladder fibrosis appears to occur in patients who receive large doses of cyclophosphamide. Further experience with intravenous cyclophosphamide therapy will be necessary to determine whether the incidence of bladder complications may be reduced.

Defective oogenesis and spermatogenesis has been reported with the use of alkylating agents, chlorambucil[683] and cyclophosphamide[686], and with methotrexate[670] and sulfasalazine[687]. Reduced ovarian function and azoospermia both appear to be dose-related but prediction of which patients are likely to develop these complications is not possible, although older women appear to be at greater risk of premature menopause with cyclophosphamide[684,685]. Recovery of spermatogenesis is unpredictable but is probably related to the total dose and length of time cyclophosphamide has been discontinued[685]. Males who have had temporary azoospermia with cyclophosphamide have subsequently had normal children[688,689]. Likewise, some women who have previously been treated with cyclophosphamide have subsequently had normal pregnancies following cessation of therapy[690].

NSAIDs and slow-acting antirheumatic drugs (SAARDs) have the potential to do much harm as well as provide significant benefit. Care should be taken, particularly with the frail elderly and those people with underlying organ dysfunction such as previous or current renal, hepatic, or gastrointestinal disease. Therapy should be frequently reviewed, with careful monitoring of patients for potential toxicity. With care, serious toxicity can be reduced to a minimum and the potential benefits of these treatments can be maximized.

References

1. Weber, J. C. P. (1984). Epidemiology of adverse reactions to nonsteroidal anti-inflammatory drugs. In *Advances in Inflammation*, Rainsford, K. D. and Velo, G. P. (eds.) Vol. 6, pp. 1–7. (New York: Raven Press)
2. Roth, S. H. (1988). NSAID and gastropathy: a rheumatologist's review. *J. Rheumatol.*, **15**, 912–919
3. Mistilis, S. P. (1985). Current concepts in gastric cytoprotection. *Med. J. Aust.*, **142** (Suppl.), 2–28
4. Rainsford, K. D. (1988). Current concepts of the mechanisms of side effects of non-steroidal anti-inflammatory drugs as a basis for establishing research priorities. An experimentalist's view. *J. Rheumatol.* (Suppl. 17), **15**, 63–70
5. Huskisson, E. C. and Wojyulewski, J. A. (1974). Measurements of side effects of drug. *Br. Med. J.*, **2**, 698–699
6. Fossgreen, J. (1976). Ketoprofen: a survey of current publications. *Scand. J. Rheumatol.* (Suppl.), **14**, 7–32
7. Caruso, I. and Porro, G. B. (1980). Gastroscopic evaluation of anti-inflammatory agents. *Br. Med. J.*, **1**, 75–78
8. Coles, L. S., Fries, J. F., Kraines, R. G. et al. (1983). From experiment to experience: side effects of non-steroidal anti-inflammatory drugs. *Am. J. Med.*, **74**, 820–828
9. Lanza, F. L. (1984). Endoscopic studies of gastric and duodenal injury after the use of ibuprofen, aspirin and other non-steroidal anti-inflammatory agents. *Am. J. Med.*, **77**, 19–24
10. Graham, D. Y., Smith, J. L., Holmes, G. I. et al. (1985). Non-steroidal anti-inflammatory effects of sulindac sulfoxide and sulfide on gastric mucosa. *Clin. Pharmacol. Ther.*, **38**, 65–70
11. Semble, E. H. and Wu, W. C. (1987). Anti-inflammatory drugs and gastric mucosal damage. *Semin. Arthritis Rheum.*, **16**, 271–286
12. Capell, H. A., Rennie, J. A. N., Rooney, P. J. et al. (1979). Patient compliance: a novel method of testing non-steroidal anti-inflammatory analgesics in rheumatoid arthritis. *J. Rheumatol.*, **6**, 584–593
13. Rejholec, V. (1975). Long term ibuprofen therapy of rheumatic disease in patients with a past history of peptic ulceration. *Curr. Med. Res. Opin.*, **3**, 522–524
14. Capell, H. A., Rennie, J. A. N., Rooney, P. J., Murdoch, R. M., Hale, D. J., Dick, W. C. and Buchanan, W. W. (1979). Patient compliance: a novel method of testing non-steroidal anti-inflammatory analgesics in rheumatoid arthritis. *J. Rheumatol.*, **6** 584–593
15. Pullar, T., Zoma, A. A., Madhok, R., Hunter, J. A. and Capell, H. A. (1985). Have the newer NSAIDs contributed to the management of rheumatoid arthritis? *Scott. Med. J.*, **30**, 161–163
16. Meisel, A. D. (1986). Clinical benefits and comparative safety of piroxicam: analysis of worldwide clinical trials data. *Am. J. Med.*, **81** (Suppl. 5B), 15–21
17. Graham, D. Y., Agrawal, N. M. and Roth, S. H. (1988). Prevention of NSAID-induced gastric ulcer with misoprostol: multicentre, double-blind, placebo-controlled trial. *Lancet*, **2**, 1277–1280
18. Dromgoole, S. H., Furst, D. E. and Paulus, H. E. (1981). Rational approach to the use of salicylates in the treatment of rheumatoid arthritis. *Semin. Arthritis Rheum.*, **11**, 257–283
19. Silvoso, G. R., Ivey, K. J., Butt, J. H., Lockard, O. O., Holt, S. D., Sisk, C. et al. (1979). Incidence of gastric lesions in patients with rheumatic disease on chronic aspirin therapy. *Ann. Intern. Med.*, **91**, 517–520
20. Lanza, F., Royer, G. L., Nelson, R. S., Chen, T. T., Seckman, C. E. and Rack, M. F. (1981). A comparative endoscopic evaluation of the damaging effects on non-steroidal anti-inflammatory agents on the gastric and duodenal mucosa. *Am. J. Gastroenterol.*, **175**, 17–21
21. Collins, A. J., Davies, J. and Dixon, A. St.J. (1986). Contrasting presentation and findings between patients with rheumatic complaints taking non-steroidal anti-

inflammatory drugs and a general population referred for endoscopy. *Br. J. Rheumatol.*, **25**, 50–53
22. Dawes, P. T. and Haslock, I. (1986). The importance of gastrointestinal symptoms in arthritis patients. *Br. J. Rheumatol.*, **25**, 315–316
23. Graham, D. J. and Smith, J. L. (1986). Aspirin and the stomach. *Ann. Intern. Med.*, **104**, 390–398
24. Roth, S. J. and Bennet, R. E. (1987). Non-steroidal anti-inflammatory drug gastropathy: recognition and response. *Arch. Intern. Med.*, **147**, 2093–2100
25. Double, A. and Morris, A. (1988). Non-steroidal anti-inflammatory drug-induced dyspepsia — is *Campylobacter pyloridis* implicated? *Br. J. Rheumatol.*, **27**, 110–112
26. Page, M. C., Tildesley, G. and Wood, J. R. (1988). Prevention of gastroduodenal damage induced by non-steroidal anti-inflammatory drugs: controlled trials of ranitidine. *Br. Med. J.*, **297**, 1017–1021
27. Larkai, E. N., Smith, J. L., Lidsky, M. D. and Graham, D. Y. (1987). Gastroduodenal mucosa and dyspeptic symptoms in arthritic patients during chronic non-steroidal anti-inflammatory drug use. *Am. J. Gastroenterol.*, **82**, 1153–1158
28. Upadhyay, R., Howatson, A., McKinlay, A., Danesh, B. J. Z., Sturrock, R. D. and Russell, R. I. (1988). *Campylobacter pylori* associated gastritis in patients with rheumatoid arthritis taking non-steroidal anti-inflammatory drugs. *Br. J. Rheumatol.*, **27**, 113–116
29. Hazleman, B. L. (1989). Incidence of gastropathy in destructive arthropathies. *Scand. J. Rheumatol.*, **78** (Suppl.), 1–4
30. Geczy, M., Peltier, L. and Wolbach, R. (1987). Naproxen tolerability in the elderly: a summary report. *J. Rheumatol.*, **14**, 348–354
31. Muir, A. (1963). Salicylates, dyspepsia and peptic ulceration. In *Salicylates. An International Symposium.* Dixon, A., Martin, B. K., Smith, M. J. H. and Wood, P. H. N. (eds.) p. 230. (Boston: Brown)
32. Rainsford, K. D. (1982). An analysis of the gastrointestinal side effects of non-steroidal anti-inflammatory drugs, with particular reference to comparative studies in man and laboratory species. *Rheumatol. Int.*, **2**, 1–10
33. Strand, L. J. (1982). Upper gastrointestinal effects of newer non-steroidal anti-inflammatory agents. In Pfeiffer, C. J. (ed.) *Drugs and Peptic Ulcer: Pathogenesis of Ulcer Induction Revealed by Drug Studies in Humans and Animals*, pp. 8–24. (Boca Raton, Fl: CRC Press)
34. Holt, L. P. J. and Hawkins, C. F. (1965). Indomethacin: studies of absorption and of the use of indomethacin suppositories. *Br. Med. J.*, **1**, 1354–1356
35. Lanza, F. L., Umbenhauer, E. R., Nelson, R. S., Rack, M. F., Daurio, C. P. and White, L. A. (1982). A double-blind randomized placebo controlled gastroscopic study to compare the effects of indomethacin capsules and indomethacin suppositories on the gastric mucosa of human volunteers. *J. Rheumatol.*, **9**, 415–419
36. Percy, J. S. (1982). Gastric mucosa, epigastric distress and anti-inflammatory agents. *J. Rheumatol.*, **9**, 351–352
37. Green, J. A. (1984). Indomethacin sustained-release? *Drug Intell. Clin. Pharm.*, **18**, 1004–1007
38. Duggan, D. E., Hogans, A. F., Kwan, D. C. and McMahon, F. G. (1981). The metabolism of indomethacin: a double-blind comparison of indomethacin suppositories. *N.Z. Med. J.*, **93**, 261–262
39. Batterman, R. D. (1958). Comparison of buffered and unbuffered acetylsalicylic acid. *N. Engl. J. Med.*, **258**, 213–219
40. Cronk, G. A. (1958). Laboratory and clinical studies with buffered and non-buffered acetylsalicylic acid. *N. Engl. J. Med.*, **258**, 219–222
41. Goldenberg, A., Rudnicki, R. D. and Koonce, M. L. (1978). Clinical comparison of efficacy and safety of choline magnesium trisalicylate and indomethacin in treating osteoarthritis. *Curr. Ther. Res.*, **24**, 245–259
42. Nevinny, D. and Gowans, J. C. D. (1960). Observations in the usefulness of a new liquid salicylate in arthritis. *Int. Rec. Med.*, **173**, 242–247

43. Orozco-Alcola, J. J. and Baum, J. (1979). Regular and enteric coated aspirin: a re-evaluation. *Arthritis Rheum.*, **22**, 1034–1037
44. Halla, J. T., Fallahi, S., and Hardin, J. G. (1981). Acute and chronic salicylate intoxication in a patient with gastric outlet obstruction. *Arthritis Rheum.*, **24**, 1205–1207
45. Bijlsma, J. W. J. (1988). Treatment of endoscopy-negative NSAID-induced upper gastrointestinal symptoms with cimetidine: an international multicentre collaborative study. *Aliment. Pharmacol. Ther.*, **2** (Suppl.), 75–83
46. Bijlsma, J. W. J. (1988). Treatment of NSAID-induced gastrointestinal lesions with cimetidine: an international multicentre collaborative study. *Aliment. Pharmacol. Ther.*, **2** (Suppl.), 85–96
47. Caldwell, J. R., Roth, S. H., Wu, W. C., Semble, E. L., Castell, D. O., Heller, M. D. and Marsh, W. H. (1987). Sucralfate treatment of non-steroidal anti-inflammatory drug-induced gastrointestinal symptoms and mucosal damage. *Am. J. Med.*, **83** (Suppl. 3B), 74–82
48. van Saase, J., van Denbroucke, J., Valkenburg, H., Boersma, J., Cats, A., Feslen, J., Hartman, A., Huber-Bruning, O., Rasker, J. and Weber, J. (1987). Changing pattern of drug use in relation to disease duration of rheumatoid arthritis. *J. Rheumatol.*, **14**, 476–478
49. Camarri, E., Chirone, E. and Benevenuti, D. (1980). Double-blind placebo controlled cross-over study on cimetidine prophylactic effect in patients under steroid treatments. Preliminary data. *J. Clin. Pharmacol. Ther. Toxicol.*, **18**, 258–260
50. Sum, D. C., Roth, S. H., Mitchell, C. S. *et al.* (1974). Upper gastrointestinal disease in rheumatoid arthritis. *Am. J. Dig. Dis.*, **19**, 405–410
51. Domschke, W., Domschke, S., Huber, W. *et al.* (1977). Glucocorticoid and mineralocorticoid actions on gastric secretion in man. *Acta Hepato-Gastroenterol.*, **23**, 34–37
52. Cohen, M. M. and MacDonald, W. C. (1983). Protection against aspirin-induced gastric mucosa damage in humans with enprosil (RS-84135): a double-blind endoscopic study. Abstract. *Ann. Roy. Coll. Phys. Surg. Can.*, **16**, 390.
53. Scott, J. T., Porter, I. H., Lewis, S. M. *et al.* (1961). Studies of gastrointestinal bleeding caused by corticosteroids, salicylates and other analgesics. *Q. J. Med. N.S.*, **30**, 167–188
54. Lockie, L. M., Gomez, E. and Smith, D. M. (1983). Low dose adrenocorticosteroids in the management of elderly patients with RA: selected examples and summary of efficacy in the long-term treatment of 97 patients. *Semin. Arthritis Rheum.*, **12**, 373–381
55. Stein, H. B., Patterson, A. C., Offer, R. C. *et al.* (1980). Adverse effects of D-penicillamine in rheumatoid arthritis. *Ann. Intern. Med.*, **92**, 24–29
56. Kean, W. F., Dwosh, I. L., Anastassiades, T. P. *et al.* (1980). The toxicity pattern of D-penicillamine therapy. *Arthritis Rheum.*, **23**, 158–164
57. Co-operative Systematic Studies of Rheumatic Disease Group. (1987). Toxicity of long term low dose D-penicillamine therapy in rheumatoid arthritis. *J. Rheumatol.*, **14**, 67–73
58. Multicenter Trial Group. (1973). Controlled trial of D-penicillamine in severe rheumatoid arthritis. *Lancet*, **1**, 275–280
59. Williams, H. J., Ward, J. R. and Reading, J. C. (1983). Low-dose D-penicillamine in rheumatoid arthritis: A controlled double-blind clinical trial. *Arthritis Rheum.*, **26**, 581–592
60. Situnayake, R. D., Grindulis, K. A. and McConkey, B. (1987). Long term treatment of rheumatoid arthritis with sulphasalazine, gold or penicillamine: a comparison using life-table methods. *Ann. Rheum. Dis.*, **46**, 177–183
61. Nielson, O. H. (1982). Sulfasalazine intolerance. A retrospective survey of the reasons for discontinuing treatment in patients with chronic inflammatory bowel disease. *Scand. J. Gastroenterol.*, **17**, 389–393
62. Amos, R. S., Pullar, T., Bax, D. E. *et al.* (1986). Sulphasalazine for rheumatoid arthritis: toxicity in 774 patients monitored for one to 11 years. *Br. Med. J.*, **293**, 420–423

63. Farr, M., Scott, D. G. I. and Bacon, P. A. (1986). Side effect profile of 200 patients with inflammatory arthritis treated with sulphasalazine drugs. *Drugs*, **32** (Suppl. 1), 49-53
64. Pinals, R. S. (1988). Sufasalazine in the rheumatic disease. *Semin. Arthritis Rheum.*, **17**, 246-259
65. MacKenzie, A. H. and Scherbel, A. L. (1980). Chloroquine and hydroxychloroquine in rheumatological therapy. *Clin. Rheum. Dis.*, **6**, 545-566
66. Maksymowych, W. and Russell, A. S. (1987). Antimalarials in rheumatology: efficacy and safety. *Semin. Arthritis Rheum.*, **16**, 206-221
67. Furst, D. E. and Kremer, J. M. (1988). Methotrexate in rheumatoid arthritis. *Arthritis Rheum.*, **31**, 305-314
68. Huskisson, E. C. (1984). Azathioprine. *Clin. Rheum. Dis.*, **10**, 325-332
69. Kovarsky, J. (1983). Clinical pharmacology and toxicology of cyclosphosphamide: emphasis on use in rheumatic diseases. *Semin. Arthritis Rheum.*, **12**, 359-372
70. Friedman, O. M., Myles, A. and Colvin, M. (1979). Cyclophosphamide and related phosphoramide mustards: current status and future prospects. *Adv. Cancer Chemother.*, **1**, 143-204
71. Weinblatt, M. E., Coblyn, J. S., Fraser, P. A., Anderson, R. J., Spragg, J., Trentham, D. E. and Austen, K. F. (1987). Cyclosporin. A treatment of refractory rheumatoid arthritis. *Arthritis Rheum.*, **30**, 11-17
72. Szabo, S., Spill, W. F. and Rainsford, K. D. (1989). Non-steroidal anti-inflammatory drug-induced gastropathy. *Med. Toxicol. Adv. Drug Exper.*, **4**, 77-94
73. Davenport, H. W. (1967). Salicylate damage to the gastric mucosal barrier. *N. Engl. J. Med.*, **276**, 1307-1312
74. Bahari, H., Ross, M. M. and Turnberg, L. A. (1982). Demonstration of a pH gradient across the mucus layer on the surface of human gastric mucosa in vitro. *Gut*, **23**, 513-516
75. Lichtenberg, L. M., Grazian, L. A. and Dial, E. J. (1983). Role of surface-active phospholipids in gastric cytoprotection. *Science*, **219**, 1227-1229
76. Dial, E. J. and Lichtenberger, L. M. (1984). A role for milk phospholipids in protection against stomach acid. Studies in adult and suckling rats. *Gastroenterology*, **87**, 379-385
77. Guth, P. H. (1984). Local metabolism and circulation in mucosal disease. In Allen, A., Flemstrom, G., Garner, A. et al. (eds.), *Mechanisms of Mucosal Protection in the Upper Gastrointestinal Tract*, pp. 235-258. (New York: Raven Press)
78. Turnberg, L. A. and Ross, J. N. (1984). Studies of the pH gradient across gastric mucus. *Scand. J. Gastroenterol.*, **19** (Suppl. 92), 48-50
79. Rainsford, K. D. (1989). Mechanisms of gastrointestinal toxicity of non-steroidal anti-inflammatory drugs. *Scand. J. Gastroenterol.*, **24** (Suppl. 163), 9-16
80. Vane, J. R. (1971). Inhibition of prostaglandin synthesis as a mechanism of action of aspirin-like drugs. *Nature*, **231**, 232-235
81. Takagi, K. and Kawahiwa, K. (1969). Effects of some anti-inflammatory drugs on capillary permeability of the gastric mucosa in the rat. *Jpn. J. Pharmacol.*, **19**, 431-437
82. Karim, S. M., Carter, D. C., Bhana, D. et al. (1973). Effect of orally administered prostaglandin, E_2 and its 15-methyl analogues on gastric secretion. *Br. Med. J.*, **1**, 143-146
83. Cohen, M. M. and Pollett, J. M. (1976). Prostaglandin E_2 prevents aspirin and indomethacin damage to human gastric mucosa. *Surg. Forum*, **27**, 400-401
84. Gerkens, J. F., Shand, D. G., Flexner, C., Nies, A. S., Oates, J. A. and Data, J. L. (1977). Effect of indomethacin and aspirin on gastric blood flow and acid secretion. *J. Pharmacol. Exp. Ther.*, **203**, 646-652
85. Whittle, B. J. R. (1977). Mechanisms underlying gastric mucosal damage induced by indomethacin and bile salts and the actions of prostaglandins. *Br. J. Pharmacol.*, **60**, 455-460
86. Johannson, C. and Kollberg, B. (1979). Stimulation by intragastrically administered E_2 prostaglandins in human gastric mucus output. *Eur. J. Clin. Invest.*, **9**, 229-232
87. Konturek, S. J., Obtulowicz, W., Sito, E., Olesky, J., Wilkin, S. and Kiec-Dembinski,

A. (1981). Distribution of prostaglandins in gastric and duodenal mucosa of healthy subjects and duodenal ulcer patients: effect of aspirin and paracetamol. *Gut*, **22**, 283-289

88. Konturek, S. J., Piastucki, I., Brzozowski, T. *et al.* (1981). Role of prostaglandins in the formation of aspirin-induced ulcers. *Gastroenterology*, **80**, 4-9

89. Cloud, W. G. and Ritchie, W. P. (1982). Evidence for cytoprotection of endogenous prostaglandins in gastric mucosa treated with bile acid. *Surg. Forum*, **33**, 150-152

90. Kauffman, G. L. and Whittle, B. J. R. (1982). Gastric vascular actions of prostanoids and the dual effect of arachidonic acid. *Am. J. Physiol.*, **242**, 582-587

91. Feldman, M. (1983). Gastric bicarbonate secretion in humans. Effects of pentagastrin, bethanecol and 11,16,16-trimethyl prostaglandin E_2. *J. Clin. Invest.*, **82**, 295-303

92. Hurst, B. C., Rees, W. D. W. and Garner, A. (1984). Cell shedding by the stomach and duodenum. In *Mechanisms of Gastric Mucosal Protection in the Upper Gastrointestinal Trace*, Allen, A., Flemstrom, G., Garner, A. *et al.* (eds.), pp. 21-26. (New York: Raven Press)

93. Levene, R. A. and Schwarzel, E. H. (1984). Effect of indomethacin on basal and histamine stimulated human gastric acid secretion. *Gut*, **25**, 718-722

94. Rees, W. D. W., Gibbons, L. C., Warhurst, G. *et al.* (1984). Studies of bicarbonate secretion by the normal human stomach *in vivo*. Effect of aspirin, sodium taurocholate and prostaglandin E_2. In Allen, A., Flemstrom, G., Garner, A. *et al.* (eds.) *Mechanisms of Gastric Mucosal Protection in the Upper Gastrointestinal Tract*, pp. 119-124. (New York: Raven Press)

95. Whittle, B. R. J. and Vane, J. R. (1984). A biochemical basis for the gastrointestinal toxicity of non-steroid anti-rheumatoid drugs. *Arch. Toxicol.*, **7** (Suppl.), 315-322

96. Hawkey, C. J. and Ramptom, D. S. (1985). Prostaglandins and the gastrointestinal mucosa: are they important in its function, disease or treatment? *Gastroenterology*; **89**, 1162-1188

97. Garner, A. and Allen, A. (1987). Gastroduodenal mucosal defense mechanisms and the action of non-steroidal anti-inflammatory agents. *Scand. J. Gastroenterol.*, **22** (Suppl. 127), 29-34

98. Fromm, D. (1987). Mechanisms involved in gastric mucosal resistance to injury. *Ann. Rev. Med.*, **38**, 119-128

99. Robert, A. (1979). Cytoprotection by prostaglandins. *Gastroenterology*, **77**, 761-767

100. Cohen, M. M., McCready, D., Clark, L. and Sevilius, H. (1984). Prostaglandin analogue averts gastric mucosal injury. *Gastroenterology*, **3**, 1-2

101. Gilbert, D. A., Suwitz, C. M., Silverstein, F. E. *et al.* (1984). Prevention of acute aspirin induced mucosal injury by 15-R-15 methyl prostaglandin E_2: an endoscopic study. *Gastroenterology*, **86**, 339-345

102. Cohen, M. M., McCreasy, D. R., Clark, L. *et al.* (1985). Protection against aspirin-induced antral and duodenal damage with enprostil. A double-blind endoscopy study. *Gastroenterology*, **88**, 382-386

103. Lanza, F. L. (1987). A double-blind study of prophylactic effect of misoprostol on lesions of gastric and duodenal mucosa induced by oral administration of tolmetin in healthy subjects. *Dig. Dis. Sci.*, **31** (Suppl.), 131-136

104. Silverstein, F. E., Kimmey, M. B., Saunders, D. R. and Levene, D. S. (1986). Gastric protection by misoprostol against 1300 mg of aspirin: an endoscopic study. *Dig. Dis. Sci.*, **31** (Suppl.), 137-141

105. Agrawal, N. M., Godiwala, T., Arimura, A. and Dajani, E. Z. (1986). Cytoprotection by a synthetic prostaglandin against ethanol-induced gastric mucosal damage. A double-blind endoscopic study in human subjects. *Gastrointestinal Endoscopy*, **32**, 67-70

106. Lanza, F., Robinson, M., Bowers, T. *et al.* (1988). A multicenter double-blind comparison of ranitidine versus placebo in the prophylaxis of NSAID induced lesions in gastric and duodenal mucosa. (Abstract) *Gastroenterology*, **94**, 250

107. Lanza, F., Peace, K., Gustitus, L., Rack, M. F. and Dickson, B. (1988). A blinded endoscopic comparative study of misoprostol versus sucralfate and placebo in the prevention of aspirin-induced gastric and duodenal ulceration. *Am. J. Gastroenterol.*, **83**, 143-146

108. Lanza F. L. (1989). A review of mucosal protection by synthetic prostaglandin E

analogs against injury by non-steroidal anti-inflammatory agents. *Scand J. Gastroenterol.* **24** (Suppl. 163): 36–43
109. Roth, S., Agrawal, N., Mahowald, M., Montoya, H., Robbins, D., Miller, S., Nutting, F., Woods, E., Crager, M., Missen, C. and Swabb, E. (1989). Misoprostol heals gastroduodenal injury in patients with rheumatoid arthritis receiving aspirin. *Arch. Intern. Med.,* **149**, 775–779
110. Whittle, B. J. R. (1981). Temporal relationship between cyclooxygenase inhibition, as measured by prostacyclin biosynthesis, and the gastrointestinal damage induced by indomethacin in the rat. *Gastroenterology*, **80**, 94–98
111. Ligumsky, M., Golanska, E. M., Hansen, D. G. and Kauffman, G. L. (1984). Aspirin can inhibit gastric mucosal cyclooxygenase without causing lesions in the rat. *Gastroenterology*, **84**, 756–761
112. Redfern, J. S., Lee, E. and Feldman, M. (1987). Effect of indomethacin on gastric mucosal prostaglandins in humans. Correlations with mucosal damage. *Gastroenterology*, **92**, 969–977
113. Rainsford, K. D. (1988). Comparative irritancy of oxaprozin on the gastrointestinal tract of rats and mice — relationship to drug uptake and effects *in vivo* on eicosanoid metabolism. *Aliment. Pharmacol. Ther.,* **2**, 439–450
114. Peskar, B. M., Kleien, A., Pyras, F. and Muller, M. K. (1986). Gastrointestinal toxicity. Role of prostaglandins and leukotrienes. *Med. Toxicol.,* **1** (Suppl. 1), 39–43
115. Rainsford, K. D. (1987). The effects of 5-lipoxygenase inhibitors and leukotriene antagonists on the development of gastric lesions induced by nonsteroidal anti-inflammatory drugs in mice. *Agents and Actions,* **21**, 316–319
116. Morris, G. P. (1986). Prostaglandins and cellular restitution in the gastric mucosa. In Thomson, A. B. R. (ed.) *Protective and Therapeutic Effects of Gastrointenstinal Prostaglandins. Am. J. Med.* **81** (Suppl. 2A), 23–29
117. O'Brien, P., Schults, C., Gannon, B. and Browning, J. (1986). Protective effects of the synthetic prostaglandin enprostil on the gastric microvasculature after ethanol injury in the rat. In Thomson, A. B. R. (ed.) *Protective and Therapeutic Effects of Gastrointestinal Prostaglandins. Am. J. Med.,* **81** (Suppl. 2A), 12–17
118. Clinch, D., Bamerjee, A. K., Levy, D. W., Ostick, G. and Feracher, E. B. (1987). Non-steroidal anti-inflammatory drugs and peptic ulceration. *J. Roy. Coll. Physicians Lond.,* **21**, 183–187
119. Boyd, E. J. S. and Wormsley, K. G. (1987). Gastrointestinal side effects of prostaglandins. In Rainsford, K. D. and Velo, G. P. (eds.) *Side Effects of Anti-Inflammatory Drugs,* Vol. II, pp. 143–149. (Lancaster: MTP)
120. St. John, D. J. B. and McDermott, F. J. (1970). Influence of achlorhydria on aspirin-induced occult gastrointestinal blood loss: studies in Addisonian pernicious anaemia. *Br. Med. J.,* **2**, 450–452
121. Winawer, S. J., Bejar, J., McCray, R. S. and Zamcheck, N. (1971). Aspirin and atrophic gastritis. *Arch. Intern. Med.,* **127**, 129–133
122. MacKercher, P., Ivey, K. J., Baskin, W., Krause, W. and Jeffrey, G. (1976). Effect of cimetidine on aspirin-induced human gastric mucosal damage. *Gastroenterology,* **70**, 912–916
123. Crocker, J. R., Cotton, P. B. and Boyle, A. C. (1980). Cimetidine for peptic ulcer in patients with arthritis. *Ann. Rheum. Dis.,* **39**, 275–278
124. Loludice, T. A., Saleem, T. and Lang, J. A. (1981). Cimetidine in the treatment of gastric ulcer induced by steroidal and non-steroidal anti-inflammatory agents. *Am. J. Gastroenterol.,* **75**, 104–110
125. Marks, I. M., Lucke, W., Wright, J. P. *et al.* (1981). Ulcer healing and relapse rates after initial treatment with cimetidine in sucralfate. *J. Clin. Gastroenterol.,* **3**, 163–165
126. O'Laughlin, J. C., Silvoso, G. K. and Ivey, K. J. (1982). Resistance to medical therapy of gastric ulcers in rheumatic disease patients taking aspirin: a double-blind study with cimetidine and follow-up. *Dig. Dis. Sci.,* **27**, 926–980
127. Konturek, S. J., Kwiecien, N., Obtulowicz, W. *et al.* (1983). Comparison of prostaglandin E_2 and ranitidine in prevention of gastric bleeding in man. *Gut,* **24**, 89–93
128. Berkowitz, J. M., Adler, S. N., Sharp, J. T. and Warner, C. W. (1987). Reduction of

aspirin-induced gastroduodenal mucosal damage with ranitidine. *J. Clin. Gastroenterol.*, **8**, 377
129. Zoli, G., Pasquinelli, G., Bonvicini, F., Gasbarrini, G. and Laschi, R. (1986). SEM Study II: Protective effect of ranitidine against gastric and duodenal lesions induced by non-steroidal anti-inflammatory drugs. *Int. J. Tissue Reactions*, **8**, 71–77
130. Berkowitz, J. M., Rogenes, P. R., Sharp, J. T. and Warner, C. W. (1987). Ranitidine protects against gastroduodenal mucosal damage associated with chronic aspirin therapy. *Arch. Intern. Med.*, **147**, 2137–2139
131. Kimmey, M. B., Silverstein, F. E., Saunders, D. R. and Chapman, R. C. (1987). Reduction of endoscopically assessed acute aspirin-induced gastric mucosal injury with cimetidine. *Dig. Dis. Sci.*, **32**, 851–856
132. Robinson, M. G., Griffin, J. W. Jr, Bowers, J., Kogan, F. J., Kogut, D. G., Lanza, F. L. and Warner, C. W. (1989) Effect of ranitidine gastroduodenal mucosal damage induced by non-steroidal anti-inflammatory drugs. *Dig. Dis. Sci.*, **34**, 424–428
133. Stalnikowicz, R., Goldin, E., Fich, A., Wengrower, D., Eliakim, R., Ligumsky, M. and Rachmilewitz, D. (1989). Indomethacin-induced gastroduodenal damage is not affected by cotreatment with ranitidine. *J. Clin. Gastroenterol.*, **11**, 178–182
134. Roth, S. H., Bennett, R. E., Mitchell, C. S. and Harman, R. J. (1987). Cimetidine therapy in non-steroidal anti-inflammatory drug gastropathy: double-blind long-term evaluation. *Arch. Intern. Med.*, **147**, 1798–1801
135. Nagashima, R. (1981). Mechanisms of action of sucralfate. *J. Clin. Gastroenterol.*, **3** (Suppl. 2), 117–127
136. Roth, S. H., Caldwell, J. R., Marsh, W. H. *et al.* (1981). Long term sucralfate therapy in patients with rheumatoid arthritis. An endoscopic assessment. *Scand. J. Gastroenterol.*, **67** (Suppl.), 131–135
137. Shea-Donohue, T., Steel, L., Montcalm, E. and Dubois, A. (1986). Gastric protection by sucralfate. Role of mucus and prostaglandins. *Gastroenterology*, **91**, 660–666
138. Douthwaite, A. H. and Lintott, G. A. M. (1938). Gastroscopic observation of the effect of aspirin and certain other substances on the stomach. *Lancet*, **2**, 1222–1225
139. O'Laughlin, J. C., Silvoso, G. R. and Ivey, K. J. (1981). Healing of aspirin-associated peptic ulcer disease despite continued salicylate ingestion. *Arch. Intern. Med.*, **141**, 781–783
140. Ivey, K. J. (1984). Aspirin gastrointestinal toxicity. *Adv. Ther.*, **1**, 190–206
141. Graham, D. Y., Smith, J. L. and Dobbs, S. M. (1983). Gastric adaptation occurs with aspirin administration in man. *Dig. Dis. Sci.*, **28**, 1–6
142. Baskin, W. N., Ivey, K. J., Krause, W. J. *et al.* (1976). Aspirin-induced ultrastructural changes in human gastric mucosa: correlation with potential difference. *Ann. Intern. Med.*, **85**, 299–303
143. Piper, D. W., Gellatly, R. and McIntosh, J. (1982). Analgesic drugs and peptic ulcer: human studies. In Pfeiffer, D. J. (ed.),: *Drugs and Peptic Ulcer*, Vol. 2, pp. 76–93. (Boca Raton, Fla.: CRC Press)
144. Gleeson, M. H. (1982). Gastrointestinal complications of NSAIDs. *Eur. J. Rheum. Inflamm.*, **5**, 308–312
145. Akdamar, K., Ertan, A., Agrawal, N. N. *et al.* (1986). Upper gastrointestinal endoscopy in normal asymptomatic volunteers. *Gastrointestinal Endoscopy*, **32**, 78–80
146. Rahbek, I. (1976). Gastroscopic evaluation of the effect of a new antirheumatic compound, ketoprofen, on the human gastric mucosa: a double-blind crossover trial against acetyl salicylic acid. *Scand. J. Rheumatol.*, **14** (Suppl.), 63–72
147. Loebl, D. H., Craig, R. M., Culic, D. D., Ridolfo, A. S., Falk, J. and Schmid, F. R. (1977). Gastrointestinal blood loss: effect of aspirin, fenoprofen and acetaminophen in rheumatoid arthritis as determined by sequential gastroscopy and radioactive fecal markers. *J. Am. Med. Assoc.*, **237**, 976–981
148. Lanza, F. L., Royer, G. L., Nelson, R. S., Chen, T. T., Seekman, C. E. and Rack, M. F. (1979). The effects of ibuprofen, indomethacin, aspirin, naproxen and placebo in the gastric mucosa of normal volunteers. A gastroscopic and photographic study. *Dig. Dis. Sci.*, **24**, 923–928
149. Lanza, Royer, G. L., Nelson, R. S., Chen, T. T., Seckman, C. E. and Rack, M. F. (1979). The effects of ibuprofen, indomethacin, aspirin, naproxen and placebo on

the gastric mucosa of normal volunteers. A gastroscopic and photographic study. *Dig. Dis. Sci.*, **24**, 823-828
150. Prichard, P. J., Daneshmend, T. K., Milns, P. J., Edmonds, T. J., Bhaskar, N. K. and Hawkey, C. J. (1988). The use of endoscopy and blood loss measurement to slow dose dependent protection of human gastric mucosa by famolidine against aspirin (abstract). *Gut*, **29**, 729
151. Cameron, A.-J. (1975). Aspirin and gastric ulcer. *Mayo Clin. Proc.*, **50**, 565-570
152. Murray, H. S., Strottman, M. P. and Cooke, A. R. (1974). Effect of several drugs on gastric potential difference in man. *Br. Med. J.*, **1**, 19-21
153. Caruso, I. and Bianchi Porro, G. (1980). Gastroscopic evaluation of anti-inflammatory agents. *Br. Med. J.*, **280**, 75-78
154. Lanza, F. L., Royer, G. L. and Nelson, R. S. (1975). An endoscopic evaluation of the effects of non-steroidal anti-inflammatory drugs on the gastric mucosa. *Gastrointestinal Endoscopy*, **21**, 103-105
155a. Duggan, J. M. (1972). Aspirin ingestion and perforated peptic ulcer. *Gut*, **13**, 631-633
155b. Chernish, S. M., Rosenak, B. D., Brunelle, R. L. *et al.* (1979). Comparison of gastrointestinal effects of aspirin and fenoprofen: a double-blind crossover study. *Arthritis Rheum.*, **22**, 376-383
156. Lanza, F. L., Royer, G. L. Jr, Nelson, R. S. *et al.* (1981). A comparative endoscopic evaluation of the damaging effects of non-steroidal anti-inflammatory agents in the gastric and duodenal mucosa. *Am. J. Gastroenterol.*, **75**, 17-21
157a. Lanza, F. L., Nelson, R. S. and Ruck, M. F. (1984). A controlled endoscopic study comparing the toxic effects of sulindac, naproxen, aspirin and placebo in the gastric mucosa of healthy volunteers. *J. Clin. Pharmacol.*, **24**, 89-95
157b. Glarborg, J. (1977). Drug consumption before perforation of a peptic ulcer. *Br. J. Surg.*, **64**, 247-249
158. Rainsford, K. D. (1985). Anti-inflammatory drugs and the gastro-intestinal mucosa. *Gastroenterol. Clin. Biol.*, **9**, 98-101
159. Gedda, P. O. and Moritz, U. (1959). Peptic ulcer during treatment of rheumatoid arthritis with cortisone derivatives. *Acta Rheumatol. Scand.*, **4**, 249-256
160. Morris, A. D., Holt, S. D., Silvos, G. R. *et al.* (1981). Effect of anti-inflammatory drug administration in patients with rheumatoid arthritis. An endoscopic assessment. *Scand. J. Gastroenterol.*, **16** (Suppl. 67), 131-135
161. Rainsford, K. D. (1987). Toxicity of currently used anti-inflammatory and anti-rheumatic drugs. In Lewis, A. J. and Furst, D. E. (eds.) *Newer Anti-inflammatory Drugs*, pp. 215-244. (New York: Marcel Dekker)
162. Ivey, K. J. (1986). Gastrointestinal intolerance and bleeding with non-narcotic analgesics. *Drugs*, **32** (Suppl. 4), 71-89
163. Goodman, M. J., Kent, P. W. and Truelove, S. C. (1977). Inhibition of glucosamine synthesis by salicylates, hydrocortisone and two non-ulcerogenic drugs. *Arch. Int. Pharmacodyn. Ther.*, **226**, 4-10
164. Avila, M. H., Walker, A. M., Romieu, I., Perera, D. R., Spiegelman, D. L. and Jick, H. (1988). Choice of non-steroidal anti-inflammatory drug in persons treated with dyspepsia. *Lancet*, **2**, 556-559
165. Graham, D. Y. and Smith, J. L. (1985). Effects of aspirin and an aspirin–acetaminophen combination on the gastric mucosa in normal subjects. *Gastroenterology*, **88**, 1922-1925
166. Stern, Hogan, A. I., Kahm, L. H. and Isenberg, J. I. (1984). Protective effect of acetaminophen against aspirin and ethanol induced damage to the human gastric mucosa. *Gastroenterology*, **86**, 728-733
167. Lanza, F.-L., Royer, G. L. and Nelson, R. S. (1980). Endoscopic evaluation of the effects of aspirin, buffered aspirin and enteric coated aspirin on gastric and duodenal mucosa. *N. Engl. J. Med.*, **303**, 136-138
168. Lanza, F. L., Royer, G. L., Jr and Nelson, R. S. (1980). Endoscopic evaluation of the effects of aspirin, buffered aspirin, and enteric-coated aspirin on the gastric and duodenal mucosa. *N. Engl. J. Med.*, **303**, 136-138

169. Hoftiezer, J. W., Burks, M., Silvoso, G. F. and Ivey, K. J. (1980). Comparison of the effects of regular and enteric-coated aspirin on gastroduodenal mucosa in man. *Lancet*, **2**, 609–612
170. Kilander, A. and Doterall, G. (1983). Endoscopic evaluation of the comparative effects of acetylsalicylic acid and choline magnesium trisalicylate on human and gastric duodenal mucosa. *Br. J. Rheumatol.*, **22**, 36–40
171. Cohen, A. (1979). Fecal blood loss and plasma salicylate study of salicylsalicylic acid and aspirin. *J. Clin. Pharmacol.*, **19**, 242–247
172. Anslow, J. A., Balm, T. K., Hooper, J. W. et al. (1985). Minimization of gastric damage with enteric-coated aspirin granules compared to buffered aspirin. *Pharmacology*, **30**, 40–44
173. Lanza, F. L., Rack, M. F., Wagner, G. S. et al. (1985). Reduction in gastric mucosal hemorrhage and ulceration with chronic high-level dosing of enteric-coated aspirin granules two and four times a day. *Dig. Dis. Sci.*, **30**, 509–512
174. Trondstadt, Aadland, R. I., Holler, E. T. et al. (1985). Gastroscopic findings after treatment with enteric-coated and plain naproxen tablets in healthy subjects. *Scand. J. Gastroenterol.*, **20**, 239–242
175. Petroski, D. (1989). Endoscopic comparison of various aspirin preparations — gastric mucosal adaptability to aspirin restudied. *Curr. Ther. Res.*, **45**, 945–954
176. Osmes, M., Larsen, S., Eidsaunet, W. and Thom, E. (1979). Effect of diclofenac and naproxen on gastroduodenal mucosa. *Clin. Pharmacol. Therapy*, **26**, 399–405
177a. Konturek, S. J., Kwiecien, M. and Obtulowitz, W. (1982). Effect of cartrofen and indomethacin on gastric function, mucosal integrity and generation of prostaglandins. *Hepatogastroenterology*, 267–270
177b. Kurata, J. H., Elashoff, J. F. and Grossman, M. J. (1982). Inadequacy of the literature on the relationship between drugs, ulcers and gastrointestinal bleeding. *Gastroenterology*, **82**, 373–376
178. Lanza, F. L., Nelson, R. S. and Greenburg, G. (1983). Effects of fenbufen, indomethacin, naproxen and placebo on the gastric mucosa of normal volunteers. A comparative and photographic evaluation. *Am. J. Med.* (Suppl.), 75–83
179. Lanza, F. L., Panagides, J. and Salom, I. L. (1986). Etodolac compared with aspirin: an endoscopic study of the gastrointestinal tracts of normal volunteers. *J. Rheumatol.*, **13**, 299–303
180. Lanza, F. L., Royer, G. L., Rack, M. F., Seckman, C. E., Germatt, C. M., Schwartz, J. H. and Potter, C. C. (1986). Gastro-intestinal effects of ibuprofen, naproxen and aspirin in normal volunteers. *Clin. Tri. J.*, **23**, 168–177
181. Lanza, F. L., Rack, M. F., Lynn, M., Wolf, B. S. and Sanda, M. (1987). An endoscopy comparison of the effects of etodolac, indomethacin, ibuprofen, naproxen, and placebo on the gastrointestinal mucosa. *J. Rheumatol.*, **14**, 338–341
182. Carson, J. L., Strom, B. L., Soper, K. A., West, S. L. and Lec Morse, M. (1987). The association of nonsteroidal anti-inflammatory drugs with upper gastrointestinal tract bleeding. *Arch. Intern. Med.*, **147**, 85–88
183. Collins, A. J., Davies, J. and Dixon, A. St. J. (1988). A prospective endoscopic study of the effect of Orudis and Oruvail on the upper gastrointestinal tract, in patients with osteoarthritis. *Br. J. Rheumatol.*, **27**, 106–109
184. Ivey, K. J., Paome, D. B. and Krause, W. J. (1980). Acute effects of systemic aspirin on gastric mucosa in man. *Dig. Dis. Sci.*, **25**, 97–99
185. Hansen, T. M., Matzen, P. and Madsen, P. (1954). Endoscopic evaluation of the effect of indomethacin capsules and suppositories on the gastric mucosa in rheumatic patients. *J. Rheumatol.*, **11**, 484–487
186. Phillips, S. F. (1973). Gastric and duodenal ulceration associated with aspirin ingestion. *Gastrointestinal Endoscopy*, **19**, 160–163
187. Douglas, R. A. and Johnson, E. D. (1961). Aspirin and chronic gastric ulcer. *Med. J. Aust.*, **2**, 893–897
188. Gilles, M. and Skyring, A. (1968). Gastric ulcer, duodenal ulcer and gastric carcinoma: a case-control study of certain social and environmental factors. *Med. J. Aust.*, **2**, 1132–1136

189. Chapman, B. L. and Duggan, J. M. (1969). Aspirin and uncomplicated peptic ulcer. *Gut*, **10**, 443-450
190. Emmanuel, J. H. and Montgomery, R. D. (1971). Gastric ulcer and the anti-arthritic drugs. *Postgrad. Med. J.*, **47**, 227-232
191. Duggan, J. M. (1972). Aspirin ingestion and perforated peptic ulcer. *Gut*, **13**, 631-635
192. MacDonald, W. C. (1973). Correlation of mucosal histology and aspirin intake in chronic gastric ulcer. *Gastroenterology*, **65**, 381-389
193. Duggan, J. M. (1980). Gastrointestinal toxicity of minor analgesics. *Br. J. Clin. Pharmacol.*, **10**, 407S-410S
194. Duggan, J. M. (1976). Aspirin in chronic gastric ulcer: an Australian experience. *Gut*, **17**, 378-384
195. Duggan, J. M., Dobson, A. J., Johnson, H. and Fahey, P. (1986). Peptic ulcer and non-steroidal anti-inflammatory agents. *Gut*, **27**, 929-939
196. Malone, D. E., McCormick, P. A., Daly, L., Jones, B., Long, A., Bresnihan, B. Molony, J. and O'Donoghue, D. P. (1986). Peptic ulcer in rheumatoid arthritis — intrinsic or related to drug therapy? *Br. J. Rheumatol.*, **25**, 342-344
197. Bianchi Porro, G. and Pace, F. (1988). Ulcerogenic drugs and upper gastrointestinal bleeding. *Baillière's Clin. Gastroenterol.*, **2**, 309-327
198. Farah, D., Sturrock, R. D. and Russell, R. I. (1988). Peptic ulcer in rheumatoid arthritis. *Ann. Rheum. Dis.*, **47**, 478-480
199. O'Laughlin, J. C., Hoftiezer, J. W. and Ivey, K. J. (1981). The effect of aspirin in the human stomach in normals: endoscopic comparison of damage produced 1 hour, 24 hours, and 2 weeks after administration. *Scand. J. Gastroenterol.*, **16** (Suppl. 67), 211-214
200. Eastwood, G. L. and Quimby, G. E. (1982). Effect of chronic aspirin ingestion on epithelial proliferation in rat fundus, antrum, and duodenum. *Gastroenterology*, **82**, 852-856
201. Graham, D. Y., Smith, J. L. and Dobbs, S. M. (1983). Gastric adaptation occurs with aspirin administration in man. *Dis. Sci.*, **28**, 1-6
202. Smith, J. L., Spjut, H. J., Torres, E. *et al.* (1984). Mechanism of gastric mucosal adaptation to aspirin induced injury to man (abstract). *Gastroenterology*, **86**, 1257
203. Graham, D. Y., Smith, J. L., Spjut, H. J. and Torres, E. (1988). Gastric adaptation studies in human during continuous aspirin administration. *Gastroenterology*, **95**, 327-333
204. Scott, J. T., Denman, A. M. and Dorling, J. (1964). Renal irritation caused by salicylates. *Lancet*, **1**, 344-348
205. Leonards, J. R., Levy, G. and Miemczura, R. (1973). Gastrointestinal blood loss during prolonged aspirin administration. *N. Engl. J. Med.*, **289**, 1020-1022
206. Gerber, L. H., Rooney, P. J. and McCarthy, D. M. (1981). Healing of peptic ulcers during continuing anti-inflammatory drug therapy in rheumatoid arthritis. *J. Clin. Gastroenterol.*, **3**, 7-11
207. O'Laughlin, J. C., Hoftiezier, J. W. and Ivey, K. J. (1981). Healing of aspirin associated peptic ulcer disease despite continued salicylate ingestion. *Arch. Intern. Med.*, **141**, 781-783
208. Gow, P. J. and Stewart, J. T. (1982). The arthritic ulcer: a retrospective study of peptic ulceration in patients with rheumatoid arthritis. *N.Z. Med. J.*, **95**, 387-389
209. O'Laughlin, J. C., Silvoso, G. K. and Ivey, K. J. (1982). Resistance to medical therapy of gastric ulcers in rheumatic disease patients taking aspirin. A double-blind study with cimetidine and followup. *Dig. Dis. Sci.*, **27**, 976-980
210. Manniche, C., Malchow-Moller, A., Andersen, J. R. *et al.* (1987). Randomized study of the influence of non-steroidal anti-inflammatory drugs on the treatment of peptic ulcer in patients with rheumatic disease. *Gut*, **28**, 226-229
211. Piper, D. W., McIntosh, J. H., Arvotti, D. E., Fenton, B. H. and McLennan, R. (1981). Analgesic ingestion and chronic peptic ulcer. *Gastroenterology*, **80**, 427-432
212. Conn, H. O. and Blitzer, B. L. (1976). Nonassociation of adrenocorticosteroid therapy and peptic ulcer. *N. Engl. J. Med.*, **294**, 473-479

213. Messer, J., Reitman, D., Sacks, H. S. *et al.* (1983). Association of adrenocorticosteroid therapy and peptic ulcer disease. *N. Engl. J. Med.*, **309**, 21–24
214. Spiro, H. M. (1983). Is the steroid ulcer a myth? *N. Engl. J. Med.*, **309**, 45–47
215. Conn, H. O. and Poynard, T. (1985). Adrenocorticosteroid administration and peptic ulcer: a critical analysis. *J. Chron. Dis.*, **38**, 457–458
216. Domschke, W. and Domschke, S. (1977). Glucocorticoid and mineralocorticoid actions on gastric secretion in man. *Acta Hepato-Gastroenterol.*, **23**, 34–37
217. Scott, J. T., Porter, I. H., Lewis, S. M. *et al.* (1961). Studies of gastrointestinal bleeding caused by corticosteroids, salicylates and other analgesics. *Q. J. Med.*, **30**, 167–188
218. Chung, R. S. K., Field, M. and Silen, W. (1978). Effects of methyl-prednisolone on hydrogen ion absorption in the canine stomach. *J. Clin. Invest.*, **62**, 262–270
219. Borsch, G. and Schmidt, G. (1985). What's new in steroid and non-steroid drug effects on gastroduodenal mucosa? *Pathol. Res. Pract.*, **180**, 437–444
220. Howard-Lock, H., Lock, C. J., Mewa, A. and Kean, W. F. (1986). D-Penicillamine: chemistry and clinical use in rheumatic disease. *Semin. Arthritis Rheum.*, **15**, 261
221. Lussier, A., Arsenault, A., Varady, J., de Medicis, R., Lussier, Y. and LeBel, E. (1988). The use of a ^{51}Cr technique to detect gastrointestinal microbleeding associated with nonsteroidal anti-inflammatory drugs. *Semin. Arthritis Rheum.*, **17**, 40–45
222. Simon, J. B. (1985). Occult blood screening for colorectal carcinoma: a critical review. *Gastroenterology*, **88**, 820–837
223a. Wood, P. H. N. (1962). Salicylates and gastrointestinal bleeding (acetyl-salicylic acid and aspirin derivatives). *Br. Med. J.*, **1**, 669–671
223b. Domschlke, S. and Domschke, W. (1984). Gastroduodenal damage due to drugs, alcohol and smoking. *Clin. Gastroenterol.*, **13**, 405–436
224. Wood, P. H. N., Harvey-Smith, E. A. and Dixon, A. J. (1962). Salicylates and gastrointestinal bleeding: acetylsalicylic acid and aspirin derivatives. *Br. Med. J.*, **1**, 669–675
225. Croft, D. N. and Wood, P. H. N. (1967). Gastric mucosa and susceptibility to occult gastrointestinal bleeding caused by aspirin. *Br. Med. J.*, **1**, 137–141
226. Parry, D. J. and Wood, P. N. H. (1967). Relationship between aspirin taking and gastroduodenal hemorrhage. *Gut*, **8**, 301–305
227. Summerskill, W. H. F. and Alvarez, A. S. (1958). Salicylate anaemia. *Lancet*, 925–928
228. Pierson, R. N., Holt, P. R., Watson, R. M. and Keating, R. P. (1961). Aspirin and gastrointestinal bleeding. *Am. J. Med.*, **31**, 259–265
229. Leonards, J. R. and Levy, G. (1969). Reduction or prevention of aspirin-induced occult gastrointestinal blood loss in man. *Clin. Pharmacol. Ther.*, **10**, 571–575
230. Konturek, S. J., Kwiecien, N., Obtuowicz, W., Hebzda, Z. and Oleksy, J. (1988). Effects of colloidal bismuth subcitrate on aspirin-induced gastric nuerobleeding, DNA loss and prostaglandin formation in humans. *Scand. J. Gastroenterol.*, **23**, 861–866
231. Mielants, H., Veys, E. M., Verbruggen, G. *et al* (1979). Salicylate-induced gastrointestinal bleeding: comparison between soluble buffered, enteric-coated and intravenous administration. *J. Rheumatol.*, **6**, 210–218
232. Leonards, J. R. (1969). Absence of gastrointestinal bleeding following administration of salicylsalicylic acid. *J. Lab. Clin. Med.*, **74**, 911–914
233. Leonards, J. R. and Levy, G. (1972). Gastrointestinal blood loss from aspirin and sodium salicylate tablets in man. *Clin. Pharmacol. Ther.*, **14**, 62–66
234. Leonards, J. R. and Levy, G. (1972). Effects of pharmaceutical formulation on gastrointestinal bleeding from aspirin tablets. *Arch. Intern. Med.*, **129**, 457
235. Cohen, A. and Garber, H. E. (1978). Comparison of choline magnesium trisalicylate and acetylsalicylic acid in relation to fecal blood loss. *Curr. Ther. Res.*, **23**, 187–193
236. Meilants, H., Veys, E. M., Verbruggen, G. *et al.* (1981). Comparison of serum salicylate levels and gastrointestinal blood loss between salsalate (disalcid) and other forms of salicylates. *Scand. J. Rheumatol.*, **10**, 169–173
237. Prichard, P. J., Poniatowska, T. J., Willars, J. E., Ravenscroft, A. T. and Hawkey,

C. J. (1988). Effect in man of aspirin, standard indomethacin and sustained release indomethacin preparation on gastric bleeding. *Br. J. Clin. Pharmacol.*, **26**, 167-172
238. Lussier, A., Davis, A., Lussier, Y. and Lebel, E. (1989). Comparative gastrointestinal blood loss associated with placebo, aspirin and nabumetone as assessed by radio-chromium (^{51}Cr). *J. Clin. Pharmacol.*, **29**, 225-229
239. Ranlov, P. J., Nielsen, S. P. and Barenholdt, O. (1983). Faecal blood loss during administration of acetylsalicylic acid, ketoprofen and two new ketoprofen sustained-release compounds. *Scand. J. Rheumatol.*, **12**, 280-284
240. Johnson, P. C. (1982). Gastrointestinal consequences of treatment with drugs in elderly patients. *J. Am. Geriatr. Soc.*, **30** (Suppl.), 52-57
241a. Marcolongo, R., Bageli, P. F. and Montagnami, M. (1979). Gastrointestinal involvement in rheumatoid arthritis: a biopsy study. *J. Rheumatol.*, **6**, 426-440
241b. Kurata, J., Elashoff, J. and Grossman, M. I. (1982). Inadequacy of the literature on the relationship between drugs, ulcers and gastrointestinal bleeding. *Gastroenterology*, **82**, 373-382
242. Prichard, P. J., Kitchingman, G. K., Walt, R. P., Daneshmend, T. K. and Hawkey, C. J. (1989). Human gastric mucosal bleeding induced by low dose aspirin but not warfarin. *Br. Med. J.*, **298**, 493-496
243. Daneshmend, T. K., Stein, A. G., Bhaskar, N. K. and Hawkey, C. J. (1989). Failure of ethamsylate to reduce aspirin-induced gastric mucosal bleeding in humans. *Br. J. Clin. Pharmacol.*, **28**, 109-112
244. Weber, J., Werre, J. M., Julius, H. W. and Marx, J. J. M. (1988). Decreased iron absorption in patients with active rheumatoid arthritis, with and without iron deficiency. *Ann. Rheum. Dis.*, **47**, 404-409
245. Baragar, F. D. and Duthie, J. J. R. (1960). Importance of aspirin as a cause of anemia and peptic ulcer in rheumatoid arthritis. *Br. Med. J.*, **1**, 1106-1108
246. New Zealand Rheumatism Study. (1974). Aspirin and the kidney. *Br. Med. J.*, **1**, 593-600
247. Stephens, F. O. and Lawrenson, K. B. (1967). Cr excretion in bile. *Lancet*, **1**, 158
248. Slater, T. F. and Delaney, V. B. (1970). Liver adenosine triphosphate content and the bile flow in the rat. *Biochem. J.*, **116**, 303-308
249. Cooper, M. J. and Williamson, R. C. N. (1983). The action of salicylates on bile flow in man. *Br. J. Clin. Pharmacol.*, **16**, 570-572
250. Fries, J. F., Miller, S. R., Spitz, P. W., Williams, C. A., Hubert, H. B. and Bloch, D. A. (1989). Toward an epidemiology of gastropathy associated with non-steroidal anti-inflammatory drugs and hospitalization for upper gastrointestinal bleeding. *Gastroenterology*, **96**, 647-55
251. Jick, H., Field, A. D. and Perera, D. R. (1985). Certain non-steroidal anti-inflammatory drugs and hospitalization for upper gastrointestinal bleeding. *Pharmacotherapy*, **5**, 280-284
252. Beard, K., Walker, A. M., Perera, D. R. and Jick, H. (1987). Non-steroidal anti-inflammatory drugs and hospitalization for gastroesophageal bleeding in the elderly. *Arch. Intern. Med.*, **147**, 1621-1623
253. Carson, J. L. (1988). A case study: nonsteroidal anti-inflammatory drugs and gastrointestinal bleeding. *J. Rheumatol.*, **15** (Suppl. 17), 24-27
254. Faulkner, G., Prichard, P., Somerville, K. and Langman, M. J. (1988). Aspirin and bleeding peptic ulcers in the elderly. *Br. Med. J.*, **297**, 1311-1313
255. Roth, S. H. (1988). Naproxen: antirheumatic efficacy and safety in patients with pre-existing gastrointestinal disease. *Semin. Arthritis Rheum.*, **17** (Suppl. 2), 36-39
256. Prichard, P. J., Kitchingman, G. K. and Hawkey, C. J. (1987). Gastric mucosal bleeding: what dose of aspirin is safe? (Abstract) *Gut*, **28**, 1401
257. Sigler, J. W., Ridolfo, A. S. and Bluhm, G. B. (1976). Comparison of benefit-to-risk ratios of aspirin and fenoprofen: controlled multicenter study of rheumatoid arthritis. *J. Rheumatol.*, **3**, 49-60
258. Ward, K. and Weir, D. G. (1982). Piroxicam and upper gastrointestinal hemorrhage. *Ir. Med. J.*, **75**, 10-11
259. Fok, K. H., George, P. J. M. and Vicary, F. R. (1985). Peptic ulcers induced by piroxicam. *Br. Med. J.*, **290**, 117

260. Venning, G. R. (1983). Identification of adverse reactions to new drugs. II: How were 18 important reactions discovered and with what delays? Br. Med. J., 286, 365-368
261. Laake, K., Kjeldaas, K. and Borchgrevink, C. F. (1984). Side effects of piroxicam (Feldene): a one-year material of 103 reports from Norway. Acta Med. Scand., 215, 81-83
262. Weber, J. C. P. (1984). Epidemiology of adverse reactions to non-steroidal anti-inflammatory drugs. In Rainsford, K. D. and Velo, J. P. (eds.) Advances in Inflammation Research, Vol. 6, pp. 1-7. (New York: Raven Press)
263. Committee on Safety of Medicines Update. (1986). Non-steroidal anti-inflammatory drugs and serious gastrointestinal reactions. Br. Med. J., 292, 1190-1191
264. Beerman, B. (1985). Peptic ulcers induced by piroxicam. Br. Med. J., 290, 789-791
265. Ivey, K. J., Silvoso, G. R. and Krause, W. J. (1978). Effect of paracetamol on gastric mucosa. Br. Med. J., 1, 1586-1588
266. Coggan, D., Langman, M. J. S. and Spiegelhalter, D. (1982). Aspirin, paracetamol and hematemesis and melena. Gut, 23, 340-344
267. McIntosh, J. H., Byth, K. and Piper, D. W. (1985). Environmental factors in aetiology of chronic gastric ulcer: a case-control study of exposure variables before the first symptoms. Gut, 26, 789-798
268. Levy, M., Miller, D. R., Kaufman, D. W., Siskind, V. et al. (1988). Major gastro-intestinal tract bleeding. Relation to use of aspirin and other non-narcotic analgesics. Arch. Intern. Med., 148, 281-285
269. Collier, D. St. J. and Pain, J. A. (1985). Anti-inflammatory drugs and upper gastrointestinal ulcer perforation. Editorial. Clin. Rheumatol., 4, 389-391
270. Bartle, W. R., Gupta, A. K. and Lazor, J. (1986). Non-steroidal anti-inflammatory drugs and gastrointestinal bleeding. A case-control study. Arch. Intern. Med., 146, 2365-2367
271. Somerville, K., Faulkner, G. and Langman, M. (1986). Non-steroidal anti-inflammatory drugs and bleeding peptic ulcer. Lancet, 1, 462-464
272. Armstrong, C. P. and Blower, A. L. (1987). Non-steroidal anti-inflammatory drugs and life threatening complications of peptic ulceration. Gut, 28, 527-532
273. Henry, D. A., Johnston, A., Dobson, A. and Duggan, J. (1987). Fatal peptic ulcer complications and the use of non-steroidal anti-inflammatory drugs, aspirin and corticosteroids. Br. Med. J., 295, 1227-1229
274. Levy, M. (1974). Aspirin use in patients with major upper gastrointestinal bleeding and peptic ulcer disease. N. Engl. J. Med., 290, 1158-1162
275. Jick, S. S., Perera, D. R., Walker, A. M. and Jick, H. (1987). Non-steroidal anti-inflammatory drugs and hospital admission for perforated peptic ulcer. Lancet, 2, 380-382
276. Griffin, M. R., Ray, W. A. and Schaffner, W. (1988). Non-steroidal anti-inflammatory drug use and death from peptic ulcer in elderly persons. Ann. Intern. Med., 109, 359-363
277. Belcon, M. C., Rooney, P. J. and Tugwell, P. (1985). Aspirin and gastrointestinal hemorrhage: a methodologic assessment. J. Chron. Dis., 38, 101-111
278. Henry, D. A. (1988). Epidemiological assessment of the association between NSAIDs and peptic ulcer complications. Agents and Actions 24 (Suppl.), 85-94
279. Lawson, D. H. (1988). Scientific problems in collecting and analysing safety data in non-experimental studies. Drug. Inform. J., 22, 11-18
280. Barrier, C. H. and Hirschowitz, B. I. (1989). Controversies in the detection and management of non-steroidal anti-inflammatory drug-induced side effects of the upper gastrointestinal tract. Arthritis Rheum., 31, 926-932
281. Kafetz, K. (1988). Gastrointestinal hemorrhage in elderly people. Br. J. Hosp. Med., 40, 207-209
282. Rooney, P. J. and Kean, W. F. (1987). Reinforcement of bias in the medical literature: nonsteroidal anti-inflammatory drugs and the stomach — a case in point. (Letter) Br. J. Rheumatol., 26, 231-233
283. Jick, H. and Porter, J. (1978). Drug-induced gastrointestinal bleeding. Lancet, 2, 87-89

284. Banerjee, A. K., Ostick, G. and Leroy, D. W. (1983). Nonsteroidal anti-inflammatory drugs and gastrointestinal side effects. *J. Coll. Physicians, Lond.*, **17**, 228-230
285. Booker, J. A. (1983). Hematemesis and melaena in the elderly. *Age and Aging*, **12**, 49-54
286. Alverez, A. S. and Summerskill, W. H. J. (1985). Gastrointestinal hemorrhage and salicylates. *Lancet*, **1**, 920-925
287. Clinch, D. (1986). *Peptic Ulcer Disease and its Drug Causation. The Role of Non-steroidal Anti-inflammatory Drugs.* (London: Croom Helm)
288. Doherty, M., Hunt, R. H., Langman, M. J. S., Pounder, R. E., Russell, R. I., Sturrock, R. D. and Thould, A. K. (1987). Management of NSAID induced gastrointestinal disturbance. *Ann. Rheum. Dis.*, **46**, 640-643
289. Mitchell, D. M., Spitz, P. W., Young, D. Y., Block, D. A., McShane, D. J. and Fries, J. F. (1986). Survival, prognosis and causes of death in rheumatoid arthritis. *Arthritis Rheum.*, **29**, 706-714
290. Brown, R. C., Langman, M. J. S. and Lambert, P. M. (1976). Hospital admissions for peptic ulcer during 1958-72. *Br. Med. J.*, **1**, 35-37
291. Coggan, D., Lambert, P. and Langman, M. J. S. (1981). 20 years of hospital admissions for peptic ulcer in England and Wales. *Lancet*, **1**, 1302-1304
292. Emery, P. and Grahame, R. (1982). Gastrointestinal blood loss and piroxicam. *Lancet*, **1**, 1302-1303
293. Ward, K. and Weir, D. G. (1982). Piroxicam and upper gastrointestinal hemorrhage. *Ir. Med. J.*, **75**, 10-11
294. Berry, A. R., Collin, J., Frostick, S. P., Dudley, N. E. and Morris, P. J. (1984). Upper gastrointestinal hemorrhage in Oxford. *J.R. Coll. Surg. Edin.*, **29**, 134-138
295. Caradoc-Davies, T. H. (1984). Nonsteroidal anti-inflammatory drugs, arthritis, and gastrointestinal bleeding in elderly in-patients. *Age and Aging*, **13**, 295-298
296. Alexander, A. M. A., Veitch, G. B. A. and Wood, J. B. (1985). Anti-rheumatic and analgesic drug usage and acute gastrointestinal bleeding in elderly patients. *J. Clin. Hosp. Pharm.*, **10**, 89-93
297. O'Brien, J. D. and Burnham, W. R. (1985). Bleeding from peptic ulcers and use of non-steroidal anti-inflammatory drugs in the Romford area. *Br. Med. J.*, **291**, 1609-1610
298. Walker, A. J. and Dewar, A. P. (1985). Emergency peptic ulcer surgery — an association with NSAIDs (Abstract). *Gut*, **26**, 1118
299. Llewellyn, J. G. and Pritchard, M. H. (1988). Influence of age and disease state in nonsteroidal anti-inflammatory drug associated gastric bleeding. *J. Rheumatol.*, **15**, 691-694
300. Somerville, K., Faulkner, G. and Langman, M. (1986). Non-steroidal anti-inflammatory drugs and bleeding peptic ulcer. *Lancet*, **1**, 462-464
301. Skander, M. P. and Ryan, F. P. (1988). Non-steroidal anti-inflammatory drugs and pain free peptic ulceration in the elderly. *Br. Med. J.*, **297**, 833-834
302. Rosen, A. M. and Fleischer, D. E. (1989). Upper GI bleeding in the elderly: diagnosis and management. *Geriatrics*, **44**, 25-40
303. Walt, R., Katschinski, B., Logan, R. *et al.* (1986). Rising frequency of ulcer perforation in elderly people in the United Kingdom. *Lancet*, **2**, 489-492
304. McDermott, F. T. (1985). Mortality from bleeding peptic ulcer. Alfred Hospital, Melbourne, 1976-1980. *Med. J. Aust.*, **142**, 11-14
305. Kafetz, K. (1988). Gastrointestinal hemorrhage in elderly people. *Br. J. Hosp. Med.*, **40**, 207-209
306. Boardman, P. L., Burke, M. J., Camp, A. V. *et al.* (1983). Treatment of osteoarthritis with piroxicam. *Eur. J. Rheumatol. Inflamm.*, **6**, 73-83
307. Langloh, N. (1983). Experience with piroxicam in general practice. Results of a German multicentre study on 18,888 patients. *Eur. J. Rheumatol. Inflamm.*, **6**, 84-89
308. Brogden, R. N., Heel, R. C., Speight, T. M. and Avery, G. S. (1984). Piroxicam: A reappraisal of its pharmacology and therapeutic efficacy. *Drugs*, **28**, 292-323
309. Konturek, S. J. (1990). Role of growth factors in gastroduodenal protection and

healing of peptic ulcers. In Hunt, R. H. (ed.) *Peptic Ulcer Disease, Gastroenterol. Clin. N. Am.*
310. Konturek, J. W., Bielanski, W., Konturek, S. J. *et al.* (1989). Distribution and release of epidermal growth factors in humans. *Gut*, **30**, 1194
311. Konturek, S. J. (1988). Role of epidermal growth factor in gastro protection and ulcer healing. *Scand. J. Gastroenterol.*, **23**, 129-133
312. Whaley, K., Williamson, J., Chisholm, D. M., Webb, J., Mason, D. K. and Buchanan, W. W. (1973). Sjogren's syndrome I Sicca components. *Q. J. Med.*, **42**, 279-304
313. Ehrlich, G. E. (1984). Other NSAIDs of choice for rheumatoid arthritis. *Drug Intell. Clin. Pharm.*, **18**, 39-41
314. Inman, W. H. W. and Rawson, N. S. B. (1987). Prescription-event monitoring of five nonsteroidal anti-inflammatory drugs. In Rainsford, K. D. and Velo, J. P. (eds.) *Side Effects of Anti-inflammatory Drugs*, Part I, *Clinical and Epidemiological Aspects*, pp. 55-70. (Lancaster: MTP)
315. Blechman, W. J., Smid, F. R., April, P. A., Wilson, C. H. and Brooks, C. D. (1975). Ibuprofen and aspirin in rheumatoid arthritis therapy. *J. Am. Med. Assoc.*, **233**, 336-340
316. Mikulaschek, W. M. (1980). Long-term safety of benoxaprofen. *J. Rheumatol.*, **7** (Suppl. 6), 100-107
317. Blechman, W. J. and Lechner, B. L. (1979). Clinical comparative evaluation of choline magnesium trisalicylate and acetyl salicylic acid in rheumatoid arthritis. *Rheumatol. Rehabil.*, **18**, 119-124
318. Preston, S. J., Arnold, M. H., Beller, E. M. *et al.* (1989). Comparative analgesic and anti-inflammatory properties of sodium salicylate and acetylsalicylic acid (aspirin) in rheumatoid arthritis. *Br. J. Clin. Pharmacol.*, **27**, 607-611
319. The Multicentre Salsalate/Aspirin Comparison Study Group. (1989). Does the acetyl group of aspirin contribute to the anti-inflammatory efficacy of salicylic acid in the treatment of rheumatoid arthritis? *J. Rheumatol.*, **16**, 321-327
320. Paulus, H. E. (1989). Aspirin versus nonacetylated salicylate. (Editorial) *J. Rheumatol.*, **16**, 264-265
321. Aselton, P. and Jick, H. (1983). Short-term follow-up of wax matrix potassium chloride in relation to gastrointestinal bleeding. *Lancet*, **1**, 184-186
322. Zinny, M. A. (1987). Single-blinded endoscopic evaluation of varying formulations of 80 mg potassium chloride in normal volunteers. *Today's Therapeutic Trends*, **5**, 9-14
323. Patterson, D. J., Weinstein, G. S. and Jefferies, G. H. (1983). Endoscopic comparison of solid and liquid potassium chloride supplements. (Letter to Editor) *Lancet*, **2**, 1077-1078
324. Conn, H. O. and Poynard, T. (1985). Adrenocorticosteroid administration and peptic ulcer: a critical analysis. *J. Chron. Dis.*, **38**, 457-468
325. Beaumont, W. (1833). *Experiments and Observations on the Gastric Juice and the Physiology of Digestion.* (Plattsburgh, New York: J. P. Allen)
326. Fromm, D. and Robertson, R. (1976). Effects of alcohol on ion transport by isolated gastric and esophageal mucosa. *Gastroenterology*, **70**, 220-225
327. Burbidge, E. J., Lewis, R. D. and Halsted, C. H. (1984). Alcohol and the gastrointestinal tract. *Med.Clin. N. Am.*, **68**, 77-89
328. Needham, C. D., Kyle, J., Jones, P. F., Johnson, S. J. and Kerridge, D. F. (1971). Aspirin and alcohol in gastrointestinal hemorrhage. *Gut*, **12**, 819-821
329. Falaye, J. M. and Odutola, T. A. (1978). The economic potential and the role of aspirin and alcohol ingestion to haematemesis and malaena. *Nigerian Med. J.*, **8**, 526-530
330. Friedman, G. D., Siegelaub, A. B. and Seltzer, C. C. (1974). Cigarettes, alcohol, coffee and peptic ulcer. *N. Engl. J. Med.*, **290**, 469-473
331. Tariq, M., Parmar, N. S. and Ageel, A. M. (1986). Effect of nicotine and alcohol pretreatment on the gastric mucosal damage by aspirin, phenylbutazone and reserpine in rats. *Alcoholism*, **10**, 213-216
332. Goulston, K. and Cooke, A. R. (1978). Alcohol, aspirin and gastrointestinal bleeding. *Br. Med. J.*, **4**, 664-665

333. Quick, A. J. (1967). Acetylsalicylic acid as a diagnostic aid in hemostasis. *Am. J. Med. Sci.*, **254**, 392-396
334. Willoughby, J. M. T., Essigman, W. K., Weber, J. C. P. and Pinerva, R. F. (1986). Smoking and peptic ulcer in rheumatoid arthritis. *Clin. Exp. Rheumatol.*, **4**, 31-35
335. Grossman, M. I., Matsomoto, K. K. and Lichter, R. S. (1961). Fecal blood loss produced by oral and intravenous administration of various salicylates. *Gastroenterology*, **40**, 383-388
336. Bowen, R., Mayne, J. G., Cain, J. C. *et al.* (1960). Peptic ulcer in rheumatoid arthritis and relationship to steroid treatment. *Proc. Mayo Clin.*, **35**, 537-544
337. Atwater, E. C., Mongan, E. S., Weiche, D. R. and Jacox, R. F. (1965). Peptic ulcer and rheumatoid arthritis: a prospective study. *Arch. Intern. Med.*, **115**, 184-189
338. Pemberton, R. E. and Strand, L. J. (1979). A review of upper gastrointestinal effects of the newer non-steroidal anti-inflammatory agents. *Dig. Dis. Sci.*, **24**, 53-64
339. Collins, A. J. and Dutoit, J. A. (1987). Upper gastrointestinal findings and faecal occult blood in patients with rheumatic diseases taking non-steroidal anti-inflammatory drugs. *Br. J. Rheumatol.*, **26**, 295-298
340. O'Laughlin, J. C., Hoftiezer, J. W., Mahoney, J. and Ivey, K. J. (1981). Does aspirin prolong bleeding from gastric biopsies in man? *Gastrointestinal Endoscopy*, **27**, 1-5
341. Agdal, N. (1979). Drug-induced oesophageal damage: a review and report of a fatal case of indomethacin-induced ulceration. *Ugesler Laeger*, **141**, 3019-3021
342. Bataille, C., Soumagne, D., Loly, J. and Brassine, A. (1982). Oesophageal ulceration due to indomethacin. *Digestion*, **24**, 66-68
343. Heller, S. R., Fellows, I. W., Ogilvie, A. L. and Atkinson, M. (1982). Non-steroidal anti-inflammatory drugs and benign oesophageal stricture. *Br. Med. J.*, **285**, 167-168
344. Wilkins, W. E., Ridley, M. G. and Pozniak, A. L. (1984). Benign stricture of the oesophagus: role of non-steroidal anti-inflammatory drugs. *Gut*, **25**, 478-480
345. De Caestecker, J. S. and Heading, R. C. (1988). Iatrogenic oesphageal ulceration with massive hemorrhage and stricture formation. *Br. J. Clin. Pract.*, **42**, 212-214
346. Mason, S. J. and O'Meara, T. F. (1981). Drug-induced esophagitis. *J. Clin. Gastroenterol.*, **3**, 115-120
347. Beeley, L. and Stewart, P. (1987). Drug-induced disorders of the gastrointestinal tract. *Pharmaceutical J.*, **239**, 395-397
348. Bjarnason, I., So, A., Levi, A. J. *et al.* (1984). Intestinal permeability and inflammation in rheumatoid arthritis: effects of non-steroidal anti-inflammatory drugs. *Lancet*, **2**, 1171-1174
349. Bjarnason, I., Peters, T. J. and Levi, A. J. (1986). Intestinal permeability: clinical correlates. *Dig. Dis.*, **4**, 83-92
350. Rooney, P. J., Jenkins, R. T., Smith, K. M. and Coates, G. (1986). Indium-labelled polymorphonuclear leucocyte scans in rheumatoid arthritis — an important clinical cause of false positive results. *Br. J. Rheumatol.*, **25**, 167-170
351. Bjarnason, I., Zanelli, G., Smith, T., Prouse, P., Williams, P., Smethurst, P., Delacey, G., Gumpel, M. J. and Levi, A. J. (1987). Nonsteroidal anti-inflammatory drug-induced intestinal inflammation in humans. *Gastroenterology*, **93**, 480-489
352. Mielants, H. and Veys, E. M. (1985). NSAID and the leaky gut. (Letter) *Lancet*, **1**, 218
353. Cuvelier, C., Barbatis, C., Mielants, H., de Vos, M., Roels, H. and Veys, E. (1987). Histopathology of intestinal inflammatory related to reactive arthritis. *Gut*, **28**, 394-401
354. Bjarnason, I., Williams, P., Smethurst, P., Peters, T. J. and Levi, A. J. (1986). The effect of non-steroidal anti-inflammatory drugs and prostaglandins on the permeability of the human small bowel. *Gut*, **27**, 1292-1297
355. Jenkins, R. T., Rooney, P. J., Jones, D. B., Bienenstock, J. and Goodacre, R. L. (1987). Increased permeability in patients with rheumatoid arthritis: a side effect of oral nonsteroidal anti-inflammatory drug therapy? *Br. J. Rheumatol.*, **26**, 103-107
356. Debenham, G. P. (1966). Ulcer of the cecum during oxyphenbutazone (tanderil) therapy. *Can. Med. Assoc. J.*, **94**, 1182-1184
357. Bravo, A. J. and Lowman, R. M. (1968). Benign ulcer of the sigmoid colon. *Radiology*, **90**, 113-115

358. Somogyi, A., Kovacs, K. and Selye, H. (1969). Jejunal ulcers produced by indomethacin. *J. Pharm. Pharmacol.*, **21**, 122–123
359. Sturges, H. F. and Krone, C. L. (1973). Ulceration and stricture of the jejunem in a patient on long-term indomethacin therapy. *Am. J. Gastroenterol.*, **59**, 162–169
360. Heffernan, S. J. and Murphy, J. J. (1975). Ulceration of small intestine and slow-release potassium tablets. *Corr. Br. Med. J.*, **2**, 746
361. Fang, W. -F., Broughton, A. and Jacobson, E. D. (1977). Indomethacin-induced intestinal inflammation. *Dig. Dis.*, **22**, 749–760
362. Coutrot, S., Roland, D., Barbier, J., van der Marq, P., Alcalay, M. and Matuchansky, C. (1978). Acute perforation of colonic diverticula associated with short-term indomethacin. *Lancet*, 1055–1056
363. Nagaraj, H. S., Sandhu, A. S., Cook, L. N., Buchina, J. J. and Groff, D. B. (1981). Gastrointestinal perforation following indomethacin therapy in very low birth weight infants. *J. Pediatr. Surg.*, **16**, 1003–1007
364. Schwartz, J. A. (1981). Lower gastrointestinal side effects of nonsteroidal anti-inflammatory drugs. *J. Rheumatol.*, **8**, 952–954
365. Neoptolemos, J. P. and Locke, T. J. (1983). Recurrent small bowel obstruction associated with phenylbutazone. *Br. J. Surg.*, **70**, 244–245
366. Alpan, G., Eyal, F., Vinograd, I., Udassin, R., Amir, G., Mogle, P. and Glick, B. (1985). Localized intestinal perforations after enteral administration of indomethacin in premature infants. *J. Pediatr.*, **106**, 277–281
367. Charuzi, L., Ovnat, A., Zirkin, H., Peiser, J. and Sukenik, S. (1985). Ibuprofen and benign caecal ulcer. *J. Rheumatol.*, **12**, 188–189
368. Langman, M. J. S., Morgan, L. and Worrall, A. (1985). Use of anti-inflammatory drugs by patients admitted with small or large bowel perforations and hemorrhage. *Br. Med. J.*, **290**, 347–349
369. Marshall, T. A. (1985). Intestinal perforation following enteral administration of indomethacin. *J. Pediatr.*, **107**, 484–485
370. Stewart, J. T., Pennington, C. R. and Pringle, R. (1985). Anti-inflammatory drugs and bowel perforations and hemorrhage. *Br. Med. J.*, **290**, 787–788
371. Madhok, R., Mackenzie, A. and Lee, F. D. (1986). Small bowel ulceration in patients receiving non-steroidal anti-inflammatory drugs for rheumatoid arthritis. *Q. J. Med.*, **255**, 53–58
372. Savery, Muttu, S. H., Thomas, A., Grundy, A. and Maxwell, J. D. (1986). Ileal stricturing after long-term indomethacin treatment. *Postgrad. Med. J.*, **62**, 967–968
373. Sukumar, L. (1987). Recurrent small bowel obstruction associated with piroxicam. *Br. J. Surg.*, **74**, 186
374. Aabakken, L. and Osnes, M. (1989). Non-steroidal anti-inflammatory drug-induced disease in the distal ileum and large bowel. *Scand. J. Gastroenterol.*, **24** (Suppl. 163), 48–55
375. Bjarnason, J. and MacPherson, A. (1989). The changing side effect profile of non-steroidal anti-inflammatory drugs. A new approach for the prevention of a new problem. *Scand. J. Gastroenterol.*, **24** (Suppl. 163), 48–55
376. Duggan, D. E., Hooke, K. F., Noll, R. M. and Kwann, K. C. (1975). Enterohepatic circulation of indomethacin and its role in intestinal irritation. *Biochem. Pharmacol.*, **25**, 1749–1754
377. Terhaag, B. and Hermann, U. (1986). Biliary elimination of indomethacin in man. *Eur. J. Pharmacol.*, **29**, 691–695
378. Brune, K., Dietzel, K., Nuernberg, B. and Schneider, H. Th. (1987). Recent insight into the mechanism of gastrointestinal tract ulceration. *Scand. J. Rheumatol.* (Suppl.), **65**, 135–140
379. Brooks, P. M., Stephens, W. H., Stephens, M. E. D. and Buchanan, W. W. (1975). How safe are antirheumatic drugs? A study of possible iatrogenic deaths in patients with rheumatoid arthritis. *Health Bull.*, **33**, 108–111.
380. Leach, R. D. and Callum, K. C. (1981). Salicylates, steroids and benign gastrocolic fistula. *Br. J. Clin. Pract.*, **35**, 338
381. Levy, N. and Gaspar, E. (1975). Rectal bleeding and indomethacin suppositories. *Lancet*, **1**, 577
382. Hobbin, E. and Champion, G. (1986). Indomethacin suppositories. (Letter) *J. Am. Geriatr. Soc.*, **34**, 325–326

383. Marks, J. S. and Gleeson, M. H. (1975). Steatorrhea complicating therapy with mefenamic acid. *Br. Med. J.*, **4**, 442
384. Chadwick, R. G., Hossenbocus, A. and Colin-Jones, D. G. (1975). Steatorrhea complicating therapy with mefenamic acid. *Br. Med. J.*, **1**, 397
385. Bandilla, K., Gross, D., Gross, W. *et al.* (1982). Oral gold therapy with auranofin. *J. Rheumatol.* (Suppl 9), 154–159
386. van Riel, P. L. C. M., Gribnau, F. W. J., van de Putte, L. B. A. and Tap, S. H. (1983). Loose stools during auranofin treatment: clinical study and some pathogenetic possibilities. *J. Rheumatol.*, **10**, 222–226
387. Behrens, R., Devereaux, M., Hazelman, B., Szaz, K., Calvin, J. and Neale, G. (1986). Investigation of auranofin-induced diarrhoea. *Gut*, **27**, 59–65
388. Gotlieb, N. L. (1982). Comparative pharmacokinetics of parenteral and oral gold compounds. *J. Rheumatol.* (Suppl. 9), 99–109
389. Langer, H. E., Harmann, G., Heinemann, G. and Richter, K. (1987). Gold colitis induced by auranofin treatment of rheumatoid arthritis: case report and review of the literature. *Ann. Rheum. Dis.*, **46**, 787–792
390. Marcuard, S. P., Ehrinpreis, M. N. and Fitter, W. F. (1987). Gold induced ulcerative proctitis: report and review of the literature. *J. Rheumatol.*, **14**, 142–144
391. Hickling, P. and Fuller, J. (1979). Penicillamine causing acute colitis. *Br. Med. J.*, **2**, 367
392. Assini, J. F., Hamilton, R. and Strosberg, J. M. (1986). Adverse reactions to azathioprine mimicking gastroenteritis. *J. Rheumatol.*, **13**, 1117–1118
393. Hood, K., Ruppin, D. C., Gleeson, D. and Dowling, R. H. (1988). Prevention of gallstone recurrence by non-steroidal anti-inflammatory drugs. *Lancet*, **2**, 1223–1225
394. Cucala, M., Bauerfeind, P., Emde, C., Gonvers, J. J., Koelz, H. R. and Blum, A. L. (1987). Is it wise to prescribe NSAIDs with modern gastroprotective agents? *Scand. J. Rheumatol.* (Suppl. 65), 141–154
395. Whaley, K. and Webb, J. (1977). Liver and kidney disease in rheumatoid arthritis. *Clin. Rheum. Dis.*, **3**, 527–547
396. Mydick, I., Yang, J., Stollerman, G. H., Wroblewski, F. and La Due, J. S. (1955). The influence of rheumatic fever on serum concentrations of the enzyme glutamic oxalacetic transaminase. *Circulation*, **12**, 795
397. Russell, A. S., Sturge, R. A., and Smith, M. A. (1971). Serum transaminases during salicylate therapy. *Br. Med. J.*, **2**, 428–429
398. Iancu, T. (1972). Serum transaminases and salicylate therapy. *Br. Med. J.*, **2**, 167
399. Athreya, B. H., Gorske, A. L. and Myers, A. R. (1973). Aspirin-induced abnormalities of liver function. *Am. J. Dis. Child.*, **126**, 638–641
400. Rich, R. R. and Johnson, J. S. (1973). Salicylate hepatotoxicity in patients with juvenile rheumatoid arthritis. *Arthritis Rheum.*, **16**, 1
401. Athreya, B. A., Moser, G., Cecil, H. S. and Myers, A. R. (1975). Aspirin-induced hepatotoxicity in juvenile rheumatoid arthritis. *Arthritis Rheum.*, **18**, 347–353
402. Goldenberg, D. L. (1974). Aspirin hepatotoxicity. *Ann. Intern. Med.*, **80**, 773
403. Seaman, W. E. and Plotz, P. H. (1976). Effect of aspirin on liver tests in patients with rheumatoid arthritis or SLE and in normal volunteers. *Arthritis Rheum.*, **19**, 155–160
404. Seaman, W. E., Ishak, K. G. and Plotz, P. H. (1974). Aspirin-induced hepatotoxicity in patients with systemic lupus erythematosus. *Ann. Intern. Med.*, **80**, 1
405. Wolfe, J. D., Metzger, A. L. and Goldstein, R. C. (1974). Aspirin hepatitis. *Ann. Intern. Med.*, **80**, 74
406. Ricks, W. B. (1976). Salicylate hepatotoxicity in Reiter's syndrome. Letter. *Ann. Intern. Med.*, **84**, 52–53
407. Paulus, H. E. and Furst, D. E. (1989). Aspirin and other non-steroidal anti-inflammatory drugs. In McCarty, D. J. (ed.) *Arthritis and Allied Conditions. A Textbook of Rheumatology*, 1th edn, Chap. 11, pp. 507–543. (Philadelphia: Lea & Febiger)
408. Paulus, H. E. (1982). Government affairs: FDA Arthritis Advisory Committee meeting. *Arthritis Rheum.*, **25**, 1124–1125
409. Gitlin, N. (1980). Salicylate hepatotoxicity: the potential role of hypoalbuminemia. *J. Clin. Gastroenterol.*, **2**, 281–285

410. Zimmerman, H. J. (1981). Effects of aspirin and acetaminophen on the liver. *Arch. Intern. Med.*, **141**, 333–342
411. Tolman, K. G., Peterson, P., Gray, P. and Hammar, S. P. (1978). Hepatotoxicity of salicylates in monolayer cell cultures. *Gastroenterology*, **74**, 205–208
412. Garber, E., Craig, R. M. and Bahu, R. M. (1975). Aspirin hepatitis. *Ann. Intern. Med.*, **82**, 592–593
413. Rachelefsky, G. S. (1976). Serum enzyme abnormalities in juvenile rheumatoid arthritis. *Pediatrics*, **48**, 730–736
414. Whaley, K., Goudie, R. B., Williamson, J., Nuki, G., Dick, W. C. and Buchanan, W. W. (1970). Liver disease in Sjogren's syndrome and rheumatoid arthritis. *Lancet*, **1**, 861–863
415. Webb, J., Whaley, K., MacSween, R. N. M., Nuki, G., Dick, W. C. and Buchanan, W. W. (1975). Severe disease in rheumatoid arthritis and Sjogren's syndrome: prospective study using biochemical and serological markers of hepatic dysfunction. *Ann. Rheum. Dis.*, **34**, 70–80
416. Reye, R. D. K., Morgan, G. and Baral, J. (1963). Encephalopathy and fatty degeneration of the viscera: a disease entity in childhood. *Lancet*, **2**, 749–752
417. Johnson, G. M., Scurletis, T. D. and Carroll, N. B. (1963). A study of 16 fatal cases of encephalitis-like disease in North Carolina children. *N. C. Med. J.*, **24**, 464–473
418. Halpin, T. J., Holtzhauer, F. J., Campbell, R. J. *et al.* (1982). Reye's syndrome and medication use. *J. Am. Med. Assoc.*, **248**, 687–691
419. Hurwitz, E. S., Nelson, D. B., Davis, C., Morens, D. and Schonberger, L. B. (1982). Maternal surveillance for Reye's syndrome: a five year review. *Pediatrics*, **70**, 895–900
420. Lichtenstein, P. K., Heub, J. E. and Daugherty, C. C. (1983). Grade I Reye's syndrome: a frequent cause of vomiting and liver dysfunction after varicella and upper respiratory-tract infection. *N. Engl. J. Med.*, **309**, 133–139
421. Luscombe, F. A., Monto, A. S. and Baublis, J. V. (1980). Mortality due to Reye's syndrome in Michigan: distribution and longitudinal trends. *J. Infect. Dis.*, **142**, 363–371
422. Orlowski, J. P. (1984). Aspirin and Reye's syndrome. *Postgrad. Med.*, **75**, 47–54
423. Stillman, A., Gitter, H., Shillington, D., Sobonya, R., Payne, C. M., Ettinger, D. and Lee, S. M. (1983). Reye's syndrome in the adult: case report and review of the literature. *Am. J. Gastroenterol.*, **78**, 365–368
424. Starko, K. M. and Mullick, F. G. (1983). Hepatic and cerebral pathology findings in children with fatal salicylate intoxication: further evidence for a causal relation between salicylate and Reye's syndrome. *Lancet*, **1**, 326–329
425. Partin, J. C., Schubert, W. K. and Partin, J. S. (1971). Mitochondrial ultrastructure in Reye's syndrome (encephalopathy and fatty degeneration of the viscera). *N. Engl. J. Med.*, **285**, 1339–1343
426. Daugherty, C. C., McAdams, J. A. and Partin, J. S. (1983). Aspirin and Reye's syndrome. Letter to the Editor. *Lancet*, **2**, 104
427. Rennebohm, R. M., Heubi, J. E., Daughety, C. C. *et al.* (1985). Reye's syndrome in children receiving salicylate therapy for connective tissue disease. *J. Pediatr.*, **107**, 877–880
428. Trauner, D. A., Horvath, E. and Davis, L. E. (1988). Inhibition of fatty acid beta oxidations by influenza B virus and salicylic acid in mice: implications for Reye's syndrome. *Neurology*, **38**, 239–241
429. Martens, M. E. and Lee, C. P. (1984). Reye's syndrome: salicylates and mitochondrial functions. *Biochem. Pharmacol.*, **33**, 2869–2876
430. Martens, M. E., Chang, C. H. and Lee, C. P. (1986). Reye's syndrome: mitochondrial swelling and Ca^{2+} release induced by Reye's plasma, allantoin and salicylate. *Arch. Biochem. Biophys.*, **224**, 773–786
431. Trauner, D. A., Myhan, W. L. and Sweetman, L. (1975). Short-chain organic acidemia and Reye's syndrome. *Neurology*, **25**, 296–298
432. Sinatra, F., Yoshida, T., Applebaum, M. N., Mason, W., Hoogengrad, N. J. and Sunshine, P. (1975). Abnormalities of carbamyl phosphate synthetase and ornithine transcarbamylase in liver of patients with Reye's syndrome. *Pediatric Res.*, **9**, 829–832
433. Snodgrass, P. J. and De Long, G. R. (1976). Urea cycle deficiencies and an increased

nitrogen load producing hyperammonemia in Reye's syndrome. *N. Engl. J. Med.*, **294**, 855–857

434. Robinson, B. H., Taylor, J., Cutz, E. and Gall D. G. (1978). Reye's syndrome: preservation of mitochondrial enzymes in brain and muscle compared with liver. *Pediatric Res.*, **12**, 1045–1047
435. You, K. (1983). Salicylate and mitochondrial injury in Reye's syndrome. *Science*, **221**, 163–165
436. Tomasova, H., Nevoral, J., Pachl, J. and Kincl, V. (1984). Aspirin esterase activity and Reye's syndrome. (Letter), *Lancet*, **2**, 43
437. Starko, K. M., Ray, C. G., Dominguez, L. B. *et al*. (1980). Reye's syndrome and salicylate use. *Pediatrics*, **66**, 859–864
438. Waldman, R. J., Hall, W. N., McGee, H. *et al*. (1982) Aspirin as a risk factor in Reye's syndrome. *J. Am. Med. Assoc.*, **247**, 3089–3094
439. Hurwitz, E. S., Barrett, M. J., Bregman, D. *et al*. (1985). Public Health Service study on Reye's syndrome and medications: report of the pilot phase. *N. Engl. J. Med.*, **313**, 849–857
440. Hurwitz, E. S., Barrett, M. J., Bregman, D. *et al*. (1987). Public Health Service study of Reye's syndrome and medications: report of the main study. *J. Am. Med. Assoc.*, **257**, 1905–1911
441. Christoffersen, F., Faarup, P., Geertinger, P. and Krogh, P. (1980). Reye's syndrome in a child on long-term salicylate medication. *Forensic Sci. Int.*, **15**, 129–133
442. Hurwitz, E. S. (1988). The changing epidemiology of Reye's syndrome in the United States: further evidence for a public health success. Editorial. *J. Am. Med. Assoc.*, **260**, 3178–3180
443. Barrett, M. J., Hurwitz, E. S., Schomberger, L. B. *et al*. (1986). Changing epidemiology of Reye's syndrome in the United States. *Pediatrics*, **77**, 598–602
444. Remington, P. L., Rawley, D., McGee, H. *et al*. (1986). Decreasing trends in Reye's syndrome and aspirin in Michigan, 1979–1984. *Pediatrics*, **77**, 93–98
445. Sienko, D., Anda, R. F., McGee, H. *et al*. (1987). Reye's syndrome and salicylates. Letter to the Editor. *J. Am. Med. Assoc.*, **258**, 3119
446. Rowe, P. C., Valle, D. and Bruislow, S. W. (1988). Inborn errors of metabolism in children referred with Reye's syndrome. A changing pattern. *J. Am. Med. Assoc.*, **260**, 3168–3171
447. Roe, C. R., Millington, D. S. and Conway, H. T. (1986). Reye's syndrome: need for mass spectrometry. *J. Natl. Reye's Syndrome Found.*, **6**, 94–101
448a. Remington, P. L., Shabino, C. L., McGee, H. *et al*. (1985). Reye's syndrome and juvenile rheumatoid arthritis in Michigan. *Am. J. Dis. Child.*, **139**, 870–872
448b. Rennebohm, R. M., Heubi, J. E., Dougherty, C. C. and Daniels, S. R. (1985). Reye's syndrome in children receiving salicylate therapy for connective tissue disease. *J. Pediatr.*, **107**, 877–880
449. Sullivan, K. M., Remington, P. L., Hurwitz, E. S. and Halpin, T. J. (1988). Reye's syndrome among patients with juvenile rheumatoid arthritis. (Letter). *J. Am. Med. Assoc.*, **260**, 3434–3435
450. Hollister, J.-R. (1985). Aspirin in juvenile rheumatoid arthritis. *Am. J. Dis. Child.*, **139**, 866–867
451. British Paediatric Surveillance Unit. (1987). Reye's syndrome surveillance scheme: Fourth summary surveillance report. *Communicable Dis. Rep.*, **33**, 3–6
452. Anonymous. Reye's syndrome and aspirin. *Drug Ther. Bull.*, **22**, 79–80
453. Katyare, S. S. and Satav, J. G. (1989). Impaired mitochondrial oxidative energy metabolism following paracetamol-induced hepatotoxicity in the rat. *Br. J. Pharmacol.*, **96**, 51–58
454. Hannequin, J. R., Doffoel, M. and Schmutz, G. (1988). Les hepatites secondaires aux anti-inflammatoires non steroidiens recents. *Rev. Rheum.*, **55**, 983–988
455. Llorca, G., Larbe, J. P., Collet, Ph., Ravault, A. and Lejeune, F. (1988). Changing the class of NSAID in cases of hepatotoxicity. (Correspondence). *Ann. Rheum. Dis.*, **47**, 791
456. Paulus, H. E. (1982). Government affairs: FDA arthritis advisory committee meeting. *Athritis Rheum.*, **25**, 1124–1125

457. Letendre, P. W., De Jong, D. J. and Miller, D. R. (1985). The use of methotrexate in rheumatoid arthritis. *Drug Intell. Clin. Pharm.*, **19**, 349-358
458. Gispen, J. G., Alarcon, G. S., Johnson, J. J., Acton, R. T., Barger, B. O. and Koopman, W. J. (1987). Toxicity to methotrexate in rheumatoid arthritis. *J. Rheumatol.*, **14**, 74-79
459. Health and Public Policy Committee, American College of Physicians. (1987). Methotrexate in rheumatoid arthritis. *Ann. Intern. Med.*, **107**, 418-419
460. Aponte, J. and Petrelli, M. (1988). Histopathologic findings in the liver of rheumatoid arthritis patients treated with long-term bolus methotrexate. *Arthritis Rheum.*, **31**, 1457-1464
461. Bjorkman, D. J., Hammond, E. H., Lee, R. G., Clegg, D. O. and Tolman, K. G. (1988). Hepatic ultrastructure after methotrexate therapy for rheumatoid arthritis. *Arthritis Rheum.*, **31**, 1465-1472
462. Furst, D. E. and Kremer, J. M. (1988). Methotrexate in rheumatoid arthritis. *Arthritis Rheum.*, **31**, 305-314
463. Kremer, J. M. and Lee, J. K. (1988). A long-term prospective study of methotrexate in rheumatoid arthritis. *Arthritis Rheum.*, **31**, 577-584
464. Kremer, J. M., Lee, R. G. and Tolman, K. G. (1989). Liver histology in rheumatoid arthritis in patients on long term methotrexate therapy. *Arthritis Rheum.*, **32**, 121-127
465. Robinson, J. K., Baughman, R. D., Auerbach, R. and Cimis, R. J. (1980). Methotrexate hepatotoxicity in psoriasis: consideration of liver biopsies at regular intervals. *Arch. Dermatol.*, **116**, 413-415
466. Zachariae, H., Kragballe, K. and Sogaard, H. (1980). Methotrexate-induced liver cirrhosis: studies including serial liver biopsies during continued treatment. *Br. J. Dermatol.*, **102**, 407-412
467. Alarcon, G. S., Tracy, I. C. and Blackburn, W. D., Jr. (1989). Methotrexate in rheumatoid arthritis: toxic effects as the major factor in limiting long-term treatment. *Arthritis Rheum.*, **32**, 671-681
468. Kremer, J. M. and Lee, J. K. (1986). The safety and efficacy of the use of methotrexate in long-term therapy for rheumatoid arthritis. *Arthritis Rheum.*, **29**, 822-831
469. Tugwell, P., Bennett, K. and Gent, M. (1987). Methotrexate in rheumatoid arthritis: indications, contraindications, efficacy and safety. *Ann. Intern. Med.*, **107**, 358-366
470. Wallace, C. A., Bleyer, W. A., Sherry, D. D., Salmonson, K. L. and Wedgwood, R. J. (1989). Toxicity and serum levels of methotrexate in children with juvenile rheumatoid arthritis. *Arthritis Rheum.*, **32**, 677-681
471. Morgan, S. L., Saway, A. and Alarcon, G. S. (1989). Folic acid treatment in methotrexate-treated rheumatoid arthritis patients: comment on the article by Furst and Kremer. (Letter to the Editor). *Arthritis Rheum.*, **32**, 113-114
472. Buckley, L. M., Cooper, S. M. and Vacek, P. M. (1989). The use of leucovorin after low dose methotrexate in patients with rheumatoid arthritis. (Abstract). *Arthritis Rheum.*, **31** (Suppl.), R3
473. Weinstein, G., Roenigk, H. H., Maibach, H., Cosmides, J., Halprin, K. and Millard, M. (1973). Psoriasis-liver methotrexate interactions. *Arch. Dermatol.*, **108**, 36-42
474. Van Ness, M. M. and Diehl, A. M. (1989). Is liver biopsy useful in the evaluation of patients with chronically elevated liver enzymes? *Ann. Intern. Med.*, **111**, 473-478
475. Podurgiel, B. J. (1973). Liver injury associated with methotrexate therapy for psoriasis. *Mayo Clin. Proc.*, **48**, 787-792
476. Miller, J. A. (1985). Ultrasound as a screening procedure for methotrexate-induced hepatic damage in severe psoriasis. *Br. J. Dermatol.*, **113**, 699-705
477. Huskisson, E. C. (1984). Azathioprine. *Clin. Rheum. Dis.*, **10**, 325-332
478. Zarday, Z., Veith, F. J., Guideman, M. L. *et al.* (1972). Irreversible liver damage after azathioprine. *J. Am. Med. Assoc.*, **222**, 660-661
479. Munro, D. D. (1973). Azathioprine in psoriasis. *Proc. Roy. Soc. Med.*, **66**, 747-748
480. Sparberg, M., Simon, N. and Del Greco, F. (1969). Intrahepatic cholestasis due to azathioprine. *Gastroenterology*, **57**, 439-441

481. Du Vivier, A., Munro, D. D. and Verbov, J. (1974). Treatment of psoriasis with azathioprine. *Br. Med. J.*, **1**, 49-51
482. Schein, P. S. and Winokur, S. H. (1975). Immunosuppressives and cytotoxic chemotherapy long-term complications. *Ann. Intern. Med.*, **82**, 84-95
483. DePhinho, R. A., Goldberg, C. S. and Lefkowitch, J. H. (1984). Azathioprine and the liver. Evidence favouring idiosyncratic mixed cholestatic-hepato cellular injury in humans. *Gastroenterology*, **86**, 162-165
484. Clements, P. J. and Davis, J. (1986). Cytotoxic drugs; their clinical application to the rheumatic diseases. *Semin. Arthritis Rheum.*, **15**, 231-254
485. Farr, M., Symmons, D. P. M. and Bacon, P. A. (1985). Raised serum alkaline phosphatase and aspartate transaminase levels in two rheumatoid patients treated with sulphasalazine. *Ann. Rheum. Dis.*, **44**, 798-800
486. Mitrane, M. D., Singh, A. and Seibold, J. R. (1986). Cholestasis and fatal agranulocytosis complicating sulfasalazine therapy. *J. Rheumatol.*, **13**, 969-972d
487. Pinals, R. S. (1988). Sulfasalazine in the rheumatic disease. *Semin. Arthritis Rheum.*, **17**, 246-259
488. Aubery, D. A. (1970). Massive hepatic necrosis after cyclophosphamide. (Letter). *Br. Med. J.*, **3**, 588
489. Walters, D., Robinson, R. G., Dick-Smith, J. B. *et al.* (1972). Poor response in two cases of juvenile rheumatoid arthritis to treatment with cyclophosphamide. *Med. J. Aust.*, **2**, 1070
490. Bacon, A. M. and Rosenberg, S. A. (1982). Cyclophosphamide hepatotoxicity in a patient with systemic lupus erythematosus. *Ann. Intern. Med.*, **97**, 62-63
491. Kovarsky, J. (1983). Clinical pharmacology and toxicology of cyclophosphamide: emphasis on use in rheumatic diseases. *Semin. Arthritis Rheum.*, **12**, 359-372
492. Barzilai, D., Dickstein, G., Enat, R. *et al.* (1978). Cholestatic jaundice caused by D-penicillamine. *Ann. Rheum. Dis.*, **37**, 98-100
493. Wollheim, F. A. and Lindstrom, C. G. (1979). Liver abnormalities in penicillamine treated patients with rheumatoid arthritis. *Scand. J. Rheumatol.*, **28**, 100-107
494. Multz, C. V. (1981). Cholestatic hepatitis caused by penicillamine. *J. Am. Med. Assoc.*, **246**, 674-675
495. Rodger, R. S. C., Turney, J. H., Haines, I., Michael, J., Adu, D. and McMaster, P. (1983). Cyclosporin and liver function in renal allograft recipients. *Transplant. Proc.*, **15**, 2754-2756
496. Lowthian, P. J., Cleland, L. G. and Vernon-Roberts, B. (1984). Hepatotoxicity with aurothioglucose therapy. *Arthritis Rheum.*, **27**, 230-232
497. Ben-Yehuda, O., Tomer, Y. and Shoenfeld, Y. (1988) Advances in therapy of autoimmune diseases. *Semin. Arthritis Rheum.*, **17**, 206-220
498. O'Callaghan, J. W. and Brooks, P. M. (1986). Disease-modifying agents and immunosuppressive drugs in the elderly. *Clin. Rheum. Dis.*, **12**, 275-289
499. Prescott, L. F. (1983). Paracetamol overdosage. Pharmacological considerations and clinical management. *Drugs*, **25**, 290-314
500. Prescott, L. F. (1986). Effects of non-narcotic analgesics on the liver. *Drugs*, **32** (Suppl. 4), 129-147
501. Goulding, R., Volans, G. N. and Crome, P. (1976). Paracetamol hepatotoxicity (Letter). *Lancet*, **1**, 358
502. Batterman, R. C. and Grossman, J. A. (1955). Analgesic effectiveness and safety of N-acetyl-para-amino-phenol. *Fed. Proc.*, **14**, 316-317
503. Barker, J. D., De Carle, D. J. and Anuras, S. (1977). Chronic excessive acetaminophen use and liver damage. *Ann. Intern. Med.*, **87**, 299-301
504. Johnson, G. K. and Tolman, K. G. (1977). Chronic liver disease and acetaminophen. *Ann. Intern. Med.*, **87**, 302-304
505. Bonkowsky, H. L., Mudge, G. H. and McMurtry, R. J. (1978). Chronic hepatic inflammation and fibrosis due to low doses of paracetamol. *Lancet*, **1**, 1016-1018
506. Rosenburg, D. M. and Neelon, F. A. (1978). Acetaminophen and liver disease (Letter). *Ann. Intern. Med.*, **88**, 129-30
507. Ware, A. J., Upchurch, K. S., Eigenbrodt, E. H. and Norman, D. A. (1978). Acetaminophen and the liver (Letter). *Ann. Intern. Med.*, **88**, 267-268

508. Holzbach, R. T. (1981). Drug-induced liver disease. *Primary Care*, **8**, 231–250
509. Zimmerman, H. J. (1981). Effects of aspirin and acetaminophen on the liver. *Arch. Intern. Med.*, **141**, 333–42
510. Dahlin, D. C., Miwa, G. T., Lu, A. Y. H. and Nelson, S. D. (1984). N-acelyl-*p*-benzoquinone imine: a cytochrome P-450-mediated oxidation product of acetaminophen. *Proc. Natl. Acad. Sci. USA*, **81**, 1327–1331
511. Pirotte, J. H. (1984). Apparent potentiation by phenobarbital of hepatotoxicity from small doses of acetaminophen (Letter). *Ann. Intern. Med.*, **101**, 403
512. Cupit, G. C. (1982). The use of non-prescription analgesics in an older population. *J. Am. Geriatr. Soc.*, **30** (Suppl.), 76–80
513. Benson, G. D. (1983). Acetaminophen in chronic liver disease. *Clin. Pharm. Ther.*, **33**, 95–101
514. Prescott, L. F. and Critchley, J. A. J. H. (1983). Drug interactions affecting analgesic toxicity. *Am. J. Med.*, **75** (Suppl. 5A), 113–116
515. Regal, R. E. (1986). Acetaminophen chronic toxicity (Letter). *Drug Intell. Clin. Pharm.*, **20**, 507
516. Schlegel, S. I. and Paulus, H. E. (1986). Non-steroidal and analgesic therapy in the elderly. *Clin. Rheum. Dis.*, **12**, 245–273
517. Henrich, W. L. (1983). Nephrotoxicity of nonsteroidal anti-inflammatory agents. *Am. J. Kidney Dis.*, **2**, 478.
518a. Garella, S. and Matarese, R. A. (1984). Renal effects of prostaglandins and clinical adverse effects of non-steroidal anti-inflammatory agents. *Medicine (Baltimore)*, **63**, 165–181
518b. Clive, D. M. and Stoff, J. S. (1984). Renal syndromes associated with non-steroidal anti-inflammatory drugs. *N. Engl. J. Med.*, **310**, 563–572
519. Dunn, M. J. (1987). The role of arachidonic acid metabolites in renal homeostatis: non-steroidal anti-inflammatory drugs renal function and biochemical, histological and clinical effects and drug interactions. *Drugs*, **33** (Suppl. 1), 56–66
520. Stillman, M. T., Napier, J. and Blackshear, J. L. (1984). Adverse effects of non-steroidal anti-inflammatory drugs on the kidney. *Med. Clin. N. Am.*, **68**, 371–385
521. Blackshear, J. L., Napier, J. S., Davidman, M. and Stillman, M. T. (1985). Renal complications of non-steroidal anti-inflammatory drugs: identification and monitoring of those at risk. *Semin. Arthritis Rheum.*, **14**, 163–175
522. Adams, D. H., Michael, J., Bacon, P. A., Howie, A. J., McConkey, B. and Adu, D. (1986). Non-steroidal anti-inflammatory drugs and renal failure. *Lancet*, **2**, 57–60
523. Bulpitt, C. J. (1986). Pharmaco-epidemiological considerations in patients with arthritis and vascular disease of the kidney. *Scand. J. Rheumatol.* (Suppl. 62), 4–13
524. Hart, D., Ward, M. and Lifschitz, M. D. (1987). Suprofen-related nephrotoxicity. A distinct clinical syndrome. *Ann. Intern. Med.*, **106**, 235–238
525. Levenson, D. J., Simmons, C. E. and Brenner, B. M. (1982). Arachidonic acid metabolism, prostaglandins and the kidney. *Am. J. Med.*, **72**, 354–374
526. Dunn, M. J. (1984). Clinical effects of prostaglandin in renal disease. *Hosp. Pract.*, **19**, 99–113
527. Dunn, M. J. (1984). Non-steroidal anti-inflammatory drugs and renal function. *Ann. Rev. Med.*, **35**, 411–428
528. Pugliese, F. and Ciabattoni, G. (1984). The role of prostaglandins in the control of renal function: renal effects of non-steroidal anti-inflammatory drugs. *Clin. Exp. Rheumatol.*, **2**, 345–352
529. Carmichael, J. and Shankel, S. W. (1985). Effects of non-steroidal anti-inflammatory drugs on prostaglandins and renal function. *Am. J. Med.*, **78**, 992–1000
530. Arroyo, V., Gines, P., Rimolo, A. and Gaha, J. (1986). Renal function abnormalities, prostaglandins and effects of nonsteroidal anti-inflammatory drugs in cirrhosis and ascites. An overview with emphasis on pathogenesis. *Am. J. Med.*, **81** (Suppl. 2B), 104–122
531. Cannon, P. J. (1986). Prostaglandins in congestive heart failure and the effects of non-steroidal anti-inflammatory drugs. *Am. J. Med.*, **81** (Suppl. 2B), 123–132
532. Patrono, C. (1986). Inhibition of renal prostaglandin synthesis in man: methodological and clinical implications. *Scand. J. Rheumatol.*, Suppl. 62, 14–25

533. Patrono, C. and Pierucc, A. (1986). Renal effects of non-steroidal anti-inflammatory drugs in chronic glomerular disease. *Am. J. Med.*, **81** (Suppl. 2B), 71-83
534. Scharschmidt, L., Simonson, M. and Dunn, M. J. (1986). Glomerular prostaglandins, angiotensin II and nonsteroidal anti-inflammatory drugs. *Am. J. Med.*, **81** (Suppl. 2B), 30-42
535. Schlondorff, D. (1986). Renal prostaglandin synthesis: sites of production and specific actions of prostaglandins. *Am. J. Med.*, **81** (Suppl. 2B), 1-11
536. Zipser, R. D. (1986). Role of renal prostaglandins and the effects of non-steroidal anti-inflammatory drugs in patients with liver disease. *Am. J. Med.*, **81** (Suppl. 2B), 95-103
537. Brooks, P. M., Cossum, P. A. and Boyd, G. W. (1980). Rebound rise in renin concentrations after cessation of salicylates. *N. Engl. J. Med.*, **303**, 562-564
538. Donker, A. J. M., Arisz, L., Brentjens, J. R. H., van de Hem, G. K. and Hollemans, H. J. G. (1976). The effect of indomethacin on renal function and plasma renin activity in man. *Nephron*, **17**, 288-296
539. Romero, J. C., Dunlap, C. L. and Strong, C. G. (1976). The effect of indomethacin and other anti-inflammatory drugs on the renin-angiotensin system. *J. Clin. Invest.*, **58**, 282-288
540. Lamy, P. P. (1986). Renal effects of nonsteroidal anti-inflammatory drugs. Heightened risk to the elderly? *J. Am. Geriatr. Soc.*, **34**, 361-367
541. Kleinknecht, C., Broyer, R. M., Gubler, M. C. *et al.* (1980). Irreversible renal failure after indomethacin in steroid-resistant nephrosis. (Letter). *N. Engl. J. Med.*, **302**, 691
542. Arisz, L., Donker, A. J. M., Brentjens, J. R. H. *et al.* (1976). The effect of indomethacin on proteinuria and kidney function in the nephrotic syndrome. *Acta Med. Scand.*, **199**, 121-125
543. Boyer, T. D., Zia, P. and Reynolds, T. B. (1979). Effect of indomethacin and prostaglandin A_1 on renal function and plasma renin activity in alcoholic liver disease. *Gastroenterology*, **77**, 215-222
544. Rowe, J. W., Andres, R., Tobin, J. D., Norris, A. H. and Shock, N. W. (1976). The effects of age on creatinine clearance in man: a cross-sectional and longitudinal study. *J. Gerontol.*, **31**, 155-163
545. Dybkaer, R., Lauritzen, M. and Krakhauer, R. (1981). Relative reference values for clinical chemical and haematological quantities in 'healthy' people. *Acta Med. Scand.*, **209**, 1-9
546. Henrich, W. L. (1981). Role of prostaglandins in renin secretion. *Kidney Int.*, **19**, 822-830
547. Tan, S. Y., Shapiro, R., Franco, R. *et al.* (1979). Indomethacin-induced prostaglandin inhibition with hyperkalemia: a reversible cause of hyporeninemic hypoaldosteronism. *Ann. Intern. Med.*, **90**, 783-785
548. Galler, M., Folkert, V. W. and Schlondorff, M. (1981). Reversible acute renal insufficiency and hyperkalemia following indomethacin therapy. *J. Am. Med. Assoc.*, **246**, 154-155
549. Blackshear, J. L., Davidman, M. and Stillman, T. (1983). Identification of risk for renal insufficiency from non-steroidal anti-inflammatory drugs. *Arch. Intern. Med.*, **143**, 1130-1134
550a. Torres, V. E. (1982). Presence and future of non-steroidal anti-inflammatory drugs in nephrology. *Mayo Clin. Proc.*, **57**, 389-392
550b. Schlegel, S. I. and Paulus, H. E. (1986). Non-steroidal and analgesic therapy in the elderly. *Clin. Rheum. Dis.*, **12**, 245-273
551. Meier, D. E., Myers, W. M., Swensen, R. *et al.* (1983). Indomethacin-associated hyperkalaemia in the elderly. *J. Am. Geriatr. Soc.*, **31**, 271
552. Brown, J., Dollery, C. and Valdes, G. (1986). Interaction of non-steroidal anti-inflammatory drugs with antihypertensive and diuretic agents. Control of vascular reactivity by endogenous prostanoids. *Am. J. Med.*, **81** (Suppl. 2B), 43-57
553. Skinner, M. H., Mutterperl, D. O. and Zeitz, H. J. (1987). Sulindac inhibits bumetanide-induced sodium and water excretion. *Clin. Pharmacol. Ther.*, **42**, 542-546
554. Dixey, J. J., Noormohamed, F. H., Lant, A. F. and Brewerton, D. A. (1987). The

effects of naproxen and sulindac on renal function and their interaction with hydrochlorothiazide and piretanide in man. *Br. J. Clin. Pharmacol.*, **23**, 55-63

555. Ciabattoni, G., Pugliese, F., Cinotti, G. A. and Patrono, C. (1980). Renal effects of anti-inflammatory drugs. *Eur. J. Rheum. Inflamm.*, **3**, 210-221
556. Bunning, R. D. and Barth, W. F. (1982). Sulindac, a potentially renal sparing non-steroidal anti-inflammatory drug. *J. Am. Med. Assoc.*, **248**, 2864-2867
557. Ciabattoni, G., Cinotti, G., Pierucci, A. *et al.* (1984). Effects of sulindac and ibuprofen in patients with chronic glomerular disease. *N. Engl. J. Med.*, **310**, 279-283
558a. Sedor, J. R., Davidson, E. W. and Dunn, M. J. (1986). Effects of nonsteroidal anti-inflammatory drugs in healthy subjects. *Am J. Med.*, **81** (Suppl. 2B), 58-70
558b. Sedor, J. R., Williams, S. L., Chremos, A. N., Johnson, C. L. and Dunn, M. J. (1984). Effect of sulindac and indomethacin on renal prostaglandin synthesis. *Clin. Pharmacol. Ther.*, **36**, 85-91
559. Beermann, B., Eriksson, L. O. and Kallner, M. (1986). A double blind comparison of naproxen and sulindac in female patients with heart failure. *Scand. J. Rheumatol.*, Suppl. 62, 32-35
560. Ebel, D. L., Rhymer, A. R., Stahl, E. and Tipping, R. (1986). Effect of clinoril (Sulindac, MSD), piroxicam and placebo in the hypotensive effect of propranolol in patients with mild to moderate essential tension. *Scand. J. Rheumatol.*, Suppl. 62, 41-49
561. Lewis, R. V., Toner, J. M., Jackson, P. R. and Ramsay, L. E. (1986). Effects of indomethacin and sulindac on blood pressure of hypertensive patients. *Br. Med. J.*, **292**, 934-935
562. Spence, J. D. (1986). The arthritic patient with hypertension: selection of an NSAID. *Scand. J. Rheumatol.*, Suppl. 62, 36-40
563. Wong, D. G., Spence, J. D., Lamki, L., Freeman, D. and McDonald, J. W. D. (1986). Effect of non-steroidal anti-inflammatory drugs on control of hypertension by beta-blockers and diuretics. *Lancet*, **1**, 997-1000
564. Mitnick, P. D. (1983). Sulindac and renal failure (Letter). *J. Am. Med. Assoc.*, **250**, 34
565. Brater, D. C., Anderson, S., Baird, B. and Campbell, W. B. (1984). Sulindac does not spare the kidney. Abstract. *Clin. Pharmacol. Ther.*, **35**, 229
566. Roberts, D. G., Gerber, J. G. and Nies, A. S. (1984). Comparative effects of sulindac and indomethacin in humans. *Clin. Pharmacol. Ther.*, **35**, 269
567. Svendsen, U. G., Gerstoft, J., Hansen, T. M., Christensen, P. and Lorenzen, J. B. (1984). The renal excretion of prostaglandins and changes in plasma renin during treatment with either sulindac or naproxen in patients with rheumatoid arthritis and thiazide treated heart failure. *J. Rheumatol.*, **11**, 779-782
568. Berg, K. J. and Talseth, T. (1985). Acute renal effects of sulindac and indomethacin in chronic renal failure. *Clin. Pharmacol. Ther.*, **37**, 447-452
569. Roberts, D. G., Gerber, J. G., Barnes, J. S., Zerbe, G. O. and Nies, A. S. (1985). Sulindac is not renal sparing in man. *Clin. Pharmacol. Ther.*, **38**, 258-265
570. Swainson, C. P. and Griffiths, P. (1985). Acute and chronic effects of sulindac on renal function in chronic renal disease. *Clin. Pharmacol. Ther.*, **37**, 298-300
571. Whelton, A., Bender, W., Vaghaiwalla, F., Hall-Craggs, M. and Solez, K. (1983). Sulindac and renal impairment. (Letter). *J. Am. Med. Assoc.*, **249**, 2892
572. Klatt, L. and Koss, F. W. (1973). Human pharmacokinetische untersuchungen mid ^{14}C-Azapropazon-dihydrat. *Arzneimittel Forschung*, **23**, 920-921
573. Ritch, A. E. S., Perera, W. N. R. and Jones, C. J. (1982). Pharmacokinetics of azapropazone in the elderly. *Br. Clin. Pharmacol.*, **14**, 116-119
574. Elion, G. B., Yu, T. F., Gutman, A. B. *et al.* (1968). Renal clearance of oxypurinol, the chief metabolite of allopurinol. *Am. J. Med.*, **45**, 69-77
575. Wood, M. H., Sebel, E. and O'Sullivan, W. J. (1972). Allopurinol and thiazides. (Letter.) *Lancet*, **1**, 751
576. Young, J. L., Boswell, R. B. and Nies, A. S. (1974). Severe allopurinol hyper-sensitivity. *Arch. Intern. Med.*, **134**, 553-558
577. Elion, G. B., Benezra, F. M., Beardmore, T. D. *et al.* (1980). Studies with allopurinol in patients with impaired renal function. *Adv. Exp. Med. Biol.*, **122A**, 263-267
578. Hande, K. R., Noone, R. M. and Stone, W. J. (1984). Severe allopurinol toxicity:

description and guidelines for prevention in patients with renal insufficiency. *Am. J. Med.*, **76**, 47–56
579. Singer, J. Z. and Wallace, S. L. (1986). The allopurinol hypersensitivity syndrome: unnecessary morbidity and morbidity. *Arthritis Rheum.*, **29**, 82–87
580. Puig, J. G., Casas, E. A., Ramos, T. H., Michan, A. A. and Mateos, F. A. (1989). Plasma oxypurinol concentration in a patient with allopurinol hypersensitivity. *J. Rheumatol.*, **16**, 842–844
581. Emmerson, B. T., Hazelton, R. A. and Fraser, I. H. (1988). Some adverse reactions to allopurinol may be mediated by lymphocyte reactivity to oxypurinol. *Arthritis Rheum.*, **31**, 436–440
582. Verbeeck, R., Tjandramaga, T. B., Mullie, A. *et al.* (1989). Biotransformation of diflunisal and renal excretion of its glucuronides in renal insufficiency. *Br. J. Clin. Pharmacol.*, **7**, 273–282
583. Stafanger, G., Larson, H. W., Hansen, H. and Sorensen, K. (1981). Pharmacokinetics of ketoprofen in patients with chronic renal failure. *Scand. J. Rheumatol.*, **10**, 189–192
584. Faed, E. (1980). Decreased clearance of diflunisal in renal insufficiency — an alternative explanation. *Br. J. Clin. Pharmacol.*, **10**, 185–186
585. Upton, R. A., Williams, R. L., Buskin, J. N. and Jones, R. M. (1982). Effects of probenecid on ketoprofen kinetics. *Clin. Pharmacol. Ther.*, **31**, 705–712
586. Muther, R. S. and Bennett, W. M. (1980). Effects of aspirin on glomerular filtration rate in normal humans. *Ann. Intern. Med.*, **92**, 386–387
587. Emskey, R. D. and Mills, J. A. (1982). Aspirin and analgesic nephropathy. *J. Am. Med. Assoc.*, **247**, 55–57
588. Staessen, J., Fagard, R., Lijnen, P., Moerman, E., De Schaepdryver, A. and Amery, A. (1983). Effects of prostaglandin synthesis inhibition on blood pressure and humoral factors in exercising, sodium-deplete normal man. *J. Hypertension*, **1**, 123–130
589. Brooks, P. M. and Cossum, P. (1978). Salicylates and creatinine clearance re-evaluated. *Med. J. Aust.*, **8**, 660–661
590. Bonney, S. L., Northington, R. S., Hedrich, D. A. and Walker, B. R. (1986). Renal safety of two analgesics used over the counter: ibuprofen and aspirin. *Clin. Pharmacol. Ther.*, **40**, 373–377
591. Unsworth, J., Sturman, S., Lunec, J. and Blake, D. R. (1987). Renal impairment associated with non-steroidal anti-inflammatory drugs. *Ann. Rheum. Dis.*, **46**, 233–236
592. Berg, K. J. (1977). Acute effects of acetylsalicylic acid in patients with chronic renal insufficiency. *Eur. J. Clin. Pharmacol.*, **11**, 111–116
593a. Kimberly, R. P. and Plotz, P. H. (1977). Aspirin-induced depression of renal function. *N. Engl. J. Med.*, **296**, 418–424
593b. Kimberly, R. P. and Plotz, P. H. (1977). Aspirin and renal function. (Correspondence). *N. Engl. J. Med.*, **296**, 1169–1170
594. Kimberly, R. P., Bowden, R. E., Keiser, H. R. and Plotz, P. H. (1978). Reduction in renal function by newer non-steroidal anti-inflammatory drugs. *Am. J. Med.*, **64**, 804–807
595. Kimberly, R. P., Sherman, R. L., Mouradian, J. and Lockshin, M. D. (1979). Apparent acute renal failure associated with therapeutic aspirin and ibuprofen administration. *Arthritis Rheum.*, **22**, 281–285
596. Plotz, P. H. and Kimberly, R. P. (1981). Acute effects of aspirin and acetaminophen on renal function. *Arch. Intern. Med.*, **141**, 343–348
597. Russel, G. I., Bing, R. F., Walls, J. and Pettigrew, N. M. (1978). Interstitial nephritis in a case of phenylbutazone hypersensitivity. *Br. Med. J.*, **1**, 1322
598. Brezin, J. H., Katz, S. M., Schwartz, A. B. and Chinitz, J. L. (1979). Reversible renal failure and nephrotic syndrome associated with non-steroidal anti-inflammatory drugs. *N. Engl. J. Med.*, **301**, 1271–1273
599. Cartwright, K. C., Trotter, T. L. and Cohen, M. L. (1979). Naproxen nephrotoxicity. *Arizona Med.*, **36**, 124–126
600. Chan, L. K., Winearls, C. G., Oliver, D. O. and Dunnill, M. S. (1980). Acute

interstitial nephritis and erythroderma associated with diflunisal. *Br. Med. J.*, **1**, 84–85

601. Curt, G. A., Kaldany, A., Whitley, L. G. *et al.* (1980). Reversible rapidly progressive renal failure and nephrotic syndrome due to fenoprofen calcium. *Ann. Intern. Med.*, **92**, 72–73
602. Linton, A. L., Clark, W. F., Driedger, A. A., Turnbull, D. I. and Lindsay, R. M. (1980). Acute interstitial nephritis due to drugs. *Ann. Intern. Med.*, **93**, 735–741
603. Chatterjee, G. P. (1981). Nephrotic syndrome induced by tolmetin. *J. Am. Med. Assoc.*, **246**, 1589
604. Katz, S. M., Capaldo, R., Everts, E. A. and Digregoria, J. G. (1981). Tolmetin associated with reversible renal failure and acute interstitial nephritis. *J. Am. Med. Assoc.*, **246**, 243–245
605. Lomvardias, S., Pinn, V. W., Wadhwa, M. L., Koshy, K. M. and Heller, M. (1981). Nephrotic syndrome associated with sulindac. (Correspondence). *N. Engl. J. Med.*, **304**, 424
606. Finkelstein, A., Fraley, D. S., Stachura, I. *et al.* (1982). Fenoprofen nephropathy: lipoid nephrosis and interstitial nephritis. A possible T-lymphocyte disorder. *Am. J. Med.*, **55**, 103–107
607. McCarty, J. T., Schartz, G., Blair, T. J., Pierides, A. M. and Van Den Berg, C. J. (1982). Reversible nonoliguric acute renal failure with zomepirac therapy. *Mayo Clin. Proc.*, **57**, 351–354
608. Mease, P. J., Ellsworth, A. J., Killen, P. D. and Willkens, R. F. (1982). Zomepirac, interstitial nephritis and renal failure. *Ann. Intern. Med.*, **97**, 454
609. Stillman, M. T., Davidman, M. and Abraham, P. A. (1982). Fenoprofen associated nephrotic syndrome with renal insufficiency. (Abstract). *Arthritis Rheum.*, **25**, 5136
610. Stachura, I., Jayakumar, S. and Bourke, E. (1983). T and B lymphocyte subsets in fenoprofen nephropathy. *Am. J. Med.*, **75**, 9–16
611. Abraham, P. A. and Keane, W. F. (1984). Glomerular and interstitial diseases induced by non-steroidal anti-inflammatory drugs. *Am. J. Nephrol.*, **4**, 1–6
612. Bender, W. L., Whelton, A., Beschorner, W. E., Darwish, M. O., Hall-Craggs, M. and Solez, K. (1984). Interstitial nephritis, proteinuria and renal failure caused by non-steroidal anti-inflammatory drugs. *Am. J. Med.*, **76**, 1006–1012
613. Lofgren, R. P., Nelson, A. E. and Ehlers, S. M. (1981). Fenoprofen-induced acute interstitial nephritis presenting with the nephrotic syndrome. *Minn. Med.*, 287–290
614. Wendland, M. L., Wagoner, R. D. and Holley, K. E. (1980). Renal failure associated with fenoprofen. *Mayo Clin. Proc.*, **55**, 103–107
615a. O'Brien, W. M. (1983). Long-term efficacy and safety of tolmetin sodium in treatment of geriatric patients with rheumatoid arthritis and osteoarthritis: a retrospective study. *J. Clin. Pharmacol.*, **23**, 309–323
615b. O'Brien, W. M. (1983). Pharmacology of non-steroidal anti-inflammatory drugs: practical view for clinicians. *Am. J. Med.*, **75** (Suppl.), 32–39
616. Shelley, J. H. (1967). Phenacetin, through the looking glass. *Clin. Pharmacol. Ther.*, **8**, 427–471
617. Bell, D., Kerr, D. N. S., Swinney, J. and Yeates, W. K. (1969). Analgesic nephropathy: clinical course after withdrawal of phenacetin. *Br. Med. J.*, **3**, 378–382
618. Krishnaswamy, S. and Nanra, R. S. (1976). "Phenacetin" nephropathy without phenacetin. (Abstract). *Aust. N.Z. J. Med.*, **6**, 88
619. Husserl, F. E., Lange, R. K. and Kantrow, C. M. Jr. (1979). Renal papillary necrosis and pyelonephritis accompanying fenoprofen therapy. *J. Am. Med. Assoc.*, **242**, 1896–1898
620. Anonymous. (1981). Analgesic nephropathy. (Leading Article). *Br. Med. J.*, **282**, 339–340
621. Wilson, D. R. and Gault, M. H. (1982). Declining incidence of analgesic nephropathy in Canada. *Can. Med. Assoc. J.*, **127**, 500–502
622. Nanra, R. S. (1983). Renal effects of antipyretic analgesics. *Am. J. Med.*, **75** (Suppl.), 70–81
623. Kincaid-Smith, P. (1986). Effects of non-narcotic analgesics and the kidney. *Drugs*, **32** (Suppl. 4), 109–128

624. Morales, A. and Steyn, J. (1971). Papillary necrosis following phenylbutazone ingestion. *Arch. Surg.*, **103**, 420–421
625. Nanra, R. S. and Kincaid-Smith, P. (1975). Renal papillary necrosis in rheumatoid arthritis. *Med. J. Aust.*, **1**, 194–197
626. Wiseman, E. H. and Reinert, H. (1975). Anti-inflammatory drugs and papillary necrosis. *Agents and Actions*, **5**, 322–325
627. Jackson, B. and Lawrence, J. R. (1978). Renal papillary necrosis associated with indomethacin and phenylbutazone treated rheumatoid arthritis patients. *Aust. N.Z. J. Med.*, **8**, 165–167
628. Nanra, R. S., Stuart-Taylor, J., de Leon, A. H. *et al.* (1978). Analgesic nephropathy: etiology, clinical syndrome and clinico pathologic correlations in Australia. *Kidney Int.*, **13**, 79–92
629. Prescott L. F. (1979). The nephrotoxicity and hepatotoxicity of antipyretic analgesics. *Br. J. Clin. Pharmacol.*, **7**, 453–462
630. Robertson, C. E., Van Someren, V., Ford, M. J. *et al.* (1980). Mefenamic acid and nephropathy. *Lancet*, **2**, 232–233
631. Shah, G. M., Muhalwas, K. K. and Winer, R. L. (1981). Renal papillary necrosis due to ibuprofen. *Arthritis Rheum.*, **24**, 1208–1210
632. Munn, E., Lynn, K. L. and Bailey, R. R. (1982). Renal papillary necrosis following regular consumption of non-steroidal anti-inflammatory drugs. *N.Z. Med. J.*, **95**, 213–214
633. Prescott, L. F. (1982). Analgesic nephropathy: a reassessment of the role of phenacetin and other analgesics. *Drugs*, **23**, 75–149
634. Caruana, R. J. and Semble, E. L. (1984). Renal papillary necrosis due to naproxen. *J. Rheumatol.*, **11**, 90–91
635. Shelley, J. H. (1978). Pharmacological mechanisms of analgesic nephropathy. *Kidney Int.*, **13**, 15–26
636. Elliott, G., Whited, B. A., Purmalis, A., Davis, J. P., Field, S. O., Lancaster, C. and Robert, A. (1986). Effect of 16,16-dimethyl PGE_2 on renal papillary necrosis and gastro-intestinal ulcerations (gastric, duodenal, intestinal) produced in rats by mefenamic acid. *Life Sci.*, **39**, 423–432
637. New Zealand Rheumatism Association Study. (1974). Aspirin and the kidney. *Br. Med. J.*, **1**, 593–596
638. Macklon, A. F., Craft, A. W., Thompson, M. and Kerr, D. N. S. (1974). Aspirin and analgesic nephropathy. *Br. Med. J.*, 597–600
639. Akyol, S. M., Thompson, M. and Kerr, D. N. S. (1982). Renal function after prolonged consumption of aspirin. *Br. Med. J.*, **284**, 631–632
640. Bengtsson, U., Angervall, L., Ekman, H. and Lehmann, L. (1968). Transitional cell tumours of the renal pelvis in analgesic abusers. *Scand. J. Urol. Nephrol.*, **2**, 145–150
641. Taylor, J. S. (1972). Carcinoma of the urinary tract and analgesic abuse. *Med. J. Aust.*, **1**, 407–409
642. McCredie, M. (1982). Analgesics in cancer of the renal pelvis in New South Wales. *Cancer*, **49**, 2617–2625
643. Hall, C. L. (1983). Gold and D-penicillamine induced renal disease In Bacon, P. A. and Hadler, N. M. (eds.) *The Kidney and Rheumatic Disease*, Chapter 15, pp. 246–266. (London: Butterworth Scientific)
644. Palosuo, T., Provost, I. T. and Milgrom, F. (1976). Gold nephropathy serologic data suggesting an immune complex disease. *Clin. Exp. Immunol.*, **25**, 311–318
645. Ainsworth, S. K., Watanabe, N., Webb, C. M., Stokes, D. K. and Hennigar, G. R. (1981). Gold nephropathy: ultrastructural, fluorescent and energy-dispersive x-ray microanalysis study. *Arch. Pathol. Lab. Med.*, **105**, 373–378
646. Silverberg, D. S., Kidd, E. G., Shmitka, T. H. and Ulan, R. A. (1970). Gold nephropathy: a clinical and pathological study. *Arthritis Rheum.*, **13**, 812–825
647. Watanabe, I., Whithier, F. C., Moore, J. and Cuppage, F. E. (1976). Gold nephropathy. *Arch. Pathol. Lab. Med.*, **101**, 632–635
648. Chevallard, M., Carrabba, M., Venegoni, C., Imbasciati, E., Banfi, G. and Mihatsch, M. J. (1985). Gold nephropathy and renal amyloidosis in a patient with rheumatoid arthritis. *Clin. Exp. Rheumatol.*, **3**, 161–171

649. Bacon, P. A., Tribe, C. R., MacKenzie, J. C. et al. (1976). Penicillamine nephropathy in rheumatoid arthritis. *Q. J. Med.*, **45**, 661-684
650. Dische, F. E., Swinson, D. R., Hamilton, E. B. D. et al. (1976). Immunopathology of penicillamine-induced glomerular disease. *J. Rheumatol.*, **3**, 145-154
651. Neild, G. H., Gartner, H. V. and Bohle, A. (1979). Penicillamine-induced membranous glomerulonephritis. *Scand. J. Rheumatol.*, **28** (Suppl.), 79-90
652. Ross, J. H., McGinty, F. and Brewer, D. G. (1980). Penicillamine nephropathy. *Nephron*, **26**, 184-186
653. Sternlieb, I., Bennett, B. and Scheinberg, I. H. (1975). D-Penicillamine induced Goodpasture's syndrome. *Ann. Intern. Med.*, **82**, 673-676
654. Gibson, T., Burry, H. C. and Chisholm, O. (1976). Goodpasture's syndrome and D-Penicillamine. *Ann. Intern. Med.*, **84**, 100
655. McCormick, J. N., Wood, P. and Bell, D. (1977). D-Penicillamine-induced Goodpasture's syndrome. In Munthe, E. (ed.), *Penicillamine Research in Rheumatoid Disease*, pp. 268-278. (Oslo, Fabritius)
656. Matloff, D. S. and Kaplan, M. M. (1980). D-Penicillamine-induced Goodpasture's-like syndrome in primary biliary cirrhosis — successful treatment with plasmapheresis and immunosuppressives. *Gastroenterology*, **78**, 1046-1049
657. Gavaghan, T. E., McNaught, P. J., Ralson, M. et al. (1981). Penicillamine-induced "Goodpasture's syndrome": successful of a fulminant case. *Aust. N.Z. J. Med.*, **11**, 261-265
658. Swainson, C. P., Thomson, D., Short, A. I. K. et al. (1982). Plasma exchange in the successful treatment of drug-induced renal disease. *Nephron*, **30**, 244-249
659. Sadjadi, S. A., Seelig, M. S., Berger, A. R. et al. (1985). Rapidly progressive glomerulonephritis in a patient with rheumatoid arthritis during treatment with high-dosage D-penicillamine. *Am. J. Nephrol.*, **5**, 212-216
660. Devogelaer, J. P., Pirson, Y., Van den Broucke, J. M., Cosyns, J. P., Brichard, S. and Nagant de Deuxchaisnes, C. (1987). D-Penicillamine induced crescentic glomerulonephritis: report and review of the literature. *J. Rheumatol.*, 1036-1041
661. Bennett, W. M. and Norman, D. J. (1986). Action and toxicity of cyclosporine. *Ann. Rev. Med.*, **77**, 652-656
662. Kahan, B. D. (1986). Cyclosporine nephrotoxicity: pathogenesis, prophylaxis, therapy and prognosis. *Am. J. Kidney Dis.*, **8**, 323
663. Ben-Yehuda, O., Tomer, Y. and Shoenfeld, Y. (1988). Advances in therapy of autoimmune diseases. *Semin. Arthritis Rheum.*, **17**, 206-220
664. Tugwell, P., Bombardier, C., Gent, M., Bennett, K., Ludwin, D., Grace, E., Buchanan, W. W., Bensen, W. G., Bellamy, N., Murphy, G. F. and von Graffenreid, B. (1987). Low dose cyclosporine in rheumatoid arthritis: a pilot study. *J. Rheumatol.*, **14**, 1108-1114
665. Berg, K. J., Forre, O., Bjerkhoel, F. et al. (1986). Side-effects of cyclosporine A treatment in patients with rheumatoid arthritis. *Kidney Int.*, **29**, 1180-1187
666. Van Rijthoven, A. W. A. M., Dijkmans, B. A. C., Goeithe, H. S., Harmans, J., Montnor-Beckers, L. M. B., Jacobs, P. C. J. and Cats, A. (1986). Cyclosporin treatment for rheumatoid arthritis. A placebo controlled, double-blind, multicentre study. *Ann. Rheum. Dis.*, **45**, 726-731
667. Forre, O., Bjerkhoel, F., Salveson, C. F., Berg, K. J., Rugstad, H. E., Saelid, G., Mellbye, O. J. and Kass, E. (1987). An open, controlled, randomized comparison of cyclosporine and azathioprine in the treatment of rheumatoid arthritis. A preliminary report. *Arthritis Rheum.*, **30**, 88-92
668. Weinblatt, M. E., Coblyn, J. S., Fraser, P. A., Anderson, R. J., Spragg, J., Trentham, D. E. and Austen, K. F. (1987). Cyclosporin: a treatment of refractory rheumatoid arthritis. *Arthritis Rheum.*, **30**, 11-17
669. Huskisson, E. C. (1984). Azathioprine. *Clin. Rheum. Dis.*, **10**, 325-332
670. Seldin, M. F. and Steinberg, A. D. (1988). Immunoregulatory agents. In Gallin, J. I., Goldstein, I. M. and Snyderman, R. (eds.) *Inflammation: Basic Principles and Clinical Correlates*, pp. 911-935. (New York: Raven Press)
671. Gispen, J. G., Alarcon, G. S., Johnson, J. J., Acton, R. T., Barger, B. O. and

Koopman, W. J. (1987). Toxicity to methotrexate in rheumatoid arthritis. *J. Rheumatol.*, **14**, 74-79
672. Johnson, W. W. and Meadows, D. C. (1971). Urinary bladder fibrosis and telangiectasia associated with long-term cyclophosphamide therapy. *N. Engl. J. Med.*, **284**, 290-294
673. Aptekar, R. G., Atkinson, J. P., Decker, J. L., Wolff, S. M. and Chu, S. M. (1973). Bladder toxicity with chronic oral cyclosphosphamide therapy in non-malignant disease. *Arthritis Rheum.*, **16**, 461-467
674. Schein, P. S. and Winokur, S. H. (1975). Immunosuppressive and cytotoxic chemotherapy: long-term complications. *Ann. Intern. Med.*, **82**, 84-95
675. Wall, R. L. and Clausen, K. P. (1975). Carcinoma of the urinary bladder in patients receiving cyclophosphamide. *N. Engl. J. Med.*, **293**, 271-273
676. Richtsmeier, A. J. (1975). Urinary bladder tumors after cyclophosphamide. (Letter). *N. Engl. J. Med.*, **293**, 1045-1046
677. Plotz, P. H., Klippel, J. H., Decker, J. L., Grauman, D., Wolff, B., Brown, B. C. and Rutt, G. (1979). Bladder complications in patients receiving cyclophosphamide for systemic lupus erythematosus or rheumatoid arthritis. *Ann. Intern. Med.*, **91**, 221-223
678. Colvin, M. and Hilton, J. (1981). Pharmacology of cyclosphosphamide and metabolites. *Cancer Treat. Rep.*, **66** (Suppl. 3), 89-95
679. Cox, P. J. (1979). Cyclosphosphamide cystitis — identification of acrolein as the causative agent. *Biochem. Pharmacol.*, **28**, 2045-2049
680. De Fronzo, R. A., Braine, H., Colvin, O. M. and Davis, P. J. (1973). Water intoxication in man after cyclophosphamide therapy. Time course and relation to drug activation. *Ann. Intern. Med.*, **78**, 861-869
681. Austin, H. A., Klippel, J. H., Balow, J. E., Leriche, N. G. H., Steinberg, A. D., Plotz, P. H. and Decker, J. L. (1986). Therapy of lupus nephritis. Controlled trial of prednisone and cytotoxic drugs. *N. Engl. J. Med.*, **314**, 614-619
682. McCune, W. J., Golbus, J., Zeldes, W., Bohlke, P., Dunne, R. and Fox, D. A. (1988). Clinical and immunologic effects of monthly administration of intravenous cyclophosphamide in severe systemic lupus erythematosus. *N. Engl. J. Med.*, **318**, 1423-1431
683. Lazowski, Z., Janczewski, Z. and Polowiec, Z. (1982). The effect of alkylating agents in the reproductive and hormonal testicular function in patients with rheumatoid arthritis. *Scand. J. Rheumatol.*, **11**, 49-54
684. Warne, G. L., Fairley, K. F., Hobbs, J. B. and Martin, F. I. R. (1973). Cyclophosphamide-induced ovarian failure. *N. Engl. J. Med.*, **289**, 1159-1162
685. Schilsky, R. L., Lewis, B. J., Sherins, R. J. and Young, R. C. (1980). Gonadal dysfunction in patients receiving chemotherapy for cancer. *Ann. Intern. Med.*, **93**, 109-114
686. Trompeter, R. S., Evans, P. R. and Barratt, T. M. (1981). Gonadal function in boys with steroid-responsive nephrotic syndrome treated with cyclophosphamide for short periods. *Lancet*, **1**, 1177-1179
687. Levi, A. J., Fisher, A. M., Hughes, K. *et al.* (1979). Male infertility due to sulphasalazine. *Lancet*, **2**, 276-278
688. Hinkes, E. and Plotkin, D. (1973). Reversible drug-induced sterility in a patient with acute leukemia. *J. Am. Med. Assoc.*, **223**, 1490-1491
689. Blake, D. A., Heller, R. H., Hsu, S. H. *et al.* (1976). Return of fertility in a patient with cyclosphosphamide-induced azoospermia. *Johns Hopkins Med. J.*, **139**, 20-22
690. Fairley, R. F., Barrie, J. U. and Johnson, W. (1972). Sterility and testicular atrophy related to cyclophosphamide therapy. *Lancet*, **1**, 568-569

19
New concepts in prognosis of rheumatic diseases for the 1990s

T. PINCUS

INTRODUCTION

Prognosis in rheumatic diseases remains uncertain in individual patients, as is the case in all diseases. However, the capacity to estimate prognosis in rheumatic diseases has advanced considerably during the 1980s, perhaps as much as in the three previous decades together, particularly in rheumatoid arthritis (RA). New concepts in prognosis provide a basis toward further understanding of RA in the 1990s, to advance management of this important chronic disease.

In this chapter, ten advances in the prognosis in RA which appear pertinent to all rheumatic diseases, will be reviewed:

1. The prognosis of RA includes severe morbidity in most patients with disease longer than 2 years, who usually experience radiographic progression and functional declines, as well as frequent work disability.
2. The prognosis of RA includes increased mortality rates in all series from clinical centers.
3. Comorbidities are important in the prognosis of RA; comorbidities are seen in most patients, resulting in predisposition to increased mortality rates.
4. Prognosis of individual RA patients may be assessed effectively according to clinical markers that identify patients at high risk for earlier mortality.
5. Prognosis for mortality in RA may be compared to prognosis for mortality in cardiovascular and neoplastic diseases, not only to recognize certain patients with risks of 5-year survivals less than 50% but also to provide markers for identification of optimal therapies in relation to baseline clinical status.
6. Optimal estimation of prognosis results from quantitative measures, rather than from empirical impressions.

7. Prognosis appears more effectively estimated according to measures of functional status, including questionnaires, rather than radiographic and laboratory measures, *at this time*.
8. Estimation of long-term prognosis in RA appears more effectively achieved from long-term observational studies than from clinical trials.
9. Classification criteria and population-based studies have important limitations in estimation of long-term prognosis of individual RA patients.
10. Prognosis in RA may be affected as much by patient behaviors and lifestyles as by treatments and other actions of health-care providers and the health-care system.

The reader is referred to chapters in this volume regarding data concerning other rheumatic diseases as well as to an earlier review that includes some of the data presented here[1].

1 THE PROGNOSIS OF RA INCLUDES SEVERE MORBIDITY IN MOST PATIENTS WITH DISEASE LONGER THAN 2 YEARS, WHO USUALLY EXPERIENCE RADIOGRAPHIC PROGRESSION AND FUNCTIONAL DECLINES, AS WELL AS FREQUENT WORK DISABILITY

The conventional view of prognosis of RA until the last few years may be epitomized in statements in the 1985 editions of the two major American textbooks of rheumatology that "RA is, in the majority of instances a disease with a good prognosis"[2] and "the majority of patients can control RA satisfactorily with well-accepted conservative regimens"[3]. These views have changed considerably over the last 5 years with the comment in the 1989 edition of Kelley's text that, "RA is a chronic and progressive disease, and it is likely that once it is active and chronic in a given individual it will become progressively worse"[4].

The newer views of prognosis in RA are based in part on analyses of long-term disease course in clinical settings, discussed here, as well as recognition of limitations of clinical trials and classification criteria regarding long-term prognosis, discussed below (Sections 8 and 9). The findings regarding the long-term course of RA are more extensively presented in Chapter 3.

In this section, studies regarding the severe morbidity of RA over 5–20 years, including radiographic progression, functional declines, and work disability, are briefly summarized.

Radiographic progression

All reports in which radiographs of RA patients have been quantitatively scored for erosion, joint-space narrowing, or global changes indicate significant associations with duration of disease[5-8],

Table 1 Analyses of studies in which slowing of radiographic progression in RA is reported. Number of studies providing different levels of support for this concept

	Strong support	Probable support	Doubtful support	No support	Total
Gold salts	1	2	—	3	6
Penicillamine	—	—	1	1	2
Antimalarials	—	—	1	4	5
Azathioprine	—	—	—	1	1
Cyclophosphamide	1	—	1	2	4
	2	2	3	11	18

Adapted from Iannuzzi, L., Dawson, N., Zein, N. and Kushner, I. (1983). Does drug therapy slow radiographic deterioration in rheumatoid arthritis? *N. Engl. J. Med.*, **309**, 1023-1028.

including longitudinal analyses of individual patients[9,10]. Reports that radiographic progression may be modified in clinical trials have been reinterpreted (Table 1) to indicate that this finding is actually *unusual*[11], and certainly not applicable to the long-term course of disease. Furthermore, evidence of joint-space narrowing and erosion, indicating permanent articular damage, is seen in almost 50% of patients within the first 2 years of disease[8,12-14]. Although sedimentation rates may be improved in most patients over 1 year of treatment, almost all experience radiographic progression (Figure 1)[10]. Therefore, radiographic progression is usual, rather than exceptional, in most RA patients.

Functional declines

Analyses of functional status over 5-20 years have also indicated meaningful declines in most patients. Duthie[15] and Rasker and Cosh[16] found that most patients showed significant declines in global functional status over a decade. Scott *et al.* found that some improvement might have been apparent after 11 years of observations[17], but recognized significant declines by 20 years[18]. Wolfe and Hawley found that 18% of 485 patients treated with gold or penicillamine showed evidence of a short-term remission, but this remission was sustained for longer than 3 years in fewer than 10% of these patients – only 1.8% of all patients[19]!

Analysis of functional capacity in 75 RA patients 9 years apart indicated severe declines in almost all patients in capacities to perform physical tests of function such as grip strength and the button test, as well as according to questionnaires regarding activities of daily living[20] (Figure 2). Many patients showed improvement in morning stiffness over 9 years, suggesting that the disease process may "burn-out" over time but leave an individual patient with significant losses in functional capacity. In this study, all 75 patients studied at baseline were reviewed 9 years later.

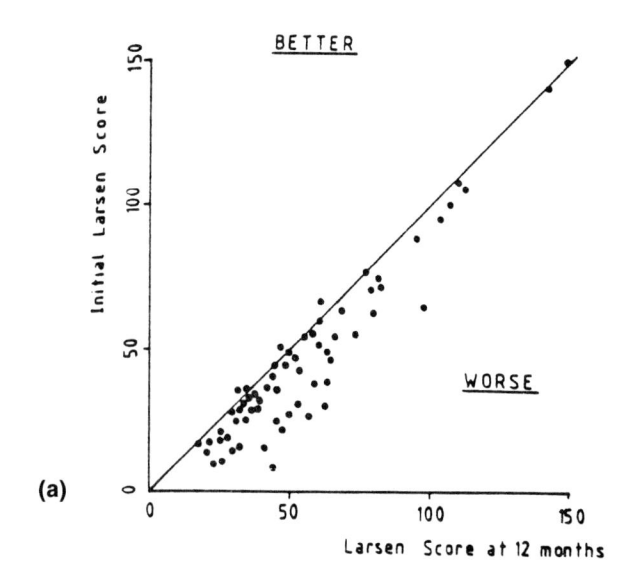

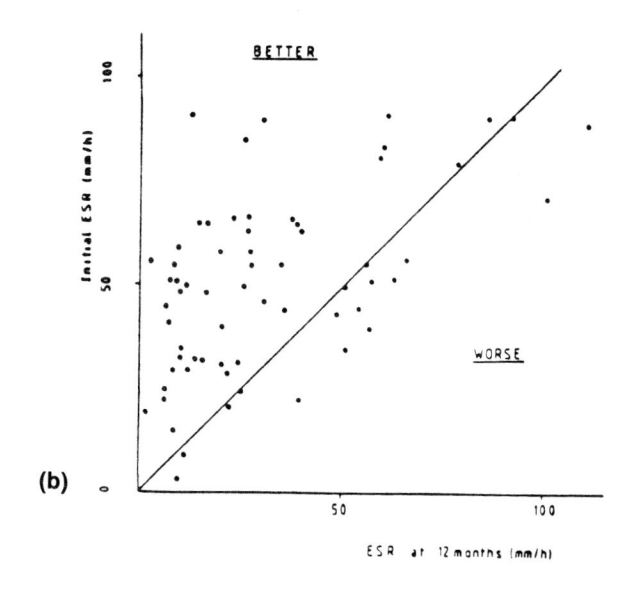

Figure 1 Changes in erythrocyte sedimentation rate and radiographic score in 50 rheumatoid arthritis patients over 1 year. (a) Short-term study. Scatter diagram showing changes in Larsen score during 1 year of treatment with second-line drugs. A 45-degree no-change line is indicated. (b) Short-term study. Similar scatter diagram showing changes in ESR during 1 year of treatment with second-line drugs. Note that approximately 75% of patients show improvement in the sedimentation rate, but all patients show Larsen radiographic scores 12 months later which indicate unchanged status or progression, despite treatment with various second-line drugs. (From ref. 10).

FUTURE PERSPECTIVES

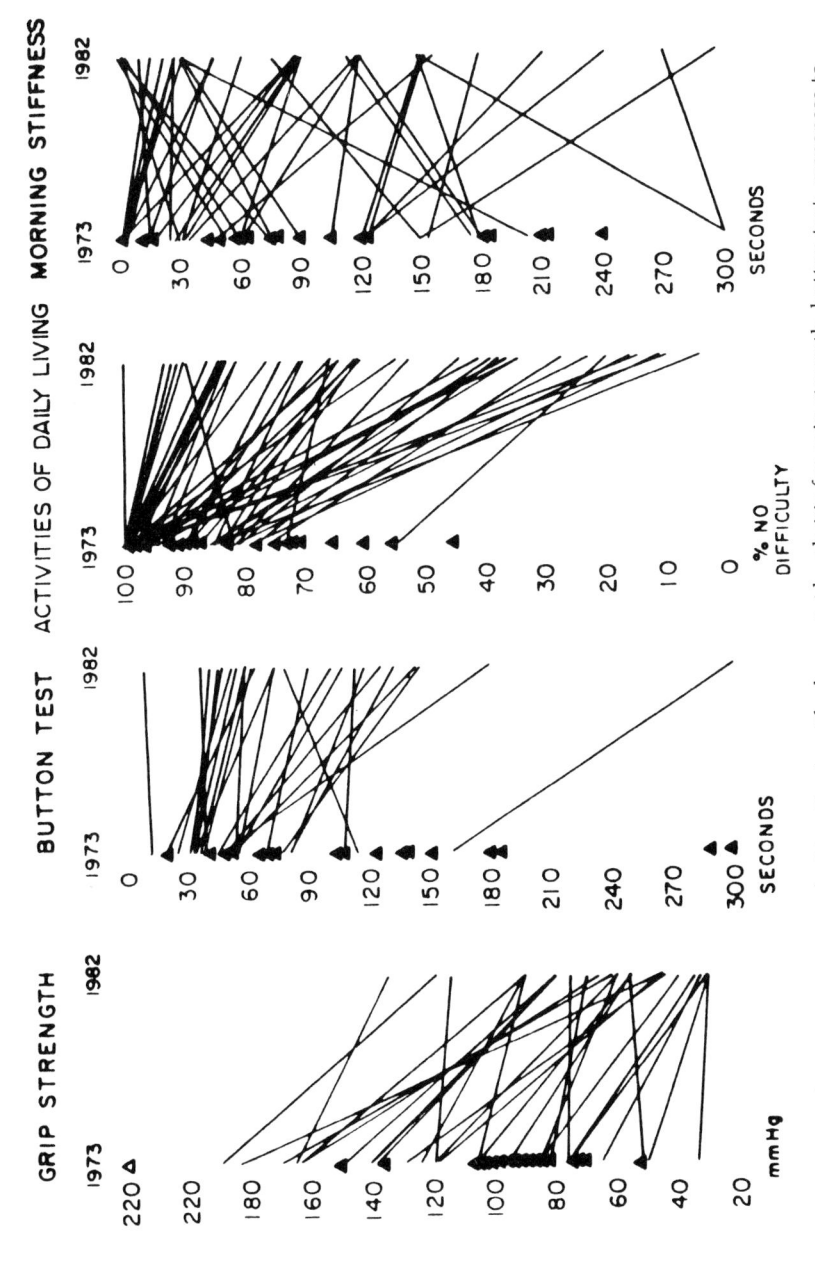

Figure 2 Changes over 9 years in 50 patients with rheumatoid arthritis for grip strength, button test, responses to questions about activities of daily living, and morning stiffness. Patients who had died over the 9 years are depicted by triangles. Note that only one patient shows improvement and a few have maintained functional capacity over the 9 year interval, while most patients show significant functional declines. Morning stiffness had improved in half of the patients, suggesting that the disease process may "burn-out" over time, but leaving an individual severely dysfunctional.

Table 2 Disability and work status of people with symmetric polyarthritis aged 18-64 in 1978 US population[a]

Category of individuals	Total number (thousands)	Percent of population	Disability status			Work status		
			Percent Not disabled	Percent Moderately disabled	Percent severely disabled	Percent working	Percent not working	Total earnings
Females								
No arthritis	51 520	80.5	90.1	5.4	4.5	61.6	38.4	$ 8 006
Symmetric polyarthritis	1 511	2.4	22.2	26.8	51.0	31.0	69.0	$ 2 122 (26.5%)
Males								
No arthritis	54 033	86.2	90.6	5.8	3.7	89.4	10.6	$19 360
Symmetric polyarthritis	855	1.4	29.7	23.3	47.0	56.1	43.9	$ 9 198 (47.5%)

Adapted from Mitchell, J. M., Burkhauser, R. V. and Pincus, T. (1988). The importance of age, education and comorbidity in the substantial earnings losses of individuals with symmetric polyarthritis. *Arthritis Rheum.*, **31**, 348-357.
[a] Data derived from 1978 United States Social Security Survey of Disability and Work, weighted to be representative of the US working-age population age 18-64.

Work disability

All analyses of clinical RA patients over 5-20 years indicate work disability in 60-70% of patients less than 65 years of age who had been working at onset of disease[20-22]. Work disability was only weakly associated with radiographic stage, and appeared to be as effectively explained by demographic variables as by disease variables[21].

Clinical analyses of the progression of RA in treatment centers leave concern that only unusually severe patients might be selected for inclusion. Hence, population-based study of work disability was performed in individuals with symmetric polyarthritis, a surrogate for RA[23]. Among men aged 18-64 in 1978, 87% were working, including 89% of those with no arthritis, versus only 56% of those with symmetric polyarthritis. Similar findings were seen for women, although fewer women were working. However, more women were affected by symmetric polyarthritis than men, and earnings were lower both for individuals with symmetric polyarthritis and for those with no arthritis (Table 2). In econometric analyses, women with symmetric polyarthritis (2.4% of all women) had only 26.5% of the earnings of women with no arthritis, while men with symmetric polyarthritis had only about half of the earnings of men with no arthritis. The 1.9% of the working-age population with symmetric polyarthritis experienced earnings losses of $17.6 billion, indicating major economic consequences of RA in addition to the substantial direct and indirect costs of disease and its treatment[23].

These studies were conducted using data from a subset of the 1978

US Health Interview Survey designed to be representative of the entire US population. The findings indicate that work disability in RA is a problem throughout the population, not only in secondary or tertiary rheumatology care settings.

The data derived from the above studies provide a picture of prognosis in RA that differs considerably from the traditional view of an easily controlled disease. RA is a progressive disease, in which most patients experience radiographic progression, severe functional declines, and work disability.

2 THE PROGNOSIS OF RA INCLUDES INCREASED MORTALITY RATES IN ALL SERIES FROM CLINICAL CENTERS

While an earlier view suggested that RA is not a "fatal" disease, all of 13 studies from rheumatology clinical settings indicate that RA patients die at an earlier age than would be expected for individuals of similar age and sex in the general population[24]. Ten studies from such diverse locations as Massachusetts[25,26], Canada[27,28], Sweden[29], England[16], the Netherlands[30], Finland[31], Minnesota[32] and Tennessee[33] include actuarial life-table analyses to examine survival and mortality (Figure 3). All of these studies indicate accelerated mortality rates in RA patients compared to the general population (one study depicts comparisons with osteoarthritis patients rather than with the general population[26] — Figure 3A — and two depict comparisons of different RA patients[16,32] — Figures 3E and 3I).

The life tables show several striking similarities: (a) Mortality trends require at least 2–3 years of observation (periods longer than those found in clinical trials and most clinical studies). (b) Higher life expectancies are seen for females than for males in both the general population and RA patients. (c) The most substantial increases in mortality rates among RA patients versus the general population appear between the third and tenth years after baseline observation. Mortality rates of RA patients have remained higher compared to those in the general population over the last 35 years, although mortality rates in both groups are lower today than 35 years ago[24].

One explanation for underestimation of accelerated mortality rates in RA involves the fact that the attributed immediate causes of death are similar to those in the general US population (Table 3). Among 2262 deaths of RA patients from 13 locations in North America and Europe[34], cardiovascular disease was the major attributed cause of death, seen in about 40% of RA patients, as in the general US population. RA patients are more likely to have their acute cause of death attributed to infection, renal disease, respiratory disease, or gastrointestinal disease than are individuals in the general population. However, the overall frequency patterns of various attributable causes of death in RA patients are not recognized to differ meaningfully from those in the general population when patients are viewed one at a time.

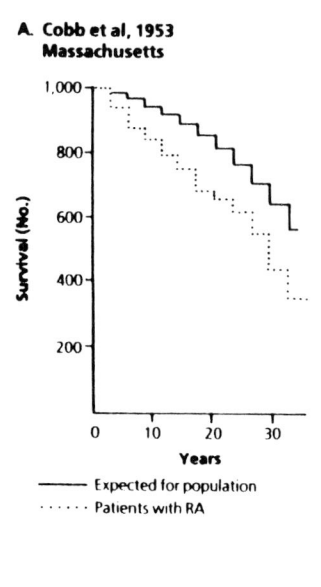

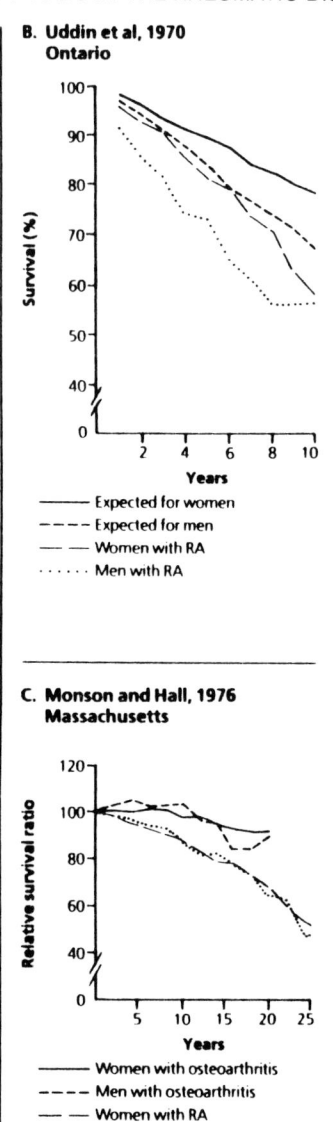

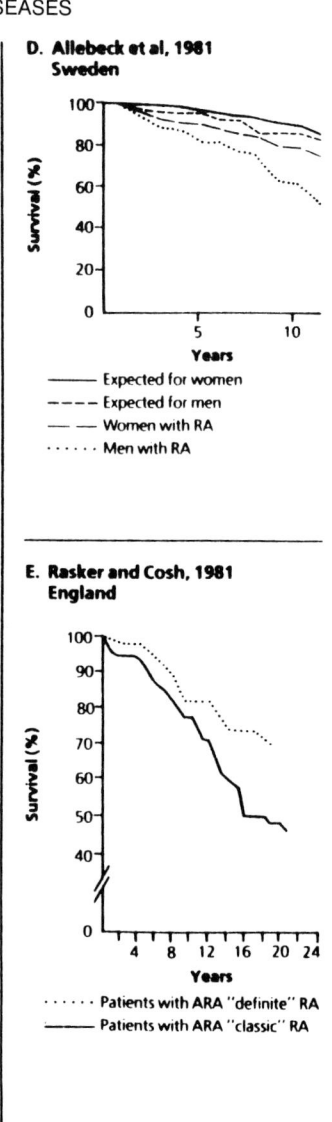

PROGNOSIS IN THE RHEUMATIC DISEASES

A. Cobb et al, 1953
Massachusetts

— Expected for population
····· Patients with RA

B. Uddin et al, 1970
Ontario

— Expected for women
---- Expected for men
— — Women with RA
····· Men with RA

C. Monson and Hall, 1976
Massachusetts

— Women with osteoarthritis
---- Men with osteoarthritis
— — Women with RA
····· Men with RA

D. Allebeck et al, 1981
Sweden

— Expected for women
---- Expected for men
— — Women with RA
····· Men with RA

E. Rasker and Cosh, 1981
England

····· Patients with ARA "definite" RA
— Patients with ARA "classic" RA

NEW CONCEPTS

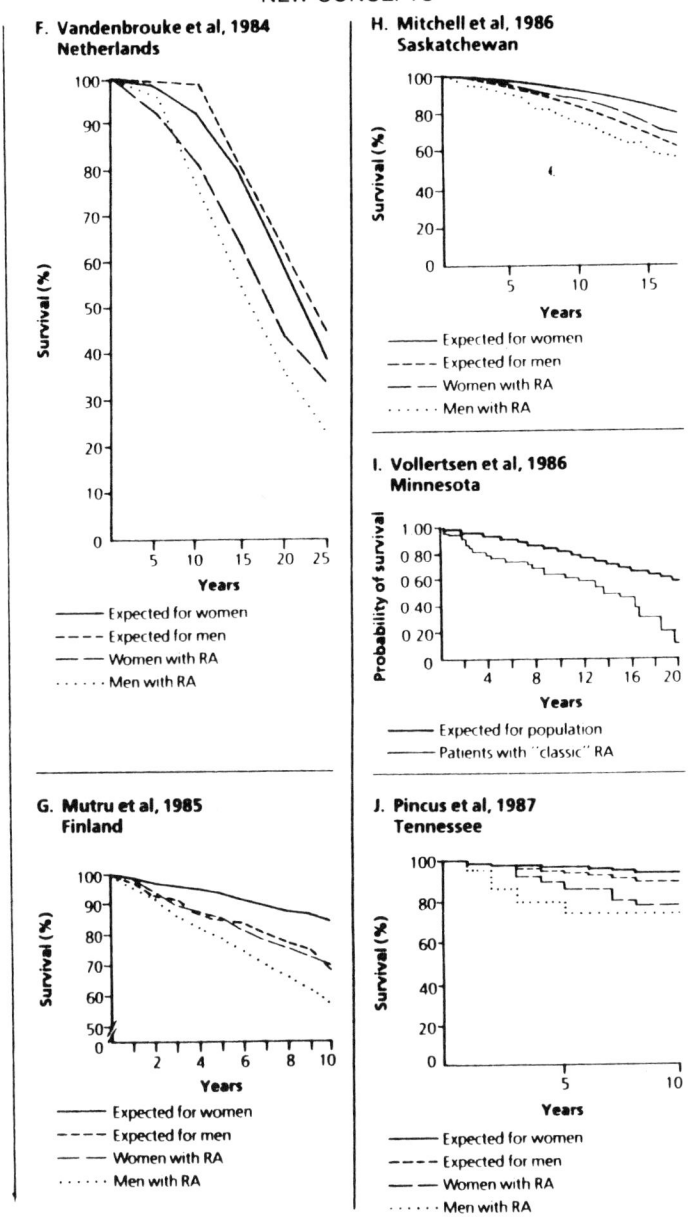

Figure 3 Survival analyses of patients with rheumatoid arthritis (RA) compared with general population (exceptions: in C, RA patients are compared with osteoarthritis patients; in E, two different groups of RA patients are compared). Note the increased mortality rates in RA patients over more than 35 years of study from ten diversely located centers in North America and Europe, including the United States (Boston, Mass. A and C; Rochester, Minn. I; Nashville, Tenn., J), Canada (Ontario, B; Saskatchewan, H), Scandinavia (Sweden, D; Finland, G), England (E), and the Netherlands (F). (From ref. 24; A, ref. 25; B, ref. 27, C. ref. 26, D, ref 29; E, ref. 16; F, ref. 30; G, ref. 31; H, ref. 23; I, ref. 32; J, ref. 33.)

459

RA is not listed anywhere on the death certificate in more than half of the patients who die with this disease[21,29].

3 COMORBIDITIES ARE IMPORTANT IN THE PROGNOSIS OF RA AS THEY OCCUR IN MOST PATIENTS RESULTING IN PREDISPOSITION TO INCREASED MORTALITY RATES

The observation that mortality rates in RA patients are increased, while acute identified causes of death involve primarily cardiovascular and other types of diseases, suggests a considerable level of comorbidity in RA patients. Analyses of 254 consecutive RA patients at Vanderbilt University indicated extensive comorbidities, including hypertension in 36%, allergies in 22%, peptic ulcer disease in 21%, diabetes in 5%, chronic bronchitis in 13% (Table 4(a)), figures considerably higher than those reported in the US population (Table 4(b)).

A major concern in the analysis of comorbidities involves "Berkson's bias"[35], i.e., the concept that comorbidities are more likely to be detected in individuals seen in medical settings as compared to the general population. This possibility could be analyzed according to population-based data representative of the US population. Individuals with symmetric polyarthritis, the surrogate for RA described above[22], could be compared to individuals with no arthritis. The frequencies of comorbidities in individuals with symmetric polyarthritis identified in the survey (Table 4(c)) were remarkably similar to those seen in the Nashville clinical RA population (Table 4(a)). Significantly higher frequencies of comorbidities were seen in individuals with symmetric polyarthritis or clinical RA than in individuals with no arthritis[36] (Table 4(d)).

These findings may be explained in part on the basis of higher age and lower formal education level in clinical patients with RA[37], as well as in individuals with symmetric polyarthritis identified in surveys[23,34]. However, odds ratios for the presence of various comorbidities, adjusted for age, formal education level, sex, and race (Table 4(e)), indicate that individuals with symmetric polyarthritis have substantially higher odds to develop most common chronic diseases, compared to individuals with no arthritis. Therefore, RA may be viewed as a marker for development of many comorbid chronic conditions, possibly explaining in part higher mortality rates in RA patients.

4 PROGNOSIS OF INDIVIDUAL RA PATIENTS MAY BE ASSESSED EFFECTIVELY ACCORDING TO CLINICAL MARKERS, THAT IDENTIFY PATIENTS AT HIGH RISK FOR EARLIER MORTALITY

Recognition of increased mortality rates in RA is of considerable interest. However, prognosis for individual RA patients is best

NEW CONCEPTS

Table 3 Attributed causes of death in 2262 patients with RA in 13 series

Series	Cobb et al. 1953	Van Dam et al. 1961	Duthie et al. 1964	Uddin et al. 1970	Monson and Hall 1976	Lewis et al. 1980	Allbeck et al. 1981	Rasker and Cosh 1981	Vanden-broucke et al.	Pincus et al. 1984	Prior et al. 1984	Mutra et al. 1985	Mitchell et al. 1986	Cumulative total	1977 US population
Ref.	25		15	27	26		29	16	38	10		31	28		
Number of deaths:	130	229	75	94	570	46	84	43	165	20	199	356	251	2 262	
Attributed cause of death	Percentage of deaths in each series attributed to listed causes															
Cardiovascular disease	24.6	38.5	36.0	51.0[a]	43.3	41.3	48.8	41.9	43.0	40.0	31.2	46.6	42.6	42.1	41.0
Cancer	11.5	15.2	13.3	7.4	12.6	28.3	23.8	11.6	19.5	25.0	15.1	11.8	13.1	14.1	20.4
Infection	24.6	12.6	14.7	19.1	NL[b]	13.0	2.4	18.6	2.4	20.0	2.0	2.0	13.5	9.4[c]	1.0
Renal disease	13.1	7.8	17.3	4.2	4.4	NL	0	9.3	5.5	0	3.0	20.5	3.2	7.8	1.1
Respiratory disease	3.1	NL	4.0	4.2	10.0	6.5	1.2	NL	12.1	5.0	14.6	8.1	4.8	7.2	3.9
RA	NL	NL	NL	NL	6.7	2.2	4.8	NL	10.3	5.0	17.1	NL	10.0	5.3	NL
Gastrointestinal disease	6.2	6.5	8.0	2.1	4.0	2.2	6.0	NL	5.5	5.0	5.5	NL	6.0	4.2	2.4
CNS disease	9.2	NL	5.3	NL	11.2	NL	6.0	18.6	NL	0	0	NL	1.0	4.2	9.6
Accidents	0	NL	1.3	NL	NL	NL	NL	NL	0.6	0	0	4.0	4.0	1.0	5.4
Miscellaneous	7.7	16.9	NL	3.2	7.8	6.5	7.1	NL	1.2	0	3.5	7.9	2.0	6.4	15.2
Unknown	NL	2.2	NL	8.5	NL	NL	NL	NL	0	0	0	0	0	0.6	NL

[a] Pulmonary embolus classified as "Cardiovascular Disease."
[b] NL — This cause of death not listed in this series.
[c] Percentage calculation does not include Monson and Hall's 570 cases, as infection was not listed as a cause of death.

461

Table 4 Comorbidities in individuals with symmetric polyarthritis in various populations

	Percentage of individuals reporting conditions				
	(a)	(b)	(c)	(d)	(e)
Health condition	250 clinical RA patients	Total US population[a]	Symmetrical polyarthritis survey population[a]	Survey non-arthritis population[a]	Odds & ratio: Symmetrical polyarthritis vs non-arthritis[b]
Hypertension	36	11.1	41.2	7.8	3.4 : 1
Allergies	22	4.2	15.0	3.2	5.1 : 1
Stomach ulcer	21	3.6	6.5	2.7	2.9 : 1
Diabetes	5	2.5	11.3	1.8	3.0 : 1
Kidney disease	5	1.9	4.6	1.1	4.7 : 1
Chronic bronchitis	13	1.6	6.9	0.9	4.3 : 1
Heart attack	8	1.4	6.6	0.7	4.3 : 1
Cancer	4	0.7	1.3	0.5	2.4 : 1

Adapted from Pincus, T., Callahan, L. F. and Mitchell, J. M. (1987). Increased mortality in rheumatoid arthritis is explained in part on the basis of extensive comorbidity with other diseases. *Arthritis Rheum.*, **30**, S12.

[a] Data from the 1976 Health Interview Survey for US population aged 18–64.
[b] Adjusted for age, sex, race, and formal educational level.

advanced by identification of baseline markers for a subsequent good or poor outcome. The classical studies of Duthie and colleagues[15], Rasker and Cosh[38], and others indicated that poor baseline functional status was predictive of earlier mortality. Gordon et al.[39] found that RA patients with rheumatoid factor and extra-articular disease (excluding nodules only) had a 5-year mortality of about 40%, compared to a 5-year mortality of about 12% in the subgroup with no rheumatoid factor or extra-articular disease (Figure 4).

We have analyzed quantitative functional and articular measures as potential markers of subsequent mortality in RA over 9 years[24,33] (Figure 5). Age was an important predictive marker, as expected (Figure 5A), while duration of disease was not discriminatory for predicting increased risk of mortality (Figure 5B). The number of involved joints (Figure 5C), presence of comorbid cardiovascular disease (beyond hypertension) (Figure 5D), baseline functional status in activities of daily living (Figure 5E), physical measures of functional status, including modified walking time (Figure 5F) and button test (Figure 5G), were significant predictors of higher mortality rates over the next 9 years[24,33]. Five-year survivals were in the range of 85–95% in individuals with favorable values, versus 45–55% in patients with unfavorable baseline values for most of these measures.

Significant correlations were seen between baseline values for questionnaire and physical measures of functional capacity, as expected. Therefore, mortality patterns were analyzed according to whether patients showed 0, 1, 2, or 3 severely dysfunctional values at

[Figure: Mortality (%) vs Years chart showing three curves]

— Patients with RA and extra-articular disease
••••• All patients with RA
- - - Patients with seronegative RA or RA without extra-articular disease

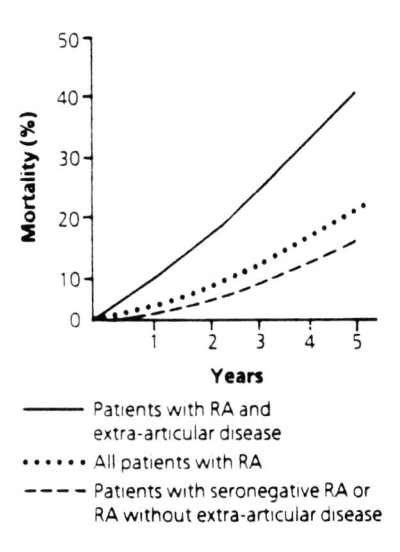

Figure 4 Analyses of mortality over 5 years in 116 patients with rheumatoid arthritis. Two subgroups were identified: (a) patients with no rheumatoid factor and no extra-articular disease, in which mortality was 14% at 5 years, (b) patients with extra-articular disease, in which mortality was 40% at 5 years. (From ref. 39.).

baseline for questions regarding activities of daily living, walking time or the button test. Dysfunctional values were defined as activities of daily living scores of less than 80% "with ease," modified walking time of more than 30 seconds, and button test of more than 120 seconds (Figure 5H). The only two patients with three severely dysfunctional values at baseline were not alive 4 years later. The seven patients with two severely dysfunctional values showed 5-year survivals of about 40%. The nine patients with one severely dysfunctional value showed 5-year survivals of about 70%. Patients who had no severely dysfunctional values showed 5-year survivals of about 95% — not significantly different from expected mortality in the general population.

These studies indicate that increased mortality rates in RA are predicted effectively by quantitative measures indicative of more severe clinical status, including functional status measures. Evidence for "dose–response" relationships can be seen in the incremental risk of subsequent mortality according to the number of baseline values of severely dysfunctional status.

A. Age

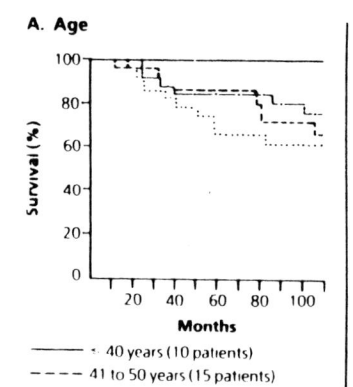

- ≤ 40 years (10 patients)
- 41 to 50 years (15 patients)
- 51 to 60 years (26 patients)
- >60 years (24 patients)

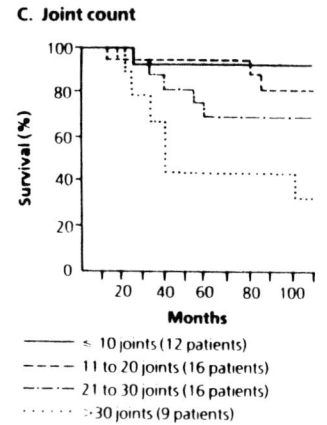

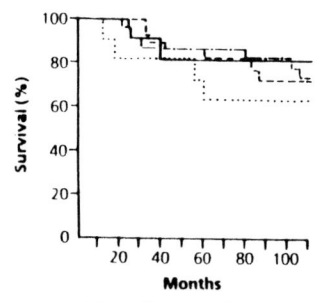

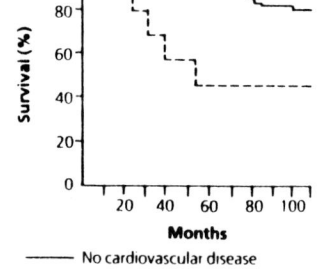

B. Duration of disease

- ≤ 5 years (11 patients)
- 6 to 10 years (30 patients)
- 11 to 15 years (23 patients)
- >15 years (11 patients)

C. Joint count

- ≤ 10 joints (12 patients)
- 11 to 20 joints (16 patients)
- 21 to 30 joints (16 patients)
- >30 joints (9 patients)

D. Cardiovascular disease

- No cardiovascular disease (64 patients)
- Cardiovascular disease (9 patients)

Activities of daily living *

— >90% (39 patients)
---- 81% to 90% (19 patients)
—·— 71% to 80% (7 patients)
······ ≤70% (6 patients)

* "With ease"

G. Button test

— ≤ 40 seconds (15 patients)
---- 41 to 80 seconds (36 patients)
—·— 81 to 120 seconds (9 patients)
······ >120 seconds (12 patients)

I. Formal education level

— >12 years (21 patients)
---- 9 to 12 years (34 patients)
—·— ≤ 8 years (20 patients)

F. Modified walking time

— ≤ 10 seconds (27 patients)
---- 11 to 20 seconds (29 patients)
—·— 21 to 30 seconds (7 patients)
······ >30 seconds (8 patients)

H. Measures indicating severe dysfunction*

— None (50 patients)
---- One (9 patients)
—·— Two (7 patients)
······ Three (2 patients)

* Activities of daily living score ≤70% "with ease," modified walking time >30 seconds, button test >120 seconds

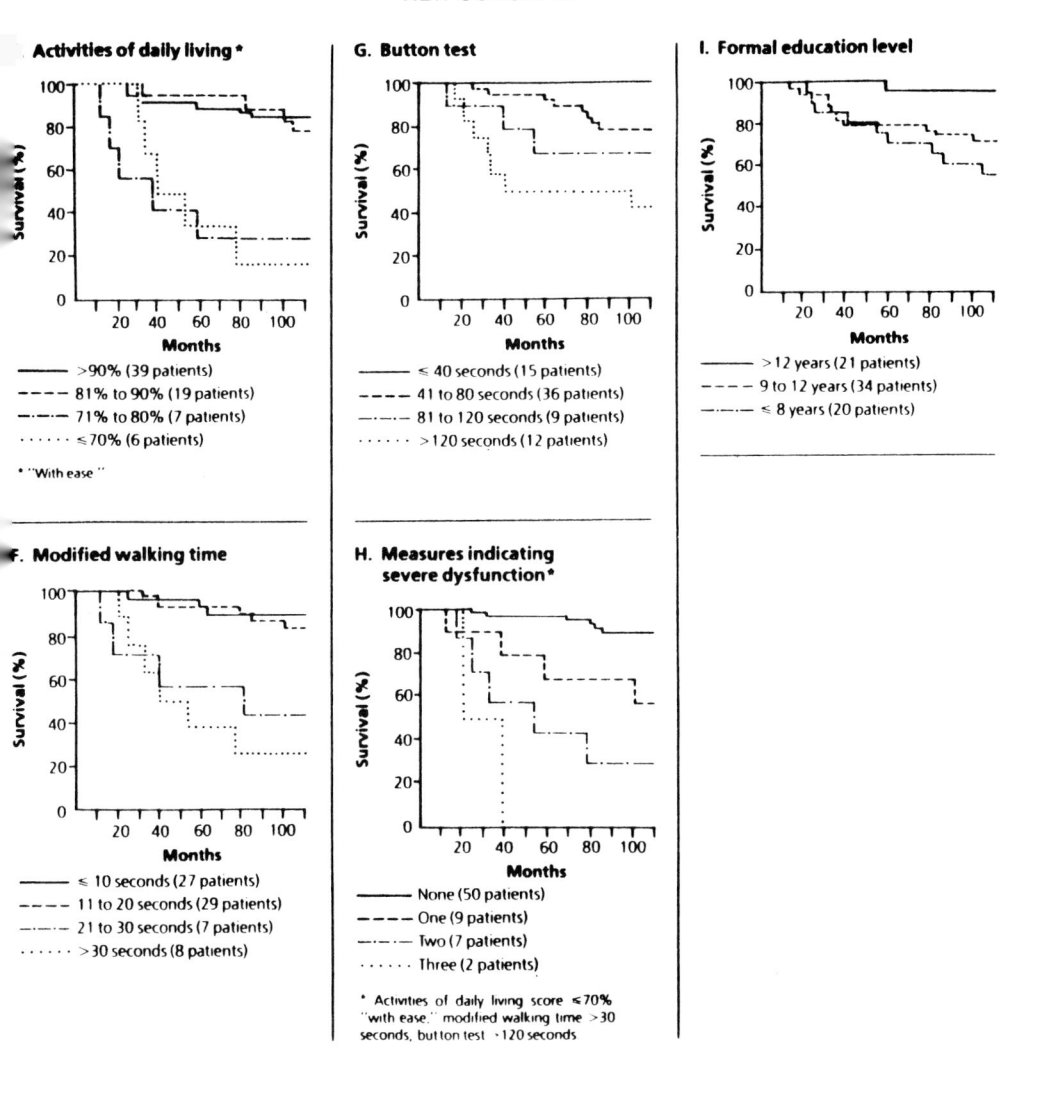

Figure 5 Analyses of survival in 75 patients with rheumatoid arthritis based on various quantitative measures available at baseline. Note significant differences according to age (A), joint count (C), cardiovascular disease (D), questionnaire scores for activities of daily living (E), modified walking time score (F), button test (G), and formal education level (I). The only variable depicted that does not significantly predict differences in mortality rates is duration of disease (B).

The most explanatory variable in these analyses was questionnaire scores for activities of daily living. Although different measures of functional capacity were correlated, there was evidence of dose–response relations for mortality rates and the presence of none, one, two, or three measures of severe dysfunction (H) for activities of daily living questionnaire responses, modified walking time, and button test. (From refs. 24, 33.)

5 PROGNOSIS FOR MORTALITY IN RA MAY BE COMPARED TO PROGNOSIS FOR MORTALITY IN CARDIOVASCULAR AND NEOPLASTIC DISEASES, NOT ONLY TO RECOGNIZE CERTAIN PATIENTS WITH RISKS OF 5-YEAR SURVIVALS LESS THAN 50%, BUT ALSO TO PROVIDE MARKERS FOR IDENTIFICATION OF OPTIMAL THERAPIES IN RELATION TO BASELINE CLINICAL STATUS

Prognosis estimates of mortality over 5–10 years according to baseline markers have been most effectively applied in cardiovascular and neoplastic diseases. Two examples are seen in studies of coronary artery disease according to coronary arteriograms and Hodgkin's disease according to clinical staging (Figure 6). These studies provide a model for analysis of subsequent mortality in chronic diseases according to baseline markers.

Mortality in coronary artery disease[40] was analyzed in a review published in 1978 prior to the era of coronary artery bypass surgery, in 601 nonoperative patients seen at the Cleveland Clinic (Figure 6A). The number of involved coronary arteries in a baseline arteriogram predicted 5-year survivals of approximately 85% in individuals with one involved vessel, 65% in those with two involved vessels, and 45% in those with three involved vessels or left coronary artery involvement. Identification of a simple quantitative marker, number of involved vessels, allowed clinicians and patients to assess prognosis more accurately than without this measure, including potential risks and benefits of coronary bypass surgery versus the natural history of disease[40].

Studies of mortality in Hodgkin's disease[41] from Stanford University published in 1972, prior to widespread use of chemotherapy and linear accelerator therapy (Figure 6B), indicated 5-year survivals of about 85% in patients with Stage I or II disease, 60% in those with Stage III disease, and 45% in those with Stage IV disease. Again, the use of a quantitative predictive marker, anatomic stage of disease, facilitated assessment of aggressive chemotherapy and other treatments for Hodgkin's disease by patients and their physicians. Since 1972, results of treatment for Hodgkin's disease have improved, in part because of availability of prognostic quantitative staging data.

Analyses in RA indicate that the joint count (Figure 6C) or activities of daily living questionnaire scores (Figure 6D) predict that certain patients will show 5-year survival patterns in the range of patients with three-vessel coronary artery disease or Stage IV Hodgkin's disease[39,40]. It must be emphasized that a smaller proportion of RA patients appear in the poorest prognostic category compared to patients with cardiovascular or neoplastic diseases, and that many coronary artery disease and Hodgkin's disease patients were studied earlier in disease course than the RA patients. Nonetheless, certain RA patients have a poor prognosis for survival comparable to those seen for certain patients

9-10 YEAR SURVIVAL ACCORDING TO QUANTITATIVE MARKERS IN THREE CHRONIC DISEASES

A. CORONARY ARTERY DISEASE
Number of Involved Vessels

Proudfit et al 1978

B. HODGKIN'S DISEASE
Anatomic Stage

Kaplan et al 1972

C. RHEUMATOID ARTHRITIS
Joint Count

Pincus et al 1987

D. RHEUMATOID ARTHRITIS
Activities of Daily Living Score

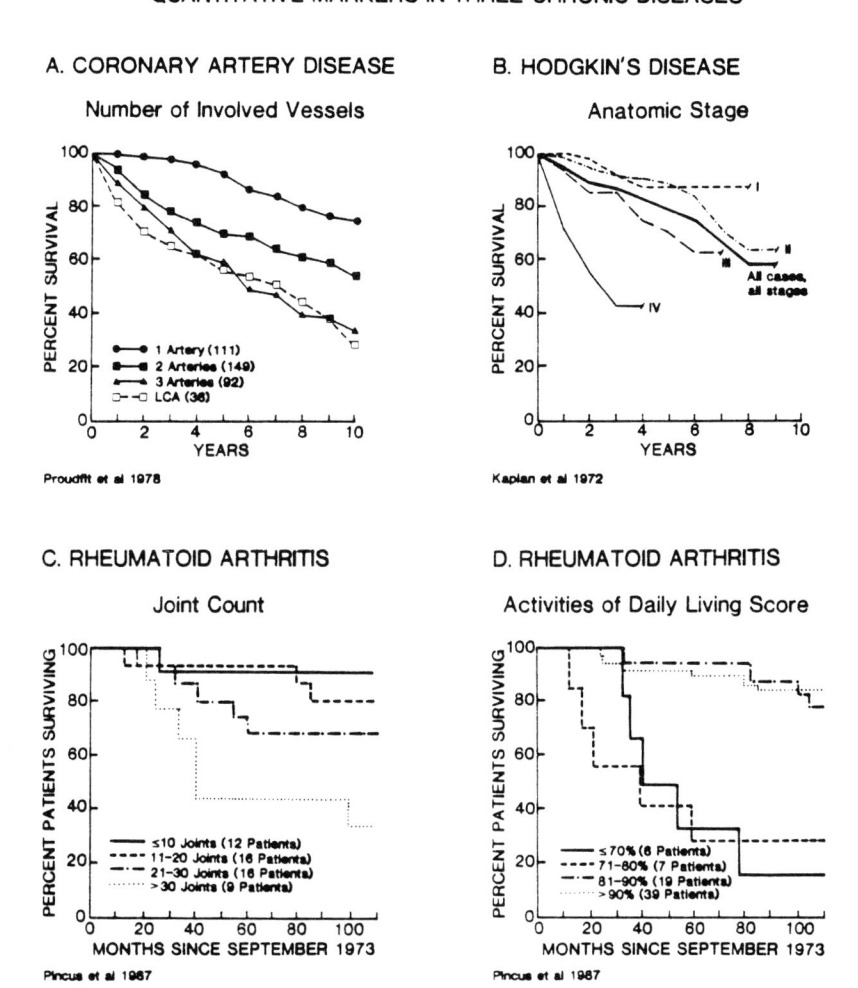

Pincus et al 1987

Figure 6 Survival analyses in three chronic diseases, including cardiovascular, neoplastic and rheumatic, based on specific disease markers, for example, the number of coronary arteries involved in coronary artery disease, the anatomic stage in Hodgkin's disease, and the joint count and activities of daily living questions in rheumatoid arthritis. (From refs. 24, 33, 34.)

with cardiovascular and neoplastic diseases, including 50% mortality over 5 years.

Many RA patients are not seen until long after disease is established, and not treated aggressively until irreversible damage is present. Earlier recognition and treatment of RA may prevent the progression of clinical status to levels projecting 5-year survivals of less than 50%, comparable to those seen in three-vessel coronary artery disease or Stage IV Hodgkin's disease. These data suggest that prognosis for disease might justify risks of aggressive therapy much earlier than has been traditional, with evidence that earlier therapies are being implemented[42,43]. A rationale for earlier therapies is available primarily from quantitative prognostic data.

6 OPTIMAL ESTIMATION OF PROGNOSIS RESULTS FROM QUANTITATIVE MEASURES, RATHER THAN FROM EMPIRICAL IMPRESSIONS

The value of quantitative measures, rather than empirical impressions, in the prognosis of RA is documented above. A brief discussion is presented below concerning the methods used to develop quantitative prognostic indicators in RA, including joint counts, radiographs, laboratory tests, questionnaires, and physical measures of functional status such as grip strength, walking time, and the button test.

Joint count

Quantitative assessment of the number of involved joints would appear an optimal method to develop a prognosis for an RA patient. However, a consensus does not exist regarding a single standardized method for assessment of the joint count, including the optimal number of joints to be scored, the number of abnormalities among tenderness, pain on motion, swelling, limited motion, and deformity, for scoring, and whether joint count scores should be recorded according to a graded linear scale or simply as normal or abnormal.

The most widely used method for assessing the joint count is the Ritchie Index, in which 52 peripheral joints are scored for tenderness or pain on motion[44]. A method used in studies conducted by the Co-operating Clinics of the American Rheumatism Association (ARA) have included 68 peripheral joints, scored for pain on motion, tenderness, and/or swelling[45]. Lansbury and Haut described a method termed the Lansbury Index[46] in which 86 peripheral joints are assessed, with scoring weighted for the relative surface area of each joint. An ARA Glossary Committee has proposed an examination[47] which included 80 peripheral joints, evaluated according to five graded scales for swelling, tenderness, pain on motion, limited motion, and deformity. Egger et al.[48] have described a simplified reduced joint index involving 36 joints, with evidence that information was comparable to that obtained with more elaborate examinations. Our group[49] have described a 28-joint index which appeared as effective as a traditional 70-joint index in comparison with other measures of clinical status. The 28-joint index includes 10 metacarpophalangeal (MCP) and 10 proximal interphalangeal (PIP) joints, as well as two shoulder, elbow, wrist, and knee joints.

Studies of our group[49] indicated a strong correlation between joint count scores for tenderness and pain on motion, as well as between scores for deformity and limitation of motion, but scores for tenderness or pain on motion were only weakly correlated with those for limitation of motion and deformity. Joint count scores for swelling were correlated at higher levels with joint tenderness and pain on motion scores than with joint limitation of motion and deformity scores. A simple normal/abnormal index was found to be as effective as a graded index for each of these abnormalities. The joint count was correlated significantly with other measures of clinical status[49].

The number of involved joints appeared quite predictive of survival in 75 RA patients over 9 years after a baseline assessment (see Figures 5C and 6C). Survival over 5 years was almost 50% in patients with 30 or more involved joints, compared to 70% in patients with 20–30 involved joints, and 95% patients with fewer than 20 involved joints. A simplified joint count involving only 12 joints, i.e., eight metacarpal phalangeal (MCP) joints, knees and shoulders, provided greater discriminatory power for mortality over 5 years than the complete joint count (Pincus, unpublished data). These data are consistent with clinical studies which indicate that exclusion of feet and other joints may not result in loss of meaningful information, possibly because findings in the feet are not necessarily correlated with other aspects of the rheumatoid process.

The Cooperating Clinics of the Rheumatic Diseases have used the joint count measure as the primary determinant of clinical improvement in RA. Generally, a 50% improvement in the joint count is regarded as evidence of a favorable response to a therapy under study. A patient may continue to show considerable disease and be regarded as a "responder" according to this criterion.

Quantitative assessment of radiographs

Radiographs provide an excellent permanent record of clinical status in RA, but generally are not read quantitatively. An initial method to analyze radiographs quantitatively was provided by the Steinbrocker Radiographic Stage, involving a scale of 1–4[50]. This stage is useful for a rapid quantitative score, but is quite limited in its global nature. For example, Larsen pointed out that a patient with ankylosis of the wrist joint might be capable of running to a bus and yet be Stage IV, while another patient may be confined to a wheelchair and yet be Stage III[51]. Therefore, a need for more detailed quantitative scales was recognized.

Detailed quantitative radiographic scoring systems have been described by Larsen[52], Sharp[53,54], Genant[55], and Kaye[56,57] and colleagues over the last decade. The Larsen scale is most widely used in European centers; each joint is scored on a scale of 1-4 for radiographic changes[52]. The most widely used scale in American studies involves that of Sharp, in which separate readings are scored for erosions and joint-space narrowing[53,54]. A modified version of the scale of Sharp et al. was reported by Kaye and colleagues[56], which includes a score for malalignment in addition to erosion and joint-space narrowing scores.

Radiographic scores are correlated significantly with duration of disease[5-10]. However, many patients show erosions and joint-space narrowing within the first 2 years of disease[8,12-14]. Malalignment is seen in fewer than 50% of patients within the first 2 years, and is unusual during the first 5 years of disease[8]. Malalignment is the most easily observed long-term change. However, joint-space narrowing and erosions indicate permanent damage, with disruption of the normal joint architecture.

Articular abnormalities seen on physical examination in the joint count and in the radiograph are often considered equivalent. However, analyses of correlations between the two types of articular measures indicate related and unrelated findings[58]. Joint count tenderness, an extremely useful measure of clinical status in RA, is totally independent of radiographic score at a given point ($r = 0.01$). Joint count swelling scores are correlated at relatively weak, though statistically significant, levels with the radiographic score ($r = 0.19$). Joint count deformity and limitation of motion are quite highly significantly correlated with the radiographic score ($r = 0.69$ and $r = 0.68$, respectively). These findings suggest expected correlations of joint deformity and limited motion with radiographs, and a somewhat unexpected absence of correlation of joint tenderness with radiographs[58].

The observation that most RA patients show significant erosion and joint-space narrowing within the first 2 years of disease without malalignment[8] may provide an important message to both the medical community and the public at large. Many physicians and many patients do not recognize severe disease unless there is deformity and malalignment. Most rheumatologists see patients with a disease duration of more than 2 years; the mean duration of disease is 5 years. If treatment is to benefit RA patients, it may be optimal if started early, before evidence of permanent damage is seen.

Laboratory measures

The two most widely used indices of acute inflammation are the erythrocyte sedimentation rate (ESR) and C-reactive protein (CRP)[59]. These indices are elevated in most RA patients, but they may be normal in the face of active disease. Recent studies have suggested the possibility that serum levels of interleukin 2 (Il-2) receptors may provide useful data for monitoring clinical status[60].

Identification of rheumatoid factor (RF) in RA in 1948[61] was an important milestone in the history of clinical rheumatology, in that it established an immunologic association with RA. Studies by Olsen and colleagues indicate that the level of RF production by peripheral blood lymphocytes may be a useful indicator of clinical response to second-line therapy. About 50% of RA patients produce RF in culture conditions, compared to very few normal individuals[62]. Patients who respond to gold, penicillamine, or methotrexate show significant reductions in RF production concomitant with clinical improvement[63].

An association of RA with the major histocompatibility locus antigen HLA-DR4 was described about a decade ago[64]. Individuals who bear the HLA-DR4 haplotype show a 3.5-fold relative risk of developing RA, and those with the subtype of HLA-DR4 DW4 show 5-fold relative risk for RA, compared to the general population. The DW4 locus differs from other subtypes of HLA-DR4 by only one amino acid, coded for by only a single base, at position 71 in the third hypervariable region of the HLA beta-chain. Differences at this one locus are associated with substantial differences in the relative risk of developing RA[65].

Prognostic associations of outcome in RA according to HLA-DR4 haplotype have been described in some studies and not in others[66]. The conclusion appears to depend on which indicator of clinical outcome is studied. HLA-DR4 is associated with the prevalence of RF, severity of radiographic changes, and limited motion and deformity in the joint count (which are significantly correlated with radiographic changes) as noted above. However, swelling and tenderness in the joint count, self-report questionnaire measures, and physical measures of functional status are not correlated significantly with HLA-DR4 in individual RA patients[66].

These observations suggest that two categories of prognostic measures may be seen in RA; measures within one category are correlated at much higher levels with one another than with measures in the other category. The two categories include: (a) radiographic scores, duration of disease, ESR, HLA-DR4, rheumatoid factor positivity and joint limited motion and joint deformity; and (b) age, joint swelling, joint tenderness, American Rheumatism Association (ARA) functional class, and other measures of patient functional status, including questionnaires. The finding that measures within each category appear to be more highly correlated with one another than with those from the other category suggests that two different types of pathogenetic mechanisms may be seen in the progression of RA[18].

Questionnaires to assess functional status and pain

Questionnaires are used to provide information concerning the functional status of the patient to perform activities of daily living (ADL), as well as the patient's level of pain. Most rheumatologists and patients agree that ADL and pain levels are the most important concerns in RA[67]. These concerns cannot be measured directly through any physical measure, radiography, or laboratory tests.

Among potential predictors of outcome in RA, the patient's history is still referred to as "subjective," in contrast to physical examination, radiographs, and laboratory tests, which are considered to be "objective." In this view, a statement that "My knee hurts" is regarded as subjective, while observations that physical examination suggests a knee effusion, that a radiograph suggests early medial compartment narrowing, or that the ESR is 24 are regarded as "objective." However, the most reproducible information here is the "subjective" data. A patient asked ten times, "Does your knee hurt?," replies ten times that the knee does hurt. In contrast, ten physicians asked to assess a mild knee effusion, or ten radiologists asked to interpret a marginally abnormal X-ray, may provide widely different interpretations[68]. Therefore, the term "subjective" applied to patient responses may be inappropriate, since "subjective" implies that the data are not reproducible, and these are very reproducible data.

The major considerations in a questionnaire as a measure of clinical status in RA are identical to those regarding any quantitative measure in clinical medicine, including: (a) reliability — is the measure reproducible; (b) validity — is what is measured what is thought to be measured; and (c) feasibility — is it practical to obtain the measure in clinical settings? Over the last decade, it has been found that self-report questionnaires, in which the patient provides the data, have greater reliability than those involving a health professional. The explanation appears to involve the fact that removal of another individual, including a health professional, eliminates a source of variability in patient response.

A number of self-report questionnaires have been found to be useful in prognosis and clinical monitoring of RA. The most prominently used questionnaires include the Health Assessment Questionnaire (HAQ)[69], the Arthritis Impact Measurement Scales (AIMS)[70], the Modified Health Assessment Questionnaire (MHAQ)[33], and MACTAR[71]. All of these questionnaires have been found to be valid, reliable, and feasible for the administration in clinical settings. Questionnaire data appear to provide as effective information as traditional measures to predict mortality[33] and health services utilization[72] in RA. Self-report questionnaire data have been found as effective as any other data in clinical trials to detect changes in clinical status in RA[73].

Questionnaire scores are highly correlated with traditional measures in RA, including joint count, radiographs, and laboratory tests (Table 5). For example, in patients with a joint count greater than 10 joints, 11% had a questionnaire score of 1, 37% had a score of 1–1.5, 67% of 1.5–2, 70% of 2–3 and 100% of 3–4, indicating a strong association between higher joint counts and higher dysfunction. Furthermore, among all measures to best explain variation in other measures (Table 6) the questionnaire score was most explanatory of the joint count,

Table 5 Percentage of 259 patients with rheumatoid arthritis who had poor clinical status according to various traditional clinical status measures in different categories of activities of daily living activities questionnaire responses

	\multicolumn{5}{c}{Range of activities of daily living scores}
	1.00	1.01–1.50	1.51–2.00	2.01–3.00	3.01–4.00
Percentage of all patients:	6	20	32	33	9
Clinical status measure					
Sedimentation rate > 20	29	49	64	74	85
X-ray erosion score > 0.5	63	80	83	83	100
Grip strength < 100	19	29	57	83	100
Walking time > 8 s	6	29	42	69	100
Button test > 40 s	31	53	71	88	100
Joint count > 10 joints	11	37	67	79	100

Adapted from Pincus, T., Callahan, L. F., Brooks, R., Fuchs, J. A., Olsen, N. J. and Kaye, J. J. (1989). Self-report questionnaires are in rheumatoid arthritis compared with traditional physical, radiographic, and laboratory measures. *Ann. Intern. Med.*, **110**, 259–266

ARA Functional Class, and global self-assessment, and second most explanatory of grip strength and walking time. Therefore, questionnaire scores appear most representative of all other measures, and self-report questionnaire score may be the single most representative measure of clinical status in RA patients. If physicians wish to monitor an individual RA patient quantitatively, and can choose only a single measure, the questionnaire would appear the optimal measure.

All validated self-report questionnaires have been found useful in clinical assessment[73]. Over the past 5 years at the Vanderbilt University Clinic, patients have been given a simple MHAQ questionnaire at each visit to provide a quantitative recording of clinical status at the time. This procedure is well-accepted by patients, and provides the capacity to document quantitatively clinical responses to various therapies.

Physical measures of musculoskeletal function: grip strength, walking time and button test

Physical measures of musculoskeletal function may be viewed as complementary to self-report questionnaire measures[74]. These measures of functional status, including the grip strength[75], walking time[76], and button test[77], are widely used in clinical trials but not in clinical practice.

The grip strength[74,75] is measured by inflating a blood-pressure cuff to 30 mmHg and asking the patient to squeeze as hard as he can. The walking time involves a measured course of 25 or 50 feet, in which the

Table 6 Explanatory variables for measures of clinical status in patients with rheumatoid arthritis based on regression models[a]

Measure of clinical status analyzed	Most explanatory variable		Second most explanatory variable		Variation explained by model
	Variable	Partial R^2	Variable	Incremental R^2	(Total R^2)
Self-report questionnaire score[b]	Global self-assessment	0.44	Walking time	0.08	0.59
Joint count	Questionnaire score	0.29	Radiographic score	0.08	0.38
Radiographic scores	Duration of disease	0.38	Grip strength	0.11	0.52
Erythrocyte sedimentation rate	Formal educational level	0.05	ARA functional class[c]	0.02	0.07
Grip strength	Radiographic score	0.24	Questionnaire score	0.14	0.40
Walking time	ARA functional class	0.26	Questionnaire score	0.04	0.34
ARA functional class	Questionnaire score	0.30	Walking time	0.09	0.47
Global self-assessment	Questionnaire score	0.44	Age	0.03	0.51

Adapted from ref. 78.
[a] The variables of clinical status in the left column were analyzed in regression models as dependent variables. The possible explanatory independent variables examined included all of the other variables of clinical status in the left column, as well as age, duration of disease, and formal educational level. The most explanatory and second most explanatory independent variables for variation in each dependent variable are indicated. The total R^2 indicates the proportion of variation for each dependent variable explained by all the dependent variables in the regression.
[b] Patients answered an activities-of-daily-living questionnaire.
[c] ARA = American Rheumatism Association.

patient is asked to walk at a normal pace from a starting point to a measured stopping point, timing the walk with a stopwatch[74,76]. The button test involves a standard button board; the patient is asked to unbutton five buttons and then button them as quickly as he can with the score recorded in seconds[74,77].

When these measures are assessed using standardized instructions, they provide excellent interobserver and intraobserver reliabilities ($r = 0.797$, $p < 0.001$) (Callahan, Brooks, and Pincus, unpublished data). Physical measures of functional status are correlated with joint count, radiographic, and laboratory measures, though highest correlations are seen with questionnaire measures[78]. Furthermore, the walking time and button test have been shown to be excellent predictors of mortality in RA, as patients with poor results show survivals lower than 50% when the button test result is greater than 120 seconds (see above[33]). These data suggest potential utility of physical measures of functional status in usual rheumatologic care. These measures may overcome problems associated with self-report measures, including differences in languages and inability of certain patients to complete questionnaires, although self-report questionnaires appear most explanatory of all quantitative measures in RA.

7 PROGNOSIS APPEARS MORE EFFECTIVELY ESTIMATED ACCORDING TO MEASURES OF FUNCTIONAL STATUS, INCLUDING QUESTIONNAIRES, RATHER THAN RADIOGRAPHIC AND LABORATORY MEASURES, AT THIS TIME

Traditional approaches to prognosis in rheumatic diseases have involved emphasis on data derived from high-technology sources such as laboratory tests or radiographs. In some inflammatory rheumatic diseases, this approach has been quite effective. For example, in systemic lupus erythematosus, evidence has suggested that the levels of DNA antibodies and serum complement are useful prognostic indicators, and normalization of these indicators is associated with a good outcome, while failure to normalize these values predicts a poor outcome[79]. Reports that certain drugs may modify radiographic progression (see ref. 27) and laboratory tests[80] have been the primary basis for the term "disease-modifying."

In RA, however, surveys of expert rheumatologists suggest that measures of functional status in activities of daily living (ADL) and pain, assessed using questionnaires, appear as valuable as traditional radiographic or laboratory measures to depict clinical status in RA[67,73,81]. The search for laboratory markers in RA has not yielded evidence that classical "objective"[82] indicators of clinical status are effective in prognosis. ADL and pain questionnaires have been shown to be useful in recent clinical trials[73,83,84], but were not included in any of the classical reports concerning therapies in RA, e.g., studies documenting the value of gold salts[80,85]. The two indisputably undesirable outcomes in RA —

work disability and death — have not been analyzed in any clinical trials.

If the discriminatory power for survival or death in RA depicted in Figure 5E for functional markers were reported for a laboratory measure (e.g., a new T lymphocyte cell-surface antigen, DNA restriction fragment, or elaborate imaging procedure) it would likely be introduced widely into the assessment of all RA patients. However, the most effective predictors of mortality in RA identified to date — functional capacity in activities of daily living, measured by questionnaire or physical measures such as walking time or the button test — are regarded as "subjective," and not likely to be as valuable as laboratory tests. Clinicians recognize that a patient history generally provides 60-80% of the information needed to make a diagnosis or recognize the clinical status of a patient. A well-designed questionnaire may be regarded as an "objective" form of history-taking, with data as reproducible as laboratory tests, radiographs, and other high-technology procedures[73].

Questionnaire data have been documented to provide the most valuable information to predict morbidity, work disability, health-care utilization, and mortality in RA, compared to radiographs, laboratory tests, or any data available to date[73]. Furthermore, scores on functional-status questionnaires are highly correlated with traditional measures such as the joint count, radiographic scores, erythrocyte sedimentation rate, and physical measures of function such as grip strength and walking time[78].

Current management of individual RA patients remains based primarily on empirical dialogue between providers and patients. While such dialogues are clearly the most important component of patient care, the introduction of simple functional status questionnaires into routine clinical practice could provide quantitative, cost-effective data to document and monitor the course of RA. Such procedures could facilitate quantitative comparisons of individual patients from one visit to the next in the same clinical setting, and of patients seen in different rheumatology clinical settings, according to the same data. Standardized data collection in RA patients could promote comparison of patient status according to quantitative data, comparable to Anatomic Stage of Hodgkin's disease or number of involved vessels in coronary arteriography.

Research in rheumatic diseases may some day identify laboratory or imaging markers predictive of the course of RA more effective than currently available measures. However, *at this time*, data obtained from patients appear more effective than traditional laboratory or radiographic data to predict the long-term course of RA. Therefore, it might be desirable at present for clinicians to acquire standard functional data as a component of usual patient care.

NEW CONCEPTS

8 ESTIMATION OF LONG-TERM PROGNOSIS IN RA APPEARS MORE EFFECTIVELY ACHIEVED FROM LONG-TERM OBSERVATIONAL STUDIES THAN FROM CLINICAL TRIALS

One source of incorrect impressions concerning the long-term prognosis of RA is the assumption that data from clinical trials may be applied effectively to analysis of the long-term course of RA. While the randomized clinical trial has great attraction, based on the model of a "scientific" experiment[85,86], a number of important limitations to clinical trials exist, including the following:

Exclusion criteria

Exclusion criteria are necessary for any clinical trial, to circumvent variables such as comorbidities, prior treatment with the study drug, etc., which might confound the comparison of two treatment programs[85,86]. However, a greater proportion of RA patients than patients with other diseases may be ineligible for clinical trials as a result of exclusion criteria. In five of seven clinical trials conducted at Vanderbilt University over the last 5 years, fewer than 5% of 1200 identified RA patients were eligible for participation; in two trials, fewer than 0.5% of these 1200 patients were eligible[86].

Most RA patients do not present to treatment centers until after several years of disease, and many have already received several treatments, including second-line drugs, that were unsuccessful. Such patients are ineligible for excellently designed trials, ironically most often on the basis of past or present use of therapies believed to affect the disease process (for which the evidence appears considerably overstated, as discussed above). Exclusion of patients in whom various previous therapies have been unsuccessful may favorably bias results of clinical trials.

Adjustments for "drop-outs"

Patients who "drop out" of clinical trials because of drug toxicities or even mortality are often excluded from analyses of results. In trials involving RA patients, at least one-third of patients generally "drop out" within 6 months. Analyses in which "drop-outs" are excluded may give exaggerated impressions of efficacy.

The time frame of observation in clinical trials is relatively short

Most clinical trials in RA patients have been conducted over 2–12 months, and no published trial has been conducted over a period longer than 24 months. Many clinical trials indicate improvement in RA patients over 2–24 months. These trials are excellently designed and

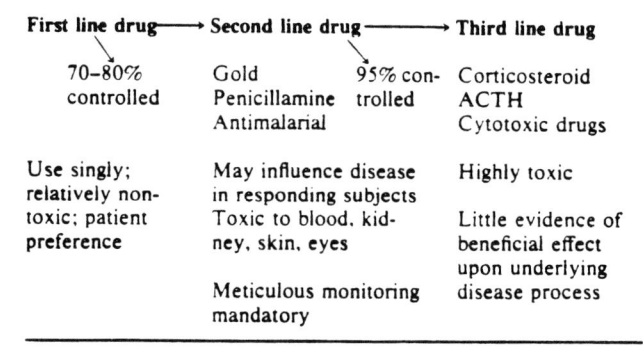

First line drug →	Second line drug →	Third line drug
70–80% controlled	Gold 95% con- Penicillamine trolled Antimalarial	Corticosteroid ACTH Cytotoxic drugs
Use singly; relatively non-toxic; patient preference	May influence disease in responding subjects Toxic to blood, kidney, skin, eyes Meticulous monitoring mandatory	Highly toxic Little evidence of beneficial effect upon underlying disease process

Figure 7 Schema entitled "Drug treatment of rheumatoid arthritis" from 1981 edition of Kelley textbook[87].

well-executed, with scrupulous attention to methodological requirements such as random allocation, double-blind treatments, concurrent controls, proper statistical tests, etc.[85,86], but these trials themselves may have contributed to important misconceptions regarding the long-term course of RA.

An example of potential misconceptions concerning the course of RA emerging from clinical trials, as well as population-based studies, is seen in the comment in the 1981 edition of Kelley's textbook that "70–80% of RA patients are controlled with first-line nonsteroidal anti-inflammatory drugs" (Figure 7)[87]. This concept may be valid if applied to all individuals who meet ARA criteria for RA, many of whom have a self-limited process rather than a progressive disease, as discussed above. While first-line therapies have been documented to be effective in hundreds of clinical trials, these therapies do not "control" RA in most patients over extended periods[8,10,11,18,20-22,24,28,33,34,88].

Exaggeration of efficacy based on significant differences between treatment and placebo

In the rheumatology literature, second-line drugs, including gold salts, penicillamine, hydroxycholoroquine, corticosteroids, methotrexate, azathioprine, and cyclophosphamide are frequently described as "remission-inducing"[89]. Evidence that this term is inappropriate includes the following points:

1. *Marginal benefits are often exaggerated.* Ianuzzi et al.[11] reviewed the 18 published studies of second-line drugs which have been suggested to document slowing of radiographic progression in RA (Table 1). Only four studies were found to provide probable support for this concept, while 11 showed no support whatsoever[11]. Radiographic progression does not appear to be affected reproducibly in most RA patients by drug therapy.

2. *A sustained remission longer than 3 years is seen in about 1% of patients treated with second-line agents.* Wolfe and Hawley[19] reviewed 485 patients who

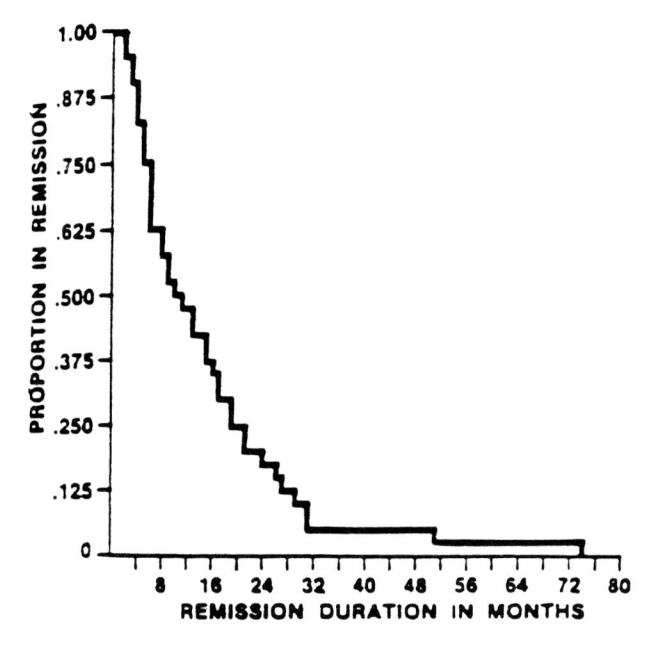

Figure 8 Analysis of duration of remission in RA patients in a clinical practice. The initial survey involved 485 patients of whom 86 (18%) appeared to have a clinical remission. Of these remissions, 80% ended by 24 months and 90% by 36 months. Therefore, fewer than 2% of patients treated with second-line agents experienced remissions longer than 3 years. (From ref. 19.)

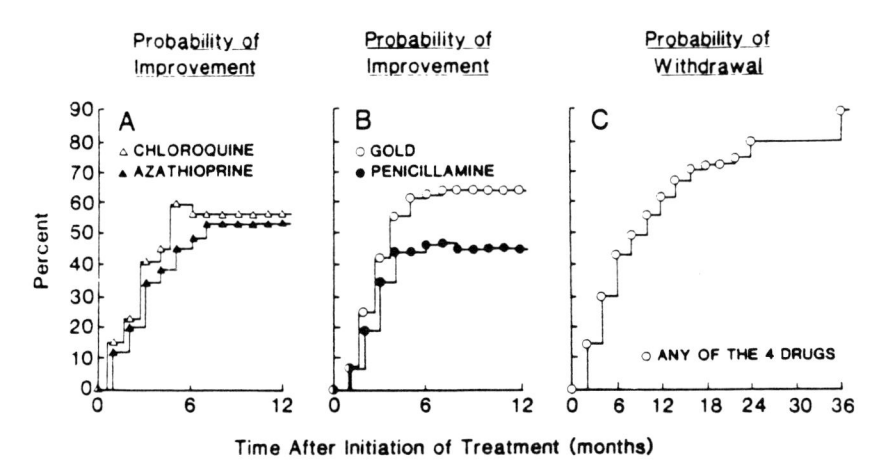

Figure 9 Analysis of results of treatment with chloroquine, azathioprine, gold, and penicillamine. At 6 months, about 50% of patients responded to each of the agents, without significant differences among the agents (A, B). However 50% of patients have withdrawn from treatment by 12 months, 80% by 24 months, and 90% by 36 months (C). These data indicate relatively poor clinical responses over prolonged periods using these second-line agents. (From ref. 90).

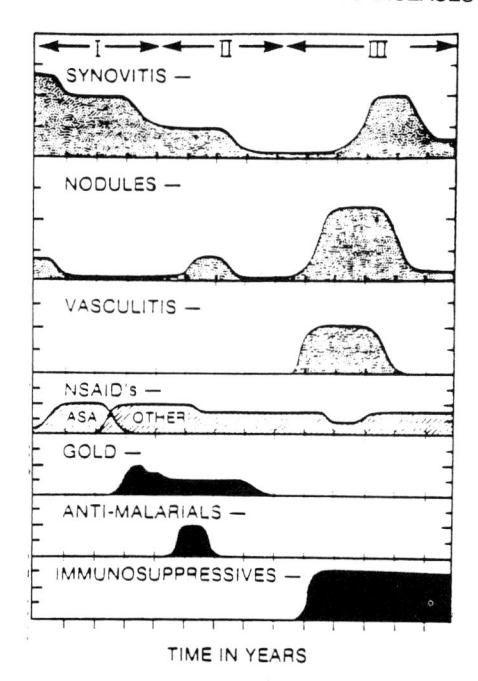

Figure 10 Scheme entitled "Management choices in hypothetical [RA] patient over several years." from 1985 edition of McCarty textbook[3]. Note that initiation of gold is not projected until after 2.5 years, antimalarials until after 4.5 years, and immunosuppressives until after 8.5 years.

were treated with second-line drugs. Evidence of remission was seen in only about 18% of these patients. Equally importantly, fewer than 50% of these remissions were sustained for even 1 year, and fewer than 10% for more than 3 years (Figure 8). Therefore, fewer than 1.8% of patients treated with second-line agents in a rheumatology practice experienced a sustained remission lasting longer than 3 years[19]. These data appear applicable to most rheumatology care settings. No data have been reported to suggest better results from other locales.

3. *Fewer than one in five patients begun on therapies with second-line agents continues to take these agents 2 years later.* Thompson et al.[90] studied 251 courses of therapy with four second-line drugs, gold salts, penicillamine, azathioprine, or hydroxychloroquine, in 154 patients (Figure 9). Clinical efficacy within the first 6 months was reported by patients for 57% of these courses of therapy, reflecting documented benefit in clinical trials (Figure 9A and 9B). However, fewer than 50% of individuals who began a course of these drugs completed 1 year, fewer than 20% completed 2 years, and fewer than 10% completed 3 years of therapy (Figure 9C). Most discontinuations were based on inefficacy or toxicity, and not on remission[90]. Similar findings have been reported by Amor et al.[91] and Situnayake et al.[92].

These data suggest that long-term results in actual practice indicate that remission is unusual, sustained remission is rare, and loss of efficacy with time is frequent. There is loss of efficacy after 3–12 months even in most patients who respond to second-line agents, based on possible tachyphylaxis, regression toward the mean, etc.[85]. This phenomenon has not been extensively studied.

Results in actual clinical use of second-line agents in RA are disappointing, possibly in part because the drugs may not be initiated sufficiently early in disease course. In the 1985 edition of the McCarty textbook, it was suggested that gold might be initiated after 2¾ years, antimalarials after 4½ years, and immunosuppressive drugs after 9 years (Figure 10). Clinical trials inevitably exclude patients who have received multiple prior therapies, thereby selecting for patients with both short duration of disease and/or milder disease. The usual office RA patient is not seen until disease has been present for several years.

Recognition of the progressive nature of RA over 5–20 years in most patients may have contributed to the current practice of using second-line drugs earlier in disease course[42]. Clearly, the accurate assessment of the prognosis of RA requires recognition that "remission-induction" is rare with use of currently available drugs.

9 CLASSIFICATION CRITERIA AND POPULATION-BASED STUDIES HAVE IMPORTANT LIMITATIONS IN ESTIMATION OF LONG-TERM PROGNOSIS OF INDIVIDUAL RA PATIENTS

Classification criteria for RA have proven of great value in differentiating patients with RA from those with other rheumatic diseases, but may have contributed misconceptions regarding prognosis. The 1958 American Rheumatology Association (ARA) Criteria for RA[93] were used in all studies over 30 years, and were revised in 1987[94]. Textbook discussions of RA include an assumption that people who meet criteria for RA are relatively homogeneous with respect to pathogenesis and prognosis. However, analyses of individuals defined as having RA in population-based versus clinical settings suggest that is not the case. On the contrary, most individuals identified in clinical settings as meeting ARA Criteria for RA appear to have a severe progressive disease, while most individuals identified in population-based studies as meeting these criteria appear to have a self-limited process. The evidence for this suggestion includes the following:

Re-evaluation of individuals who meet ARA Criteria for RA 3–5 years later

Only two studies are available in which almost all individuals in a population were examined to identify those who met ARA Criteria for RA, and these same individuals were then re-examined 3–5 years later. In both studies, fewer than 30% of those who met criteria at baseline also met criteria at later review[95,96]. In Sudbury, Massachusetts, 118 of

Table 7 Follow-up evaluation of individuals who met 1958 ARA Criteria for rheumatoid arthritis[a]

Category	Initial evaluation	Number reexamined	Evaluation 3-5 years later		
			Probable	Definite	No evidence of RA
Definite RA	40 (0.9%)	36	7 (19.4%)	12 (33.3%)	17 (47.2%)
Probable RA	79 (1.7%)	73	7 (9.6%)	4 (5.7%)	2 (84.9%)
Total	118 (2.6%)	109	14 (12.8%)	16 (14.7%)	79 (72.5%)

Adapted from O'Sullivan, J. B. and Cathcart, E. S. (1972). The prevalence of RA: follow-up evaluation of the effect of criteria on rates in Sudbury, Massachusetts. *Ann. Intern. Med.*, **76**, 573-577

[a] Evaluations were performed in 4552 individuals at baseline. The 1958 ARA Criteria were met by 118 individuals (2.6%). A review 3-5 years later was performed on 109 of the 118 individuals who met ARA Criteria for RA according to 1958 ARA Criteria.

4522 individuals (2.6%) examined at baseline met the 1958 ARA Criteria for definite or probable RA. When 109 of these 118 individuals were re-examined 3-5 years later, only 30 (27.5%) still met the criteria for definite or probable RA[95] (Table 7). In Tecumseh, Michigan, only 109 of 402 (26.6%) individuals who met ARA Criteria for RA at baseline met the Criteria four years later[96], figures remarkably similar to the Sudbury data. In the only long-term "inception cohort" study of 50 patients with disease for less than 6 months who met ARA Criteria for definite or probable RA, most patients did not show evidence of a progressive disease[97].

By contrast, almost all individuals seen in rheumatology clinical settings who meet ARA Criteria for RA show evidence of disease 3-5 years later, generally with substantial progression[8,10,11,18,20-22,24,28,33,34,88,98] as discussed above[3,99,100].

Rheumatoid factor prevalence in individuals meeting ARA Criteria for RA in population-based versus clinical studies

Four studies have been conducted in which individuals were analyzed for both whether they met the 1958 ARA Criteria for RA and whether they had rheumatoid factor, from such diverse locations as Tecumseh, Michigan[101], Wensleydale, England[102], Jerusalem, Israel[103], and Arizona[104]. These studies all indicated that rheumatoid factor was seen in only about 25% of individuals who met ARA Criteria for RA (Table 8).

By contrast, about 75-80% of individuals who meet ARA Criteria for RA in clinical settings have rheumatoid factor in their serum[59,105], and no published report indicates a prevalence less than 70% in a clinically identified group of RA patients.

These observations suggest that the 1958 ARA Criteria for RA identify individuals with at least two types of pathogenetic process:

NEW CONCEPTS

Table 8 Prevalence of rheumatoid factor in individuals identified in entire populations who met 1958 ARA Criteria for rheumatoid arthritis

	Wensleydale, England (1960)[102]	Tecumseh, Michigan (1959–60)[101]	Jerusalem, Israel (1962–64)[103]	Blackfoot Indians, Montana (1961)[102]
Rheumatoid factor test and titer	Latex fix. $>1:80$	Latex fix. $>1:20$	Latex fix. $>1:320$	Bentonite floc. $>1:128$
Number tested	870	6590	1602	1049
Prevalence RA (def. & prob.)	4.9%	6.0%	2.4%	3.8%
Sensitivity	24%	19%	25%	25%
Specificity	91%	98%	96%	98%

1. Individuals identified in the general population as meeting ARA Criteria for RA are most likely not to have evidence of disease 3–5 years later. Only about 25% have rheumatoid factor in their sera. Many of these individuals may never see a physician for their symptoms, but may be over-represented in clinical trials[85,106].
2. Individuals identified in clinical rheumatology settings as meeting ARA Criteria for RA, at least 75% of whom have rheumatoid factor in their sera, are most likely to have evidence of disease 3–5 years later, generally with progression[3,99,100].

The likelihood of a progressive disease rather than a self-limited process appears substantially greater when symptoms have been present for longer than 6 months, although some patients may experience an indolent course over many years.

In the 1987 revision of the ARA Criteria for RA[94], a requirement for joint swelling, rather than tenderness alone, may provide greater stringency than the 1958 Criteria to identify progressive, sustained disease. However, both the 1958[93] and 1987[94] ARA Criteria were established on the basis of individuals seen in rheumatology office settings, and not in the general population. It is not known how the 1987 Criteria for RA might function in population-based studies, but results would appear intermediate between those found using the 1958 Criteria and those in rheumatology office settings, not dissimilar to the inception cohort study[97]. Recognition that ARA Criteria for RA may identify a heterogenous group of individuals with very different outcomes would appear to clarify some apparently contradictory statements regarding the prognosis of RA.

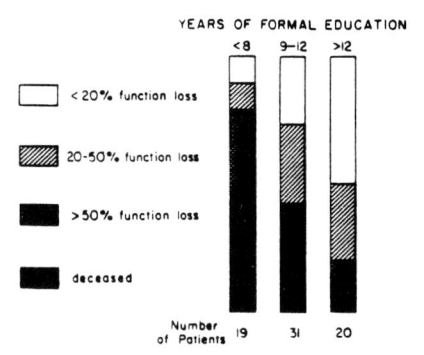

Figure 11 Analysis of morbidity and mortality in 70 rheumatoid arthritis patients over 9 years. Note evidence of biologic dose–response curve among three groups according to formal education level: patients with fewer than 8 years of education included almost half who did not survive and very few good courses; patients with more than 12 years of formal education included almost half with relatively good courses. (From ref. 37.).

10 PROGNOSIS IN RA MAY BE AFFECTED AS MUCH BY PATIENT BEHAVIORS AND LIFESTYLES AS BY TREATMENTS AND OTHER ACTIONS OF HEALTH-CARE PROVIDERS AND THE HEALTH-CARE SYSTEM

An underlying assumption in modern health care is that difficult outcomes in different patients result from differences in health care system variables, e.g., differences between drugs in clinical trials. This concept is most valid in short-term studies, e.g., treatment of pneumonia or myocardial infarction over a few days, in which the health care system is in control of the situation. However, as the observation period is lengthened, patient characteristics appear to show increasing importance. For example, recent studies in RA suggest that formal education level as a marker of differences in patient characteristics is highly predictive of morbidity and mortality (Figure 11) over 9 years. The associations between formal education level and outcome are not explained by treatments used, nor by age, duration of disease, functional status measures, or any other baseline variable[37].

Further analyses of 385 RA patients seen at a University Clinic, Veterans Administration Hospital, and private practice settings, indicate poorer clinical status in individuals with low levels of formal education according to all indicators examined (Table 9), including joint count, erythrocyte sedimentation rate, grip strength, walking time, and questionnaire self-assessment measures[107]. These findings are also not explained by age, duration of disease, race, or clinical setting.

These studies in RA patients are consistent with data from the cardiovascular literature indicating associations between formal education level and clinical status. In a clinical trial involving prevention of mortality after myocardial infarction with use of propranolol versus placebo (B-HAT study), it was observed that formal educational level, life stress, and social isolation were more predictive of subsequent mortality than whether the patient was randomized to drug or

Table 9 Mean values for laboratory, physical, and self-report measures of disease status in 385 rheumatoid arthritis patients, classified according to level of formal education

		Patients classified according to formal education level				
Disease status measure[a]	All patients	Grade school	Some high school	High school graduate	Some college or more	P value[b]
Laboratory measures						
ESR (mm/h)	40.1	48.3	49.4	34.7	31.2	0.002[c]
Joint count (number of painful joints)	12.1	16.3	15.1	9.1	9.8	0.001[d]
Physical measures						
Grip strength (mmHg)	98.8	93.7	92.1	97.9	109.8	0.079
Walking time (s)	10.3	11.2	10.0	10.6	9.4	0.424[c]
Button test (s)	62.5	80.5	61.3	60.8	49.8	0.003[c]
Self-report measures						
ADL difficulty scale (1–4)	1.97	2.26	2.04	1.86	1.77	<0.00
ADL pain scale (1–4)	2.37	2.62	2.56	2.26	2.13	0.001[d]
ADL dissatisfaction scale (1–4)	2.26	2.54	2.41	2.12	2.05	0.006
Visual analog pain scale (0–10)	5.12	5.75	5.85	4.89	4.34	0.074
Global self-assessment (1–4)	2.68	3.09	2.70	2.55	2.44	<0.00

Adapted from Callahan, L. F. and Pincus, T. (1988). Formal educational level as a significant marker of clinical status in rheumatoid arthritis. *Arthritis Rheum.*, **31**, 1346–1357.
[a] ESR = erythrocyte sedimentation rate; ADL = activities of daily living.
[b] By analysis of covariance, after controlling for age, sex, clinical setting, and disease duration.
[c] $P < 0.05$ after adjustment for multiple comparisons.
[d] $P < 0.01$ after adjustment for multiple comparisons.

placebo[108]. Analyses of London, England, civil servants have indicated that employment grade as a marker of socioeconomic status explained patterns of cardiovascular mortality considerably more effectively than recognized physiologic risk factors such as smoking, blood pressure, and cholesterol.[109]

Formal education level may be regarded as a marker for overall socioeconomic status. The data may be interpreted to suggest that differences in patients according to socioeconomic status variables such as formal education level may identify important, though relatively neglected, variables associated with different outcomes in patients with RA and other chronic diseases.

Studies indicating associations between formal education level and morbidity and mortality in chronic diseases[37,107-109] have been extended to recognize that the prevalence of most common diseases in the VS population, including arthritis, back pain, hypertension and other cardiovascular diseases, peptic ulcer, diabetes, chronic lung disease, and many others, vary directly with years of formal education (Table 10)[34,110]. The relative odds for individuals to develop most chronic

Table 10 Percentage of individuals in the 1978 US population aged 18-64 reporting health conditions according to level of formal education[1]

Condition	Total number (thousands) (percent of total population) aged 18-64 reporting condition		Percentage of individuals reporting condition according to years of formal education				Odds ratios according to years of formal education			
			1-8	9-11	12	>12	1-8	9-11	12	>12
Arthritis	14 215	(11.3%)	26.4	13.1	11.0	6.8	5.0	2.1	1.7	1.0
Hypertension	14 015	(11.1%)	26.1	15.1	9.5	7.2	4.6	2.3	1.4	1.0
Allergies	5 313	(4.2%)	3.6	3.3	4.6	4.4	0.8	0.8	1.1	1.0
Stomach ulcer	4 568	(3.6%)	6.9	5.7	3.4	2.1	3.4	2.8	1.6	1.0
Diabetes	3 205	(2.5%)	5.2	3.6	2.5	1.4	3.9	2.6	1.8	1.0
Thyroid disease	3 015	(2.4%)	1.9	2.5	3.0	1.9	1.0	1.3	1.6	1.0
Kidney disease	2 354	(1.9%)	5.1	2.4	1.4	1.3	4.2	1.9	1.1	1.0
Chronic bronchitis	2 033	(1.6%)	4.0	2.3	1.6	0.7	5.6	3.2	2.2	1.0
Heart attack	1 805	(1.4%)	4.9	2.0	1.2	0.6	8.8	3.4	2.0	1.0
Cancer	837	(0.7%)	1.5	0.6	0.6	0.5	2.7	1.1	1.1	1.0
Tuberculosis	261	(0.2%)	0.3	0.4	0.1	0.2	1.8	2.2	0.6	1.0
Multiple sclerosis	148	(0.1%)	0.0	0.1	0.1	0.2	0.2	0.4	0.7	1.0

Adapted from Pincus, T., Callahan, L. F. and Burkhauser, R. V. (1987). Most chronic diseases are reported more frequently by individuals with fewer than 12 years of formal education in the age 18-64 United States population. *J. Chron. Dis.*, **40**, 865-874.

diseases range from 3 : 1 to 6 : 1 for those with fewer than 9 years versus those having more than 12 years of formal education. These findings are explained in part by differences in age, sex, race, or smoking according to education level[110], and exist independently of these explanatory variables. Differences in disease frequencies according to formal education level are seen for 27 of 37 conditions recorded for the US population. Among the 20 diseases seen in 1% of the population, only thyroid disease, allergies, and asthma do not differ significantly in prevalence according to level of education. An inverse pattern, with higher frequencies in more educated individuals, is seen for one condition — multiple sclerosis[110]. Lower formal education level is therefore associated with a higher prevalence, morbidity, and mortality of many chronic diseases.

Similar observations have been made in surveys in Italy[111] and Great Britain[112,113]. Formal education level is not included in most clinical investigations, as most physicians are unaware of associations between formal education and health. The associations may be regarded as nonexplanatory, as they are seen in many diseases and may be regarded as merely the result of limited access to medical care for individuals of lower socioeconomic status. However, recent data indicate that medical services are utilized as much or more by individuals of lower socioeconomic class as by those of higher socioeconomic class[114].

A hypothesis has been proposed that low formal education level is a composite/surrogate variable that identifies behavioral risk factors predisposing to the etiology and poor outcomes of most chronic diseases[115]. Some of these behaviors include diet, smoking, compliance, efficiency in using medical services, problem-solving capacity, sense of personal responsibility, capacity to cope with stress, life stress[108], social isolation[108], health locus of control[116], and learned helplessness[117]. The data strongly suggest that associations between poor outcomes and low formal education levels are not likely to be explained simply on the basis of limited access to medical care for individuals of lower education levels, as the frequencies of disease could not be explained on this basis. Further studies of these associations might lead to new understanding of disease prevention and outcomes.

References

1. Pincus, T. and Callahan, L. F. (1989). Reassessment of twelve traditional paradigms concerning the diagnosis, incidence, morbidity and mortality of rheumatoid arthritis. *Scand. J. Rheumatol.* (Suppl.), **79**, 67-95
2. Kelley, W. N., Harris, E. D., Jr., Ruddy, S. and Sledge, C. (eds.) (1985). *Textbook of Rheumatology*, p. 979. (Philadelphia: W. B. Saunders)
3. McCarty, D. J. (1985). *Arthritis and Allied Conditions: A Textbook of Rheumatology*, p. 675. (Philadelphia: Lea & Febiger)
4. Kelley, W. N., Harris, E. D., Jr, Ruddy, S. and Sledge, C. B. (1989). *Textbook of Rheumatology*. (Philadelphia: W. B. Saunders)
5. Sharp, J. T. (1989). Scoring radiographic abnormalities in rheumatoid arthritis. *J. Rheumatol.*, **16**, 568-569
6. Luukkainen, R., Kajander, A. and Isomaki, H. (1977). Effect of gold on progression of erosions in rheumatoid arthritis: better results with early treatment. *Scand. J. Rheumatol.*, **6**, 189-192
7. Salaffi, F. and Ferraccioli, G. F. (1989). Progress of the anatomical damage in rheumatoid hands. Radiography of the natural course of the disease or of the course during treatment? *Scand. J. Rheumatol.*, **18**, 119-120
8. Fuchs, H. A., Kaye, J. J., Callahan, L. F., Nance, E. P. and Pincus, T. (1989). Evidence of significant radiographic damage in rheumatoid arthritis within the first 2 years of disease. *J. Rheumatol.*, **16**, 585-591
9. Luukkainen, R., Kaarela, K., Isomaki, H. *et al.* (1983). The prediction of radiological destruction during the early stage of rheumatoid arthritis. *Clin. Exp. Rheumatol.*, **1**, 295-298
10. Scott, D. L., Grindulis, K. A., Struthers, G. R., Coulton, B. L., Popert, A. J. and Bacon, P. A. (1984). Progression of radiological changes in rheumatoid arthritis. *Ann. Rheum. Dis.*, **43**, 8-17
11. Iannuzzi, L., Dawson, N., Zein, N. and Kushner, I. (1983). Does drug therapy slow radiographic deterioration in rheumatoid arthritis? *N. Engl. J. Med.*, **309**, 1023-1028
12. Thould, A. K. and Simon, G. (1966). Assessment of radiological changes in the hands and feet in rheumatoid arthritis: their correlation with prognosis. *Ann. Rheum. Dis.*, **25**, 220-228
13. Brook, A. and Corbett, M. (1977). Radiographic changes in early rheumatoid disease. *Ann. Rheum. Dis.*, **36**, 71-73
14. Scott, D. L., Coulton, B. L., Bacon, P. A. and Popert, A. J. (1985). Methods of X-ray assessment in rheumatoid arthritis: a re-evaluation. *Br. J. Rheumatol.*, **24**, 31-39
15. Duthie, J. J. R., Brown, P. E., Truelove, L. H., Baragar, F. D. and Lawrie, A. J. (1964). Course and prognosis in rheumatoid arthritis: a further report. *Ann. Rheum. Dis.*, **23**, 193-204
16. Rasker, J. J. and Cosh, J. A. (1981). Cause and age at death in a prospective study of 100 patients with rheumatoid arthritis. *Ann. Rheum. Dis.*, **40**, 115-120

17. Scott, D. L., Coulton, B. L., Chapman, J. H., Bacon, P. A. and Popert, A. J. (1983). The long-term effects of treating rheumatoid arthritis. *J. R. Coll. Physicians. Lond.*, **17**, 79–85
18. Scott, D. L., Symmons, D. P. M., Coulton, B. L. and Popert, A. J. (1987). Long-term outcome of treating rheumatoid arthritis: results after 20 years. *Lancet*, **1**, 1108–1111
19. Wolfe, F. and Hawley, D. J. (1985). Remission in rheumatoid arthritis. *J. Rheumatol.*, **12**, 245–252
20. Pincus, T., Callahan, L. F., Sale, W. G., Brooks, A. L., Payne, L. E. and Vaughn, W. K. (1984). Severe functional declines, work disability, and increased mortality in seventy-five rheumatoid arthritis patients studied over nine years. *Arthritis Rheum.*, **27**, 864–872
21. Yelin, E. H., Meenan, R., Nevitt, M. and Epstein, W. (1980). Work disability in rheumatoid arthritis: effects of disease, social, and work factors. *Ann. Intern. Med.*, **93**, 551–556
22. Meenan, R. F., Yelin, E. H., Nevitt, M. and Epstein, W. V. (1981). The impact of chronic disease: a sociomedical profile of rheumatoid arthritis. *Arthritis Rheum.*, **24**, 544–549
23. Mitchell, J. M., Burkhauser, R. V. and Pincus, T. (1988). The importance of age, education, and comorbidity in the substantial earnings losses of individuals with symmetric polyarthritis. *Arthritis Rheum.*, **31**, 348–357
24. Pincus, T. (1988). Is mortality increased in rheumatoid arthritis (RA)? *J. Musculoskel. Med.*, **5**, 27–46
25. Cobb, S., Anderson, F. and Bauer, W. (1953). Length of life and cause of death in rheumatoid arthritis. *N. Engl. J. Med.*, **249**, 553–556
26. Monson, R. R. and Hall, A. P. (1976). Mortality among arthritics. *J. Chron. Dis.*, **29**, 459–467
27. Uddin, J., Kraus, A. S. and Kelly, H. G. (1970). Survivorship and death in rheumatoid arthritis. *Arthritis Rheum.*, **13**, 125–130
28. Mitchell, D. M., Spitz, P. W., Young, D. Y., Bloch, D. A., McShane, D. J. and Fries, J. F. (1986). Survival, prognosis, and causes of death in rheumatoid arthritis. *Arthritis Rheum.*, **29**, 706–714
29. Allebeck, P., Ahlbom, A. and Allander, E. (1981). Increased mortality among persons with rheumatoid arthritis, but where RA does not appear on death certificate: eleven year follow-up of an epidemiological study. *Scand. J. Rheumatol.*, **10**, 301–306
30. Vandenbroucke, J. P., Hazevoet, H. M. and Cats, A. (1984). Survival and cause of death in rheumatoid arthritis: A 25-year prospective follow-up. *J. Rheumatol.*, **11**, 158–161
31. Mutru, O., Laakso, M., Isomaki, H. and Koota, K. (1985). Ten-year mortality and causes of death in patients with rheumatoid arthritis. *Br. Med. J.*, **290**, 1797–1799
32. Vollertsen, R. S., Conn, D. L., Ballard, D. J., Ilstrup, D. M., Kazmar, R. E. and Silverfield, J. C. (1986). Rheumatoid vasculitis: survival and associated risk factors. *Medicine (Baltimore)*, **65**, 365–375
33. Pincus, T., Callahan, L. F. and Vaughn, W. K. (1987). Questionnaire, walking time and button test measures of functional capacity as predictive markers for mortality in rheumatoid arthritis. *J. Rheumatol.*, **14**, 240–251
34. Pincus, T. and Callahan, L. F. (1986). Taking mortality in rheumatoid arthritis seriously — predictive markers, socioeconomic status and comorbidity. (Editorial.) *J. Rheumatol.*, **13**, 841–845
35. Berkson, J. (1946). Limitations of the application of fourfold table analysis to hospital data. *Biomet. Bull.* **2**, 47–53
36. Pincus, T., Callahan, L. F. and Mitchell, J. M. (1987). Increased mortality in rheumatoid arthritis is explained in part on the basis of extensive comorbidity with other diseases. *Arthritis Rheum.*, **30** (Suppl. 4), S12
37. Pincus, T. and Callahan, L. F. (1985). Formal education as a marker for increased mortality and morbidity in rheumatoid arthritis. *J. Chron. Dis.*, **38**, 973–984
38. Rasker, J. J. and Cosh, J. A. (1981). The natural history of rheumatoid arthritis: a fifteen year follow-up study: the prognostic signification of features noted in the first year. *Clin. Rheumatol.*, **3**, 11–20

39. Gordon, D. A., Stein, J. L. and Broder, I. (1973). The extra-articular features of rheumatoid arthritis: a systematic analysis of 127 cases. *Am. J. Med.*, **54**, 445-452
40. Proudfit, W. L., Bruschke, A. V. G. and Sones, F. M. Jr. (1978). Natural history of obstructive coronary artery disease: ten-year study of 601 nonsurgical cases. *Progr. Cardiovasc. Dis.*, **21**, 53-78
41. Kaplan, H. S. (1972). Survival as related to treatment. In Kaplan, H. S. (ed.) *Hodgkin's Disease*, pp. 360-388. (Cambridge: Harvard University Press)
42. Spector, T. D., Thompson, P. W., Evans, S. J. W. and Scott, D. L. (1988). Are slow-acting antirheumatic drugs being given earlier in rheumatoid arthritis? (Letter.) *Br. J. Rheumatol.*, **27**, 498-499
43. Wilske, K. R. and Healey, L. A. (1989). Remodeling the pyramid — a concept whose time has come. *J. Rheumatol.*, **16**, 565-567
44. Ritchie, D. M., Boyle, J. A., McInnes, J. M. *et al.* (1968). Clinical studies with an articular index for the assessment of joint tenderness in patients with rheumatoid arthritis. *Q. J. Med.*, **147**, 393-406
45. Cooperating Clinics Committee of the American Rheumatism Association (1965). A seven-day variability study of 499 patients with peripheral rheumatoid arthritis. *Arthritis Rheum.*, **8**, 302-335
46. Lansbury, J. and Haut, D. D. (1956). Quantitation of the manifestations of rheumatoid arthritis. 4. Area of joint surfaces as an index to total joint inflammation and deformity. *Am. J. Med. Sci.*, **232**, 150-155
47. American Rheumatism Association. (1982). *Dictionary of the Rheumatic Diseases Vol. I: Signs and Symptoms.* (New York: Contact Associates International)
48. Egger, M. J., Huth, D. A., Ward, J. R., Reading, J. C. and Williams, H. J. (1985). Reduced joint count indices in the evaluation of rheumatoid arthritis. *Arthritis Rheum.*, **28**, 613-619
49. Fuchs, H. A., Brooks, R. H., Callahan, L. F. and Pincus, T. (1989). A simplified 28-joint quantitative articular index in rheumatoid arthritis. *Arthritis Rheum.*, **32**, 531-537
50. Steinbrocker, O., Traeger, C. H. and Batterman, R. C. (1949). Therapeutic criteria for rheumatoid arthritis. *J. Am. Med. Assoc.*, **140**, 659-662
51. Larsen, A. (1974). A radiological method for grading the severity of rheumatoid arthritis. *Academic dissertation*.
52. Larsen, A. and Dale, K. (1977). Radiographic evaluation of rheumatoid arthritis and related conditions by standard reference films. *Acta Radiol. Diag.*, **18**, 481-491
53. Sharp, J. T., Lidsky, M. D., Collins, L. C. and Moreland, J. (1971). Methods of scoring the progression of radiologic changes in rheumatoid arthritis: correlation of radiologic, clinical and laboratory abnormalities. *Arthritis Rheum.*, **14**, 706-720
54. Sharp, J. T. (1983). Radiographic evaluation of the course of articular disease. *Clin. Rheum. Dis.*, **9**, 541-557
55. Genant, H. K. (1983). Methods of assessing radiographic change in rheumatoid arthritis. *Am. J. Med.*, **75** (Suppl. 6A), 35-47
56. Kaye, J. J., Nance, E. P., Callahan, L. F. *et al.* (1987). Observer variation in quantitative assessment of rheumatoid arthritis: part II. A simplified scoring system. *Invest. Radiol.*, **22**, 41-46
57. Kaye, J. J., Callahan, L. F., Nance, E. P. Jr., Brooks, R. and Pincus, T. (1987). Bony ankylosis in rheumatoid arthritis: associations with longer duration and greater severity of disease. *Invest. Radiol.*, **22**, 303-309
58. Fuchs, H. A., Callahan, L. F., Kaye, J. J., Brooks, R. H., Nance, E. P. and Pincus, T. (1988). Radiographic and joint count findings of the hand in rheumatoid arthritis: related and unrelated findings. *Arthritis Rheum.*, **31**, 44-51
59. Baum, J. and Ziff, M. (1985). Laboratory findings in rheumatoid arthritis. In McCarty D. J. (ed.) *Arthritis and Allied Conditions: A Textbook of Rheumatology*, pp. 643-659. (Philadelphia: Lea & Febiger)
60. Symons, J. A., Wood, N. C., Di Giovine, F. S. and Duff, G. W. (1988). Soluble IL-2 receptor in rheumatoid arthritis: correlation with disease activity and IL-1 and IL-2 inhibition. *J. Immunol.*, **141**, 2612-2618
61. Rose, H. M., Ragan, C., Pearce, E. and Lipman, M. O. (1949). Differential agglutina-

tion of normal and sensitized sheep erythrocytes by sera of patients with rheumatoid arthritis. *Proc. Soc. Exp. Biol. Med.*, **68**, 1
62. Olsen, N., Ziff, M. and Jasin, H. E. (1984). Spontaneous synthesis of IgM rheumatoid factor by blood mononuclear cells from patients with rheumatoid arthritis: effect of treatment with gold salts or D-penicillamine. *J. Rheumatol.*, **11**, 17-21
63. Olsen, N. J., Callahan, L. F. and Pincus, T. (1987). Immunologic studies of rheumatoid arthritis patients treated with methotrexate. *Arthritis Rheum.*, **30**, 481-488
64. Stastny, P. (1978). Association of B-cell alloantigen DRW4 with rheumatoid arthritis. *N. Engl. J. Med.*, **298**, 869-871
65. Stastny, P., Ball, E. J., Khan, M. A., Olsen, N. J., Pincus, T. and Gao, X. (1988). HLA-DR4 and other genetic markers in rheumatoid arthritis. *Br. J. Rheumatol.*, **27** (Suppl. II), 132-138
66. Olsen, N. J., Callahan, L. F., Brooks, R. H. *et al.* (1988). Associations of HLA-DR4 with rheumatoid factor and radiographic severity in rheumatoid arthritis. *Am. J. Med.*, **84**, 257-264
67. Buchanan, W. W. and Smythe, H. A. (1982). Can clinicians and statisticians be friends? (Editorial.) *J. Rheumatol.*, **9**, 653-654
68. Koran, L. M. (1975). The reliability of clinical methods, data and judgements. *N. Engl. J. Med.*, **293**, 642-46, 695-701
69. Fries, J. F., Spitz, P., Kraines, R. G. and Holman, H. R. (1980). Measurement of patient outcome in arthritis. *Arthritis Rheum.*, **23**, 137-145
70. Meenan, R. F., Gertman, P. M. and Mason, J. H. (1980). Measuring health status in arthritis: the Arthritis Impact Measurement Scales. *Arthritis Rheum.*, **23**, 146-152
71. Tugwell, P., Bombardier, C., Buchanan, W. W., Goldsmith, C. H., Grace, E. and Hanna, B. (1987). The MACTAR patient preference disability questionnaire – an individualized functional priority approach for assessing improvement in physical disability in clinical trials in rheumatoid arthritis. *J. Rheumatol.*, **14**, 446-451
72. Nevitt, M. C., Yelin, E. H., Henke, C. J. and Epstein, W. V. (1986). Risk factors for hospitalization and surgery in patients with rheumatoid arthritis: implications for capitated medical payment. *Ann. Intern. Med.*, **105**, 421-428
73. Meenan, R. F. and Pincus, T. (1987). The status of patient status measures. (Editorial.) *J. Rheumatol.*, **14**, 411-414
74. Pincus, T., Callahan, L. F. and Brooks, R. H. (1986). Quantitative nonlaboratory measures to monitor and predict the course of rheumatoid arthritis. In Ehrlich, G. E. (ed.) *Rehabilitation Management of Rheumatic Conditions*, pp. 45-63. (Baltimore: Williams & Wilkins)
75. Lee, P., Baxter, A., Dick, W. C. and Webb, J. (1973). Assessment of grip strength measurement in rheumatoid arthritis. *Scand. J. Rheumatol.*, **3**, 17-23
76. DeCeulaer, K. and Dick, W. C. (1981). The clinical evaluation of antirheumatic drugs. In Kelley, W. N., Harris, E. D. Jr., Ruddy, S. and Sledge, C. B. (eds.), *Textbook of Pheumatology*, pp. 729-739. (Philadelphia: W. B. Saunders)
77. Clawson, D. K., Souter, W. A., Carthum, C. J. and Hymen, M. L. (1971). Functional assessment of the rheumatoid hand. *Clin. Orthop.*, **77**, 203-210
78. Pincus, T., Callahan, L. F., Brooks, R. H., Fuchs, H. A., Olsen, N. J. and Kaye, J. J. (1989). Self-report questionnaire scores in rheumatoid arthritis compared with traditional physical, radiographic, and laboratory measures. *Ann. Intern. Med.*, **110**, 259-266
79. Laitman, R. S., Glicklich, D., Sablay, L. B., Grayzel, A. I., Barland, P. and Bank, N. (1989). Effect of long-term normalization of serum complement levels on the course of lupus nephritis. *Am. J. Med.*, **87**, 132-138
80. Research Sub-Committee of the Empire Rheumatism Council. (1960). Gold therapy in rheumatoid arthritis. Report of a multi-centre controlled trial. *Ann. Rheum. Dis.*, **19**, 95-119
81. Bombardier, C., Tugwell, P., Sinclair, A., Dok, C., Anderson, G. and Buchanan, W. W. (1982). Preference for endpoint measures in clinical trials: results of structured workshops. *J. Rheumatol.*, **9**, 798-801
82. Weed, L. L. (1968). Medical records that guide and teach. *N. Engl. J. Med.*, **278**, 593-600, 652-57

83. Meenan, R. F., Anderson, J. J., Kazis, L. E. et al. (1984). Outcome assessment in clinical trials: evidence for the sensitivity of a health status measure. *Arthritis Rheum.*, **27**, 1344-1352
84. Bombardier, C., Ware, J., Russell, I. J. et al. (1986). Auranofin therapy and quality of life in patients with rheumatoid arthritis. Results of a multicenter trial. *Am. J. Med.*, **81**, 565-578
85. Pincus, T. (1988). Rheumatoid arthritis: disappointing long-term outcomes despite successful short-term clinical trials. (Editorial.) *J. Clin. Epidemiol.*, **41**, 1037-1041
86. Feinstein, A. R. (1983). An additional basic science for clinical medicine: II. The limitations of randomized trials. *Ann. Intern. Med.*, **99**, 544-550
87. Kelley, W. N., Harris, E. D, Jr, Ruddy, K. S. and Sledge, C. B. (1981). *Textbook of Rheumatology* (Philadelphia: W. B. Saunders), p. 779
88. Sherrer, Y. S., Bloch, D. A., Mitchell, D. M., Young, D. Y. and Fries, J. F. (1986). The development of disability in rheumatoid arthritis. *Arthritis Rheum.*, **29**, 494-500
89. Kelley, W. N., Harris, E. D. Jr, Ruddy, S. and Sledge, C. B. (eds.) (1985). *Textbook of Rheumatology* (Philadelphia: W. B. Saunders), p.987
90. Thompson, P. W., Kirwan, J. R. and Barnes, C. G. (1985). Practical results of treatment with disease-modifying antirheumatoid drugs. *Br. J. Rheumatol.*, **24**, 167-175
91. Amor, B., Herson, D., Cherot, A. and Delbarre, F. (1981). Polyarthrites rheumatoides evoluant depuis plus de 10 ans (1966-1978). *Ann. Med. Interne. (Paris)*, **132**, 168-173
92. Situnayake, R. D., Grindulis, K. A. and McConkey, B. (1987). Long term treatment of rheumatoid arthritis with sulphasalazine, gold, or penicillamine: a comparison using life-table methods. *Ann. Rheum. Dis.*, **46**, 177-183
93. Ropes, M. W., Bennett, G. A., Cobb, S., Jacox, R. F. and Jessar, R. A. (1958). Revision of diagnostic criteria for rheumatoid arthritis. *Bull. Rheum. Dis.*, **9**, 175-176
94. Arnett, F. C., Edworthy, S. M., Block, D. A. et al. (1988). The American Rheumatism Association 1987 revised criteria for the classification of rheumatoid arthritis. *Arthritis Rheum.*, **31**, 315-324
95. O'Sullivan, J. B. and Cathcart, E. S. (1972). The prevalence of rheumatoid arthritis: follow-up evaluation of the effect of criteria on rates in Sudbury, Massachusetts. *Ann. Intern. Med.*, **76**, 573-577
96. Mikkelsen, W. M. and Dodge, H. (1969). A four year follow-up of suspected rheumatoid arthritis: the Tecumseh, Michigan, Community Health Study. *Arthritis Rheum.*, **12**, 87-91
97. Masi, A. T., Feigenbaum, S. L. and Kaplan, S. B. (1983). Articular patterns in the early course of rheumatoid arthritis. *Am. J. Med.*, **75** (Suppl. 6A), 16-26
98. Ragan, C. and Farrington, E. (1962). The clinical features of rheumatoid arthritis: prognostic indices. *J. Am. Med. Assoc.*, **181**, 663-667
99. Paulus, H. E., Furst, D. E. and Dromgoole, S. H. (1987). *Drugs for Rheumatic Disease*, (New York: Churchill Livingstone), pp. 203-226
100. Kirwan, J. R. and Currey, H. L. F. (1983). Rheumatoid arthritis: disease-modifying antirheumatic drugs. *Clin. Rheum. Dis.*, **9**, 581-599
101. Mikkelsen, W. M., Dodge, H. J., Duff, I. F. and Kato, H. (1967). Estimates of the prevalence of rheumatic diseases in the population of Tecumseh, Michigan, 1959-1960. *J. Chron. Dis.*, **20**, 351-369
102. Valkenberg, H. A., Ball, J., Burch, T. A., Bennett, P. H. and Laurence, J. S. (1966). Rheumatoid factors in a rural population. *Ann. Rheum. Dis.*, **25**, 497-507
103. Adler, E., Abramson, J. H., Elkan, Z., Ben Hador, S. and Goldberg, R. (1967). Rheumatoid arthritis in a Jerusalem population: 1. Epidemiology of the disease. *Am. J. Epidemiol.*, **85**, 365-367
104. Burch, T. A., O'Brien, W. M., Lawrence, J. S., Bennett, P. H. and Bunim, J. J. (1963). A comparison of the prevalence of rheumatoid arthritis (R.A.) and rheumatoid factor (R.F.) in Indian tribes living in Montana mountains and in Arizona desert. *Arthritis Rheum.*, **6**, 765
105. Carson, D. A. (1985). Rheumatoid factor. In Harris, E. D. Jr, Ruddy, S. and Sledge, C. B. (eds.) *Textbook of Rheumatology*, pp. 664-676. (Philadelphia: W. B. Saunders)

106. Bunch, T. W. and O'Duffy, T. D. (1980). Disease-modifying drugs for progressive rheumatoid arthritis. *Mayo Clin. Proc.*, **55**, 161-179
107. Callahan, L. F. and Pincus, T. (1988). Formal education level as a significant marker of clinical status in rheumatoid arthritis. *Arthritis Rheum.*, **31**, 1346-1357
108. Ruberman, W., Weinblatt, E., Goldberg, J. D. and Chaudhary, B. S. (1984). Psychosocial influences on mortality after myocardial infarction. *N. Engl. J. Med.*, **311**, 552-559
109. Marmot, M. G., Rose, G., Shipley, M. and Hamilton, P. J. S. (1978). Employment grade and coronary heart disease in British civil servants. *J. Epidemiol. Community Health*, **32**, 244-249
110. Pincus, T., Callahan, L. F. and Burkhauser, R. V. (1987). Most chronic diseases are reported more frequently by individuals with fewer than 12 years of formal education in the age 18-64 United States population. *J. Chron. Dis.*, **40**, 865-874
111. LaVecchia, C., Negri, E., Pagano, R. and Decarli, A. (1987). Education, prevalence of disease, and frequency of health care utilization. The 1983 Italian National Health Survey. *J. Epidemiol. Community Health*, **41**, 161-165
112. Blazter, M. (1987). Evidence of inequality in health from a national survey. *Lancet*, **2**, 30-33
113. Marmot, M. G. and McDowall, M. E. (1986). Mortality decline and widening social class inequalities. *Lancet*, **2**, 274-276
114. Epstein, A., Stern, R. S., Tognetti, J. *et al.* (1988). The association of patients' socioeconomic characteristics with the length of hospital stay and hospital charges within diagnosis-related groups. *N. Engl. J. Med.*, **318**, 1579-1585
115. Pincus, T. (1988). Formal educational level — a marker for the importance of behavioral variables in the pathogenesis, morbidity, and mortality of most diseases? (Editorial.) *J. Rheumatol.*, **15**, 1457-1460
116. Nicassio, P. M., Wallston, K. A., Callahan, L. F., Herbert, M. and Pincus, T. (1985). The measurement of helplessness in rheumatoid arthritis: the development of the Arthritis Helplessness Index. *J. Rheumatol.*, **12**, 462-467
117. Callahan, L. F., Brooks, R. H. and Pincus, T. (1988). Further analysis of learned helplessness in rheumatoid arthritis using a "Rheumatology Attitudes Index". *J. Rheumatol.*, **15**, 418-426

Index

acetaminophen (paracetamol) 349, 372, 376, 407, 415
  overdose 412
  side-effects 415
acute renal failure 416
adenine nucleotide degradation 98
adrenal glucocorticoids 18-20
adult-onset Still's disease 288
alcofenac 363
Alka-Seltzer (buffered aspirin) 371, 404
allopurinol 107, 348, 354, 375-6
  hypersensitivity 112, 417
aluminium hydroxide 371
American Rheumatism Association
  Cooperative Clinics 468, 474 (table)
  criteria 272, 482-3
  Medical Information System (ARAMIS) 7
aminoglycosides 368 (table)
amyloidosis 85, 87, 138-9
ampicillin 376
analgesic nephropathy 100, 112, 418
angiotensin 100
angiotensin-converting enzyme inhibitors 225
ankylosing spondylitis 133-49
  adverse prognostic factors 147 (table)
  age of onset 135
  amyloidosis associated 138-9
  anthropometric measurement 139-41
    treatment effect 141-3, 144 (fig.)
  assessment 136-7
  asymptomatic 137
  cardiovascular disease 138
  causes of death 137 (table)
  disability 147
    outcome 145-6
  discomfort/pain relief 144-5
  genetic differences 135
  Klebsiella sp., associated 134, 148
  mortality 137, 146
  natural history 134-5
  peripheral joint involvement 139
  pregnancy associated 288-9
  primary 133
    vs secondary 136
  pulmonary disease 138
  radiographic changes 139
  radiotherapy 134
  range of movement 147
  secondary 133
  sex differences 135-6
antacids 368 (table)
  NSAIDS interactions 371
anticoagulants 370 (table)
  NSAIDS interactions 371-2
antidiabetic drugs, NSAIDs interactions 374
antihypertensives 369 (table), 372-3
antimalarials
  congenital malformations due to 307 (table), 308
  in breast milk 309
  in pregnancy 306
antineutrophil cytoplasmic antibody 262
antiphospholipid antibody syndrome 296-9
antipyrine, half-life 353
antirheumatic drugs 305-11, 347-76
  congenital malformations due to 307 (table)
  disease-modifying 42
  fetal death due to 308
  in breast milk 308-11
  in pregnancy 305-11
  interactions 366-76
  meta-analysis 306
  prediction of efficacy 349-59
    NSAIDs 350-1
    pharmacokinetics 352-4
    simple analgesics 349
    slow-acting antirheumatic drugs 354-9
  removed from sale 361
  Roubenhoff data 305-306
  second-line 478-81
  side-effects 359-66, 403-20
    acute gastrointestinal

493

antirheumatic drugs, side effects (*continued*)
    haemorrhage 409-12
    acute renal failure,
        haemodynamic/functional 416
    adverse drug reactions 360
    analgesic nephropathy 418
    dyspepsia 403-5
    elderly patients 362-3
    estimation of risk 360-2
    gastric mucosa damage 405-9
    genetic control of metabolism 365-6
    genetic predisposition 363-5
    hyperkalaemia 417-18
    hypernatraemia 416-17
    in pregnancy 309 (table)
    interstitial nephritis 418
    liver 412-16
    microbleeding 405-9
    perforation 409-12
    route of administration effect 363
    slow-acting/immunoregulatory
        agents 418-20
    tablet formulations 363
    treatment *vs* placebo
        differences 478-81
    see also individual drugs
apatite-associated arthropathy 123-5
    acute arthritis 124
    destructive arthritis 124-5
    mixed pyrophosphate/apatite crystal
        disease 124
    natural history 123-5
    osteoarthritis 123-4
    prognosis 125
apheresis 348
Arteparon 29
Arthritis Impact Measurement Scales
    (AIMS) 6, 48, 53-7 (table), 472
arthrocentesis 108
aspirin 21
    buffered (Alka-Seltzer) 371, 404
    for:
        osteoarthritis 21, 22
        psoriatric arthritis 160
    in pregnancy 305, 306
    interactions 366-71
    Reye's syndrome associated 413-14
    side-effects 408, 417-18
    teratogenicity effect 306, 307 (table)
auranofin 348, 352
    side-effects 412
    see also gold
azapropazone 417
    excretion 354
    indomethacin compared 22
    interactions 367 (table)
azathioprine 359, 480 (fig.)
    congenital malformations due to 307
        (table)

    for:
        rheumatoid arthritis 71
        systemic sclerosis 224
    in breast milk 309
    in pregnancy 305, 308, 309 (table)
    NSAIDs interactions 375
    side effects 405, 412, 415, 419

barbiturates 369 (table)
basic calcium phosphate arthropathy *see*
    apatite-associated arthropathy
benoxaprofen 21, 351, 417
    drug-related deaths 360
    half-life 354
    side-effects in elderly patients 354
benzothiadiazine 100
Berkson's bias 460
beta-adrenoreceptor blockers 372-3
British National Association for
    Ankylosing Spondylitis 135
bromosulphthaline testing 415

caffeine 369 (table)
calcium channel blocking agents 222,
    224
calcium pyrophosphate dihydrate
    (CPPD/pyrophosphate) 97
captopril 348, 372
carpal tunnel syndrome in
    pregnancy 303-4
carprofen 351, 407
cauda equina syndrome 138
cephalosporins 376
Charcot-like arthropathy 19
chlorambucil 224
    congenital malformations due to 307
        (table)
    defective oogenesis/spermato-
        genesis 420
chloroquine 160, 415, 480 (fig.)
chlorothiazide 376
chondrocalcinosis 23
chlorambucil in pregnancy 306, 308
chloroquine in pregnancy 303 (table)
cholestyramine 369 (table)
choline magnesium trisalicylate 404
choline salicylate 404
chondrocalcinosis 28, 119-20
chrysotherapy *see* gold
Churg-Strauss' allergic and
    granulomatous angiitis 261; *see
    also* vasculitis
cimetidine 374, 404, 406
cisapride 224
codeine 349
colchicine, for:
    gout 103, 379
    pyrophosphate crystal-deposition
        disease 121

INDEX

collagenase 19, 118
colonic diverticula 411
connective-tissue disorders 376
coronary artery disease 466, 467 (fig.)
corticosteroids 358
  for:
    juvenile arthritis 87
    polymyositis 359
    rheumatoid arthritis 347
    systemic sclerosis 222
    vasculitis 262
  in pregnancy 305, 309 (table)
  local injection 92
  NSAIDs interactions 373–4
  side-effects 90, 408
cotrimoxazole, meningitis syndrome due to 353
C-reactive protein 87, 136, 470
CREST syndrome 217
cyclophosphamide
  congenital malformation due to 307 (table)
  for:
    lupus disease 358
    rheumatoid arthritis 348
    systemic lupus erythematosus 348
    vasculitis 262, 348
    Wegener's granulomatosis 348
  in breast milk 309
  in pregnancy 305–11
  normal pregnancy after 420
  side-effects
    azoospermia, temporary 420
    bladder 419–20
    defective oogenesis/spermatogenesis 420
    gastrointestinal 405
    liver damage 415
    premature menopause 420
cyclosporin A 160, 348
  side-effects
    gastrointestinal 405
    hepatoxicity following transplant 415
    nephrotoxicity 419

dapsone 348, 365
data, hard/soft 5–6
deflazocort 93
diabetes mellitus
  neuropathic arthropathy 23
  neuropathy 23
diclofenac sodium 21
  in breast milk 309, 310 (table)
dicouramol 376
diffuse proliferative lupus nephritis 358
diflunisal 107
  half-life 354
  in breast milk 310 (table)

digoxin 368 (table), 374
dimethyl-sulfoxide 224
Distalgesic 349, 372
diuretics 369 (table), 370 (table), 373
DNA restriction fragment 476
DR3 364

education, formal, health conditions related (US) 485–7
elderly patients, adverse drug reactions 362–3
ephamsylate 409
esophageal stricture, haemorrhage 411
esophageal varices 411
etodolac 407
etretinate 348
ethanol 372

Felty's syndrome 364
fenclofenac 351
fenemates 411
fenoprofen 21
fibromyalgia 321–30
  childhood 322
  clinical course 323–4
  Minnesota Multiphasic Personality Index scores 326
  onset 322–3
  outcome measures 324–9
    choice of 328–9
    concomitant disease 328
    costs 328
    functional ability 326–7, 328
    iatrogenic factors 327–8
    medical services utilization 328, 329
    pain 325–6
    psychological status 326, 327–8
    work disability 327
  prognosis 329, 330 (table)
  Smyth–Moldofsky criteria 321–2
  Stanford Health Assessment functional disability index 326
  trauma antecedent 323
  treatment 327–8, 329
fibromyalgia, funnel 323, 324 (fig.)
flufenamic acid 309, 310 (table)
focal proliferative lupus nephritis 358
folic acid 415
furosemide 372

gammaglobulins 348
gastrocolic fistula, benign 411
giant cell arteritis 273–5
  blindnes due to 274–5
  death due to 274
  peripheral neuropathy 274
  treatment 275
glomerulonephritis 358
glucocorticoids 375

495

glucose-6-phosphate dehydrogenase
    deficiency 365-6
glutathione deficiency 415
gold 307, 480 (fig.)
  congenital malformations due to 307
    (table)
  for:
    juvenile arthritis 87
    psoriatic arthritis 160
    rheumatoid arthritis 71, 355, 356-7
  in breast milk 309
  in pregnancy 309 (table)
  side-effects 86, 366
    diarrhea 412
    dyspepsia 405
    genetic disposition 363
    hepatitis 415
    mucocutaneous 364
    nephropathy 418-19
    neutropenia 364
    proteinuria 364
    thrombocytopenia 364
  see also auranofin
gonococcal arthritis in pregnancy 304-5
Goodpasture's syndrome 419
gout 97-117
  atypical 108-9
  bone marrow proliferation
    associated 98
  cardiovascular risk factors 107-8
  chronic gouty arthritis 108-9
  coronary heart disease associated 105,
    115-16
  diuretic-induced 109-10
  elderly patients 109
  female patients 109
  hypercholesterolemia 105
  hyperlipidemia 104-5
  hypertension associated 98, 104
  hyperuricemic factors 98-100
    alcohol 99, 105, 106
    chronic respiratory acidosis 100
    diet 98
    genetic urate overproduction 100
    hyperparathyroidism 100
    hypertriglyceridemia 99
    myocardial infarction 100
    myxedema 100
    obesity 99
    renal disease 100
    renal excretory capacity 99-100
  incidence 103-4
  in osteoarthritic joints 110
  kidney disease 113-4
    uric acid/urate as causes 113-14
  mortality rate 116
  natural history
    correctable factors recognition 407
    recent factors affecting 106-8

  untreated 101-4, 106
  obesity associated 99, 104
  primary 98
  prognosis 97-8
    literature 115-17
  renal 111-12
  renal colic associated 106
  renal stones 113, 115
  secondary 98
  tophus without acute gouty
    arthritis 110-11
  treatment 103
  vascular disease associated 98
  vertebral bone destruction 108
growth hormone, synthetic 93
guanosine 99

Health Assessment Questionnaire
  (HAQ) 6, 472
Heberden's node 110
Helicobacter pylori 404
hemolytic anemia 366
hemophilia 372
hepatic fibrosis 415
herniated lumbar disc 335-8
  follow-up 338
  surgery 336-8
HGPRT deficiency 114
histamine receptor blockers 224
HLA-B8 364
Hodgkin's disease 466, 467 (fig.)
hydralazine 365, 372
hydrocortisone acetate,
  intra-articular 19
hydrochloric acid 406
hydroxychloroquine 71, 348, 359
  side-effects 405
hyperkalemia 417-18
Hypertension Detection and Follow-Up
  Program 110
hypersensitivity hepatitis 415
hypertriglyceridemia 99
hyperuricemia 97-8; see also gout
hypoalbuminemia 412
hypoglycuric agents 370 (table)
hyponatremia 416-17

ibuprofen 21, 372, 376
  in breast milk 309, 310 (table)
  meningitis syndrome associated 353
IgG 94
IgM rheumatoid factor 84
immunosuppressive drugs for
  vasculitis 262
inappropriate ADH syndrome 420
indocid 160
indomethacin 21, 22
  azapropazone compared 22
  in breast milk 309, 310 (table)

INDEX

in pregnancy 306
  side-effects 351, 407, 411
  suppositories 411
  teratogenicity 306, 307 (table)
'indomethacin hips' 22
interferon gamma 348
interstitial nephritis 418
iridocyclitis, chronic 84
isonicotinic acid hydrazide 365

juvenile arthritis 83-94
  age of onset 83
juvenile rheumatoid arthritis (JRA) 83, 84
  assessment 89
  causes of death 85
  clinical features 84
  complications
    amyloidosis 85, 87, 91
    ankylosing spondylitis 87
    cardiac 85
    consumption coagulopathy 86
    growth retardation 89-90
    hepatic 85
    local growth discrepancies 90
    micrognathia 90
    ocular 87-9, 91
    psychological 93
    psychosocial 90-1
    uveitis 87-9
  future perspective 92-4
  management 91-2
  mortality 85-6
  psychological problems 90-1
juvenile spondylitis 84

keratan sulfate 27, 28
keratoconjunctivitis sicca 89
keratoderma blennorrhagicum 169
ketones 100
ketoprofen
  half-life 354
  in breast milk 309, 310 (table)
  side effects 407

lactate 100
Lansbury Index 468
Larsen Scale 470
lateral recess stenosis 334-5
leucovorin 415
levamisole 348, 415, 419
lithium 367 (table), 373
liver disease 412-16
low back pain 333-43
  functional impairment/disability 341-2
  in pregnancy 304
  learned behaviour 340
  outcome predictors 338-41
lupus glomerulonephritis 358

Lyme disease 167

Maalox 371
MACTAR 472
magnesium hydroxide 371
magnesium trisilicate 371
medullary cystic kidney disease 112
mefenamic acid, in breast milk 309, 310 (table)
mefopam 349
membranous disease 358
meningitis syndrome, drug-induced 353
meperidine 349
mercatopurine (t-) 375
metaclopramide 369 (table)
metalloproteinases 19
methotrexate 352, 355
  congenital malformations due to 307 (table)
  for:
    juvenile rheumatoid arthritis 94
    psoriatic arthritis 160
    rheumatoid arthritis 71, 348
  in pregnancy 305-11
  interaction with NSAIDs 367 (table), 373
  side-effects 364
    defective oogenesis/spermatogenesis 420
    hepatic 415
methylprednisolone 347
  for:
    juvenile rheumatoid arthritis 93
    osteoarthritis 18
misoprostol 404, 406, 419
mixed connective disease 301
Modified Health Assessment Questionnaire 48, 51-2 (table), 472, 473
monoarthritis multiplex 24
monosodium urate monohydrate 97
morphine 349

naproxen sodium 21, 22, 351
  half-life 354
  in breast milk 309, 310 (table)
National Health and Nutrition Examination Survey I 11
necrotising enterocolitis, acute 411
neonatal lupus syndrome 299-301
nephrotic syndrome 358, 419
Newcastle Enthesis Index 445
nonsteroidal anti-inflammatory drugs (NSAIDs) 20-2, 347
  antiprostaglandin effect 418
  chondroprotective 22
  for:
    fibromyalgia 328
    gout 107

NSAIDs for: (continued)
    polymyalgia rheumatica 272
    psoriatic arthritis 160-1
    pyrophosphate crystal deposition
        disease 121
    systemic sclerosis 222
gallstone recurrence prevention 412
in breast milk 310 (table)
in labour 306-7
in pregnancy 305-11
interactions 366-71
side-effects 62
    dyspepsia 360
    liver disease 414-16

oral hypoglycaemic agents 367 (table)
Osmosin 361, 363
osteoarthritis 11-29
    abrasion arthroplasty 26-7
    cartilage sharing 26
    chondrocyte effect 16
    disability 14-15
        patient's perception 15
        risk factors 14-15
    immunologic tests 27
    intra-articular steroids 18-20
    joint debridement 26
    joint destruction acceleration
        factors 20-3
        neurogenic 22-3
        NSAIDs 20-2
    knee instability 17
    knee pain 14
    mortality 15-16
    pain, funcional effect 13-14
    periarticular muscular weakness 14
    prevalence 11-12
    primary 18
    prognosis 13-17
        elbow 25
        hand 24
        hip 24
        interphalangeal joints 24-5
        joint replacement surgery
            effect 25-6
        knee 23-4
        pharmacological influences 28-9
    progression 16-20
    proteoglycan 17
    psychological factors 14
    reversibility 16-17
    risk factors for clinical
            progression 17-20
        adrenal glucocorticoids 18-20
        age 20
        calcium hydroxyapatite
            crystals 17-18
        calcium pyrophosphate dihydrate
            crystals 17-18

obesity 20
primary osteoarthritis 18
subchondral bone stiffness 20
synovial inflammation 18
scintigraphy 27
socioeconomic impact 12
synovial fluid 28
tidal irrigation 27
outcome 3-7
    assessment 4-7
oxyphenbutazone 367 (table), 372
oxypurinol 112, 417
    half-life 354, 417

papain injection 27-8
paracetamol *see* acetaminophen
penicillamine (D-) 480 (fig.)
    congenital malformations due to 307
        (table)
    for:
        juvenile arthritis 87
        psoriatic arthritis 160
        rheumatoid arthritis 356
        systemic sclerosis 222, 224, 225
    in pregnancy 309 (table)
    side-effects
        acute colitis 412
        dyspepsia 404-5
        genetic predisposition 363
        liver damage 415
        mucocutaneous 364
        proteinuria 364
        real 419
pentazocine 349
phenacetin 418
phenylbutazone
    aplastic anemia due to 352
    for:
        ankylosing spondylitis 139, 144
        psoriatic arthritis 160
    in breast milk 309, 310 (table)
    interactions 367 (table), 372
    side-effects 361
        hepatitis 412
phenytoin 348, 367 (table), 374
piroxicam 20
    half-life 353
    in breast milk 309, 310 (table)
    side-effects 411
polyangiitis overlap syndrome 260-1
polyarteritis nodosa *see* vasculitis
polycystic kidney disease 112
polymyalgia rheumatica 269-75
    giant cell arteritis associated 273-5
    rheumatoid arthritis associated 272-3
polymyositis-dermatomyositis 233-46
    children 240, 243
    mortality 238-40
    natural history 234-5, 236 (table)

INDEX

prognosis-affecting factors
  cardiac involvement 245
  disability 241-4
  discomfort 244
  economic status 244
  pulmonary involvement 244-5
  serology 245-6
potassium *para*-aminobenzoate
  (Potaba) 224
potassium tablets 411
prazosin 372
prednisone 347
  congenital malformations due to 307 (table)
  for:
    giant cell arteritis 275
    osteoarthritis 19-20
    polymyalgia rheumatica 269, 272
  side-effects 20
    growth reduction 90
    low dose 404
pregnancy 279-311
  antirheumatic drugs in 305-11
  see also individual diseases
probenecid 106, 369 (table), 374-5, 376
procainamide 365
process measures 5
prognosis 1-3
  prototype individual patient outcome 4 (fig.)
propoxyphene 349
prostaglandins 405, 406, 416
  derivatives 224
pseudogout 117-8, 120
PUVA 160
pyrophosphate crystal deposition disease 117-22
  acute arthritis (pseudogout) 120
  asymptomatic 121
  chondrocalcinosis in menisci 119-20
  chronic pyrophosphate arthropathy 120-1
  heredofamilial 118-19
  metabolic associated diseases 119
  natural history 120-1
  pathogenesis 118
  prognosis 122
  sporadic 119
  subacute arthritis 120
  temporomandibular joint 120
  treatment 121-2
psoriatic arthritis 153-63
  assessment 162-3
    by Latin square design 163
  associated features 157
  clinical features 154-6
    severity of joint disease 158-9
  course of disease 159
  drug-related deaths 300

HLA antigens as disease markers 157-8
  juvenile-onset 158-9
  pregnancy associated 289-90
  prognosis 159-61
  radiologic picture 154, 156, 162
  treatment 160-1
    surgical 161

ranitidine 406
rectal bleeding 411
rectovaginal fistula 411
Reiter's syndrome 167-89
  American Rheumatism Association's criteria 167
  associated conditions 175
    AIDS 174, 186-7
  childhood 186
  clinical features 168-70
  formes frustes 41
  immunosuppressive drugs contraindicated 188
  laboratory tests 170-2
    HLA-B27 170-1, 173
  microorganisms causing 167, 175 (table)
    Chlamydia trachomatis 171-2
    dysentery organisms 172
  natural history 172-5
  prognosis 172-5
  series reports 175-85
    Csonka 180-2
    Keat 183-5
    Noer 182-3
    Paronen 176-80
  synonyms 167
relapsing polychondritis, in pregnancy 303
renal clearance 99-100
renal disease 358
renal lupus 292
repetitive strain syndrome 323
retinoic acid derivatives 160
Reye-like syndrome 366
Reye's syndrome 92, 366, 413-14
rheumatoid arthritis 37-73
  abortion 284-5
  adverse reactions to treatment 60-2
  American Rheumatism Association's criteria 272, 482-3
  causes of death 461 (table)
  classical 38 (table), 41
  classification/selection 37-43
    American College of Rheumatology 42, 43 (table)
    definite 39 (table)
    New York criteria 39-40
    possible 39 (table)
    probable 39 (table), 41

rheumatoid arthritis (continued)
    revised criteria (1987)   40 (table)
    clinical trials
        'drop-outs'   477
        exclusion from   477
        time frame   477-8
    comorbidities   460, 462 (table)
    cost   57-8
    diagnostic criteria   38-9 (table)
    disability/function measurement   44-5
    drug-related deaths   360
    erythrocyte sedimentation rate   454
        (fig.), 470, 474 (table)
    familial/non-familial   65
    fertility   280-1
    fetal abnormality   285-6
    flow sheet   7
    functional capacity   47-8
    functional decline   453, 455 (fig.)
    functional instruments   48-55
    global self-assessment   474 (table)
    laboratory measures   470-1
    Larsen Index   70
    morning stiffness   38 (table), 40
        (table), 453, 455 (fig.)
    mortality   55-7, 451, 457-60, 460-3
    muscular function tests   473-5
        button test   475
        grip strength   473-5
        walking time   473-5
    natural history   44, 45 (table)
    pain   58-9
    perinatal mortality   285
    polymyalgia rheumatica
        associated   272-3
    population survey (New York,
        1966)   40 (table)
    pregnancy associated   279, 282-3, 311
        course of rheumatoid arthritis
            following   283-4
        effect of rheumatoid arthritis   284
        onset of rheumatoid arthritis   281-2
        prediction of response on rheumatoid
            arthritis   286-7
    rheumatoid factor positive   41, 42
        (fig.), 42
    prognosis   2-3, 63-73, 451-65
        access to care effect   64-5
        cardiovascular disease
            compared   466-8
        clinical markers   460-5
        clinical/laboratory measures   67
        disease severity factors   65-6
        early rheumatoid arthritis   67-8
        education effect   64
        employment effect   65
        functional status vs radiographic/
            laboratory measures   475-6
        gender effect   66-7
        genetic factors   65
        income effect   64
        joint count related   468-9
        later rheumatoid arthritis   68-70
        long term, classification, criteria/
            population bases studies   481-3
        long term, observational studies vs
            clinical trials   477-81
        neoplastic disease compared   466-8
        nonmedical factors   63-7
        patient behavior/lifestyle vs
            treatment/health care   484-7
        race effect   64
        rheumatoid factor effect   66
        social support effect   65
        socioeconomic factors effect   64
        treatment effect   70-1
    psychological measurements   59-60
    questionnaires   471-3, 476
        self-report   494 (table)
    radiographic outcome   62-3, 452-3
    radiographic quantitative
        assessment   469-70, 474 (table)
    self-assessment health status
        measures   48-55
    socioeconomic factors   43
    spectrum bias   43-4
    survival analyses   458-9 (fig.), 464-5
        (fig.)
    work disability   45, 46 (table), 456-7
rheumatoid factor   66, 482-3
Ritchie Index   468
Rumalon   29

sacrolitis   84
salazopyrine, side-effects   405
salicylates   21
    in breast milk   310 (table)
    in pregnancy   309 (table)
    protein binding   353
saliva   410
Schöber's test, modified   140-1
scleroderma see systemic sclerosis
scleroderma kidney   217
SEA syndrome   92
serotonin antagonists   224
Sjögren's syndrome   413
slow-acting antirheumatic drugs
    (SAARDs)   347 375
sodium salicylate   350
sodium valproate   368 (table)
spinal aging   339
spinal stenosis   334-5
spironolactone   372-3
spondylolisthesis   334
spondylosis   334
'squeaky clean' patients   361
Stanford Arthritis Center Health
    Assessment Questionnaire   4, 46-

INDEX

7, 48, 49–50 (table), 205
steroids *see* corticosteroids
stromelysin 27
subchondral sclerosis 20
sucralfate 404, 406
sulfadimidine 365
sulfapyridine 365
sulfasalazine 147–8
  for:
    juvenile rheumatoid arthritis 94
    rheumatoid arthritis 71, 348, 356
  in breast milk 309–10
  in pregnancy 308
  side-effects 364, 365, 419
    cholestatic jaundice 415
    defective oogenesis/spermatogenesis 420
sulfinpyrazone 107, 376
sulindac 21, 373, 417
  in breast milk 310 (table)
  meningitis syndrome due to 353
  side effects 407
systemic lupus erythematosus 193–208
  corticosteroid-induced avascular necrosis of bone 206
  cumulative survival 196 (table)
  incidence 195 (table), 195–6
  Minnesota Multiphasic Personality Interview 205
  mortality 196–7
  natural history 193–4
  physical disability 204–6
  pregnancy associated 206, 290–6
    exacerbation of SLE 291–2
    fertility effect 292–3
    fetal effects 294–6
    long-term prognosis of SLE 292
    pregnancy-related complications 293–4
    renal lupus 292
  prevalence 194 (table), 195
  prognosis factors 197–204, 207 (table)
    age 197–8
    central nervous system disease 202
    coronary artery disease 203–4
    gender 198
    infection 203
    race 198–9
    renal disease 199–202
    serology 202–3
  psychosocial adjustment 204–6
  Psychosocial Adjustment to Illness Scale 205
  Stanford Health Assessment Questionnaire 205
systemic sclerosis (scleroderma) 213–27
  anti-Scl 70 antibody 216, 223
  cardiac abnormalities 215, 217, 225
    tests 227

  cutaneous vasculitis with mononeuritis multiplex 218–19
  diffusing capacity for carbon monoxide 213, 223
  drug therapy 224–5
  early diffuse disease 214–15
  early limited disease 217
  function tests 226–7
  hand involvement/evaluation 222
  laboratory tests 227
  late diffuse disease 215–17
  late limited disease 217–19
  lung involvement 213
  outcome risk factors 222–4
  pregnancy associated 301–3
  prognosis 219–22, 224–5
  pulmonary arterial hypertension 218
  Raynard's phenomenon 213, 223
  renal biopsy 200–1
  renal crisis 224
  skin thickening monitoring 225–6
  survival studies 220 (table), 221 (fig.)

thalidomide 378
theophylline 376
thoracic duct drainage 348
thymopoietin 348
tiaprofenic acid 21
T lymphocyte cell-surface antigen 476
tolmetin sodium 21
  meningitis syndrome due to 353
total lymphoid irradiation 348
toxic nephropathy 112
transaminitis 412
triamcinolone acetonide 18
triamcinolone hexacetonide, intra-articular 19
triamterene 370 (table), 373

ulcerative colitis 411
United States Health and Nutrition Survey 8
urate 98
  genetic overproduction 100
  impaired tubular transport 111
  renal underexcretion 111
urate crystal arthropathy *see* gout
urate-lowering drugs 106–7
  hypersensitivity phenomenon 107
  NSAIDs interactions 375–6

vasculitis 251–64
  classification 251–2
  economic costs 257–8
  iatrogenic factors 257
  incapacity/physical suffering 256–7
  mortality 254–6
  natural history 252–3
  prognosis

vasculitis, clinical markers (*continued*)
　biologic/immunologic indicators　261-2
　clinical markers　258-60
　　age　258-9
　　angiographic alterations　262
　　arterial hypertension　259
　　CNS involvement　260
　　gastrointestinal involvement　260
　　heart disease　260
　　liver disease　260
　　nephropathy　259

　prognosis-modifying factors　253-4
　treatment　262-4
vasopressin　100

warfarin　372, 376, 409
Wegener's granulomatosis　251
　antineutrophil cytoplasmic antibody test　262

zomepirac sodium　361